P9-AFW-600

WITHDRAWN

POINT LOMA NAZARENE UNIVERSITY
RYAN LIBRARY
3900 LOMALAND DRIVE
SAN DIEGO, CALIFORNIA 92106-2899

NUTRITIONAL STRATEGIES for the DIABETIC & PREDIABETIC PATIENT

NUTRITION AND DISEASE PREVENTION

Editorial Advisory Board

CAROLYN D. BERDANIER, PH.D.
University of Georgia, Athens, Georgia, U.S.A.

FRANK GREENWAY, M.D.
Pennington Biomedical Research Center, Louisiana State University,
Baton Rouge, Louisiana, U.S.A.

KHURSHEED N. JEEJEEBHOY, M.D.
University of Toronto Medical School, Toronto, Canada

MULCHAND S. PATEL, PH.D.
The University at Buffalo, The State University of New York,
Buffalo, New York, U.S.A.

KATHLEEN M. RASMUSSEN, PH.D.
Cornell University, Ithaca, New York, U.S.A.

Published Titles

Genomics and Proteomics in Nutrition
Carolyn D. Berdanier, Ph.D., Professor Emerita, University of Georgia, Athens,
Watkinsville, Georgia
Naima Moustaid-Moussa, Ph.D., University of Tennessee, Knoxville, Tennessee

Perinatal Nutrition: Optimizing Infant Health and Development
Jatinder Bhatia, M.B.B.S., Medical College of Georgia, Augusta, Georgia

Soy in Health and Disease Prevention
Michihiro Sugano, Ph.D., Professor Emeritus at Kyushu University, Japan

Nutrition and Cancer Prevention
Atif B. Awad, Ph.D., Department of Exercise and Nutrition Science, State University
of New York, Buffalo, New York
Peter G. Bradford, Ph.D., Department of Pharmacology and Toxicology,
    School of Medicine and Biomedical Science, State University of New York,
Buffalo, New York

Cancer Prevention and Management through Exercise and Weight Control
Anne McTiernan, Fred Hutchinson Cancer Research Center, Seattle, Washington

Nutritional Strategies for the Diabetic & Prediabetic Patient
Jeffrey I. Mechanick, Mount Sinai School of Medicine, New York, New York
Elise M. Brett, Mount Sinai School of Medicine, New York, New York

616.462
M486n
11/06
SH

NUTRITIONAL STRATEGIES for the DIABETIC & PREDIABETIC PATIENT

Edited by
Jeffrey I. Mechanick
Mount Sinai School of Medicine,
New York, New York

Elise M. Brett
Mount Sinai School of Medicine,
New York, New York

POINT LOMA NAZARENE UNIVERSITY
WITHDRAWN
RYAN LIBRARY

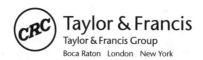

CRC Taylor & Francis
Taylor & Francis Group
Boca Raton   London   New York

A CRC title, part of the Taylor & Francis imprint, a member of the
Taylor & Francis Group, the academic division of T&F Informa plc.

Published in 2006 by
CRC Press
Taylor & Francis Group
6000 Broken Sound Parkway NW, Suite 300
Boca Raton, FL 33487-2742

© 2006 by Taylor & Francis Group, LLC
CRC Press is an imprint of Taylor & Francis Group

No claim to original U.S. Government works
Printed in the United States of America on acid-free paper
10 9 8 7 6 5 4 3 2 1

International Standard Book Number-10: 0-8247-2587-5 (Hardcover)
International Standard Book Number-13: 978-0-8247-2587-7 (Hardcover)
Library of Congress Card Number 2005052710

This book contains information obtained from authentic and highly regarded sources. Reprinted material is quoted with permission, and sources are indicated. A wide variety of references are listed. Reasonable efforts have been made to publish reliable data and information, but the author and the publisher cannot assume responsibility for the validity of all materials or for the consequences of their use.

No part of this book may be reprinted, reproduced, transmitted, or utilized in any form by any electronic, mechanical, or other means, now known or hereafter invented, including photocopying, microfilming, and recording, or in any information storage or retrieval system, without written permission from the publishers.

For permission to photocopy or use material electronically from this work, please access www.copyright.com (http://www.copyright.com/) or contact the Copyright Clearance Center, Inc. (CCC) 222 Rosewood Drive, Danvers, MA 01923, 978-750-8400. CCC is a not-for-profit organization that provides licenses and registration for a variety of users. For organizations that have been granted a photocopy license by the CCC, a separate system of payment has been arranged.

Trademark Notice: Product or corporate names may be trademarks or registered trademarks, and are used only for identification and explanation without intent to infringe.

Library of Congress Cataloging-in-Publication Data

Mechanick, Jeffrey I.
   Nutritional strategies for the diabetic/prediabetic patient / by Jeffrey I. Mechanick and Elise M. Brett.
      p. cm. -- (Nutrition and disease prevention)
   ISBN 0-8247-2587-5 alk. paper
   1. Diabetes--Nutritional aspects. I. Brett, Elise M. II. Title. III. Series.

RC662.M335 2006
616.4'620654--dc22   2005052710

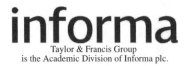

Taylor & Francis Group
is the Academic Division of Informa plc.

Visit the Taylor & Francis Web site at
http://www.taylorandfrancis.com

and the CRC Press Web site at
http://www.crcpress.com

Foreword

Nutritional Strategies for the Diabetic/Prediabetic Patient should indeed become the "Bible" on this topic for the next few years!

It contains information that is difficult to find elsewhere and is presented in an extremely scholarly manner. Each chapter contains basic information for those interested in the pathophysiology of the disease process and clinically relevant information that has practical implications regarding nutritional support for patients with diabetes.

Most importantly, the chapters are written by practicing physicians who give the book a flavor that would be absent if it was written by basic researchers or from a purely nutritionist approach.

The introductory chapter by Roubenoff elegantly explains the future of medicine, in which we will approach nutritional and, by extrapolation, pharmaceutical therapy based on genetics of the individual. This is followed by an erudite chapter on the pathophysiology and clinical management of diabetes and prediabetes by Rayfield and Valentine. This chapter sets the stage for the following chapters that focus on the nutritional aspects.

The chapter by Hensrud and the chapter by Kushner and Roth discuss the prediabetic type-2 patients and those with the metabolic syndrome, respectively, and on the whole conclude that the best approach is a reduced-calorie diet; an important conclusion in light of all the "fad diets" being propagated. Baliga and co-authors reached a similar conclusion in their chapter on medical nutrition for patients with type-2 diabetes.

In the next set of chapters on nutrition in type-1 diabetes by Weiss, gestational diabetes by Hussain and Jovanovic, carbohydrate counting by Warshaw, and nutrition with continuous insulin therapy by Drexler and Robertson, some very standard though critical aspects of these topics are covered. Their concise chapters present important practical and useful approaches to both practicing physicians and allied health professionals.

The chapter on nutritional support of hyperglycemia by Brett discusses the importance of treating hyperglycemia with intensive insulin therapy in hospitalized patients. This is an extremely topical subject because the recent published data on improved outcomes of patients, diabetic and non-diabetic, in surgical and medical ICUs and other units, include this form of therapy. The chapter also covers enteral and parenteral feedings and the balance between these types of feedings and control of blood glucose.

Vassalotti's chapter describes nutritional strategies for the patient with diabetic nephropathy, and Breit and Mechanick's chapter covers nutritional strategies for wound healing; both topics are often not foremost on the minds of the practicing health professional, and these two chapters should correct that anomaly. Exercise and diabetes are, of course, critical elements in the management of both type-1 and type-2 diabetic patients, and the nutritional support of this aspect of management is presented concisely but adequately by Rabito and co-authors.

Finally, there are two chapters by Mechanick, one on mitochondrial function, which has been shown by some elegant studies to be deranged in diabetics. His second chapter deals with dietary supplements and nutraceuticals and their potential role in treating diabetes. Both chapters are extremely well covered in a scholarly fashion. The take-home message, at this stage, is that there are few published, well-controlled trials to support the use of supplements and nutraceuticals. However, as the author points out, the health professional needs to be aware of their biological functions because many diabetics use them, and they may affect pharmaceuticals that are being used by those individuals.

Overall, the book is a compilation of chapters dealing primarily with various nutritional aspects of the management of the diabetic patient written by numerous experts. As expected there is some overlap with certain topics, though each chapter stands alone. The authors have excelled in their presentations, giving basic pathophysiological information as well as very practical advice.

Kudos to Drs. Mechanick and Brett for compiling such an outstanding group of chapters on an extremely important topic. It is a must read for health professionals dealing with patients with diabetes.

Derek LeRoith, M.D., Ph.D.
Chief, Division of Endocrinology, Diabetes and Bone Disease
Professor of Medicine
Mount Sinai School of Medicine

Preface

One of the first questions usually asked by a newly diagnosed patient with diabetes is "Doctor, what should I eat?" Many physicians would prefer not to answer this question, not only because of the time it takes to do so properly, but because they do not feel confident doing so. Most physicians have been poorly trained in nutrition, yet we are frequently asked to advise patients in this area. Clearly, there is never a simple answer to the question. Although nutrition is central to the management of diabetes, there is no one "diabetic diet." The nutritional prescription will depend on the person's type of diabetes, food preferences, lifestyle, treatment regimen, comorbidities, state of heath, and the route of caloric administration. Nutritional counseling ideally starts before the diagnosis of diabetes in the patient with prediabetes (i.e., those with metabolic syndrome or impaired glucose regulation). For these patients, diabetes may be prevented by appropriate diet and weight loss. As the prevalence of obesity continues to increase at an alarming rate, early identification of prediabetic patients and aggressive nutritional intervention become critical.

This book was written primarily for physicians to advance their knowledge in nutrition as it relates to diabetes and provide evidence-based recommendations to their diabetic patients. Dietitians and diabetes educators who desire an in-depth understanding of the pathophysiology and medical treatment of diabetes will also find this book useful. Contributors to the book include basic scientists, clinicians from various subspecialties, registered dietitians, and certified diabetes educators, each with expertise on a different aspect of diabetes care. Molecular mechanisms of disease and drug therapy are reviewed in detail. Recommendations for management are provided and the level of evidence indicated where appropriate. In areas where little research data are available, recommendations are based on extensive clinical experience. There is a particular focus on the synchronization of nutrient intake with medications. Unique clinical management tools are provided and meant to be replicated for patient use. We hope that this book will serve to fill some of the gaps in the clinician's knowledge and help to optimize care of the diabetic and prediabetic patient.

Editors

Drs. Jeffrey Mechanick and Elise Brett are in practice together in Manhattan. They are on the clinical faculty of Mount Sinai School of Medicine.

Jeffrey I. Mechanick, M.D., F.A.C.P., F.A.C.E., F.A.C.N.
Dr. Mechanick earned his M.D. degree from Mount Sinai School of Medicine in 1985 and completed his residency in internal medicine at the Baylor College of Medicine in 1988. After returning to Mount Sinai to complete his fellowship training in endocrinology, metabolism, and nutrition in 1990, Dr. Mechanick started his private practice in Manhattan in endocrinology, diabetes, and metabolic support. Since then, he has become the director of metabolic support and an associate clinical professor of medicine in the Division of Endocrinology, Diabetes, and Bone Disease at The Mount Sinai Hospital. He continues to care for many patients with diabetes and nutritional disorders, as well as train physicians in endocrinology and nutrition.

Dr. Mechanick has authored over 70 scientific publications in endocrinology and nutrition. His research interests are in the fields of parenteral nutrition support, chronic critical illness, and stress hyperglycemia. He is on the Board of Directors of the American Association of Clinical Endocrinologists and also serves as the Chairman of the AACE Nutrition and Publication Committees. Dr. Mechanick is an associate editor for *Endocrine Practice*. In addition, he is currently serving as President of the American Board of Physician Nutrition Specialists, and lectures extensively around the country in endocrinology and nutrition.

Elise M. Brett, M.D., F.A.C.E.
Dr. Brett earned her B.S. degree from the University of Michigan in 1989 and her M.D. degree from Mount Sinai School of Medicine in 1994. She completed her residency in internal medicine in 1997 and a fellowship in endocrinology and metabolism in 1999, both at The Mount Sinai Hospital. She was certified as a Nutrition Support Physician in 1998. She has been in private practice in Manhattan in endocrinology, diabetes, and metabolic support since completing her fellowship. Dr. Brett is currently assistant clinical professor of medicine at Mount Sinai and trains physicians in endocrinology and nutrition.

Dr. Brett has published in the field of general endocrinology, diabetes, metabolic support, and nutrition, and lectures regularly on these topics. She is a past member of the board of directors of the American Association of Clinical Endocrinologists and currently serves on the AACE Nutrition Committee, Diabetes Guidelines Committee, and AACE Self-Assessment Profile Nutrition Subcommittee.

Contributors

Bantwal Suresh Baliga, M.D.
Mount Sinai School of Medicine
and
North General Hospital
New York, New York

**Zachary Bloomgarden, M.D.,
  F.A.C.E.**
Mount Sinai School of Medicine
New York, New York

Neal G. Breit, M.D.
Mount Sinai School of Medicine
New York, New York

**Elise M. Brett, M.D., F.A.C.E.,
  C.N.S.P.**
Mount Sinai School of Medicine
New York, New York

Andrew Jay Drexler, M.D., F.A.C.E.
New York University School of
  Medicine
New York Diabetes Program
New York, New York

Donald D. Hensrud, M.D., M.P.H.
Mayo Clinic
Rochester, Minnesota

Zohair Hussain
Sansum Diabetes Research Institute
Santa Barbara, California

Lois Jovanovic, M.D.
University of Southern California
Los Angeles, California
and
University of California
Santa Barbara, California
and
Sansum Diabetes Research Institute
Santa Barbara, California

Robert F. Kushner, M.D.
Northwestern Memorial Hospital
Chicago, Illinois

**Jeffrey I. Mechanick, M.D.,
  F.A.C.P., F.A.C.E., F.A.C.N.**
Mount Sinai School of Medicine
New York, New York

Cathy Nonas, R.D., C.D.E.
North General Hospital
New York, New York

Philip Rabito, M.D., F.A.C.E.
Mount Sinai School of Medicine
New York, New York
and
Mount Sinai Medical Center at
  Elmhurst
Elmhurst, New York

Elliot J. Rayfield, M.D., F.A.C.E.
Mount Sinai School of Medicine
New York, New York

Carolyn Robertson, A.P.R.N., M.S.N., B.C.-A.D.M.
New York Diabetes Program
New York, New York

Julie L. Roth, M.D.
Northwestern University
Chicago, Illinois

Ronenn Roubenoff, M.D., M.H.S.
Tufts University
Boston, Massachusetts
and
Millennium Pharmaceuticals, Inc.
Cambridge, Massachusetts

Claudia Shwide-Slavin, M.S., R.D., B.C.-A.D.M., C.D.E.
Private Practice
New York, New York

Don Smith, M.D., M.P.H.
The Mount Sinai School of Medicine
New York, New York

Marilyn V. Valentine, M.D.
Pfizer Pharmaceuticals
New York, New York

Joseph A. Vassalotti, M.D., F.A.S.N.
Mount Sinai School of Medicine
New York, New York

Hope S. Warshaw, M.M.Sc., R.D., C.D.E., B.C.-A.D.M.
Dietitian and Certified Diabetes
  Educator
Alexandria, Virginia

Stuart Weiss, M.D.
New York University School of
  Medicine
New York, New York

Table of Contents

1 Foundations of Nutritional Medicine: From Basic Concepts to Genomic Medicine

Ronenn Roubenoff

CONTENTS

EVOLUTION AND CURRENT STATE OF NUTRITIONAL MEDICINE

THE UPS AND DOWNS OF NUTRITION IN MEDICINE

Nutrition played a prominent role in the education and practice of physicians from the time of Hippocrates until the mid-twentieth century. Hippocrates, for example, is noted for one of his aphorisms: "Let food be thy medicine and medicine thy food" [1]. For much of human history, undernutrition was a major cause of death, both directly through starvation and indirectly by its amplification of susceptibility to and mortality from disease, especially infectious diseases. Until the period just after World War II, most American medical schools included separate, year-long courses on nutrition in their curriculum. However, with the explosion in knowledge in biochemistry and molecular biology, coupled with the apparent triumph of antibiotics and public health laws over infectious diseases, nutrition was seen as less and less important and lost its place in the medical school curriculum. By the 1980s, most schools had either limited their students' nutrition exposure to a few weeks in the first year, or blended nutrition lectures into biochemistry and physiology, eliminating it altogether as a perceived specialty in the minds of most students.

However, the tide has turned in the past two decades. It is now clear that most of the leading causes of death in both industrialized and emerging societies have a major nutritional basis, although that basis is more likely to be overnutrition than undernutrition in most of the world (see Table 1.1). The emergence of the obesity epidemic in the 1990s has once again raised the profile of nutrition as an important medical issue, drawing research and policy attention that is urgently needed. Unfortunately, the current generation of practicing physicians is for the most part woefully ill-equipped to either diagnose or treat the nutritional aspects of most diseases, and as a result physicians are often far less interested in this aspect of medical care than are their patients. Furthermore, there is now at most medical schools a lack of faculty qualified to teach nutrition; this will take some time to redress. Thus, an important interim step in educating both students and practitioners is filled by texts such as this one.

INPATIENT NUTRITION SUPPORT

The provision of calories and protein to the sick has been recognized as a priority since antiquity, but it was also largely de-emphasized in the mid-twentieth century. In 1936, Studley showed that patients who were malnourished before surgery had higher risk of complications after surgery for peptic ulcers [2]. By the 1970s, "iatrogenic malnutrition" was rampant in inpatient settings, prompting Butterworth to call it "the skeleton in the hospital closet" [3]. Several surveys showed that malnutrition rates in excess of 70% were common even in the most sophisticated teaching hospitals, and that most house staff could not recognize malnutrition [4]. The seminal work that began reversing this indifference to feeding had been carried out a few years earlier by Dudrick et al., who showed that dogs could be kept alive for extended periods using parenteral nutrition only [5]. This led to the flowering at most large medical centers of nutrition support teams specializing in intravenous feedings. More recently, these teams have largely been disbanded because of cost constraints and the recognition that most patients who are unable to eat can be fed more safely, effectively, and cheaply using interal tube feedings. In addition, routine perioperative intravenous nutritional support was shown to be effective only in patients with severe malnutrition [6]. Today, at least some level of nutrition screening is mandated by the accredited authorities in most developed nations, although the delay between the beginning of inadequate intake and its treatment is still generally far too long, missing the golden opportunity to forestall iatrogenic malnutrition rather than to treat it.

OUTPATIENT NUTRITION SUPPORT

In the United States, outpatient nutritional services are underfunded and understaffed. Ironically, public spending on weight loss programs and nutritional supplements is enormous and growing rapidly, totaling 1–6% of gross domestic product of industrialized nations [7]. Not surprisingly, then, most of the public's interaction with nutritional services comes not from trained professionals such as dietitians or physicians, but rather from profit-seeking services of various types, ranging from authentic providers to charlatans and quacks. The obesity epidemic has focused the attention of government and private funders on obesity research and treatment, and it is likely that medical services to treat obesity will grow substantially in the next decade. The pharmaceutical industry has not failed to note this, and many companies are pursuing pharmacological treatments of obesity, recognizing that an effective and safe weight loss drug would be a blockbuster.

TABLE 1.1
Obesity and Overweight as Causes of Death in the United States, 1990–2000

Actual Cause	No. (%) in 1990	No. (%) in 2000
Tobacco	400,000 (19)	435,000 (18.1)
Poor diet and physical inactivity	300,000 (14)	400,000 (16.6)
Alcohol consumption	100,000 (5)	85,000 (3.5)
Microbial agents	90,000 (4)	75,000 (3.1)
Toxic agents	60,000 (3)	55,000 (2.3)
Motor vehicle	35,000 (2)	43,000 (1.8)
Firearms	35,000 (2)	29,000 (1.2)
Sexual behavior	30,000 (1)	20,000 (0.8)
Illicit drug use	20,000 (<1)	17,000 (0.7)
Total	1,060,000 (50.0)	1,159,000 (48.2)

Source: From Reference [53] with permission.

FUTURE DIRECTIONS

Medical nutrition is changing rapidly due to several forces. First, the public health and policy impact of the obesity epidemic and its siblings—the epidemics in diabetes, metabolic syndrome, and heart disease—has emerged as the leading health problem of both the developed and developing world. For instance, the leading cause of death in India today is heart disease, which was virtually unknown only two generations ago [8]. It is likely that the effect of the obesity epidemic on nutrition will be comparable to the effect of the human immunodeficiency virus (HIV) epidemic on infectious diseases two decades earlier: it will mobilize both research and treatment funding and recruit a new cadre of medical nutritionists to the field. Second, the availability of the human genome, proteome, kinome, and metabolome will revolutionize our understanding of the mechanisms of both macronutrient and micronutrient regulation and metabolism. Where nutrition policy in the past has focused on recommended dietary intakes for the population as a whole, in the post-genomic world it is likely that specific nutritional recommendations will be feasible for individuals depending on their genetic makeup and propensity toward various nutrition-related diseases. Third, Internet access and the informational democracy it brings are changing what patients know, how soon they know it, and what demands they make of their physicians. Often, patients today are better-informed than their doctors, but lack the scientific and medical background needed to make sense of the information they have. Nevertheless, the knowledge gap between doctor and patient will shrink faster in nutrition than in almost any other field of medicine, because the public's interest in—and stake in—nutrition is overwhelming. After all, nutrition is the ultimate environmental exposure; one shared by all living beings, and is one of the health-related behaviors that people feel they can both control and use to influence their health.

BASIC CONCEPTS

NUTRITION THROUGH THE LIFE CYCLE

Any attempts to assess nutritional status or prescribe nutritional therapy for a patient must take into account that patient's physiological status. Obviously, a growing child will metabolize and utilize nutrients differently from an elderly man or woman. The metabolic milieu in which a person exists changes on several different time scales, each with their own set of controlling hormonal and immunological regulators (see Figure 1.1). On a decades-long level, changes in sex steroids and growth hormone govern menopausal status, bone and muscle anabolic propensity, and thus the balance of calcium, nitrogen, and potassium. On a monthly scale, changes in estrogen and progesterone modulate menstrual status in premenopausal women, and thus affect iron status. On a daily basis, insulin and glucagon respond to dietary intake variations by altering the ebb and flow of glucose and fatty acids in and out of muscle, liver, brain, and other tissues. Episodically, changes in prolactin with pregnancy and lactation further alter nutrient balance [9]. Similarly, during acute illnesses inflammatory cytokines—interleukin-1 (IL-1), tumor necrosis factor-α (TNF-α), and IL-6, primarily—dramatically alter insulin sensitivity and muscle amino acid balance, as well as hepatic and leukocyte protein production and utilization. Any acute illness that causes inflammation, including trauma, surgery, myocardial infraction, systemic infections, and systemic autoimmune diseases, will activate these catabolic cytokines and cause negative energy, protein, and micronutrient balance (see Figure 1.1). Thus, any nutritional evaluation must begin with a physiological assessment of the host's ability to withstand stress.

Effect of Acute Illness

Importance of Premorbid Status

In both acute and chronic illness, the ability of the patient to withstand the physiological stress of the disease depends on two factors: the baseline reserves of essential macro- and micronutrients the patient has, and the loss rate of each. An example is a woman's risk of osteoporosis at age 70, which is a function of her peak bone mass (reached in her 20s), and the loss rate of bone after menopause (typically by age 52). If her intake of calcium and vitamin D as a teenager was inadequate, her peak bone mass may have been low, reducing her ability to withstand the rapid loss of bone which occurs with estrogen withdrawal 30–40 years later. Similarly, for the diabetic, obesity is the greatest nutritional risk, but it can be compounded by age-related sarcopenia, which leads to loss of muscle on top of the gain in fat experienced. The result is additional insulin resistance due to both excess adipose tissue and loss of muscle.

Of the three macronutrients (protein, fat, and carbohydrate), only protein becomes limiting in terms of biochemical requirements for survival. With severe catabolic illness, a healthy man's amino acid stores will be exhausted in about 3 weeks [10,11]. In general, loss of more than 40% of baseline body cell mass (somewhat arbitrarily defined as the amount a person has at age 25) is fatal [12,13]. With normal aging, there is loss of about 6% per decade, so a 70-year-old patient with acute illness has 30% less cell mass to draw on for protein stores than does a 20-year-old with the same illness. Thus, the older patient's protein reserves become substrate-limiting much sooner than in the young patient, and complications due to malnutrition—infections, bedsores, edema, poor wound healing—are much more frequent. If the patient is not given the necessary nutrients exogenously, either via the gut or the vein, these complications are often fatal.

However, protein metabolism does not occur in a vacuum. Carbohydrate stores are exhausted within 48 hours of fasting, increasing the requirement for energy from fat and protein. In diabetics, and even in nondiabetics who are stressed, insulin resistance limits the ability of fat to be metabolized, accelerating the utilization of muscle protein stores for energy via gluconeogenesis, a much less efficient and more metabolically expensive process than lipolysis [14]. The insulin resistance of acute illness, driven largely by TNF-α, causes hyperlipidemia, which is a poor prognostic sign in critically ill patients [15]. The metabolic disturbances of critical illness are severe, but aggressive control of hyperglycemia can improve survival, although the need for more insulin signals a poorer prognosis [16,17]. In less severely ill patients, these metabolic derangements occur to a lesser degree, but can still complicate the patient's treatment.

Importance of Intra-Morbid Nutritional Support

Given the above issues, there is no doubt that provision of exogenous nutrients is crucial to the care of acutely ill patients. This is just as true in obese and diabetic patients as it is in cachectic, emaciated ones. However, provision of the proper energy and protein load is complicated by end-

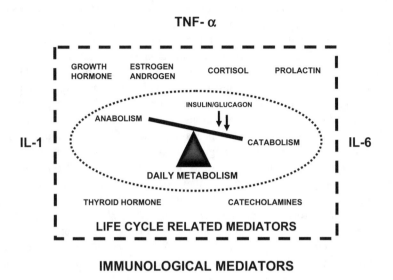

FIGURE 1.1 Mediators of metabolism on different time scales and under different physiological conditions. From Reference [54] with permission. Abbreviations: IL = interleukin; TNF-α = tumor necrosis factor.

organ limitations in the absorption or utilization of these nutrients [18]. Nevertheless, even in the morbidly obese patient, avoidance of feeding is detrimental because (a) gut integrity is weakened by the absence of food, increasing the risk of infections and possibly other complications such as ileus, hemorrhage, and perforation; (b) even in the presence of massive fat stores, protein will still be excessively oxidized unless exogenous amino acids and glucose are provided; (c) prolonged avoidance of feedings makes return to feeding more difficult, as the gut atrophies and its enzymatic digestive capabilities are reduced. Ironically, an important result of malnutrition is more malnutrition.

It is natural for clinicians to be averse to taking on additional risks perceived to derive from feeding patients: concerns about aspiration, perforation of viscus by a feeding tube, diarrhea with tube feedings; metabolic derangements, infection, volume overload, and electrolyte imbalances with intravenous feedings are all reasonable. However, it is equally important to remember that no system in the body works better starved than fed; that no clinician would avoid treatment of infection with antibiotics, arrhythmia with antiarrhythmics, or cardiac ischemia with vasodilators. Why should the provision of nutrition be any different? Presumably because nutritional support is seen as elective, that the patient can withstand no exogenous energy or protein for "a few days," and that the risks outweigh the benefits. However, these notions have not stood up to scientific inquiry: today, nutrition support can be given more safely and effectively than ever, and recognition of the risks of malnutrition has grown widespread. In effect, the argument against nutrition support is often upheld by the fact that such treatment is started after prolonged iatrogenic malnutrition, when the complications are greater and the ability of the gut to accept feedings is reduced. The result is a self-fulfilling prophecy, confirming the difficulty and intolerability of nutrition support. However, this is specious: with aggressive, early feedings, outcomes improve, complications decrease, and length of stay shortens [19,20].

Importance of Post-Illness Rehabilitation

It is a clinical truism that recovery from an illness takes three times as long as the original insult. Treating an acute exacerbation of a chronic illness, such as rheumatoid arthritis, prevents further deterioration of nutritional status, but does not in and of itself reverse muscle loss [21]. This is likely to be true after an acute illness as well, although this is less well-studied. It is crucial that patients receive both nutritional and exercise treatment to replete their protein status as they recover from an illness. There are many priorities for the clinician to balance during convalescence, including the level of frailty the patient evinces both physically and psychologically, interventions aimed at underlying causes of the acute illness or exacerbation, and measures aimed at rehabilitating the patient to a higher level of function. It is safe to say that all of these would benefit from appropriate dietary and exercise recommendations. The level of micronutrient and macronutrient intake should be assessed and corrected if necessary, and the patient should be encouraged to exercise to the point of mild to moderate fatigue but not exhaustion. Shortly after a severe illness, simply rising from bed may be exhausting, but as patients recover it is important to push the goal of their rehabilitation program forward so that they continue to progress. Exercise should include resistance training, which requires less oxygen consumption than aerobic exercise and will increase muscle mass and protein stores much more effectively [22]. Walking, on land or in the water, swimming, and stationary bicycling are the most accessible aerobic exercises for most patients. The role of exercise in the rehabilitation process is twofold: first, it imparts important benefits in terms of energy balance, muscle fitness, and insulin resistance; and second, it is the most effective way to partition nutrients toward the lean mass and away from fat.

Nutritional Assessment

In clinical practice, micronutrient status is usually measured by blood or urine. However, there is no definitive biochemical test for macronutrient status, which must also be evaluated using history and physical examination, along with selected imaging techniques when necessary. The history portion of nutritional assessment is predicated on an adequate review of recent dietary intake. This is often best done by a registered dietitian (RD). The goal is to assess whether dietary intake has been sufficient to account for any weight changes seen over the past 6–12 months. In addition, the sufficiency of micronutrient intake can be estimated. Weight loss of greater than 5% in 6 months or 10% in 1 year is a marker of nutritional risk, and should prompt investigation for a medical cause of weight loss. Conversely, weight gain increases the risk of obesity-related diabetes, osteoarthritis, cardiovascular disease, hypertension, and gallstones. While in most clinical situations weight and weight change are sufficient to assess fat and protein stores, occasionally (or for research) more precise techniques are needed. Body composition to assess lean and fat compartments, especially when the physical examination is less reliable due to the presence of anasarca, can be measured using a variety of techniques [12]. However, in most cases, tracking weight over time is the single most useful test a physician can perform.

Undernutrition

Weight loss can be classified as having three "tracks," roughly corresponding to slow, medium, and rapid loss of lean body mass (see Table 1.2) [23]. The slowest loss, which happens to everyone and is not disease-related, is sarcopenia, from the Greek for "poverty of flesh." Sarcopenia refers to the loss of muscle mass and strength that happens with aging in all persons. Sarcopenia seems to be caused by the age-related withdrawal of anabolic stimuli, such as sex steroids and growth hormone, and the commensurate increase in catabolic stimuli to muscle due to increased production of cytokines such as interleukin-6 and others with age [24]. The only known intervention to prevent or reverse sarcopenia is resistance exercise with adequate dietary intake [25].

At the opposite extreme, rapid weight loss is best called wasting, a term used since the onset of the AIDS epidemic to refer to unintentional weight loss, with loss of both lean and fat compartments. Wasting is largely driven by inadequate dietary energy and protein intake, and is fatal when body cell mass falls below 60% of baseline for healthy young adults [13,23]. Metabolic rate is

TABLE 1.2
Comparison of Cachexia, Wasting, and Sarcopenia

Feature	Cachexia	Wasting	Sarcopenia
Decreased BCM	Yes	Yes	Yes, skeletal muscle cells
Weight loss	None or little compared with loss of BCM	Yes	Not necessarily
Decreased energy intake	No	Yes	No
Elevated REE	Often	Not necessarily	No
Decreased functional status	Yes	Yes	Yes
Increased cytokine production	Yes, IL-1β, TNF-α, others	No, often decreased	Yes, IL-6
Reduced immune defense	Yes	Yes	Not necessarily
Increased mortality	Yes	Yes	?
Treatment	Anabolic hormones; progressive resistance exercise; ? anti-cytokine agents	Increased dietary intake; progressive resistance exercise	Progressive resistance exercise; ? anabolic hormones
Clinical examples	Critical illness with adequate nutritional support; end-organ failures (CHF, renal, hepatic); rheumatoid arthritis; HIV infection without opportunistic infection	Critical illness without adequate nutritional support; starvation; end-stage cancer, tuberculosis; advanced HIV infection	Normal aging

Abbreviations: REE—resting energy expenditure; BCM—body cell mass; CHF—congestive heart failure; HIV—human immunodeficiency virus; IL—interleukin; TNF-α—tumor necrosis factor.

Source: From Reference [23] with permission.

suppressed and physical activity is reduced in a compensatory fashion. The key therapeutic intervention for wasting is feeding.

Finally, there is cachexia, from the Greek for "bad condition," to describe loss of lean body mass (principally muscle) despite stable or even rising weight. Cachexia is seen in end-organ failures, such as heart, liver, or renal failure, where extracellular water increases as muscle mass falls, and in chronic inflammatory conditions like rheumatoid arthritis, where there is an increase in fat mass and a decline in muscle. In these situations, the increase in one compartment masks the decline in another, so that weight changes little and does not reveal the ongoing malnutrition. In cachexia, dietary intake can be normal or even increased, but cytokine-driven metabolic alterations favor proteolysis and spare fat [26]. The major intervention here must be aimed at the underlying disease, with judicious use of resistance exercise, as excess calories will only create greater obesity without replenishing muscle mass [27,28].

OVERNUTRITION AND OBESITY

Energy Balance

Development of obesity is a multifactorial process involving genetic, metabolic, and environmental factors. Genetic factors confer the potential for obesity, but it is the interaction between genetic and environmental factors, such as diet and level of physical activity, that result in weight gain. Gains in body weight by definition represent an imbalance between energy intake and energy expenditure; to maintain body weight, an individual must match intake and expenditure. To illustrate just how precise this regulation is, consider a small energy imbalance of +2% (or +50 kcal/day for an individual with total maintenance needs of 2500 kcal/day), an imbalance that can easily occur. That small imbalance, if persisting over one year, would result in a gain in body weight of approximately 5 lb. In epidemiological studies, the average weight gain in adults is between 0.5 and 2.0 lb/year [29,30], suggesting that most persons chronically maintain energy balance to greater than 99% tolerance. Discussion of the role of energy intake in obesity is well beyond the scope of this chapter; Schoeller [31] recently reviewed the contribution of energy intake and dietary factors to energy balance.

CNS Mechanisms of Appetite Control

There has been an explosion of knowledge about the neuroendocrine regulation of food intake in the past decade. It is now clear that obesity is not merely a failure of willpower, but a hormonally driven disorder in brain control of energy balance. Many different genetic mutations have been found to explain up to 5% of cases of childhood obesity, but in general no simple genetic explanation has emerged for obesity. The key pathways regulating dietary intake and physical activity are shown in Figure 1.2. For a more detailed discussion, please see the review by Korner and Aronne [32]. The emerging biology of obesity indicates that leptin, a hormone made by fat cells in the periphery, acts along with insulin in lean persons to reduce dietary intake by suppressing the orexigenic neuropeptide Y (NPY) and stimulating the anorexic neuropeptide melanocortin at the same time. These two peptides, with overlapping support from melanin concentrating hormone (MCH), orexins, cocaine- and amphetamine-regulated transcript (CART), and others, regulate food intake and energy expenditure to achieve energy balance. As fat mass expands, leptin levels rise, but there develops a relative resistance to both leptin and insulin in the brain which slowly limits the ability of leptin to brake positive energy balance. At the same time, insulin resistance is thought to be at least partially responsible for many of the deleterious health effects of obesity, such as diabetes, hypertension, and cardiovascular disease.

Schwartz et al. [33] have suggested that the balance of these hormones favors weight gain and failure of energy restricted diets (see Figure 1.3). They propose that in the basal state, the weight-losing (catabolic) pathways (primarily via melanocortin) are activated by leptin and insulin, while the weight-gaining (anabolic) pathways (primarily NPY) are suppressed to maintain weight. With weight loss, the reverse happens, and there is activation of the anabolic pathways and inhibition of the catabolic ones. This response is inherently stronger than the response to weight gain, which leads to the attempted further stimulation of the already basally stimulated catabolic pathways and further inhibition of the already-suppressed anabolic pathways. Thus, over time, most people tend to gain weight in developed societies where energy expenditure is relatively low and energy availability is high. Almost 50 years ago, Jean Mayer hypothesized that the mechanisms controlling energy balance are accurate at high levels of physical activity, but that there is a threshold below which these mechanisms become imprecise and this leads to obesity; recent data suggest that this hypothesis is valid, although the mechanisms underlying it are much more complex than originally proposed [34]. Thus, an important role of exercise in treating obesity may be to increase daily caloric needs to a level where the body's regulatory mechanisms are better able to function.

Physical Activity

Regular exercise seems to attenuate the increase in fat mass with age. Van Pelt et al. [35] found that postmenopausal female runners (mean age 56 years; average 28 miles/week) averaged 23.4% body fat, compared to 15% body fat in premenopausal female runners (mean age 30 years; average 38 miles/week). Although this observation suggests that fat mass increases substantially with age even among highly active runners, note how these results compare with those of sedentary women studied at the same time: the postmenopausal sedentary women (mean age 61 years) had 40% body fat while the premenopausal sedentary women (mean age 29 years) had 27% body fat. Thus, the

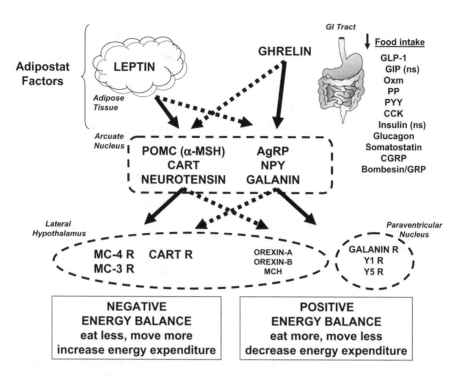

FIGURE 1.2 Pathways regulating energy balance. Dark arrows indicate positive effects; dashed arrows negative ones. Various gut peptides, many of which are involved in the incretin effect, have a suppressive effect on appetite. Abbreviations: GLP-1—glucagon-like peptide-1; GIP—glucose-dependent insulinotropic polypeptide; ns—nonspecific effect on appetite; Oxm—oxyntomodulin; PP—pancreatic polypeptide; PYY— peptide YY; CCK—cholecystokinin; CGRP—calcitonin gene-related peptide, GRP—gastrin-releasing peptide, POMC—proopiomelanocortin; α-MSH—alpha-melanocyte stimulating hormone; CART—cocaine- and amphetamine-regulated transcript; CART R—CART receptor; MC-4 R—melanocortin 4 receptor; MC-3 R— melanocortin 3 receptor; AgRP—agouti-related peptide; NPY—neuropeptide Y; Y1 R—Y1 receptor; Y5 R— Y5 receptor; galanin R—galanin receptor.

athletes had an age-related difference in their adiposity of 8.4%, while the sedentary women had a difference of 13.0%. These data suggest that habitual exercise reduced the age-related increase in body fatness by about 35%. In addition, the habitual exercisers were also significantly more fit than the sedentary women at any age ($V_{O2\ max}$ 55 ± 0.9 vs. 42 ± 1.5 mL/kg/minute). Although some caution is appropriate in interpreting cross-sectional rather than longitudinal data, these observations suggest that high levels of physical activity can prevent obesity.

While a large portion of total energy expenditure (TEE) is determined by resting energy expenditure (REE), energy spent on physical activity remains an effective way to increase total expenditure. Since eating a few cookies can overcome the caloric expenditure of an hour of exercise, it is relatively difficult to create a negative energy balance by physical activity alone. It is true that expending an extra 100 or 200 calories/day with exercise amounts to only about 10% of the day's energy intake. Nevertheless, as discussed previously, the difference between positive and negative energy balance in most individuals is relatively small, so that even a small increase in physical activity can influence whether that day's balance is positive or negative. As Figure 1.4 shows, even moderate physical activity can lead to important caloric expenditures, especially in more obese people who require more energy to perform work on their body mass (i.e., to simply move around).

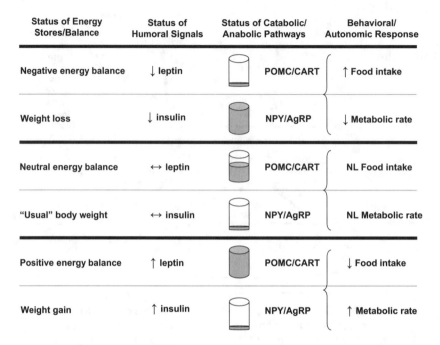

Status of Energy Stores/Balance	Status of Humoral Signals	Status of Catabolic/ Anabolic Pathways	Behavioral/ Autonomic Response
Negative energy balance	↓ leptin	POMC/CART	↑ Food intake
Weight loss	↓ insulin	NPY/AgRP	↓ Metabolic rate
Neutral energy balance	↔ leptin	POMC/CART	NL Food intake
"Usual" body weight	↔ insulin	NPY/AgRP	NL Metabolic rate
Positive energy balance	↑ leptin	POMC/CART	↓ Food intake
Weight gain	↑ insulin	NPY/AgRP	↑ Metabolic rate

FIGURE 1.3 Possible neurohormonal propensity toward weight gain. From Reference [33] with permission.

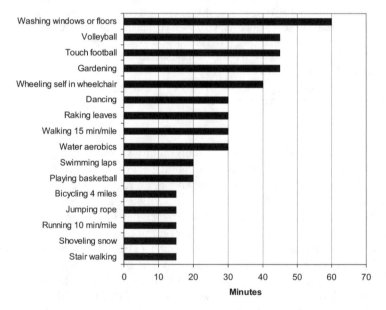

FIGURE 1.4 Time required (in minutes) for selected physical activities to burn the same number of calories. From Reference [55].

CARE OF THE DIABETIC AND PREDIABETIC PATIENT

DIET

Recognition of the importance of diet to the treatment of diabetes is attributed to Aretaeus of Cappadocia (30–90 A.D.), who both named diabetes and prescribed treatment with milk, cereal, starch, fruit, and wine [36]. Weight loss has been known to improve hyperglycemia since the eighteenth century, and before the discovery of insulin, Joslin and others pioneered the use of starvation diets for the treatment of diabetes [36,37]. With improved diets, survival after diagnosis improved from 1.3 to 2.6 years for 10-year-old diabetics; from 2.4 to 4.0 years for 25-year-olds; and from 8.5 to 10.5 years for 45-year-olds [36]. With improved pharmacotherapy, dietary treatment of diabetes has taken on a secondary role, but in recent years, it has become clear that diet and exercise are key to the treatment of diabetes and prevention of type-2 diabetes (T2DM). Indeed, the obesity epidemic that has overtaken the post-industrial nations gives rise to the diabetes epidemic, which in turn leads to cardiovascular disease with substantial morbidity and mortality [38].

The specific approaches to macronutrient and micronutrient prescription in diabetes will be discussed in detail later in this text. However, it is striking to note a recent World Health Organization (WHO) Expert Consultation on Chronic Disease Prevention, which found that a striking increase in sugar intake in the developing world, coinciding with public health efforts to lower fat intake, may have inadvertently contributed to the obesity epidemic [39]. Dietary energy intake has been increasing in the USA, with most of the increase coming from carbohydrates, specifically from high-fructose corn syrup (HFCS) (see Figure 1.5) [40,41]. Recently, it has been suggested that overconsumption of HFCS in sweetened beverages may play a role in the obesity and diabetes epidemics [40]. Theoretically, this is because fructose, unlike glucose, does not stimulate insulin secretion or enhance leptin production, but does promote *de novo* lipogenesis [41]. Clearly, the obesity epidemic has developed in the face of a 20-year attempt by the nutrition community to brand fat intake as bad. The food industry responded by developing foods that were low in fat, but were often not lower in calories than higher fat foods. On the other hand, recent publications have shown that, in the short-term, low-carbohydrate/high-fat diets can lead to weight loss comparable to those produced by low-fat diets, without dramatic increases in cardiovascular risk factors [42,43]. However, on a long-term basis, it is not known if these low-carbohydrate/high-fat diets are safe, especially if they are interpreted as being high in saturated fat, which is clearly a risk factor for atherosclerosis. Since the majority of patients with T2DM are obese and successful treatment of obesity remains elusive, dietary strategies for treatment of diabetes will have to be balanced against competing claims in the public arena regarding weight loss diets. The public will continue to be confused and unhappy with this situation, and clinicians will need more and more expertise with dietary treatment in order to stop inappropriate and even dangerous dietary practices in their patients.

FUTURE DIRECTIONS

Personalized Medicine and Personalized Nutrition

The completion of the human genome map in 2001 [44] has ushered in a new era of biomedicine, one which will affect diagnosis, treatment, and prognosis of all human diseases over the next century. Already, the diagnosis of human cancers is shifting from century-old histological description to genetic analysis of the precise biochemical mutation causing the neoplasm [45], and it is likely that most chronic diseases will be similarly redefined in the coming years. This revolution in biomedicine, which is on par with the physics and chemistry revolutions that led to the industrial age, has led to the concept of "personalized medicine," the notion that an individual's genome (his DNA), transcriptome (his RNA), proteome (his protein expression profile), and metabolome (his cellular metabolite profile) can be evaluated to determine risk of disease, optimal therapy, and risk of side effects from medications [46]. These approaches have already revolutionized medical

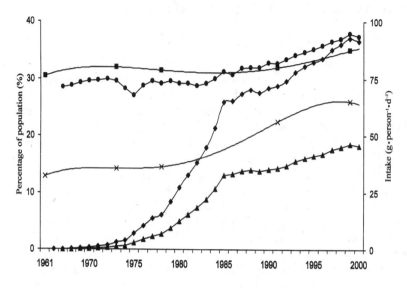

FIGURE 1.5 Estimated intakes of total fructose (●), free fructose (▲), and high fructose corn syrup (♦) in relation to trends in overweight (■) and obesity (✕) in the United States. From Reference [41] with permission.

research and drug discovery [47,48]. While such a genomic approach to medicine is still hypothetical, it is likely that information from the human genome will slowly trickle down to clinical medicine, even though this process may be excruciatingly slow [49].

Alongside the advent of "personalized medicine" will also come "personalized nutrition," the concept that we can determine which diet will work best for an individual, rather than prescribing diets across entire populations or disease groups, as is the case now with the Dietary Guidelines and Recommendations [50]. The hope is that we will be able to identify patients who respond to, for example, a high-fat diet better than to a low-fat diet for weight loss. While this is still out of reach, it is currently possible to identify high-risk mutations in genes such as the Apo-E gene, the methylene tetrahydrofolate reductase gene, and others that confer increased probability of developing Alzheimer's disease or hyperhomocysteinemia—a risk factor for atherosclerosis [51,52]. Such individuals might benefit from increased intake of vitamin E and folic acid, respectively, and thus delay or reduce their risk of expressing the clinical phenotype associated with these genes.

Over the next decade, as the prices of genetic (evaluation of specific genes) and genomic (evaluation across the entire genome) assays continue to fall, it may become practical to evaluate risk and responsiveness well ahead of the advent of clinical disease. Such an enhanced lead time would amplify the ability of long-term interventions, such as diet and exercise, to alter risk of disease. In addition, knowing their genetic risk may well motivate many individuals to make lifestyle changes that they would otherwise ignore. However, society will have to grapple with the consequences of having such information, including issues about insurance, healthcare costs, and freedom to make lifestyle choices that incur societal costs. Thus, we are entering an extremely exciting time in the annals of human nutrition, in which genetic information, coupled with the ultimate environmental exposure—diet—combine to maximize the quality and duration of human life. The potential impact of this strategy for patients with abnormal glucose tolerance is enormous.

REFERENCES

1. Adams F, *The Genuine Works of Hippocrates*, Huntington, NY: Robert E. Krueger Publishing Co., 1972.
2. Studley H, Percentage of weight loss with physical impairment: A basic indicator of surgical risk in patients with chronic peptic ulcer, *JAMA,* 106:458–460, 1936.
3. Weinsier R, Hunker E, and Krumdieck C et al., Hospital malnutrition: A prospective evaluation of general medical patients during the course of hospitalization, *Am J of Clin Nutr,* 32:418–426, 1979.
4. Roubenoff R, Roubenoff R, and Preto J et al., Malnutrition among medical inpatients: A problem of physician awareness, *Arch Intern Med,* 147:1462–1465, 1987.
5. Dudrick S, Wilmore D, and Vars H et al., Long-term total parenteral nutrition with growth, development, and positive nitrogen balance, *Surgery,* 64:134–142, 1968.
6. VA Study Group, Perioperative total parenteral nutrition in surgical patients, *N Engl J Med,* 325:525–532, 1991.
7. Baker JP, Detsky AS, and Wesson DE et al., Obesity: Preventing and managing the global epidemic, Report of a WHO consultation, Geneva: World Health Organization, 2000.
8. Mahpatra P and Rao P, *Causes of Death in Rural Areas of Andhra Pradesh,* 1998, Hyderabad: Institute of Health Systems (www.ihsnet.org.in), 2001: 20.
9. Frohman L, Diseases of the anterior pituitary, In: Felig P, Baxter JD, and Frohman LA, Eds., *Endocrinology and Metabolism,* Vol. 1, New York: McGraw-Hill, 309–311, 1995.
10. Moore F, Energy and the maintenance of body cell mass, *J Parenteral Enteral Nutr,* 4:228–260, 1980.
11. Cahill G, Starvation in man, *NEJM,* 282:668–75, 1972.
12. Roubenoff R and Kehayias J, The meaning and measurement of lean body mass, *Nutr Rev,* 46:163–175, 1991.
13. Kotler D, Tierney A, and Pierson R, Magnitude of body cell mass depletion and the timing of death from wasting in AIDS, *Am J Clin Nutr,* 50:444–447, 1989.
14. Linder M, *Nutritional Biochemistry and Metabolism,* New York: Elsevier, 1991.
15. Memon R, Feingold K, and Grunfeld C, Role of cytokines in lipid metabolism and cachexia, In: Puri R, Ed., *Human Cytokines: Their Role in Disease and Therapy,* Cambridge, MA: Blackwell Science, 239–251, 1995.
16. Finney S, Zevkeld C, and Elia A et al., Glucose control and mortality in critically ill patients, *JAMA,* 290:2041–2047, 2003.
17. Montori V, Bistrian B, and McMahon M, Hyperglycemia in acutely ill patients, *JAMA,* 288:2167–2169, 2002.
18. FAO, WHO, UNU, Energy and protein requirements, Report of a joint FAO/WHO/UNU expert consultation, Technical report series 724, Geneva: World Health Organization, 1985.
19. Chiarelli A, Enzi G, and Casadei A et al., Very early nutrition supplementation in burned patients, *Am J Clin Nutr,* 51:1035–1039, 1990.
20. Prichard C, Kyle U, and Morabia A et al., Nutritional assessment: Lean body mass depletion at hospital admission is associated with an increased length of stay, *Am J Clin Nutr,* 79:613–618, 2004.
21. Roubenoff R, Roubenoff R, and Ward L et al., Rheumatoid cachexia: Depletion of lean body mass in rheumatoid arthritis, Possible association with tumor necrosis factor, *J Rheumatol,* 19:1505–1510, 1992.
22. Franklin B, Whaley M, and Howley E, *ACSM's Guidelines for Exercise Testing and Prescription,* Philadelphia: Lippincott Williams & Wilkins, 2000:368.
23. Roubenoff R, Heymsfield S, and Kehayias J et al., Standardization of nomenclature of body composition in weight loss, *Am J Clin Nutr,* 192–196, 1997.
24. Roubenoff R and Hughes V, Sarcopenia: Current concepts, *J Gerontol Med Sci,* 55A:M716–M724, 2000.
25. Fiatarone M, O'Neill E, and Ryan N et al., Exercise training and nutritional supplementation for physical frailty in very elderly people, *N Engl J Med,* 330, 1994.
26. Rall L, Rosen C, and Dolnikowski G et al., Protein metabolism in rheumatoid arthritis and aging: Effects of muscle strength training and tumor necrosis factor-alpha, *Arthr Rheum,* 39:1115–1124, 1996.
27. Rall L, Meydani S, and Kehayias J et al., The effect of progressive resistance training in rheumatoid arthritis: Increased strength without changes in energy balance or body composition, *Arthritis Rheum,* 39, 1996.

28. Pu C, Johnson M, and Forman D et al., Randomized trial of progressive resistance training to counteract the myopathy of chronic heart failure, *J Appl Physiol,* 90:2341–2350, 2001.
29. Williamson DF, Dietary intake and physical activity as "predictors" of weight gain in observational, prospective studies of adults, *Nutr Rev,* 54:S101–S109, 1996.
30. Jeffrey RW and French SA, Preventing weight gain in adults: Design, methods, and one-year results from the pound of prevention study, *Int J Obes,* 21:457–464, 1997.
31. Schoeller D, Balancing energy expenditure and body weight, *Am J Clin Nutr,* 68:956S–961S, 1998.
32. Korner J and Aronne L, The emerging science of body weight regulation and its impact on obesity treatment, *Journal of Clinical Investigation,* 111:565–570, 2003.
33. Schwartz M, Woods S, and Seeley R et al., Is the energy homeostasis system inherently biased toward weight gain? *Diabetes,* 52:232–238, 2003.
34. Mayer J, Glucostatic mechanisms of the regulation of food intake, *N Eng J Med,* 249:13–16, 1953.
35. van Pelt RE, Davy K, and Stevenson E et al., Smaller differences in total and regional adiposity with age in women who regularly perform endurance exercise, *AJCN,* 42:983–990, 1998.
36. Davidson J, Diet therapy for non-insulin-dependent (type-2) diabetes mellitus, In: Davidson J, Ed., *Clinical Diabetes Mellitus: A Problem-Oriented Approach,* New York: Thieme, 241–265, 2000.
37. Joslin E, *Diabetic Metabolism with High and Low Diets,* Washington, DC: Carnegie Institution, 1923.
38. Mokdad A, Bowman B, Ford E, Vinicor F, Marks J, and Koplan J, The continuing epidemics of obesity and diabetes in the United States, *JAMA,* 286:1195–1200, 2001.
39. Joint WHO/FAO Expert Consultation on Diet, Nutrition, and the Prevention of Chronic Diseases, Diet, nutrition, and the prevention of chronic diseases, Report of a joint WHO/FAO expert consultation, Geneva: World Health Organization, 2003.
40. Anonymous, Trends in intake of energy and macronutrients—United States, 1971–2000, *MMWR,* 53:80–82, 2004.
41. Bray G, Nielsen S, and Popkins B, Consumption of high-fructose corn syrup in beverages may play a role in the epidemic of obesity, *Am J Clin Nutr,* 79:537–543, 2004.
42. Foster G, Wyatt H, and Hill J et al., A randomized trial of a low-carbohydrate diet for obesity, *N Engl J Med,* 348:2082–2090, 2003.
43. Samaha F, Iqbal N, and Seshadri P et al., A low-carbohydrate as compared with a low-fat diet in severe obesity, *N Engl J of Med,* 348:2074–2081, 2003.
44. Consortium TIHGS, Initial sequencing and analysis of the human genome, *Natural,* 409:860–921, 2001.
45. Staudt L and Wilson W, Focus on lymphomas, *Cancer Cell,* 2:363–366, 2002.
46. Ginsburg G, McCarthy J, Personalized medicine: Revolutionizing drug discovery and patient care, *Trends Biotechnol,* 19:491–496, 1999.
47. Collins F, Green E, and Guttmacher A et al., A vision for the future of genomics research, *Natural,* 422:835–847, 2003.
48. Lesko LJ, Rowland M, and Peck CC et al., Optimizing the science of drug development: Opportunities for better candidate selection and accelerated evaluation in humans, *Eur J Pharm Sci,* 10:iv–xiv, 2000.
49. Sung N, Crowley W, and Genel M et al., Central challenges facing the national clinical research enterprise, *JAMA,* 389:1278–1287, 2003.
50. RDAs SotTEot, *Recommended Dietary Allowances,* Washington, DC: National Academy Press, 1989.
51. Ma J, Stampfer M, and Hennekens C et al., Methylenetetrahydrofolate reductase polymorphism, plasma folate, homocysteine, and risk of myocardial infarction in U.S. physicians, *Circulation,* 94:2410–2416, 1996.
52. Marz W, Scharnagl H, and Kirca M et al., Apolipoprotein e polymorphism is associated with both senile plaque load and alzheimer-type neurofibrillary tangle formation, *Ann NY Acad Sci,* 777:276–280, 1996.
53. Mokdad AH, Marks J, and Stroup D et al., Actual causes of death in the United States, 2000, *JAMA,* 291:1238–1245, 2004.
54. Roubenoff R, Inflammatory and hormonal mediators of cachexia, *Journal of Nutrition,* 127:1014S–1016S, 1997.
55. Prevention CfDCa, *Nutrition & Physical Activity,* Figure 1: CDC web site at: http://www.cdc.gov/nccdphp/dnpa/physical/recommendations/adults.htm, accessed 8/11/05.

2 Pathophysiology and Clinical Management of Diabetes and Prediabetes

Elliot J. Rayfield and Marilyn V. Valentine

CONTENTS

DEFINITION OF DIABETES MELLITUS

Diabetes mellitus (DM) is a group of diseases characterized by hyperglycemia and varying degrees of an insufficient insulin effect. Chronic hyperglycemia alters the metabolism of carbohydrate, fat, and protein, and ultimately produces complications. The hydrophilic properties of the glucose molecule produce tremendous shifts in serum osmolarity, causing increased vasopressin secretion, generalized vascular dysfunction, and irreversible glycosylation of proteins resulting in protein, lipoprotein, enzymes, and DNA dysfunction. With diabetes, a diverse array of hormonal, metabolic, and molecular alterations instigates and perpetuates a pathophysiological state that can markedly compromise a patient's quality of life. In this chapter, a clinical and biochemical framework will be outlined that reveals potential sites for nutritional intervention.

DEMOGRAPHICS

According to the World Health Organization (WHO) there are approximately 177 million people with diabetes worldwide and this figure is expected to double by the year 2030 [1]. According to the National Health and Nutritional Examination Survey for 1999–2000 (NHANES 1999–2000) [2], approximately 29 million persons over age 20 years in the U.S. had DM or impaired fasting glucose (IFG), with 29% of diabetes cases undiagnosed. The overall prevalence of DM was 8.3% and IFG was 6.1% [2]. The prevalence of DM increased with age to 19.2% in persons over 60 years old [2]. Prevalence rates were comparable by sex but lower in non-Hispanic whites compared with Mexican Americans and non-Hispanic blacks [2].

Modernization and lifestyle changes in developed and developing countries have resulted in increased caloric intake and decreased physical activity across all age groups. There has also been a shift from ingesting more naturally grown or produced foods to foods that are processed to increase shelf-life and palatability. These lifestyle changes may be responsible for the increasing prevalence of diabetes.

DIAGNOSTIC CRITERIA OF DIABETES

Diabetes is diagnosed when: (1) the fasting blood glucose (FBG) is 126 mg/dL or greater on at least two different occasions or (2) there are symptoms of diabetes with a casual plasma glucose value greater than 200 mg/dL [3]. There are times when this test is not conclusive and there is a high suspicion of diabetes given the patient's family history of diabetes—or the patient's current disease state—that makes it necessary to perform an oral glucose tolerance test (OGTT). This test is performed after fasting for 8 hours. The patient is given a standardized 75 g dose of glucose orally and blood glucose is measured at 0 and 120 minutes. If the patient has a blood glucose value of 200 mg/dL or greater at 2 hours, the diagnosis of diabetes is made. If the glucose level is between 140–199 mg/dL at 2 hours, the patient has impaired glucose tolerance (IGT) [3].

CLASSIFICATION OF DIFFERENT TYPES OF DIABETES

Type-1 Diabetes Mellitus

Type-1 diabetes (T1DM) is comprised of type-1A diabetes (immune-mediated) and type-1B diabetes (other forms of diabetes with severe insulin deficiency) according to an expert committee of the American Diabetes Association (ADA) [4]. Type-1A diabetes is autoantibody positive in greater than 90% of the cases. Animal models of type-1A diabetes include the nonobese diabetic (NOD) mouse and the biobreeding (BB) rat (which differ from the human type-1A diabetes by having an autosomal recessive mutation resulting in T-cell lymphopenia) [5]. T1DM is the most dramatic form of all diabetic diseases. It can present at any age after birth although the two most common ages are 4 and those occurring with puberty [6]. The common denominator is a genetic predisposition which, when associated with certain environmental factors, triggers the invasion of the pancreas by mononuclear cells and the production of islet cell antibodies that destroy pancreatic β-cells [7].

One type of trigger pertains to food and associated gene-nutrient interactions. Khono et al. [8] have studied the humoral and mucosal responses to food antigens in patients with T1DM and in normal subjects. They have used a two-sided enzyme, immunoassay, to identify immunoglobulins and cytokines and have measured autoantibodies against glutamic acid decarboxylase (GAD), thyroglobulin (TG), and thyroid peroxidase (TPO). Patients with T1DM had a significant elevation of IgG and IgA to food antigens such as milk proteins and ovalbumin. However, milk proteins are not conclusively linked as causal agents in diabetes.

Another potential trigger for T1DM is infection. There are data from human and animal models suggesting a viral etiology of diabetes. The viruses most convincingly implicated are coxsackie, mumps, and rubella—the last being associated with the Congenital Rubella Syndrome [9]. These data are suggestive and not yet conclusive.

Type-2 Diabetes Mellitus

Type-2 diabetes (T2DM) has a multifactorial etiology resulting from a combination of multiple genetic mutations and environmental exposure. The presence of a strong family history of diabetes is enough to warrant an attempt at detection in other family members with an OGTT [10].

The early phase of T2DM is characterized by normal blood glucose in the presence of high insulin levels. The insulin responsive tissues, skeletal muscle and adipose tissue, have a decreased response to insulin with decreased disposal of glucose and fatty acids. The pancreas increases insulin production as a compensatory mechanism to maintain glucose homeostasis [11]. Concomitantly, gluconeogenesis increases in the liver and the β-cells secrete even more insulin.

Studies in knockout mice have shown that the presence of insulin resistance at the level of the β-cell could be a causative factor in diabetes [12]. Also, insulin receptor tyrosine kinase activity has been shown to be defective in insulin resistance and T2DM [13]. Genetic mutations can be at the level of the insulin receptor gene and the insulin receptor tyrosine kinase gene [13–16].

Another mechanism which results in T2DM is a defect in insulin secretion; that is, an alteration of the pancreatic sensitivity to glucose that alters the response to hyperglycemia. This insufficient response to blood glucose levels may provoke an inappropriate stimulation of glucagon secretion and an increase in hepatic glucose production with further elevated fasting plasma glucose levels.

Genetic Defects of the β-Cell

Maturity onset of diabetes of the young (MODY) is characterized by impaired insulin secretion with minimal or no defects in insulin action. It is inherited in an autosomal dominant pattern. Abnormalities are identified on six genetic loci of the chromosomes. The most common form is in a hepatic transcription factor (HNF)-1α (MODY 3; chromosome 12). Another form of MODY results from a defect in the glucokinase gene. This results in a defective "glucose sensor" for the β-cell and requires higher glycemia levels to elicit a normal insulin secretion pattern [4].

Mitochondrial Diabetes

Mitochondrial diabetes (MTDM) is one of the diseases caused by the mutation of mitochondrial DNA, the most common being the A3243G mutation [17]. This disease has a maternal form of inheritance and frequently becomes clinically manifest by the age of 35–40 years although it can present at any time before age 70. It is referred to as an age-dependent form of diabetes accompanied by rapid deterioration of the pancreatic β-cells. By the age of 40 years, most of the carriers of this mutation have IGT. MTDM may present as a T1DM or T2DM but the patients with T2DM tend to require insulin treatment within a timeframe of a couple of years. MTDM is accompanied by hearing impairment to sounds above 5 kHz in most patients.

The A3243G mutation is present in all tissues and heteroplasmy is high in tissues with low mitotic activity. The altered glucose metabolism seen with this mutation is thought to be due to the imbalance of 5-adenosine triphosphate (ATP)/5-adenosine diphosphate (ADP), low energy equivalents, stimulation of hepatic glucose production, increased lactate in the skeletal muscle, and increased hepatic gluconeogenesis. The low energy ratio of ATP/ADP is accountable for producing alteration of the pancreatic glucose sensor and reduction of insulin secretion. There is also an abnormality in the conversion of pro-insulin to insulin that was identified in some families [4].

Genetic Defects in Insulin Action

Metabolic abnormalities resulting from insulin receptor apparatus mutations range from mild hyperglycemia to severe diabetes. Some patients have hyperandrogenism, insulin resistance, and acanthosis nigricans (HAIR-AN syndrome), which can be associated with polycystic ovary syndrome or hyperthecosis [4]. Other syndromes are associated with extreme insulin resistance [4]:

- Familial lipodystrophy
- Acquired lipodystrophy
- Type A insulin resistance syndrome
- Type B insulin resistance syndrome
- Leprechaunism
- Rabson–Mendenhall syndrome
- Alström syndrome

Diseases of the Exocrine Pancreas

Processes that injure the pancreas can also cause diabetes. These include trauma to or infection of the pancreas, pancreatectomy, chronic pancreatitis, pancreatic carcinoma, cystic fibrosis, and hemochromatosis.

Diseases Associated with T2DM

T2DM may be associated with other disease entities such as obesity, dyslipidemia, hypertension, hyperuricemia, and accelerated atherosclerosis. At the time of diagnosis, each is often accompanied by diabetic complications such as coronary artery disease (CAD), peripheral vascular disease (PVD), nephropathy, neuropathy, and retinopathy [4].

Secondary Diabetes Mellitus

Secondary diabetes can result from endocrine disease in which counter-regulatory hormones are secreted in excess, such as in acromegaly, Cushing's syndrome, pheochromocytoma, and glucagonoma [4].

Drugs, Chemicals, and Toxins That Cause Hyperglycemia

Several drugs are associated with hyperglycemia due to their antagonistic effect on insulin secretion, insulin action, or impairment of glucose tolerance. Other chemicals and toxins also produce hyperglycemia including those listed below [18]:

- **Diuretics**: thiazides, chlorthalidone, furosemide, ethacrinic acid, metolazone, diazoxide
- **Antihypertensive agents**: clonidine, beta-adrenergic antagonists, alpha-adrenergic antagonists
- **Hormones**: glucocorticoids, adrenocorticotropic hormone, growth hormone, glucagon, oral contraceptives, progestational agents
- **Psychoactive drugs**: lithium, opiates, ethanol, phenothiazines, clozapine, olanzapine
- **Anticonvulsants**: diphenylhydantoins
- **Antineoplastic agents**: streptozotocin, L-asparaginase, mithramycin
- **Antiprotozoal agents**: pentamidine
- **Rodenticides**: pyriminal
- **Miscellaneous**: nicotinic acid, cyclosporine, tacrolimus, N-nitrosamines, theophylline

Post-Transplant Diabetes

Post-transplant diabetes (PTDM) is sustained hyperglycemia occurring in any patient post-organ transplant without a prior history of diabetes [19]. The incidence in the literature ranges from 2–53%. Most cases are diagnosed within the first 3 months post-transplant. In addition, PTDM resembles T2DM and is due to an underlying insulin resistant state (liver, kidney or cardiac failure) as well as the immunosuppressant drugs used after transplant. Corticosteroids increase peripheral insulin resistance whereas the calcineurin inhibitors, tacrolimus and cyclosporin, cause a reversible insulin secretory defect [19–21]. The most significant risk factors for PTDM are high body mass index (BMI) and a family history of T2DM [22]. Treatment of PTDM usually requires insulin. Newer data suggest that the thiazolidinediones (TZD) are useful in these patients and can lower insulin requirements [23].

Gestational Diabetes

Gestational diabetes (GDM) usually presents during the third trimester but it can present at any time during pregnancy. Blood glucose levels typically normalize after delivery. Since the prevalence of diabetes in the general population is expected to increase in the coming years, the prevalence of GDM should also be expected to increase.

GDM can be detected using an OGTT during the third trimester. However, individual assessment of the pregnant mother should be done as early as possible during pregnancy to determine the risk of developing GDM. Considerations must be given to the risk factors of the general population for developing diabetes such as obesity, family history of diabetes, as well as a high birth weight of the mother and a history of GDM in a prior pregnancy [4,24,25].

The goal of early detection and treatment of GDM is to prevent or reduce perinatal morbidity. Fasting blood glucose levels should be maintained between 65 and 90 mg/dL and 1 hour postprandial glucose levels should be less than 120 mg/dL. All women with GDM should receive nutritional counseling by a qualified professional.

Insulin is the pharmacological treatment of choice in GDM, when diet and exercise fail to meet the treatment goal, and in the cases of undiagnosed pregestational DM. Urinary ketones should be measured at bedtime and before breakfast to ensure adequate intake of carbohydrates.

Oral hypoglycemic agents are not recommended because they traverse the placental barrier and may affect the fetus. However, the oral hypoglycemic agent glyburide does not seem to traverse the placenta [26]. Nevertheless, most diabetes specialists are not comfortable with the use of any oral agent during pregnancy.

For pregnant women who are diabetic, frequent periodic evaluations by the obstetrician and diabetes specialist to monitor the well being of both fetus and mother are recommended. At each visit during pregnancy, tests should be done to detect proteinuria, ketones, hemoglobin A1C (A1C) levels, and glycemic status. Patients with pre-existing diabetes should have an ophthalmologic exam to detect retinal disease. Most cases of gestational diabetes resolve after delivery. However, patients should be reassessed with an OGTT 6 weeks after delivery, to determine the presence, stage, and appropriate treatment of diabetes as indicated.

Prediabetic Conditions

These clinical states reflect early stages in the pathogenesis of diabetes but do not fulfill the current diagnostic criteria for frank diabetes. Their relevance is more than simple epidemiology. With earlier detection and recognition of these stages, various preventive strategies can be implemented to reduce the risks of frank diabetes, eventual complications, compromised quality of life, and ultimately diabetes-related mortality. Over the recent years, the diagnostic criteria for these prediabetic states have become more and more subtle in an attempt to diagnose diabetes subclinically. The natural extrapolation of this public health policy and pattern of clinical screening is to one day utilize genomic medicine for risk-reduction strategies very early in life.

Risk Factors for Type-2 Diabetes

On the basis of the Expert Committee on the Diagnosis and Classification of Diabetes Mellitus [27], risk factors for T2DM are: age $\geq$ 45 years, overweight, family history of T2DM, habitual physical inactivity, race/ethnicity, previously identified impaired fasting glucose (IFG) or impaired glucose tolerance (IGT), history of gestational diabetes or delivery of a baby weighing > 9 lb, hypertension, HDL cholesterol < 35 mg/dL or a triglyceride level > 150 mg/dL, polycystic ovary syndrome, or a history of vascular disease.

Impaired Fasting Glucose

This entity, the earliest finding of the prediabetic state, is diagnosed with a history of plasma glucose, following an 8-hour period of no food or beverage other than water, of $\geq$ 100 mg/dL but < 126 mg/dL. This range for IFG is associated with a similar prevalence as IGT, according to the WHO criteria, which is based on both fasting and 2-hour oral glucose tolerance test (OGTT) values. A 7-year follow-up from the Diabetes Epidemiology: Collaborative analysis of Diagnostic criteria in Europe (DECODE) study, reveals that the 2-hour value on the OGTT was predictive of increased cardiovascular mortality, while the fasting blood glucose was not [28]. Thus, postprandial hyperglycemia is more strongly linked with cardiovascular risk and death than fasting blood glucose.

Impaired Glucose Tolerance

The diagnosis of IGT involves an OGTT using a 75-g oral glucose load. Sinha et al. [29] studied obese American children and adolescents and found a high prevalence of IGT: 25% in children 4–10 years of age and 21% in adolescents 11–18 years of age. IGT is defined as a 2-hour post-glucose load plasma glucose $\geq$ 140 mg/dL and < 200 mg/dL. IGT is treated with lifestyle changes, such as diet and exercise, though pharmacotherapy is sometimes used at the time of diagnosis as a preventive measure. The most common drugs used in patients with IGT are biguanides and TZD, though neither are currently approved by the Food and Drug Administration (FDA) for this indication. The Diabetes Prevention Program (DPP) demonstrated that the incidence of frank diabetes in people with IGT was reduced 58% with lifestyle modifications and 31% with the biguanide metformin, compared with placebo after a mean duration of 2.8 years of intervention [30]. Approximately one quarter of the beneficial effect of metformin to prevent T2DM in the DPP was due to a pharmacological effect that did not persist after cessation of the drug [30]. The use of TZD in patients with IGT is based on the TRIPOD study and is discussed later in the chapter.

PATHOPHYSIOLOGY OF DIABETES MELLITUS

Insulin Secretagogues

Metabolites, hormones and neurotransmitters stimulate insulin secretion. The most potent stimulatory metabolite is glucose. Other nutrients such as amino acids and fatty acids also stimulate insulin secretion but to a lesser degree than glucose. Gastrointestinal hormones and polypeptides also stimulate insulin secretion.

Carbohydrates

When carbohydrate is ingested, it is eventually broken down to glucose. Glucose stimulates insulin secretion and inhibits glucagon. The liver is a non-insulin-dependent organ and glucose enters the hepatocyte by the facilitated transporter glucose transporter 2 (GLUT2). It is phosphorylated to glucose-6-phosphate (G6P), which stimulates hepatic glycogen synthesis. G6P also enters the anaerobic glycolysis process. The resulting pyruvate enters the mitochondria for aerobic metabolism in the Krebs cycle, which generates nicotinamide adenine dinucleotide, reduced form (NADH) and flavin adenine dinucleotide ($FADH_2$) and, via the electron transport chain and oxidative phosphorylation (OXPHOS), ATP is formed. In pancreatic β-cells, OXPHOS is associated with ATP/K^+ channel closure, cytoplasmic membrane depolarization, voltage-dependent calcium channels opening, and exocytosis of secretory vesicles containing stored insulin.

The increased insulin and decreased glucagon stimulate pyruvate dehydrogenase which converts pyruvate to acetyl coenzyme A (CoA), which is necessary for the synthesis of free fatty acids. In cases of increased hepatic glucose uptake, such as excess carbohydrate intake, insufficient insulin secretion, and insulin resistance, there is increased synthesis of fatty acids, triglycerides, very low-density lipoproteins (VLDL), and cholesterol-causing dyslipidemia. With progressive decrease of β-cell mass in diabetes, insulin secretagogues have a diminished effect on insulin secretion and eventually, there is no endogenous insulin released.

Neurotransmitters

The vagal nerve innervates the pancreas, is stimulated during the cephalic, intestinal, and absorptive phases of digestion, and produces acetylcholine (ACh) at its postganglionic synapses. This parasympathetic ACh activates M3 muscarinic receptors stimulating glucose-dependent insulin secretion. In contrast, norepinephrine and epinephrine inhibit the first-phase insulin response to glucose with no effect on basal insulin secretion. In the presence of β-cell dysfunction and insulin deficiency, basal insulin levels are low and the response to neurological stimulation of insulin is low. In insulin resistance states, there are increased basal insulin levels, increased insulin responses to neurological stimulation, and a potential for increased synthesis of free fatty acids, triglycerides, VLDL, and cholesterol.

Hepatic Glucose Production

The liver plays an important part in glucose homeostasis. During periods of fasting the liver maintains carbohydrate metabolism by producing glucose from its glycogen stores. This is especially important during fasting when the liver is responsible for producing about 180 g/day glucose to maintain central nervous system (CNS) function [31]. In contrast, with insulin deficiency, glycogenolysis inappropriately continues despite hyperglycemia [32]. Moreover, in patients with T2DM, glucagon-induced hyperglycemia primarily results from gluconeogenesis, and to a lesser extent, glycogenolysis [32]. In normal controls, most of the glucose produced in response to glucagon is derived from glycogenolysis [32]. Using a glucose-insulin clamp technique in patients with T2DM, glucose-stimulated glucose uptake is impaired at high levels of glycemia while glucose-suppression of hepatic glucose production and gluconeogenesis is normal [32].

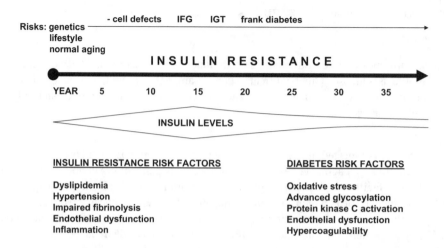

FIGURE 2.1 The natural history of prediabetes. Abbreviations: IFG—impaired fasting glucose; IGT—impaired glucose tolerance.

Insulin Resistance and Type-2 Diabetes Mellitus

Insulin resistance is a clinical state in which a given increase in plasma insulin causes less of an effect in lowering the plasma glucose then it does in normal individuals. The insulin resistant state precedes T2DM (see Figure 2.1). Historically, the euglycemic hyperinsulinemic clamp technique was initially used to assess insulin resistance. The Insulin Resistance Syndrome (IRS) is defined by the presence of hypertension, dyslipidemia (low high-density lipoprotein cholesterol [HDL-c] and hypertriglyceridemia), hyperglycemia and obesity. Biochemically, IRS patients have hyperinsulinemia, a procoagulant state (measured by increased plasminogen activator inhibitor-1 [PAI-1] and fibrinogen), endothelial dysfunction and increases in the proinflammatory C-reactive protein (CRP). Ketosis is infrequent. Decreased insulin action may be due to decreases in insulin production, insulin receptor binding, or insulin receptor signal transduction (see Figure 2.2). These defects may occur alone or in combination and are also found in association with inflammatory states. The term "mixed insulin resistance" describes the condition in which there is inhibition of gluconeogenesis (hyperglycemia) but not fatty acid oxidation (hepatic triglyceride accumulation) [35,36]. Thus, insulin resistance, with or without hyperglycemia, is a major risk factor for CAD because of its inflammatory and proatherogenic features [39].

Insulin resistance is also associated with endothelial dysfunction and vascular disease. The peroxisome proliferators activated receptor (PPAR)-γ agonists have been shown to decrease insulin resistance. The molecular mechanisms by which the PPAR-γ agonists and cytokines (tumor-necrosis factor-α [TNF-α], adiponectins) are linked to vascular disease are an active area of investigation [40].

Effects of Hyperglycemia

Hyperglycemia produces an elevation in plasma osmolarity that triggers arginine-vasopressin (AVP) secretion in the CNS. AVP produces both behavioral (polydipsia) and physiological (decreased free-water clearance) responses to maintain intracellular and extracellular compartment homeostasis. Hyperosmolarity increases the demand for AVP and there is recruitment and adaptation of hippocampal and hypothalamic neurons to produce AVP. Chronically high concentrations of AVP play a role in renal failure in diabetics. V_2 AVP receptors in the renal cortex and collecting ducts mediate the anti-diuretic response. Activation of V_2 receptors leads to insertion of aquaporin-2

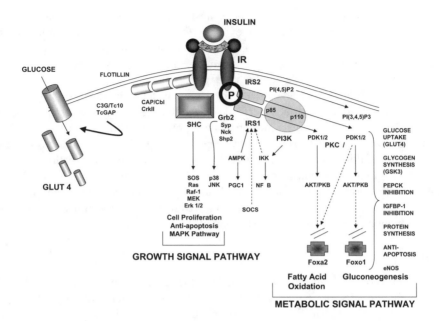

FIGURE 2.2 Insulin receptor signal cascade. Following the interaction of insulin with the insulin receptor (IR), autophosphorylation of IR occurs creating insulin receptor substrate-1 (IRS1) and -2 (IRS2) docking sites [33]. Three major pathways are activated: (1) phosphatidylinositol-3-kinase (PI3K)/protein kinase B (Akt) kinome controlling metabolism, (2) MAPK/Erk pathway controlling mitogenesis, and (3) CAP/Cbl/Tc10 pathway in the lipid raft [34] activating GLUT4. IRS exerts dominant control over Foxa2 mediated fatty acid oxidation > Foxo1 mediated control over gluconeogenesis; this accounts for mixed insulin resistance in patients with T2DM [35,36]. 5'-adenosine monophosphate activated protein kinase (AMPK) is an evolutionarily conserved fuel sensor that activates IRS1 as well as peroxisome proliferator activated receptor γ coactivator 1α (PGC1α) [37]. Suppressor of cytokine signaling (SOCS) proteins are induced by cytokines and negatively regulate IRS1. Inhibitor κB kinase (IKK) is activated by PI3K-dependent pathways, cytokines, and sepsis, via the Toll-like receptor 4 [38]. IKK inhibits IRS1 activity via serine phosphorylation and activates NF-κB. This is one mechanism of how sepsis is associated with insulin resistance.

(AQP2) water-permeable channels in the renal collecting ducts, which acutely limit the rise in serum osmolality. However, long-term hyperstimulation of V_2 receptors leads to glomerular hyperfiltration, albuminuria, and renal hypertrophy [41].

Polyphagia occurs as a result of impaired glucose utilization. There is also relative starvation in the presence of increased food intake with compensatory increases in energy-producing pathways, such as proteolysis-gluconeogenesis and lipolysis-ketogenesis. Hyperglycemia has multiple effects on all tissues in the body as circulating glucose levels increase glucosuria resulting in an osmotic diuresis with loss of water and electrolytes. The resultant dehydration results in impaired renal function, blurred vision, hypernatremia, and cognitive dysfunction.

Glucose Toxicity

Glucose toxicity typically refers to a phenomenon wherein β-cell dysfunction occurs as a result of prolonged and/or severe hyperglycemia. β-cell dysfunction and eventually apoptosis can be demonstrated *in vitro* as a result of prolonged exposure to elevated glucose. When β-cells are induced to increase glucokinase activity and intracellular glycolytic intermediates (by doxycycline exposure), the result is reduced NADH availability, cellular damage, and apoptosis [42]. Furthermore, glucose toxicity produces defective insulin gene expression that can cause deterioration of glycemic control in patients with T2DM. There is also evidence to suggest that β-cells have low antioxidant defense mechanisms, making them vulnerable to oxidative stress [43,44]. The length of time and extent required for tight glycemic control to normalize β-cell responsiveness to glucose is quite variable but is frequently reversible in the short term. Three principal metabolic pathways of hyperglycemic damage have been identified. The common denominator in each pathway is the production of excessive mitochondrial superoxide during hyperglycemic stress [45]. Reactive oxygen species (ROS) induce DNA breaks, which activate poly-ADP-ribose polymerase (PARP). The key enzyme, glyceraldehyde 3-phosphate dehydrogenase (GAPDH), is then inactivated by poly-ADP-ribosylation, resulting in diversion of glycolytic substrate to alternative pathways involved in cellular injury: [1] *de novo* synthesis of diacylglycerol (DAG) which activates protein kinase C (PKC) isoforms; [2] formation of intracellular advanced glycation endproducts (AGE); [3] stimulation of aldose reductase (AR) activity producing accumulation of sorbitol in the endothelium; and [4] augmentation of hexosamine pathway activity [46].

Nitric Oxide

The endothelium serves as a barrier between blood and the vascular wall and has multiple endocrine and paracrine functions. Its role in the regulation of the microcirculation is due to its direct secretion of various vasodilators, such as nitric oxide (NO), endothelium-derived relaxing factors, endothelial-derived polarizing factors, prostacyclins, and various vasoconstrictors such as prostaglandins and endothelin. NO is produced by nitric oxide synthase III (NOS III), also known as endothelial NOS. NOS III expression is enhanced by PKC inhibitors, hydrogen peroxide, estrogens, insulin, vascular endothelial growth factor (VEGF), 3-hydroxy-3-methylglutaryl coenzyme A (HMG CoA) reductase inhibitors, and transforming growth factor (TGF)-β. NOS III is down regulated by AGE, oxidized LDL-c, TNF-α, glucocorticoids, hypoxia and erythropoietin [47]. Under normal conditions, NO is described as having favorable effects such as anti-inflammatory, anti-apoptosis, anti-vascular smooth muscle cell proliferation, and anti-platelet aggregation. Although NO can also be produced by neutrophils, macrophages, fibroblasts, smooth muscle cells, and endothelial cells—especially in the presence of inflammation—its inability to be protective in diabetes is believed to be due to decreased synthesis and oxidative inactivation by superoxide [48].

Endothelial Dysfunction

The endothelium regulates vascular tone, vascular smooth muscle cell proliferation, trans-endothelial leukocyte migration, thrombosis and thrombolysis. In response to various mechanical and chemical stimuli, endothelial cells synthesize and release a large number of vasoactive substances, growth modulators, and other factors that mediate these functions [49]. Endothelial dysfunction is defined as an imbalance between opposing vascular states such as constriction and dilatation, pro-inflammation and anti-inflammation, growth promotion and growth inhibition, and coagulation and fibrinolysis. The complex interplay of intrinsic endothelial dysfunction, reflected by low-grade inflammation with cardiac risk factors, ROS, and the renin-angiotensin axis activation, culminate in atherogenesis [50].

The production of ROS decreases NO production, NO action, and activates the renin-angiotensin system. This releases endothelial transcription and growth factors, pro-inflammatory cytokines, chemo-attractant substances and adhesion molecules pivotal to atherogenesis [50]. Leukocytes are attracted to the vessel wall by vascular adhesion molecule-1 (VCAM-1) found in nascent atheromas. Other chemo-attractants thought to play a role *in vitro* are E and P selectin, and TNF-α. The leukocytes enter the intima by diapedesis, which can be enhanced by their secretion of monocyte chemotactic protein-1 (MCP-1). In the intima, the monocytes are transformed to foam cells by their scavenger action on modified lipoproteins. Foam cells give rise to atheromas and plaques [51].

Overall, it is the production of ROS that triggers the coordinated events of endothelial dysfunction and may be identified as a prime target for nutritional antioxidant intervention (see Figure 2.3). Hyperglycemia, insulin resistance, cytokines, and AGE fuel this process and PARP, GAPDH, diacylglycerol (DAG), protein kinase C (PKC), NO, nuclear factor (NF-κB), and prostacyclin (PGI2) serve as downstream mediator.

Evaluation of Endothelial Function

The most common tools to evaluate vascular reactivity and blood flow assess the balance between vasoconstriction and vasodilatation as well as inflammation, such as the highly sensitive CRP [52]. Other markers of endothelial dysfunction are tissue plasminogen activator-1 (tPA-1), PAI-1, fibrinogen, thrombomodulin, and adhesion molecules, such as soluble vascular cellular adhesion molecule (sVCAM), soluble intercellular adhesion molecule (sICAM), selectin-E, and selectin-P. In the early phase of endothelial inflammation, circulating monocytes and macrophages are attracted to the vascular wall after a mechanical or biochemical insult via adiponectin, von Willebrand factor, NO, endothelin-1 (ET-1), TNF-α, and interleukin-1 (IL-1) [50].

The intensive lifestyle modification arm of the DPP study, combining a balanced dietary regimen as well as an exercise program conducive to a mean loss of 5% body weight, resulted in a significant reduction in bedtime CRP, fibrinogen, and tPA in individuals with IGT [53]. In fact, dietary changes leading to weight loss have a higher impact than exercise alone on markers of inflammation, including bedtime CRP, TNF-α, and interleukin-6 (IL-6) [54]. In addition, vascular function is improved most when diet and exercise are combined [25].

Diabetic Complications

Microvascular Complications

The results of the Diabetes Control and Complications Trial (DCCT) showed a direct correlation between degree of hyperglycemia and the development of microvascular complications in patients with T1DM [56]. The same relationship was found in type-2 diabetics in the United Kingdom Prospective Diabetes Study (UKPDS) [57]. Clearly, this is evidence for a causal relationship but is not the only factor. There are presumably also genetic predispositions to the development of complications since they are frequently seen in family clusters. Complications are also due to a lack of adherance treatment.

Chronic hyperglycemia produces complications due to the deleterious effects on several organs. Non-enzymatic glycosylation of substrates is believed to be the major contributing factor of long-term diabetic complications. The main mechanisms of diabetic complications are similar to those involved in endothelial and microvascular injury described above and in Figure 2.3. These mechanisms involve oxidative stress as a proximal event, which leads to increased activity of the polyol (AR) and hexosamine pathways, increased activity of PKC, and non-enzymatic glycation of proteins giving rise to AGE [46,57]. These mechanisms also result in ROS production, thus amplifying pathway flux and promoting tissue injury (see Figure 2.4).

Aldose Reductase Pathway

Reduction of glucose by AR via the polyol pathway has long been linked to the development of diabetes microvascular complications. This was initially thought to be due to sorbitol accumulation in tissues but the clinical response to inhibitors of sorbitol formation has been disappointing. The exact mechanism of sorbitol-induced injury remains unclear.

Aldose reductase is the first rate-limiting enzyme of the polyol pathway of glucose metabolism and increases NAD^+ formation [59]. Aldose reductase activity also induces oxidative stress (via PARP activation and peroxynitrate formation) [60], contributes to PKC activation [61], and detoxifies aldehydes generated from lipid peroxidation [59]. It is now thought that it may be necessary to selectively inhibit aldose-reductase-mediated glucose metabolism without affecting aldehyde detoxification. Not only is the AR pathway important in the development of diabetic microvascular

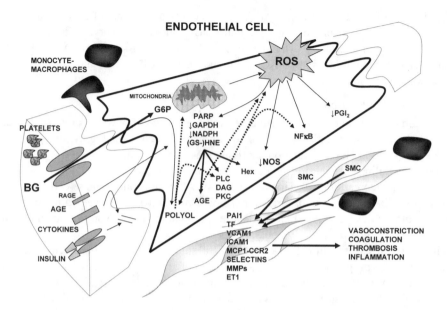

FIGURE 2.3 Endothelial dysfunction in diabetic patients. Hyperglycemia, hyperinsulinemia, insulin resistance, cytokines and AGEs act through mitochondrial pathways to augment ROS production. Increased ROS production induces DNA damage, lipid peroxidation, formation of toxic lipid adehydes (4-hydroxynonenal [HNE] and glutathione-HNE), and poly(ADP ribose) polymerase (PARP) production. PARP inhibits glyceraldehyde-3-phosphate dehydrogenase (GAPDH) diverting glycolytic intermediates to the following four pathways: (1) glucose to polyols; (2) fructose-6-phosphate to glucosamine (hexosamine pathway [Hex]); (3) glyceraldehydes-3-phosphate (GAP) to diacylglycerol (DAG) to protein kinase C (PKC) activation; and (4) GAP to methylglyoxal to AGEs. Independent of ROS generation, hyperglycemia also activates the aldose reductase (polyol) pathway, which can reduce HNE and GS-HME into products that activate the PLC-PKC-NKκB pathway. ROS participate in AGE formation, which in turn, increase ROS formation. ROS also participate in the (1) reduction of nitric oxide (NO; vasodilator) production; (2) activation of NF–κB, a transcription factor that switches on various proinflammatory genes; and (3) reduction of PGI$_2$ levels (another vasodilator). Various peptides are then produced by endothelial, inflammatory, and smooth muscle cells (SMC): plasminogen activator inhibitor-1 (PAI-1), tissue factor (TF), vascular cell adhesion molecule-1 (VCAM-1), intercellular adhesion molecule-1 (ICAM-1), monocyte chemotactic protein-1 (MCP-1; binds to the CCR2 receptor), selectins, matrix metalloproteinases (MMPs), and endothelin-1 (ET-1). Finally, these coordinated events result in inflammation, procoagulation, and thrombosis.

complications, but the C-106T polymorphism has been associated with microalbuminuria development among Finnish patients with T2DM [62]. In a multicenter, randomized, double-blind study of 101 patients with T1DM or T2DM, administration of an AR inhibitor (AS-3201) inhibited sorbitol accumulation in the sural nerve and improved sensory nerve conduction [63].

Hexosamine Pathway

Increased glucose flux into the hexosamine pathway, producing glucosamine, leads to insulin resistance, cellular injury, and microvascular complications. These effects are due to the dynamic addition and removal of a single O-linked N-acetylglucosamine residue (O-GlcNAcylation). N-acetylglucosamine brings about covalent modification of various transcription factors and nuclear proteins contributing to diabetic complications. In addition, O-GlcNAcylation impairs the metabolic arm (IR-IRS1-PI3K-Akt) and enhances the mitogenic arm (ERK-1/2 and p38 MAPK) of the insulin signaling pathway [64]. This deregulates endothelial nitric oxide synthase (eNOS) and increases matrix metalloproteinases (MMP)-2 and -9 expression [64]. The single nucleotide polymorphism

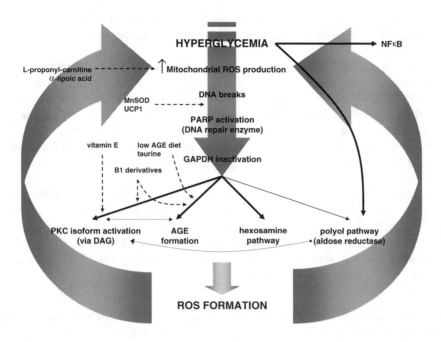

FIGURE 2.4 Amplification loop between ROS and four pathways involved in microvascular complications. Hyperglycemia may induce glucose toxicity. This results in increased mitochondrial ROS formation. ROS induces DNA damage and the activation of repair enzymes like PARP. GAPDH activity is reduced by PARP, resulting in the diversion of glycolytic intermediates into four pathways contributing to microvascular complications. These pathways eventually produce ROS, which can amplify this biochemical loop. Various nutrients and nutrient-dependent pathways exert negative (dashed line) effects on this loop [58]. Thin arrows indicate modulatory interactions among the various pathways.

A1396G in the N-acetylglucosamine-phosphate mutase (AGM$_1$, a key enzyme in the hexosamine pathway) gene may confer resistance to diabetic nephropathy and neuropathy [65]. Also, O-GlcNAcylation impairs cardiac calcium cycling via altered expression of the sarcoendoplasmic reticulum Ca^{2+} ATPase (SERCA2a) yielding diastolic dysfunction and cardiomyopathy [66]. Of interest, glucosamine ingestion for the treatment of osteoarthritis is not associated with any significant changes in glycemic control among patients with T2DM [67].

AGE Formation

The slow accumulation of AGE in tissues has also been implicated in the development of diabetic complications, although their role is not fully defined. AGEs are formed when glycated proteins undergo arrangement to an Amadori product and then undergo further autooxidation to AGE via dicarbonyl intermediates. AGE precursors that are associated with diabetic complications are methylglyoxal (MG) and N-carboxymethyl-lysine (CML). Protein crosslinking leads to AGE accumulation in the extra-cellular matrix producing capillary basement membrane thickening. These structural changes alter vascular function, electrical charge, and filtration properties. AGEs also consume NO leading to defective vasodilatation. In patients with diabetes, erythrocytes affected by AGE contain glycosylated hemoglobin and are analyzed as part of the A1C determination [68]. These erythrocytes bind to endothelial AGE receptors (RAGE) and are responsible for increases in vascular permeability and endothelial cell dysfunction. The vascular leakage of albumin and other proteins causes large and small vessel disease [69]. In the retina, AGEs increase permeability of retinal endothelial cells and are toxic to pericytes [70]. In the kidney, AGEs trap plasma proteins and contribute to thickening of the basement membrane and reduced filtration [70]. AGEs have also been shown to reduce sensory motor conduction velocity action potentials and blood flow in peripheral nerves [70].

The role of exogenous (dietary or tobacco) AGE in the pathogenesis of diabetes complications is also unclear and controversial. In a 2-week, randomized, crossover study, a diet high in rapid heat-generated AGE was associated with increased levels of inflammatory markers (CRP, VCAM-1, TNF-α, mRNA, and AGE-modified LDL) compared with a low-AGE diet where the food was prepared by steaming [71]. Interestingly, in rats, dietary taurine seems to prevent accumulation of AGE [72]. Examples of foods with AGE-bioreactive properties according to decreasing amounts of AGE precursors are: broiled chicken cubes > broiled tuna > boiled egg yolk > toasted white bread > boiled pasta [71].

Overall, the whole body AGE pool contributes to oxidative stress, inflammation, and diabetic complications. The AGE pool is in steady state with endogenous production and dietary intake. Even though dietary AGE intake correlates with serum AGE levels and markers of inflammation, there are still no clinical data demonstrating outcome benefit. There are no significant risks associated with a low-AGE diet. Further studies are required before a low-AGE diet can routinely be recommended to diabetic patients (grade C).

PKC Isoforms

Hyperglycemic activation of the DAG-PKC signal transduction pathway may also play a key role in the development of diabetes vascular complications. In fact, PKC activation may represent a final common pathway by which oxidation and glycation products exert their adverse effects. Protein kinase C constitutes a family of phospholipid-dependent serine/threonine kinases.

Glucose-induced increases in DAG levels and PKC activity have been reported in retinal endothelial cells, renal mesangial cells, aortic endothelial cells, and smooth muscle cells, but not in brain cells, demonstrating a tissue-specific effect. Preferential activation of the PKC-β isoform led to the development of LY333531, an inhibitor of the enzyme, which has been shown to reduce increased albumin excretion and prevent a decrease in motor nerve conduction velocity in rats, and to improve retinal blood flow in humans [73,74]. Vitamin E inhibits the DAG-PKC pathway and can decrease vascular complications in animal models [73]. The formation of AGE changes PKC activity. Moreover, increased PKC activity enhances the effect of AGE on glomerular basement membrane thickness in the pathogenesis of diabetic nephropathy in rats [75].

Macrovascular Disease

There are several mechanisms by which hyperglycemia promotes atherosclerosis in diabetes. The interaction of glycosylated proteins with their receptor results in PKC activation, pro-inflammatory responses, and oxidative stress [76]. These mechanisms are very similar to those occurring in the genesis of microvascular disease.

T1DM and T2DM are both independent risk factors for CAD, stroke, and PVD [77–79]. Atherosclerosis accounts for virtually 80% of all deaths among North American diabetic patients, almost threefold greater than all deaths in the general North American population. More than 75% of all hospitalizations for diabetic complications are attributable to cardiovascular disease [76]. Microalbuminuria in T1DM is a marker for renal disease as well as CAD.

Numerous studies have shown in-hospital mortality from myocardial infarction (MI) in diabetic patients is 1.5–2.0 times higher than nondiabetics. Late mortality in diabetes is mainly related to recurrent MI and the development of new chronic heart failure. It has been speculated that unique pathogenic mechanisms in diabetes operate to weaken plaque stability.

Diabetic Neuropathy

There has been debate as to the cause of diabetic neuropathy, whether it is a result of a direct effect of hyperglycemia on the nerve or a consequence of a lesion on the vasa nervorum. The answer seems to lie in the nerve. Studies by Caselli et al. [80] and Veves et al. [81] offer some clarity to the debate. Caselli et al. [80] examined the role of the C-nociceptive fibers in reflex-related vasodilatation in diabetics. They explored direct and indirect vasodilatation in the skin of diabetics, with and without neuropathy, and normal individuals. When iontophoresis with ACh was applied on the skin of normal individuals, it produced direct vasodilatation at the site of iontophoresis and indirect vasodilatation at the surrounding sites thought to be secondary to C-nociceptive fiber stimulation. When a topical anesthetic was applied to the skin, and iontophoresis with ACh applied, there was no change in the direct vasodilatory response and the indirect vasodilatation of the surrounding areas was diminished. This response was observed in the diabetics and normal subjects, suggesting that independent of diabetes, the C-nociceptive fibers play a key role in indirect reflex-related vasodilatation.

To investigate endothelial-mediated microvascular regulation, Veves et al. [81] studied patients having diabetic neuropathy with and without vascular disease, diabetics with Charcot's arthropathy, diabetics without complications, and normal subjects. They used two approaches to measuring vasodilatation: a laser Doppler iontophoresis and the laser Doppler perfusion imager which measures the response to iontophoresis with computer imaging of the erythrocyte flux [81]. They demonstrated an association between diabetic neuropathy and the alteration of endothelial-dependent and endothelial-independent vasodilatation, suggesting that neuropathy is the key factor for the compromised microvascular response [81]. These two studies suggest that diabetic neuropathy is a primary lesion of the nerves. Common neurological findings in diabetics with long-standing poorly controlled disease are dysesthesia, decreased propioception, and muscular atrophy.

TREATMENT OF DIABETES

Clinical Management of Type-1 Diabetes Mellitus

T1DM frequently presents with an acute metabolic decompensation characterized by generalized fatigue, polyuria, polydipsia, blurred vision, nocturia, severe dehydration, oliguria, and a fruity odor on their breath. The diagnosis of T1DM is made by demonstrating the presence of ketones in serum or urine, a low pH by arterial blood gases, an elevated anion gap, and high blood glucose levels > 250 mg/dL.

Acute Management

Once a diagnosis of diabetic ketoacidosis (DKA) is established, the primary focus of treatment is hydration and insulin, achieving a decrease in capillary glucose at a rate of 80–100 mg/dL per hour until a glucose level of 250 mg/dL is achieved. Initially the fluids should be normal saline, two liters intravenously over the first 2 hours, followed by 100–500 cc/hour based on the clinical response. In this setting, insulin is best administered as a regular human insulin (RHI) intravenous bolus followed by a drip starting at a rate of 5 units/hour, with hourly measurements of capillary blood glucose. The insulin infusion is then adjusted based on the results of capillary glucose measurements. Certain metabolic derangements, such as hypokalemia, hypophosphatemia, and hyperchloremia, result from the acute management of DKA and require prompt attention (see Table 2.1).

Intermediate Management

When the BG is at 250 mg/dL, then the focus shifts towards maintenance of fluid and electrolyte equilibrium. Hydration is changed to 0.45% NaCl at a rate of 100 cc/hour and the capillary blood glucose is measured every 2 hours. If the results are < 150mg/dL, IV fluids should be changed to 5% dextrose in 0.45% NaCl. Once the anion gap is closed, the glucose is < 200 mg/dL, and the patient is tolerating oral diet, the insulin drip can be discontinued. A subcutaneous injection of

TABLE 2.1
Metabolic Derangements in DKA

Derangement	Etiology	Treatment
Hyperglycemia	Severe insulinopenia	Insulin
Hypovolemia	Osmotic diuresis—glucosuria	Normal saline intravenously
Ketosis	No insulin to suppress lipolysis	Insulin and fluids to improve renal ketone clearance
Acidosis	Severely increased ketoacids	Above plus Na-bicarbonate or Na-acetate
Hypokalemia	Insulin therapy	KCl or K-acetate, IVSS or about 40 mEq/L in IVF
Hypophosphatemia	Insulin therapy and glucose uptake	Na- or K-Phos, IVSS if serum level < 1.0–1.5 mg/dL
Hyperchloremia	Non-anion gap metabolic acidosis	Decrease chloride in IV fluids (use acetate)

rapid-acting insulin must be given a half hour prior to discontinuing the insulin drip. This is preferentially done at a mealtime. Intermediate or long-acting insulin must be given at this time as well to cover basal requirements [82]. If not previously known, the total daily dose (TDD) of insulin can be calculated as 0.5 units/kg body weight. For example, in a 70 kg individual, the requirement would be 35 units/day; 17 units for the (premeal) bolus insulin (50% of the TDD divided in three parts, one for each meal), and 17 units of insulin glargine, every 24 hours, usually at bedtime.

In addition to the standing bolus of rapid-acting insulin before meals, a correction dose is also given before meals (or every 6 hours if the patient is not eating). The correction dose of insulin is individualized according to the patient's insulin sensitivity. The sensitivity factor can be calculated by dividing 1800 by the estimated insulin TDD. For instance, if the insulin TDD is 60 units/day, then the sensitivity factor is 30. Thus, each unit of insulin would be expected to result in a 30 mg/dL decrease in the blood glucose level. The target blood glucose is < 110 mg/dL preprandially and < 180 mg/dL postprandially in the hospital [83–85].

It is important to try to determine the etiology of the DKA and rule out underlying infections, myocardial infarction, or non-compliance with diabetes medication. The patient should be educated about insulin management during future illness to prevent another episode of DKA. Patients should also be provided with urine or serum ketone strips for home use.

Long-Term Management

Every patient must be given diabetes education, which discusses:

- Survival skills
- Overview of disease process and treatment options
- Nutrition
- Exercise
- How to use medications
- Glucose monitoring
- Complications
- Psychosocial issues
- Reproductive health, if applicable
- Promoting general health and well-being
- Sick day rules

Every newly diagnosed diabetic should be instructed on the use of a glucometer and provided with a regimen for glucose testing. While it is true that the more one tests the better, a bare-bones approach would include testing before each meal, at bedtime, and when the patient feels sick. The patient must be taught how to recognize and treat hypoglycemia. The symptoms of hypoglycemia often begin with a sensation of hunger; as plasma glucose continues to decline, symptoms may include shakiness, lightheadedness, tachycardia, dizziness, disorientation, confusion, numbness of the legs and tongue, blurred vision, nausea, headache, profuse sweating, drowsiness, and ultimately unconsciousness and seizures [81].

An estimate of the maintenance insulin dose of the patient with new onset T1DM is based on the body weight, as above, but varies depending on residual insulin secretory capacity and the carbohydrate content of the individual diet. The patient must be warned about the "honeymoon" period. This refers to a transient period of β-cell recovery lasting from several weeks to over a year during which insulin requirements may be minimum or not at all. In general, β-cell function is not completely compromised for 5 years. Over this period, the patient will need to gradually increase both basal and pre-meal insulins as endogenous insulin secretion diminishes.

Insulin

Insulin was discovered in 1921 by Banting and Best and is used for the treatment of T1DM or T2DM as monotherapy or in combination with oral agents. Currently available insulins are synthetic human insulins or analogs of human insulin, which vary in their rate of absorption and duration of action (see Table 2.2). There are also products that are mixtures of rapid/short-acting and intermediate-acting insulins. Purified animal insulins are no longer used.

RHI is structurally identical to human insulin and is synthesized by *E. coli* bacteria. It consists of zinc insulin crystals dissolved in clear fluid. Insulin lispro is a rapid-acting insulin analog in which the amino acids at positions 28 and 29 on the human insulin B-chain are reversed. Insulin aspart is another rapid-acting insulin analog with a substitution of aspartic acid for proline in position 28 on the B-chain. Insulin glulisine is the newest rapid-acting analog in which the aspargine at position 3 on the B-chain is replaced by lysine and the lysine at position 29 on the B-chain is replaced by glutamic acid. These amino acid changes result in a reduced propensity for insulin molecules to self-associate (form dimers and hexamers) giving them a more rapid onset and shorter duration of action than RHI. These insulins are used to cover carbohydrates at mealtimes, to correct an elevated glucose, and in insulin pumps.

Neutral pH–protamine–Hagedorn (NPH) is an intermediate-acting insulin which is a suspension of RHI with protamine which delays its absorption. This insulin can be used at bedtime to normalize fasting glucose and in combination with rapid-acting insulins during the daytime to provide basal and some carbohydrate coverage.

Insulin glargine is an insulin analog in which the asparagine residue at position A21 is replaced with glycine and two arginine residues are added to the B-chain C-terminus. Insulin glargine has a pH of 4 in solution but when injected subcutaneously and exposed to pH 7.4, it microprecipitates, delaying its absorption. It is virtually peakless with a 24-hour duration of action. Insulin detemir is a soluble long-acting human insulin analog with the threonine removed at position B30 and a 14-carbon myristoyl fatty acid acylated to lysine at position B29. This enables reversible binding of the determir molecule to tissue albumin, conferring a slow absorption into the circulation and a prolonged effect lasting up to 24 hours. These insulins are used once or twice daily to provide basal coverage.

The most physiological way of tailoring insulin therapy is to administer a dose of insulin that will provide basal insulin levels usually once daily, as well as a synchronized bolus of insulin prior to each meal, proportional to the carbohydrate consumed, to control the resultant glucose elevations. Combining a long-acting insulin to achieve basal levels and multiple rapid-acting insulin injections to control post-prandial glucose elevations will provide better glycemic control than the use of mixed insulin preparations. Carbohydrate counting is the preferred method to determine the amount of rapid-acting insulin to be administered before each meal. Patients must be instructed to have the meal ready for consumption before administering a dose of rapid-acting insulin in order to avoid hypoglycemia. Moreover, studies show that there is less hypoglycemia with bedtime administration of insulin glargine or detemir compared with NPH, because its effect is slow and sustained over a

TABLE 2.2
Commercially Available Insulins

Type	Name	Onset of Action	Time to Peak Activity	Duration of Action
Rapid-acting	Aspart	15 Minutes	1 Hour	3–4 Hours
	Glulisine	15 Minutes	½–1½ Hours	3–5 Hours
	Lispro	15 Minutes	1 Hour	3–4 Hours
Short-acting	Regular	30–60 Minutes	2–4 Hours	6–8 Hours
Intermediate-acting	NPH	1–3 Hours	6–8 Hours	12–16 Hours
Long-acting	Detemir	1 Hour	No peak	About 20–24 hours
	Glargine	1–2 Hours	No peak	About 24 hours

long period approximating 24 hours [82]. Insulin allergies are uncommon with the recombinant preparations of insulins.

Unused insulin vials, cartridges, and pens should be kept refrigerated but not frozen, and will stay potent until the expiration date. Unrefrigerated vials of the insulin analogs should be discarded after 28 days. Insulin glargine, once opened, must be changed after 28 days, whether or not refrigerated. Rapid-acting insulins in a pen should not be refrigerated and should be discarded after 28 days. Mixed analog insulins in a pen should be discarded after 10–14 days. All insulins should be kept away from direct heat or sunlight.

Amylin

Synthetic human amylin, pramlintide, recently became available as adjunctive treatment for patients who remain uncontrolled with T1DM or T2DM using mealtime insulin. Amylin is a naturally occurring hormone produced by pancreatic β-cells. Pramlintide has been shown to reduce glucose fluctuations, improve long-term glycemic control, reduce mealtime insulin requirements, and reduce body weight. Empiric reductions in mealtime insulin doses are recommended at the start of pramlintide therapy to decrease the risk for hypoglycemia. The drug is available in a disposable pen device, which must be refrigerated. Pramlintide cannot be mixed with insulin.

Use of Insulin Pumps and Continuous Glucose Monitoring Systems

Insulin pumps are devices with a subcutaneous catheter which deliver continuous subcutaneous insulin infusion (CSII). One or more basal rates are preprogrammed by the user and boluses are taken as needed whenever carbohydrates are ingested. The catheter is changed every 2–3 days and abdominal infusion sites are most commonly used. In a motivated patient, better glycemic control can be achieved with CSII—compared with multiple subcutaneous insulin injections—since CSII can provide multiple basal rates of insulin. Pumps are generally used in patients with T1DM but can also be used in patients with T2DM. A meta-analysis by Weissberg-Benchell et al. [86] of 52 studies concluded that CSII is associated with improved A1C and mean blood glucose levels. Bode et al. [87] demonstrated that mean A1C levels decreased from 8.3–7.5 %, with a significant reduction in severe hypoglycemia, in comparison to multiple insulin injections during the first year of therapy. Patients that counted carbohydrates, checked their glucoses 3 or more times a day, and recorded their glucoses in a log book had better glycemic control than those who did not [87].

Continuous glucose monitoring systems (CGMS) are available that utilize a glucose sensor to provide up to 3 days of continuous glucose monitoring in the subcutaneous tissue. The record shows glucose patterns and trends which can help in the recognition and prevention of hypoglycemia, hyperglycemia, post-prandial glucose excursions, and effects of exercise [88]. However, "normal" interstitial glucose values may be lower than realized, including some values in the "hypoglycemic range." Also, the CGMS may not always read the glucose concentrations consistently accurately [89]. Future sensors which are more accurate will obviate some of these limitations and potentially replace fingerstick monitoring.

Clinical Management of Type-2 Diabetes Mellitus

T2DM may present insidiously with a slow progression of increased thirst, urination, blurred vision, craving for sweet drinks, and weight loss, or it may be recognized on a routine blood test in an asymptomatic patient. When severe, there is acute decompensation with dehydration, fatigue, generalized weakness, and depressed mental status (nonketotic hyperosmolar state). Physical findings may include dry mucous membranes, lack of skin turgor, hypotension, and postural tachycardia.

Acute Management of Nonketotic Hyperosmolar State

The initial blood exam should include electrolytes (Na, K, Cr, CO_2, Ca, Mg, Phos), a complete blood count, blood urea nitrogen (BUN), urine analysis, ketone bodies, and anion gap.

In contrast to T1DM, the glucose levels are extremely high with a greater degree of free water deficit and hyperosmolarity. The primary focus is fluid replacement with insulin administration a secondary priority.

Intravenous hydration should be provided with normal saline, 1 liter/hour for the first 2 hours. By that time blood pressure and pulse should be stable and urine output improved. Regular insulin should be administered at a rate of 2–4 units/hour intravenously based upon the initial glucose level. Capillary glucose determinations should be done hourly with a goal of sustained decline in glucose levels until 150 mg/dL. Once a glucose level of 150 mg/dL is attained, the intravenous fluid should be changed to 0.45% NaCl at a rate of 100 cc/hour. If the etiology is not simply new-onset T2DM, then consideration should be given to determine the cause of the hyperosmolar state and rule out underlying infections, myocardial infarction, poor adherence with diabetes medication, or emotional stress. Appropriate treatment should be given if a cause is found.

Intermediate Management

Once the glucose is 150 mg/dL or less and the patient can eat, subcutaneous insulin should be administered before meals with rapid-acting insulin, and at bedtime with intermediate- or long-acting insulin. Correction doses of rapid-acting insulin, based on a sliding scale above 150 mg/dL, should be added before meals and at bedtime. Follow-up blood exams should be done every 4 hours and as appropriate. Typically, a newly diagnosed type-2 diabetic patient can be converted from insulin therapy to oral agents over the next 1–2 months as glucose toxicity resolves and β-cell function recovers.

Pharmacologic Treatment of Type-2 Diabetes Mellitus

The most important feature of a comprehensive treatment plan for T2DM is lifestyle modification, which incorporates a proper diet and regular exercise. For most patients, this is extremely difficult to implement and sustain lifelong. When glycemic targets are still not reached with lifestyle modifications alone, a pharmacologic approach is introduced. Oral agents are used depending on desired clinical responses, biochemical responses and toxicities (see Table 2.3 and Figure 2.5). The natural history of T2DM is one of progressive deterioration of β-cell function over many years, ultimately resulting in insulin-dependence.

Metformin

Metformin has been used in Europe for several decades but has only been marketed in the United States since 1995. The primary mechanism of action of metformin is to decrease hepatic glucose output by inhibiting glucose-6-dehydrogenase activity. The starting dose for metformin is 500 mg orally with dinner for 1 week and then 500 mg orally with breakfast and dinner. A sustained-release preparation is available that allows once-daily dosing. Due to its mechanism of action, there is minimal risk for hypoglycemia. This drug should not be used in renal failure or potential hypoxic states, such as congestive heart failure and severe pulmonary disease, due to the risk of lactic acidosis. The risk of lactic acidosis is low and is estimated to be 9 per 100,000 person/years. The

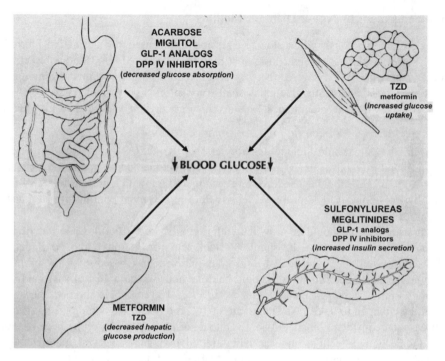

FIGURE 2.5 Target activities of various antidiabetic drugs.

TABLE 2.3
Commercially Available Oral Agents Used to Treat T2DM

Drug Class	Generic Name	Mechanism of Action	Expected A1C Reduction (%)	Daily Dose
Biguanides	Metformin	Decreases hepatic glucose output	1.0–2.0	500 mg qD to 1000 mg BID to 850 mg TID
Thiazolidinedione	Pioglitazone	PPAR α and γ agonist	1.0–1.5	15–45 mg qD
	Rosiglitazone	PPAR γ agonist	1.0–1.5	2 mg qD - BID, 8 mg qD
Sulfonylurea	Glipizide	β-cell insulin synthesis and release	1.0–2.0	2.5–20 mg qD - BID
	Glyburide			1.25–10 mg qD - BID
	Glimepiride			0.5–8 mg qD
Meglitinides	Repaglinide	β-cell insulin synthesis and release	1.0–2.0	0.5–4 mg TID
	Nateglinide		0.5–1.0	60–120 mg TID
α-glucosidase inhibitors	Acarbose	α-glucosidase inhibition (decreased carbohydrate absorption)	0.5–1.0	50–100 mg TID
	Miglitol		0.5–1.0	50–100 mg TID

most common side effects are gastrointestinal—nausea, diarrhea and abdominal pain—as well as a metallic taste. It should not be used in patients with impaired renal function (serum creatinine > 1.5 mg/dL in men and > 1.4 mg/dL in women). Caution should be exercised in prescribing metformin to the elderly. If used in patients over age 80 years, then a normal glomerular filtration rate should be documented. Metformin should be discontinued on the day patients receive an iodinated contrast material for radiographic studies, which can temporarily impair renal function as well as prior to any surgical procedure. The metformin dose can be resumed 48 hours later if the serum creatinine is in the normal range. Metformin lowers the A1C by 1–2%. Metformin can be used to treat the metabolic syndrome since it lowers serum concentrations of triglycerides, PAI-1 activity, and body weight.

Thiazolidinediones

These agents induce PPAR-γ binding to nuclear receptors in muscle and adipocytes, allowing insulin-stimulated glucose transport. Three PPARs have been identified to date: PPAR-α, PPAR-δ (also known as PPAR-β), and PPAR-γ [86]. After ligand binding, PPARs change their conformation to permit the recruitment of one or more coactivator proteins [87]. The first mechanism, transactivation, is DNA-dependent and consists of binding of PPAR components with target genes and heterodimerization with the retinoid X receptor [87]. The second mechanism, transrepression, interferes with other transcription factor pathways which are not DNA-dependent [88]. The PKC signaling pathway functions as a molecular switch that dissociates with transactivation and transrepression properties of PPAR-α [89]. PPAR-α resides mainly in the liver, heart muscle, and vascular endothelium; when it is activated, it controls genes that regulate lipoprotein levels and confers anti-inflammatory effects [90]. PPAR-γ is located mainly on adipocytes but is also found in pancreatic β-cells, vascular endothelium, and macrophages [87].

TZDs lower fasting and postprandial glucose levels as well as free fatty acid levels [91,92]. A first-generation TZD, troglitazone, is no longer available due to its hepatotoxicity. The second-generation TZDs, rosiglitazone and pioglitazone, may be used as monotherapy or in combination with insulin, sulfonylureas, or metformin, and have not been found to be hepatotoxic. TZDs are associated with weight gain due to fluid retention and proliferation of adipose tissue. However, the TZDs increase fat in the subcutaneous adipose tissue and decrease visceral adipose tissue and fat in the liver. The dose for rosiglitazone is 2–8 mg/day and for pioglitazone is 15–45 mg/day. Two side effects to be noted are peripheral tissue edema and, less frequently, congestive heart failure. TZDs are contraindicated in patients with congestive heart failure and should be used cautiously in at-risk patients.

TZDs decrease A1C levels by 1–1.5%. These agents decrease insulin resistance and possibly preserve β-cell function [86,93]. The Troglitazone in the Prevention of Diabetes (TRIPOD) study [95] was designed to investigate the preservation of pancreatic β-cell function with thiazolidinedione (TZD). Hispanic women with a prior medical history of gestational diabetes were randomized to receive troglitazone 400 mg daily or a placebo. Women who did not develop diabetes were asked to return 8 months after the trial for an OGTT and an intravenous glucose tolerance (IVGTT). The median follow up was 30 months. The troglitazone group had a 56% reduction in the incidence of T2DM for as long as 8 months after medications were stopped. This protection against earlier development of diabetes was associated with a reduction in insulin resistance [94]. Pioglitazone acts like a partial PPAR-α agonist and has beneficial effects on the lipid profile increasing HLD-c, decreasing TG and improving LDL-c subtypes. A new class of dual PPAR-α/γ agonists is in development which lowers glucose, TG, and LDL-c while raising HDL-c [95].

Sulfonylureas

Sulfonylureas (SU) are the oldest class of treatment for T2DM. The mode of action is by stimulating β-cell insulin secretion (see Figure 2.6). The β-cell SU receptor (SUR) is functionally linked to an ATP-sensitive K+ channel (K+ATP) on the cell membrane [104]. In the basal state, the K+ATP channel shifts K+ from the inside of the β-cell to the extracellular space and maintains the resting potential of the β-cell membrane. When the SU binds to the SUR, K+ efflux diminishes and the membrane depolarizes. This depolarization opens a voltage-dependent calcium channel in the same membrane which enables extracellular calcium to enter the cell. The resultant increase in intracellular calcium triggers insulin-containing secretory granule exocytosis.

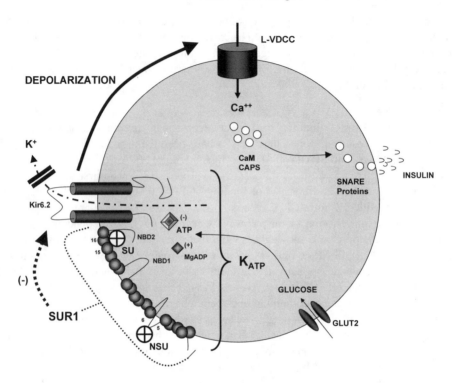

FIGURE 2.6 Mechanism of action of sulfonylureas and sulfonylurea-like insulin secretagogues. During the postprandial state when serum glucose levels increase, GLUT2 glucose transport also increases and stimulates β-cell metabolism and the ATP/mgADP ratio [100]. An increased ratio inhibits the inwardly-rectifying K⁺ channel (Kir6.2) directly or indirectly via interaction with nucleotide binding domains (NBD1 and NBD2) on the SUR1 [100,101]. Inhibition of Kir6.2 causes cell membrane depolarization and activation of the L-type voltage-dependent Ca⁺⁺ channel (L-VDCC) [102]. β-cell secretory granule recruitment is influenced by calmodulin (CaM) and the Ca⁺⁺-dependent activator protein for secretion (CAPS). Secretory granule docking with the cell membrane, exocytosis, and release of insulin are mediated by synaptotagmin and the SNARE proteins: soluble N-ethylmaleimide-sensitive fusion protein [NSF] attachment protein [SNAP] receptors, synaptobrevin-2, syntaxin-1A, and a 25-kDa synaptosomal-associated protein [SNAP-25]. The ATP-sensitive potassium channels (K_{atp}) are composed of the Kir6.2 and sulfonylurea receptor (SUR) subunits; the latter contains 17 transmembrane (TM) helices. Sulfonylurea moieties of insulin secretagogues (glipizide and glyburide) interact with the type-1 SUR (SUR1) cytoplasmic loop connecting TMs 15 and 16, whereas the nonsulfonylurea moieties of insulin secretagogues (glibenclamide, glimepiride, and their analogues, repaglinide, nateglinide, and meglitinide) interact with the SUR1 cytoplasmic loop connecting TMs 5 and 6 [100]. Repaglinide is not internalized as with sulfonylureas [99]. Nateglinide has a faster inhibition and reversal of inhibition than repaglinide [103].

The first-generation SU have a long half-life and bind ionically to plasma proteins, making them easily displaced. The major concern with these agents is hypoglycemia. The second-generation SU have a shorter half-life and bind to plasma proteins non-ionically, making them less easily displaced from proteins and available for binding to receptors. Commercially available second-generation SU are glyburide 1.25–20 mg/day; glipizide 2.5–40 mg/day, and glimepiride 1–8 mg/day. SU decrease the A1C by 1–2%.

Meglitinides

Repaglinide is a member of the meglitinide group of insulin secretagogues with a relatively short half-life of 3.7 hours. The binding site on the SUR is distinct from the binding site for sulfonylureas. The drug is taken up to 30 minutes prior to each meal. Repaglinide is particularly useful in the elderly, patients with chronic renal insufficiency, and patients who are erratic eaters. The dose varies between 0.5–4 mg before meals. Repaglinide results in a 1–2% decrease in A1C.

Nateglinide, a derivative of phenylalanine, is structurally distinct from both sulfonylureas and repaglinide. It has a quicker onset and shorter duration of action than repaglinide. Nateglinide is available as a 60–120 mg tablet taken with each meal. It is effective for lowering postprandial glucose levels. Nateglinide results in a 0.5–1.0% decrease in A1C. As with repaglinide, the dose of nateglinide should be omitted if a meal is skipped.

α-Glucosidase Inhibitors

These agents inhibit α-glucosidases in the brush border of the small intestine, delaying the absorption of complex carbohydrates, and are not systemically absorbed. They are most effective in reducing post-prandial blood glucose elevations and can be used as adjunctive therapy with other oral agents. The two available agents are acarbose, given 50–100 mg with meals, and miglitol, given 50 mg with meals. The side effects are flatulence and glycemic index (GI) discomfort. One study noted that prophylactic use of acarbose delayed the development of T2DM in patients with IGT [105]. These medications result in a 0.5–1.0% decrease in A1C levels and may be useful as an adjunct to other oral hypoglycemic agents with high-carbohydrate meals, e.g., pasta.

Incretins

The newest agents available for the treatment of T2DM belong to the class of incretin hormones. The first pharmacologic agent available in this class is the glucagon-like peptide-1 (GLP-1) analog, exenatide. Exenatide is a synthetic analog of exendin-4 derived from lizard saliva.

There is growing evidence over the past two decades that incretin hormones may play a role in the pathogenesis of DM. These hormones have a multiplicity of effects including glucose-dependent insulin secretion and β-cell proliferation [106]. The two key incretins are (GLP-1, secreted by the L cells of the distal portion of the small intestine, and gastric inhibitory peptide, or glucose-dependent insulinotropic polypeptide (GIP), secreted in the duodenal K cells. GLP-1 is derived from proglucagon along with glucagon and GLP-2 [107]. A variety of trophic intestinal effects have been attributed to GLP-2. A catalog of incretins and related therapeutic agents with antidiabetic activity is given in Table 2.4.

Both GIP and GLP-1 are decreased in T2DM. When given pharmacologically, these hormones stimulate β-cell proliferation and can prevent or delay the onset of diabetes [106]. Experiments have demonstrated that when GLP-1 is infused at physiological concentrations in patients with longstanding diabetes, there is improved glycemic control, a recuperation of the biphasic secretion pattern of insulin from the pancreas, and no evidence of hypoglycemia [108–110].

There are two approaches to utilize these hormones therapeutically in patients with T2DM. Incretin mimetics are analogs with extended half-lives and pharmacokinetic duration. Dipeptidyl peptidase IV (DPP-IV) rapidly degrades GLP-1 and GIP to inactive truncated forms. DPP-IV inhibitors retard peptide degradation of these incretins, conferring a therapeutic advantage [111]. GLP-1 analogs result in enhanced insulin secretion, decreased glucagon levels, decreased gastric emptying, decreased appetite, and weight loss. The most studied GLP-1 analog, exenetide or synthetic exendin-4, also present in lizard saliva, is naturally resistant to DPP-IV degradation. Exendin-4 stimulates the biphasic secretion of insulin and C-peptide in T2DM. It is currently available for use in T2DM uncontrolled with metformin or a sulfonylurea. It is administered as a subcutaneous injection of 5 or 10 mcg via a pen device twice daily. There are several clinical trials that are underway involving other injectable GLP-1 analogs and the oral DPP-IV inhibitor LAF-237 for the treatment of T2DM [108–110].

TABLE 2.4
Summary of Incretins with Potential Antidiabetic Activity

Incretin	Site of Production	Physiological Action	Therapeutic Potential
GLP-1	L-cells in ileum and colon proglucagon-derived	Stimulates glucose-dependent insulin secretion, β-cell proliferation, and cytoprotection; inhibits gastric emptying, glucagon secretion, and food intake	Increase insulin secretion in T2DM
GIP	K-cells in duodenum and proximal jejunum	Stimulates glucose-dependent insulin secretion, β-cell proliferation, and cytoprotection; does not inhibit gastric emptying, glucagon secretion, or food intake	Increase insulin secretion in T2DM
Exendin-4	Salivary gland venom of lizard	GLP-1 receptor agonist; IV infusion lowers fasting and postprandial glucose levels; longer acting and more potent than DPP-IV inhibitors	Increase insulin secretion in T2DM
LAF-237	—	Second-generation DPP-IV inhibitor; oral agent that lowers glucose	Increase insulin secretion in T2DM

Abbreviations: GLP-1—glucagon-like peptide-1; GIP—gastric inhibitory peptide or glucose-dependent insulinotropic polypeptide; DPP—dipeptidyl peptidase

Other Long-Term Management Issues Associated with Type-2 Diabetes Mellitus

Every patient with T2DM should be provided with diabetes education. Recommendations for glucose testing varies among individuals and depends on the current degree of control and whether the patient is taking a medication that would potentially cause hypoglycemia. It is often useful to have patients test at different times on different days, such as in the morning prior to eating ("fasting glucose"), at bedtime, before lunch or dinner, 2 hours after meals, and whenever the patient feels sick. The patient will want to know the reason for frequent testing since, unlike patients with T1DM, insulin cannot be administered to acutely lower blood glucose levels if they are receiving oral hypoglycemic agents. In order for patients to adhere to frequent testing regimens, they must understand what foods, exercise, and circumstances will have an impact on blood glucose levels, as well as how they should modify their behaviors for optimal glycemic control.

Long-term studies, like the UKPDS [112], have shown that it is beneficial to achieve tight metabolic control to significantly reduce complications such as retinopathy and nephropathy. Tight control of blood pressure has proven to significantly reduce and in some cases reverse nephropathy, and to significantly reduce retinopathy and blindness due to diabetes. Patients with T2DM are considered to have a risk factor equivalence for coronary heart disease by virtue of the diabetes alone. The National Cholesterol Education Program (NCEP) made recommendations for tight control of blood lipid levels in diabetics, especially in patients with T2DM [113].

Future Directions

Islet Cell Transplants

Whole pancreas transplants have successfully restored insulin secretion in people with advanced diabetes but are usually limited to those who are also undergoing kidney transplantation [114]. In 2000, Shapiro et al. [115] developed the Edmonton Protocol for islet transplantation, which used a larger quantity of islet cells with drugs that were less toxic to the immune system. This method infuses islet cells through a small tube into the portal vein of the liver. Patients whose islet cells fail to continue secreting insulin can be retransplanted. Islet cell transplants are still experimental and are available to people who are willing to participate in a study protocol. Also, only a small percentage of islet cell transplant recipients achieve normal blood glucose levels. It is unclear whether a transplant can stop or reverse secondary complications related to diabetes. It is also unclear whether islet cell transplantation will ultimately extend a patent's long-term survival.

Gene Therapy

T1DM is caused by T-cell mediated destruction of pancreatic insulin-producing β-cells. Tian et al. [116] have found a novel way to restore central tolerance in NOD mice using hematopoietic stem cells retrovirally transduced to express a protective form of the MHC class II β-chain. As a result, autoreactive T-cells will be killed in the thymus and never get to the pancreatic β-cells [116]. Central tolerance refers to mechanisms of tolerance acting in the thymus or bone marrow, in contrast to peripheral tolerance which occurs in immune cells after they have left the primary lymphoid organs. Pre-clinical studies must be completed before stem cells can be successfully given to humans with T1DM. Some drugs may be synthesized so that they exert their effect only within the areas of inflammation. One example is an engineered TGF-1β that can become activated locally within areas of β-cell inflammation [117,118].

Mechanical Closed-Loop Sensors

Mechanical closed-loop systems are currently under development [119]. They consist of a continuous glucose sensor and an insulin pump which can either infuse insulin subcutaneously or directly into the portal circulation. Such a device would not require immune suppression but would be potentially subject to mechanical breakdowns. In theory, these devices could provide both "basal" and synchronized "bolus" insulin requirements.

Novel Insulin Delivery Systems

Inhaled insulin systems deliver RHI to the pulmonary bed. The micron-sized particles contain 20% insulin and are loaded into an inhaler device. On deep inhalation, the insulin powder is delivered to the lungs. Oral insulin preparations use the adjuvant protein zonula occuldens toxin (ZOT), which is derived from vibrio cholera, and is thought to increase intestinal insulin transport. Both transoral and transdermal insulin patches are also under investigation. Insulin delivered by these alternative routes has the potential to provide "basal" requirements but is unable to be synchronized with oral carbohydrate ingestion and "bolus" requirements.

REFERENCES

1. World Health Organization, Diabetes: The Cost of Diabetes. http://www.who.int/mediacentre/factsheets/fs236/en/, Accessed on December 5, 2004.
2. Centers for Disease Control and Prevention, Prevalence of diabetes and impaired fasting glucose in adults—United States, 1999–2000, MMWR, 52:833–837, 2003, http://www.cdc.gov/mmwr/preview/mmwrhtml/mm5235a1.htm, Accessed on January 22, 2005.
3. Kuzuya T, Nakagawa S, and Satoh J, et al., Report of the Committee on the Classification and Diagnostic Criteria of Diabetes Mellitus, *Diabetes Res Clin Pract*, 55:65–85, 2002.
4. Diagnosis and Classification of Diabetes Mellitus, *Diabetes Care*, 27(Suppl 1):S5–10, 2004.
5. Awata T, Guberski DL, and Like AA, Genetics of the BB rat: Association of autoimmune disorders (diabetes, insulitis, and thyroiditis) with lymphopenia and major histocompatibility complex class II, *Endocrinology*, 136: 5731–5735, 1995.
6. Dahlquist G, Gustavsson KH, and Holmgren G et al., The incidence of diabetes mellitus in Swedish children 0–14 years of age, a prospective study 1977–1980, *Acta Paediatr Scand*, 71:7–14, 1982.
7. Eisenbarth GS, Type-1 diabetes mellitus: A chronic autoimmune disease, *N Engl J Med*, 314:1360–1368, 1986.
8. Khono T, Kobashiri Y, and Sugie Y et al., Antibodies to food antigens in Japanese patients with type-1 diabetes mellitus, *Diabetes Res Clin Pract*, 55:1–9, 2002.

9. Rayfield EJ and Ishimura K, Environmental factors and insulin-dependent diabetes mellitus, *Diabetes Metab Rev,* 3:925–957, 1987.

10. American Diabetes Association, Screening for type-2 diabetes, *Diabetes Care,* 27(Suppl 1):S11–14, 2004.

11. Pirola L, Johnson AM, and Van Obberghen E, Modulators of insulin action and their role in insulin resistance, *Diabetologia,* 47:170–184, 2004.

12. Kahn CR, Bruning JC, and Michael MD et al., Knockout mice challenge our concepts of glucose homeostasis and the pathogenesis of diabetes mellitus, *J Pediatr Endocrinol Metab,* 13:1377–1384, 2000.

13. Arner P, Pollare T, and Lithell H et al., Defective insulin receptor tyrosine kinase in human skeletal muscle in obesity and type-2 diabetes mellitus, *Diabetologia,* 30:437–440, 1987.

14. Le Marchand-Brustel Y, Gremeaux T, and Ballotti R et al., Insulin receptor tyrosine kinase is defective in skeletal muscle of insulin-resistant obese mice, *Natural,* 315:676–679, 1985.

15. Li S, Covino ND, and Stein EG et al., Structural and biochemical evidence for an autoinhibitory role for tyrosine 984 in the juxtamembrane region of the insulin receptor, *J Biol Chem,* 278:26007–26014, 2003.

16. Sesti G, Federici M, and Lauro D et al., Molecular mechanism of insulin resistance in type-2 diabetes mellitus: Role of the insulin receptor variant forms, *Diabetes Metab Res Rev,* 17:363–373, 2001.

17. Petersen KF, Dufour S, and Befroy D et al., Impaired mitochondrial activity in the insulin-resistant offspring of patients with type-2 diabetes, *N Engl J Med,* 350:664–671, 2004.

18. Ganda OP, Secondary forms of diabetes, In: Kahn CR and Weir GC, Eds., *Joslin's Diabetes Mellitus,* 13th ed., Lea and Febinger, Philadelphia, 1994, Table 17–1.

19. Mora PF, Post-transplantation diabetes mellitus, *Am J Med Sci,* 329:86–94, 2005.

20. Uchizono Y, Iwase M, and Nakamura U et al., Tacrolimus impairment of insulin secretion in isolated rat islets occurs at multiple distal sites in stimulus-secretion coupling, *Endocrinology,* 145:2264–2272, 2004.

21. Backman LA, Post-transplant diabetes mellitus: The last 10 years with tacrolimus, *Nephrol Dial Transplant,* 19(Suppl 6):vi13–16, 2004.

22. Romagnoli J, Citterio F, and Violi P et al., Post-transplant diabetes mellitus: A case control analysis of the risk factors, *Transplant Int,* 18:309–312, 2005.

23. Luther P and Baldwin D, Jr, Pioglitazone in the management of diabetes mellitus after transplantation, *Am J Transplant,* 4:2135–2138, 2004.

24. American Diabetes Association, Gestational diabetes mellitus, *Diabetes Care,* 27(Suppl 1):S88–93, 2004.

25. Woo KS, Chook P, and Yu CW et al., Effects of diet and exercise on obesity-related vascular dysfunction in children, *Circulation,* 27:1981–1986, 2004.

26. Elliott BD, Langer O, and Schenker S et al., Insignificant transfer of glyburide occurs across the human placenta, *Am J Obstet Gynecol,* 165:807–812, 1991.

27. The Expert Committee on the Diagnosis and Classification of Diabetes Mellitus, Followup report on the diagnosis of diabetes mellitus, *Diabetes Care,* 26:3160–3167, 2003.

28. DECODE Study Group, the European Diabetes Epidemiology Group, Glucose tolerance and cardio-vascular mortality: Comparison of fasting and 2-hour diagnostic criteria, *Arch Intern Med,* 161:397–405, 2001.

29. Sinha R, Fisch G, and Teague B, et al., Prevalence of impaired glucose tolerance among children and adolescents with marked obesity, *J Clin Endocrinol Metab,* 346:802–810, 2002.

30. Knowler WC, Barrett-Connor E, and Fowler SE et al., Diabetes Prevention Program Research Group, Reduction in the incidence of type-2 diabetes with lifestyle intervention or metformin, *N Engl J Med,* 346:393–403, 2002.

31. Ruderman NB, Aoki TT, and Cahill GF, Jr, Gluconeogenesis and its disorders in man, In: Hansom RW and Mehlman MA, Eds., *Gluconeogenesis: Its Regulation in Mammalian Species*, New York: John Wiley and Sons 515–532, 1976.

32. Dinneen S, Gerich J, and Rizza R, Carbohydrate metabolism in non-insulin dependent diabetes mellitus, *N Engl J Med,* 327:707–713, 1992.

33. Pirola L, Johnston AM, and Obberghen EV, Modulation of insulin action, *Diabetologia,* 47:170–184, 2004.

34. Bickel PE, Lipid rafts and insulin signaling, *Am J Physiol Endocrinol Metab,* 282:E1–E10, 2002.
35. Montminy M and Koo SH, Outfoxing insulin resistance? *Natural,* 432:958–9, 2004.
36. Wolfrum C, Asilmaz E, and Luca E et al., Foxa2 regulates lipid metabolism and ketogenesis in the liver during fasting and in diabetes, *Natural,* 432:1027–1032, 2004.
37. Zong H, Ren JM, and Young LH et al., AMP kinase is required for mitochondrial biogenesis in skeletal muscle in response to chronic energy deprivation, *Proc Natl Acad Sci USA,* 99:15983–15987, 2002.
38. Marik PE and Raghavan M, Stress-hyperglycemia, insulin and immunomodulation in sepsis, *Intens Care Med,* 30:748–756, 2004.
39. Lempaiainen P, Mykkanen L, and Pyorala K et al., Insulin resistance syndrome predicts coronary heart disease events in elderly nondiabetic men, *Circulation,* 100:123–128, 1999.
40. Collins AR, Pleiotropic vascular effects of PPAR-ligands, Drug News Perspectives, 2003, May, 16 (4):197–204, http://www.prous.com/journals/dnp/20031604/summary/ dn0197.cfm, Accessed on July 2, 2005.
41. Klein JP and Waxman SG, The brain in diabetes: Molecular changes in neurons and their implications for end-organ damage, *Lancet Neurol,* 2:548–554, 2003.
42. Wu L, Nicholson W, and Knobel S et al., Oxidative stress is a mediator of glucose toxicity in insulin-secreting pancreatic islet cell lines, *J Biol Chem,* 279:12126–12134, 2004.
43. Robertson R, Harmon J, and Tran P et al., β-cell glucose toxicity, lipotoxicity, and chronic oxidative stress in type-2 diabetes, *Diabetes,* 53:S119–S124, 2004.
44. Robertson P, Harmon J, and Tran P et al., Glucose toxicity in β-cells: Type-2 diabetes, good radicals gone bad, and the glutathione connection, *Diabetes,* 52:581–587, 2003.
45. Nishkawa T, Edelstein D, and Liang Du X et al., Normalizing mitochondrial superoxide production blocks three pathways of hyperglycaemic damage, *Natural,* 404:787–790, 2000.
46. Du X, Matsumura T, and Edelstein D et al., Inhibition of GAPDH activity by poly(ADP-ribose) polymerase activates three major pathways of hyperglycemic damage in endothelial cells, *J Clin Invest,* 112:1049–57, 2003.
47. Tanaka Y, Gleason C, and Tran P et al., Prevention of glucose toxicity in HIT-T15 cells and Zucker diabetic fatty rats by antioxidants, *Proc Natl Acad Sci USA,* 96:10857–10862, 1999.
48. Rubio AR and Morales-Segura MA, Nitric oxide, an iceberg in cardiovascular physiology: Far beyond vessel tone control, *Arch Med Res,* 35:1–11, 2004.
49. Vane VR, Anggard EE, and Botting RM, Regulatory functions of the vascular endothelium, *N Engl J Med,* 323:27–36, 1990.
50. Libby P, Ridker M, and Maseri A, Inflammation and atherosclerosis, *Circulation,* 105:1135–1143, 2002.
51. Libby P, Inflammation in atherosclerosis, *Natural,* 420:868–874, 2002.
52. Ridker PM, Rifai N, and Rose L et al., Comparison of C-reactive protein and low-density lipoprotein cholesterol levels in the prediction of first cardiovascular events, *N Engl J Med,* 347:1557–1565, 2002.
53. Haffner S, Temprosa M, and Crandall J et al., Diabetes Prevention Program Research Group, Intensive lifestyle intervention or metformin on inflammation and coagulation in participants with impaired glucose tolerance, *Diabetes,* 54:1566–1572, 2005.
54. Nicklas BJ, Ambrosius W, and Messier SP et al., Diet-induced weight loss, exercise, and chronic inflammation in older obese adults, *Am J Clin Nutr,* 79:544–551, 2004.
55. The Diabetes Control and Complications Trial Research Group, The effect of intensive treatment of diabetes on the development and progression of long-term complications in insulin-dependent diabetes mellitus, *N Engl J Med,* 329:977–986, 1993.
56. UK Prospective Diabetes Study (UKPDS) Group, Intensive blood-glucose control with sulphonylureas or insulin compared with conventional treatment and risk of complications in patients with type-2 diabetes (UKPDS 33), *Lancet,* 352:837–853, 1998.
57. Wautier JL and Guillausseau PJ, Advanced glycation end products, their receptors, and diabetic angiopathy, *Diabetes Metab (Paris),* 27:535–542, 2001.
58. Ceriello A, New insights on oxidative stress and diabetic complications may lead to a 'causal' antioxidant therapy, *Diabetes Care,* 26:1589–1596, 2003.

50. Srivastava SK, Ramana KV, and Bhatnagar A, Role of aldose reductase and oxidative damage in diabetes and the consequent potential for therapeutic options, *Endocr Rev,* 10:1210/er.2004–0028 [Epub ahead of print], 2005 as doi (*Endocr Rev,* 26(Suppl 3):380–392, 2005, May).

60. Obrosova IG, Pacher P, and Szabo C et al., Aldose reductase inhibition counteracts oxidative-nitrosative stress and poly(ADP-ribose) polymerase activation in tissue sites for diabetes complications, *Diabetes,* 54:234–242, 2005.

61. Ramana KV, Friedrich B, and Tammali R et al., Requirement of aldose reductase for the hyperglycemic activation of protein kinase C and formation of diacylglycerol in vascular smooth muscle cells, *Diabetes,* 54:818–829, 2005.

62. Sivenius K, Niskanen L, and Voutilainen-Kaunisto R et al., Aldose reductase gene polymorphisms and susceptibility to microvascular complications in type-2 diabetes, *Diabetic Med,* 21:1325–1333, 2004.

63. Bril V and Buchanan RA, Aldose reductase inhbition by AS-3201 in sural nerve from patients with diabetic sensorimotor polyneuropathy, *Diabetes Care,* 27:2369–2375, 2004.

64. Federici M, Menghini R, and Mauriello A et al., Insulin-dependent activation of endothelial nitric oxide synthase is impaired by O-linked glycosylation modification of signaling proteins in human coronary endothelial cells, *Circulation,* 23:466–472, 2002.

65. Pang H, Amano S, and Inagaki Y et al., N-acetylglucosamine-phosphate mutase genotype and diabetic microvascular complications, *Diabet Med,* 20:419–420, 2003.

66. Clark RJ, McDonough PM, and Swanson E et al., Diabetes and the acccompanying hyperglycemia impairs cardiomyocyte calcium cycling through increased nuclear O-GlcNAcylation, *J Biol Chem,* 278:44230–44237, 2003.

67. Scoggie DA, Albright A, and Harris MD, The effect of glucosamine-chondroitin supplementation on glycosylated hemoglobin levels in patients with type-2 diabetes mellitus: A placebo-controlled, double-blinded, randomized clinical trial, *Arch Int Med,* 163:1587–1590, 2003.

68. Vlassara H, Brownlee M, and Cerami A, Nonenzymatic glycosylation: Role in the pathogenesis of diabetic complications, *Clin Chem,* 32(Suppl 10):B37–41, 1986.

69. Zieman SJ and Kass DA, Advanced glycation endproduct crosslinking in the cardiovascular system: Potential therapeutic target for cardiovascular disease, *Drugs,* 64:459–470, 2004.

70. Ahmed N, Advanced glycation endproducts-role in pathology of diabetic complications, *Diabetes Res Clin Pract,* 67:3–21, 2005.

71. Vlassara H, Cai W, and Crandall J et al., Inflammatory mediators are induced by dietary glycotoxins, a major risk factor for diabetic angiopathy, *Proc Natl Acad Sci,* 99:15596–15601, 2002.

72. Nandhini AT, Thisunavukkarasu V, and Anuradha CV, Stimulation of glucose utilization and inhibition of protein glycation and AGE products by taurine, *Acta Physiol Scand,* 181:297–303, 2004.

73. Way KJ, Katai N, and King GL, Protein kinase C and the development of diabetic vascular complications, *Diabetic Med,* 18:945–959, 2001.

74. Shen GX, Selective protein kinase C inhibitors and their applications, *Curr Drug Targets Cardiovasc Haematol Disord,* 3:301–307, 2003.

75. Rong J, Qiu H, and Wang S, Advanced glycosylation end products, protein kinase C and renal alterations in diabetic rats, *Chin Med J,* 113:1087–1091, 2000.

76. Aronson D and Rayfield EJ, How hyperglycemia promotes atherosclerosis: Molecular mechanisms, *Cardiovasc Diabetol,* 1:1–10, 2002.

77. American Diabetes Association Consensus Statement, Role of cardiovascular risk factors in prevention and treatment of macrovascular disease in diabetes, *Diabetes Care,* 16:72–78, 1993.

78. Stamler J, Vaccaro O, and Neaton JD et al., Diabetes, other risk factors, and 12-yr cardiovascular mortality for men screened in the multiple risk factor intervention trial, *Diabetes Care,* 16:434–444, 1993.

79. Schwartz CJ, Valente AJ, and Sprague EA et al., Pathogenesis of the atherosclerotic lesion, Implications for diabetes mellitus, *Diabetes Care,* 15:1156–1167, 1992.

80. Caselli A, Rich J, and Hanane T et al., Role of C-nociceptive fibers in the nerve axon reflex-related vasodilatation in diabetes, *Neurol,* 60:297–300, 2003.

81. Veves A, Akbari C, and Primavera J et al., Endothelial dysfunction and the expression of endothelial nitric oxide synthase in diabetic neuropathy, vascular disease, and foot ulceration, *Diabetes,* 47:457–463, 1998.

82. Riddle MC, Rosenstock J, and Gerich J, Insulin Glargine 4002 Study Investigators, The treat-to-target trial: Randomized addition of glargine or human NPH insulin to oral therapy of type-2 diabetic patients, *Diabetes Care,* 26:3080–3086, 2003.

83. van den Berghe G, Wouters P, and Weekers F et al., Intensive insulin therapy in the critically ill patient, *N Engl J Med,* 345:1359–1367, 2001.

84. Clemente S, Braithwaite SS, and Magee MF et al., American Diabetes Association Diabetes in Hospitals Writing Committee, Management of diabetes and hyperglycemia in hospitals, *Diabetes Care,* 27:553–561, 2004, Erratum in: *Diabetes Care,* 27:856, 2004, Hirsh Irl B [corrected to Hirsch Irl B]; dosage error in text, *Diabetes Care,* 27:1255, 2004, May.

85. AACE, Position statement on inpatient diabetes and metabolic control, *Endocr Pract,* 10:77–82, 2004.

86. Weissberg-Benchell J, Antisdel-Lomaglio J, and Seshadri R, Insulin pump therapy: A meta-analysis, *Diabetes Care,* 26:1079–1087, 2003.

87. Bode BW, Tamborlane W, and Davidson PC, Insulin pump therapy in the 21st century, *Postgrad Med,* 111:69–77, 2002.

88. Zavalkoff S and Polychronakos C, Evaluation of conventional blood glucose monitoring as an indicator of glucose values using a continuous subcutaneous sensor, *Diabetes Care,* 25:1603–1606, 2002.

89. Larsen J, Ford T, and Lyden E et al., What is hypoglycemia in patients with well-controlled type-1 diabetes treated by subcutaneous insulin pump with use of the continuous glucose monitoring system? *Endocr Pract,* 10:324–329, 2004.

90. Yki-Jarvinem H, Thiazolidenediones, *N Engl J Med,* 351:1106–1118, 2004.

91. Willson TM, Lambert MH, and Kliewer SA, Peroxisome proliferator-activated receptor γ and metabolic disease, *Annu Rev Biochem,* 70:341–367, 2001.

92. Chinetti B, Fruchart JC, and Staels B, Peroxisome proliferator-activated receptors (PPARs): Nuclear receptors at the crossroads between lipid metabolism and inflammation, *Inflamm Res,* 49:497–505, 2000.

93. Blanquart C, Mansouri R, and Paumelle R et al., The protein kinase C signaling pathway regulates a molecular switch between transactivation and transrepression activity of the peroxisome proliferator-activated receptor α, *Mol Endocrinol,* 18:1906–1918, 2004.

94. Barbier O, Torra IP, and Duquay Y et al., Pleiotropic actions of peroxisome proliferator-activated receptors in lipid metabolism and atherosclerosis, *Arterioscler Thromb Vasc Biol,* 22:717–726, 2002.

95. Nolan JJ, Ludvik B, and Beerdsen P et al., Improvement in glucose tolerance and insulin resistance in obese subjects treated with troglitazone, *N Engl J Med,* 331:1188–1193, 1994.

96. Miyazaki Y, Glass L, and Triplitt C et al., Effect of rosiglitazone on glucose and nonesterified fatty acid metabolism in type-2 diabetic patients, *Diabetologia,* 44:2210–2209, 2001.

97. Lubber WH, Potential role of oral thiazoladinedione therapy in preserving β-cell function in type-2 diabetes mellitus, *Drugs,* 65:1–13, 2005.

98. Buchanan TA, Xiang AH, and Peters RK et al., Preservation of pancreatic β-cell function and prevention of type-2 diabetes by pharmacological treatment of insulin resistance in high-risk hispanic women, *Diabetes,* 51:2796–2803, 2002.

99. Saad MF, Greco S, and Osei K et al., for the Ragaglitazar Dose-ranging Study Group, Ragaglitazar improves glycemic control and lipid profile in type-2 diabetic subjects: A 12-week, double-blind, placebo-controlled, dose-ranging study with an open pioglitazone arm, *Diabetes Care,* 27:1324–1329, 2004.

100. Gribble FM and Reimann F, Differential selectivity of insulin secretagogues, Mechanisms, clinical implications, and drug interactions, *J Diabetes Compl,* 17:11–15, 2003.

101. Proks P, Reimann F, and Green N et al., Sulfonylurea stimulation of insulin secretion, *Diabetes,* 51:S368–S376, 2002.

102. Barg S, Mechanisms of exocytosis in insulin-secreting β-cells and glucagon-secreting A-cells, *Pharmacol Toxicol,* 92:3–13, 2003.

103. Dornhorst A, Insulinotropic meglitinide analogues, *Lancet,* 358:1709–1716, 2001.

104. Schmid-Antomarchi H, De Weille J, and Fosset M et al., The receptor for antidiabetic sulfonylureas controls the activity of the ATP-modulated K$^+$ channel in insulin-secreting cells, *J Biol Chem,* 262:15840–15844, 1987.

105. Chiasson JL, Josse RG, and Gomis R et al., STOP-NIDDM Trial Research Group, *Lancet,* 359:2072–2077, 2002.

106. Drucker DJ, Enhancing insulin action for the treatment of type-2 diabetes, *Diabetes Care,* 26:2929–2940, 2003.

107. Drucker DJ, Biological actions and therapeutic potential of the glucagon-like peptides, *Gastroenterol,* 122:531–544, 2002.

108. Ebinger M, Jehle D, and Fussgaenger R et al., Glucagon-like peptide-1 improves insulin and proinsulin binding on RINm5F cells and human monocytes, *Am J Physiol Endocrinol Metab,* 279:E88–E94, 2000.

109. Zander M, Christensen A, and Madsbad S et al., Additive effects of glucagon-like peptide 1 and pioglitazone in patients with type-2 diabetes, *Diabetes Care,* 27:1910–1914, 2004.

110. D'Alessio DA and Vahl TP, Glucagon-like peptide 1: Evolution of an incretin into a treatment for diabetes, *Am J Physiol Endocrinol Metab,* 286:E882–E890, 2004.

111. Green BD, Gault VA, and O'harte FP et al., Structurally modified analogues of glucagon-like peptide-1 (GLP-1) and glucose-dependent insulinotropic polypeptide (GIP) as future antidiabetic agents, *Curr Pharm Des,* 10:3651–3662, 2004.

112. The Diabetes Control and Complications Trial Research Group, The effect of intensive treatment of diabetes on the development and progression of long-term complications in insulin-dependent diabetes mellitus, *N Engl J Med,* 329:977–986, 1993.

113. Leiter LA, Diabetic dyslipidaemia: Effective management reduces cardiovascular risk, *Atheroscler Suppl,* 6:37–43, 2005.

114. Gruessner AC and Sutherland DE, Pancreas transplant outcomes for United States (U.S.) and non-U.S. cases as reported to the United Network for Organ Sharing (UNOS) and the International Pancreas Transplant Registry (IPTR) as of May 2003, *Clin Transplant,* 21–51, 2003.

115. Shapiro AM, Lakey JR, and Ryan EA et al., Islet transplantation in seven patients with type-1 diabetes mellitus using a glucocorticoid-free immunosuppressive regimen, *N Engl J Med,* 343:230–238, 2000.

116. Tian C, Bagley J, and Cretin N et al., Prevention of type-1 diabetes by gene therapy, *J Clin Immunol,* 114:969–978, 2004.

117. Creusot RJ and Fathman CG, Gene therapy for type-1 diabetes: A novel approach for targeted treatment of autoimmunity, *J Clin Invest,* 114:892–894, 2004.

118. Adams G, Vessillier S, and Dreja H et al., Targeting cytokines to inflammation sites, *Natural Biotechnol,* 21:1314–1320, 2003.

119. Renard E, Implantable closed-loop glucose-sensing and insulin delivery: The future for insulin pump therapy, *Curr Op Pharmacol,* 2:708–716, 2002.

3 Preventive Nutritional Strategies in Diabetic and Prediabetic Patients

Donald D. Hensrud

CONTENTS

INTRODUCTION

With the large and increasing number of people developing diabetes each year, strategies that can prevent the onset of diabetes are extremely important. Not only is nutritional management the cornerstone of treatment for diabetes, but there are nutritional factors that may prevent diabetes as well. Patients with established diabetes can benefit not only from nutritional treatment for their diabetes, but also employ nutritional strategies that will help promote health and prevent the complications of diabetes. This chapter will first briefly describe basic aspects of prevention in medicine using diabetes as an example. Following that, the specific nutritional factors that are associated with the development of type-1 diabetes (T1DM) and type-2 diabetes (T2DM) will be reviewed. Finally, an optimal nutritional pattern to help prevent diabetes and its complications as well as promote overall health will be discussed.

BASIC CONCEPTS OF PREVENTIVE MEDICINE

There are three main types of prevention in medicine [1]. Primary prevention is an action that does not allow a disease to develop. In the case of diabetes it would involve factors that would prevent or at least delay the onset. Because obesity is a major risk factor for T2DM, prevention of initial weight gain would be classified as primary prevention. Secondary prevention is detecting a disease in an early asymptomatic stage so effective treatment will delay symptoms. This includes screening, e.g., obtaining an fasting blood glucose (FBG) measurement with the intent of diagnosing and treating diabetes if the value is > 126 mg/dL. Secondary prevention would also include weight loss in subjects with obesity who are at high risk of developing diabetes, such as individuals with impaired glucose regulation. Lifestyle intervention trials, which will be discussed later, are examples of secondary prevention. Tertiary prevention is not allowing the complications of established disease to develop. By treating diabetes and obtaining tight blood glucose control, complications such as retinopathy can be prevented. In this manner, tertiary prevention overlaps with conventional treatment. Implementing dietary treatment to prevent cardiovascular complications in diabetic patients would also be considered tertiary prevention.

Preventive strategies are underutilized in clinical practice due to a variety of barriers on the part of patients, physicians, and health care systems. For example, a patient with obesity may have little motivation to prevent a condition such as diabetes that has not yet affected him. Physicians are primarily taught to function in a disease-treatment model and have little time for prevention. Furthermore, most physicians have an inadequate knowledge base in nutritional medicine. The healthcare system may not be appropriately set up to promote preventive practices and may not provide adequate reimbursement for health promotion counseling, including dietary counseling in diabetes. Despite these barriers, it is extremely important to incorporate prevention into a medical practice, as it can be effective in deterring disease and improving the quality of life [2]. Resources are available to help with the implementation of preventive measures, including nutritional strategies, in clinical practice [3,4].

NUTRITIONAL RISK FACTORS IN THE DEVELOPMENT OF TYPE-1 DIABETES

Cow's Milk Protein

The development of T1DM is an autoimmune mediated process whereby β-cell destruction occurs in genetically susceptible individuals. This process may be triggered by a limited number of dietary factors. There is evidence that exposure to cow's milk protein, particularly in the first few months of life, increases the risk of developing T1DM by approximately 50% or more [5]. However, not all data are consistent and a current study, the Trial to Reduce Insulin Dependent Diabetes in the Genetically at Risk (TRIGR), should help provide further data on this association [6].

Wheat Gluten

There is an increased prevalence of celiac disease in patients who have T1DM. This observation generated interest in wheat gluten as a trigger in subjects with a common human leukocyte antigens (HLA)-risk genotype for celiac disease and T1DM, possibly by immune or inflammatory mechanisms. Exposure to gluten or cereal before 3 months of age is associated with islet cell autoantibodies [7,8]. However, a gluten-free diet initiated at an early age does not appear to decrease islet cell autoantibodies in infants at high risk for T1DM [9]—although one small study reported temporary improvement in β-cell function [10].

Vitamin D

Studies in nonobese, diabetic mice showed that vitamin D supplementation led to a decreased risk of developing T1DM. In human studies, low vitamin D intake increased the risk of developing T1DM, and vitamin D or cod-liver oil supplementation in infancy has been associated with reduced risk of developing T1DM [11–13]. It is recommended that all infants have a minimum intake of 200 IU of vitamin D daily beginning in the first 2 months of life, mainly to prevent vitamin D deficiency and rickets [14]. It is not clear whether this is a large enough dose to decrease the risk of T1DM.

Vitamin E, Nitrites, and Nitrates

Low vitamin E intake has been linked to an increased risk of T1DM, although the data are not strong [15]. Greater consumption of nitrites and nitrates has also been associated with increased risk [16]. The adverse effect of nitrites and nitrates and the protective effect of vitamin E may be due to their opposing influences on free radicals, although much more work needs to be done to establish this.

Nicotinamide

It has been thought for quite some time that one form of niacin, nicotinamide, has the potential to prevent T1DM and many studies have been conducted using this agent. Recent randomized clinical trials among subjects at high risk have revealed negative results [17,18]. Thus, there appears to be little role for nicotinamide in the prevention of T1DM.

Summary of Nutritional Risk Factors and Type-1 Diabetes

While there is limited evidence supporting the relationship between the above-mentioned nutritional factors and T1DM, the potential for primary prevention on a population-wide basis is not clear at this point. Results from prospective studies are needed to further characterize these relationships. At this time, it is reasonable to follow established guidelines and restrict cow's milk from an infant's diet during the first year of life and also provide the recommended amount of vitamin D [19]. The evidence between nutritional factors and the development of T1DM has recently been reviewed in detail [20].

MAJOR RISK FACTORS FOR TYPE-2 DIABETES

A genetic predisposition, or in most cases the interaction between a genetic predisposition and certain environmental factors, increases the likelihood of developing T2DM. The most important acquired factor that affects the propensity to develop T2DM is increased body weight and, particularly, abdominal fat mass. Approximately 80% of people with T2DM are overweight or obese. Subjects who are obese are 3 to 7 times more likely to develop diabetes compared with those who are normal weight [21]. In people with a body mass index (BMI) >35 kg/M^2 the risk is 20 times greater [22]. It has been estimated that the risk of T2DM increases 5–9% for each kg of adult weight gain [23]. Increasing abdominal fat, as estimated by the waist measurement or the waist-to-hip ratio, may be an even stronger predisposing factor than BMI for the development of T2DM [24].

Physical activity is protective against developing T2DM, in part due to its effect on body weight, but the relationship is not as strong as with body weight per se [25]. Physical activity also has an independent effect on improving muscle insulin sensitivity. Nutritional factors can influence the risk of developing T2DM through obesity or other mechanisms. However, as in the case of physical activity, the effects of nutritional factors that are independent of body weight are far less than the influence of excess body weight.

NUTRITIONAL RISK FACTORS IN THE DEVELOPMENT OF TYPE-2 DIABETES

TOTAL CALORIE INTAKE

Body weight shows a strong relationship with T2DM. Chronic excess total calorie intake (relative to energy expenditure) that promotes weight gain is the most important overall dietary risk factor. This includes excess calories from all sources, independent of diet macronutrient composition (i.e., fat, carbohydrate, and protein). Thus, controlling total calorie intake—regardless of the source — to maintain normal body weight is the major nutritional strategy to prevent T2DM. While not all people who gain weight will develop diabetes, there are many other complications of obesity that, collectively, strongly support efforts to prevent primary weight gain in the entire population. Unfortunately, the trend over the past few decades has been progressive weight gain. Reversing this trend will require promotion of healthy diet and physical activity habits at all levels, from clinical encounters in the physician's office to public health recommendations and programs.

WEIGHT LOSS

Appropriate treatment of obesity should include three modalities: diet, physical activity, and behavior modification. For this reason, the independent effect of nutritional strategies on weight loss and the secondary prevention of T2DM is difficult and perhaps inappropriate to determine. In summarizing data from observational studies and clinical studies using a variety of different interventions including pharmacotherapy and surgery, modest weight loss improves insulin sensitivity and reduces the risk of T2DM. The response to weight loss may be less in subjects with a long duration of disease resulting in β-cell destruction. In the majority that respond, the improvement in insulin sensitivity is proportional to the degree of weight loss and benefits are seen only as long as weight loss is maintained. In general, among nondiabetics, about two thirds of weight loss is maintained at 1 year and the vast majority of people who lose weight regain it within 4–5 years [26]. Nevertheless, even in the situation where lost weight is eventually regained, the appearance of diabetes may be delayed for quite some time.

CLINICAL TRIALS OF LIFESTYLE INTERVENTION IN THE SECONDARY PREVENTION OF TYPE-2 DIABETES

The few lifestyle intervention trials that have been conducted have shown consistent results of modest weight loss and a reduction in the risk of T2DM. The Finnish Diabetes Prevention Study [27] randomized 522 subjects who were overweight and had impaired glucose tolerance (IGT) to lifestyle intervention or a control group. The goals of the lifestyle intervention group were 5% weight loss, 30 minutes of exercise daily, increased dietary fiber intake (>15 g/day), and decreased intake of fat (< 30% of calories) and saturated fat (<10% of calories). Individual counseling was provided. The trial was terminated early after just over 3 years of a planned 6 years when the intervention group experienced a 58% decreased risk of diabetes compared to the control group (6% vs. 14% absolute risk in the lifestyle and control groups, respectively). More subjects met the goal for physical activity than weight loss. At 3 years, mean weight loss was 3.5 kg in the lifestyle group compared to 0.9 kg in the control group.

The Diabetes Prevention Program [28] was a multicenter trial of 3234 subjects with a BMI > 24 kg/m^2, impaired fasting glucose, and IGT. Subjects were randomized to one of three groups: intensive lifestyle, metformin, or control. The latter two groups received standard lifestyle advice.

The intensive lifestyle group received individual and group sessions on diet (low-calorie, low-fat), exercise, and behavioral modification and had goals of 7% weight loss and 150 minutes of exercise per week. This trial was also terminated a year early after the intensive lifestyle group experienced a 58% decreased incidence of diabetes and the metformin group a 31% decreased incidence compared to the control group. As in the Finnish trial, more people met the exercise goal than the weight loss goal. Mean weight loss was 5.6 kg, 2.1 kg, and 0.1 kg in the lifestyle, metformin, and control groups, respectively, after almost 3 years.

Two previous studies found similar benefits of lifestyle intervention on reduction in diabetes risk [29,30]. Collectively, these studies provide solid evidence that lifestyle interventions including dietary change and exercise can prevent T2DM. How well these results can be translated into clinical practice is unclear, but it has been estimated that the implementation of intensive lifestyle efforts around the world would be cost-effective in most countries [31].

DIET COMPOSITION

DIETARY FAT

Some studies show a specific effect of diet composition on insulin sensitivity and the risk of developing T2DM [32]. In general, total dietary fat intake and particularly saturated fat intake have modest inverse correlations with insulin sensitivity [33]. Other dietary fats have been studied less, but available data seem to show that trans-fat has been associated with decreased insulin sensitivity and monounsaturated fats (MUFA) while polyunsaturated fats (PUFA) have been associated with increased insulin sensitivity [33,34]. Increased saturated and decreased PUFA intakes also have been associated with the risk of developing T2DM in some prospective studies [35,36].

DIETARY CARBOHYDRATE

When dietary carbohydrate is substituted isocalorically for dietary fat, there is a rise in glucose, insulin, and triglyceride levels, and a fall in high-density lipoprotein (HDL) levels in the short term [37]. Subjects with diabetes or metabolic syndrome may be particularly susceptible to these responses from dietary carbohydrate. It has been suggested that a high-carbohydrate diet leads to chronic overstimulation of β-cells leading to β-cell hypertrophy, β-cell destruction, and eventually T2DM [38]. The strongest confounding factor in this sequence is body weight. For example, in rural China in the early 1980s, carbohydrates provided on average 70–75% of calories, yet the prevalence of obesity and T2DM was quite low [39]. In this situation, it is possible that insulin sensitivity was maintained because of low body weight and regular lifestyle physical activity, while the effect of dietary carbohydrates on the development of T2DM was minor in comparison.

Similar to dietary fat, the type of carbohydrate can affect glucose and insulin levels. The risk of T2DM and the type of carbohydrate appears to be more important than the type of fat. A number of studies have reported an inverse association between dietary fiber intake and risk of T2DM [37]. Another study found that a high intake of refined carbohydrate, particularly corn syrup, and low intake of dietary fiber was associated with increased risk of T2DM [40]. In this ecologic study, these relationships were independent of total energy intake in multivariate analysis. Findings from these studies may be related, in part, to the glycemic index (GI) or other properties of foods containing these forms of carbohydrate.

The GI is the area under the glucose response curve after ingesting a standard amount of carbohydrate from a food relative to a standard amount of a reference food such as glucose. The glycemic load (GL) takes into account the amount of carbohydrate contained in a food. Observational studies have reported a positive correlation between the GI or GL of a diet and risk of T2DM [41–43]. An intervention trial in obese adolescents found that a low-GI diet led to greater weight loss than a conventional calorie-controlled diet [44]. Despite this, not all data are consistent and there are issues and challenges in applying a low-GI diet in the population [45]. It is possible the GI is correlated with confounding factors including micronutrients (such as magnesium) or other properties of foods (such as energy density) that lead to decreased body weight and maintenance of insulin sensitivity.

SPECIFIC FOODS

The risk of T2DM has been associated with the intake of specific foods or with individual nutrients contained in foods. Observational studies have found an inverse correlation between the intake of vegetables, fruits, and whole grains and the risk of T2DM [46–48]. Nuts and peanut butter have been associated with reduced risk and red meat with increased risk of T2DM [35,49]. An ecological study reported that fish and seafood consumption reduced the risk of T2DM in populations with a high prevalence of obesity [50]. Coffee intake has been protective in observational studies [51]. Several cross-sectional and prospective studies have shown that moderate consumption of alcohol, 1–2 drinks/day, is associated with reduced risk of T2DM compared with no consumption or heavy consumption [37].

MICRONUTRIENTS

Although the data are not all consistent, several observational studies have reported a protective effect of vitamin E on the risk of T2DM. One study showed that the intake of antioxidants, and vitamin E in particular, was associated with a reduced risk of developing diabetes among women [52]. A low magnesium intake has been associated with increased risk of developing T2DM [53,54], and there are other data consistent with this [55]. However, it is not clear if magnesium per se is responsible for this association or some other component in magnesium-containing foods [55].

OBSERVATIONAL STUDIES ON DIETARY PATTERNS AND TYPE-2 DIABETES

Schulze et al. [56] reviewed studies evaluating dietary patterns and the risk of T2DM. In general, dietary patterns with higher consumption of vegetables, fruits, whole grains, fish, and poultry were associated with a lower risk of T2DM. Diets high in cereal fiber and PUFA and low in trans-fat and GL were also associated with a lower risk. Increased consumption of red meat, processed meat, French fries, high-fat dairy products, refined grains, sweets, and desserts was associated with increased risk.

Many studies suggest an inverse relationship between birth weight and risk of T2DM later in life [57,58]. Large offspring born to mothers with gestational diabetes also have an increased risk [59]. Exclusive breastfeeding early in life has been protective against T2DM in some studies [60,61].

NUTRITIONAL STRATEGIES FOR TERTIARY PREVENTION IN DIABETES

Patients with T1DM or T2DM are at increased risk for coronary artery disease (CAD). In fact, patients with diabetes but no history of CAD are at a similar absolute risk for a coronary event as patients with established CAD [62]. Therefore, all coronary risk factors should be aggressively treated in patients with diabetes. Hypertension is a risk factor for CAD and often coexists with T2DM such as in the metabolic syndrome or with T1DM due to nephropathy. Dyslipidemia is also frequently present in patients with diabetes; the National Cholesterol Education Program goals for treatment of dyslipidemia are similar in patients with established CAD and patients with diabetes. Independent of the treatment of hyperglycemia, patients with diabetes should follow dietary recommendations that will also help prevent hypertension, improve lipids, and decrease the risk of CAD. Fortunately, consistency and overlap of many of these dietary recommendations exist (see Table 3.1).

TABLE 3.1
Diet and Lifestyle Recommendations for Hypertension and Dyslipidemia

---

Hypertension [68]

Dietary sodium restriction
Weight loss
Regular physical activity and exercise
Decreased intake of alcohol
DASH diet (8–10 servings of vegetables and fruits daily, low-fat dairy products, and modest decrease in meat
 consumption)

Dyslipidemia and Coronary Artery Disease [62]

Total fat 25–35%
Saturated fat < 7%
Trans-fat—minimal
Monounsaturated fat up to 20%
Polyunsaturated fat up to 10%
Cholesterol < 200 mg/day
Fiber 20–30 g/day
Total calories to maintain body weight
Fish twice per week
Plant stanol- or sterol-containing foods
Regular physical activity and exercise

OTHER GUIDELINES FOR DIABETES AND NUTRITION

The American Diabetes Association has issued nutrition recommendations for those with diabetes [63], a joint statement on lifestyle modification for diabetes prevention [64], and a joint statement on weight management through lifestyle modification for the prevention and management of T2DM [65].

Other major dietary guidelines for health promotion and disease prevention include the U.S. Dietary Guidelines and the American Cancer Society guidelines on nutrition and physical activity [66]. The United States Department of Agriculture's Dietary Guidelines Advisory Committee recently published "Nutrition and Your Health: Dietary Guidelines for Americans" [67]. These guidelines are generally consistent with the previously discussed dietary guidelines shown in Table 3.1.

SUMMARY

In summary, reducing total calorie intake, because of its effect on body weight, is the most important dietary intervention in the prevention of T2DM. Regarding the relative percentages of macronutrients in the diet, there is no clear evidence to recommend a high-carbohydrate/low-fat diet or a low-carbohydrate/high-fat diet for the prevention of T1DM or T2DM.

An optimal dietary pattern for health promotion in patients with diabetes would involve generous amounts of vegetables and fruits. There could be flexibility in the relative amounts of fat vs. carbohydrate, but the types of foods providing these macronutrients should be health-supporting. Carbohydrates should be provided by whole-grain foods (whole wheat bread, brown rice, and oatmeal) with little sugar and other refined carbohydrates. The intake of fiber, phytochemicals, and plant stanols/sterols would be naturally high from vegetables, fruits, and whole grains. Fat intake would consist largely of monounsaturated sources (nuts, olive oil, and canola oil) with some polyunsaturates (vegetable oils). Saturated fat, trans-fat, and dietary cholesterol would be minimized through a low intake of meat and processed products containing hydrogenated vegetable oil. Low-fat dairy products would be used in moderation. Plant sources of protein such as legumes would be emphasized over animal protein. Moderate amounts of fish would be included. Coffee and alcohol intake, if someone chooses to drink these beverages, would be moderate. Fast food and processed food would be minimized. Following a dietary pattern such as this would have a strong potential to prevent many chronic diseases, including T2DM.

REFERENCES

1. Hensrud DD, Clinical preventive medicine in primary care: Background and practice: 1. Rationale and current preventive practices, *Mayo Clin Proc,* 75:165–72, 2000.
2. Hensrud DD, Clinical preventive medicine in primary care: Background and practice: 2. Delivering primary preventive services, *Mayo Clin Proc,* 75:255–264, 2000.
3. Lang RS and Hensrud DD, Eds., *Clinical Preventive Medicine,* 2nd ed., Chicago, IL: *JAMA,* 2004.
4. Agency for Healthcare Research and Quality, Preventive Services, http://www.ahcpr.gov/clinic/prevenix.htm, Accessed October 15, 2004.
5. Verge CF, Howard NJ, and Irwig L et al., Environmental factors in childhood IDDM, A population-based, case-control study, *Diabetes Care,* 17:1381–1389, 1994.
6. Vendrame F and Gottlieb PA, Prediabetes: Prediction and prevention trials, *Endocrinol Metab Clin North Am,* 33:75–92, 2004.
7. Norris JM, Barriga K, and Klingensmith G et al., Timing of initial cereal exposure in infancy and risk of islet autoimmunity, *JAMA,* 290:1713–1720, 2003.
8. Ziegler AG, Schmid S, and Huber D et al., Early infant feeding and risk of developing type-1 diabetes-associated autoantibodies, *JAMA,* 290:1721–1728, 2003.
9. Hummel M, Bonifacio E, and Naserke HE et al., Elimination of dietary gluten does not reduce titers of type-1 diabetes-associated autoantibodies in high-risk subjects, *Diabetes Care,* 25:1111–1116, 2002.
10. Pastore MR, Bazzigaluppi E, and Belloni C et al., Six months of gluten-free diet do not influence autoantibody titers, but improve insulin secretion in subjects at high risk for type-1 diabetes, *J Clin Endocrinol Metab,* 88:162–165, 2003.
11. EURODIAB Substudy 2 Study Group, Vitamin D supplement in early childhood and risk for type-I (insulin-dependent) diabetes mellitus, *Diabetologia,* 42:51–54, 1999.
12. Hypponen E, Laara E, and Reunanen A et al., Intake of vitamin D and risk of type-1 diabetes: A birth-cohort study, *Lancet,* 358:1500–1503, 2001.
13. Stene LC and Joner G, Norwegian Childhood Diabetes Study Group, Use of cod liver oil during the first year of life is associated with lower risk of childhood-onset type-1 diabetes: A large, population-based, case-control study, *Am J Clin Nutr,* 78:1128–34, 2003.
14. Gartner LM and Greer FR, Section on Breastfeeding and Committee on Nutrition, American Academy of Pediatrics, Prevention of rickets and vitamin D deficiency: New guidelines for vitamin D intake, *Pediatrics,* 111:908–910, 2003.
15. Hypponen E, Micronutrients and the risk of type-1 diabetes: Vitamin D, vitamin E, and nicotinamide, *Nutr Rev,* 62:340–347, 2004.
16. Virtanen SM, Jaakkola L, and Rasanen L et al., Childhood Diabetes in Finland Study Group, Nitrate and nitrite intake and the risk for type-1 diabetes in Finnish children, *Diabetic Med,* 11:656–662, 1994.
17. Lampeter EF, Klinghammer A, and Scherbaum WA et al., DENIS Group, The Deutsche Nicotinamide Intervention Study: An attempt to prevent type-1 diabetes, *Diabetes,* 47:980–984, 1998.
18. Gale EA, Bingley PJ, and Emmett CL et al., European Nicotinamide Diabetes Intervention Trial (ENDIT) Group, European Nicotinamide Diabetes Intervention Trial (ENDIT): A randomised controlled trial of intervention before the onset of type-1 diabetes, *Lancet,* 363:925–931, 2004.
19. American Academy of Pediatrics, Work Group on Breastfeeding, Breastfeeding and the use of human milk, *Pediatrics,* 100:1035–1039, 1997.
20. Vaarala O, Environmental causes: Dietary causes, *Endocrinol Metab Clin North Am,* 33:17–26, 2004.
21. Mokdad AH, Ford ES, and Bowman BA et al., Prevalence of obesity, diabetes, and obesity-related health risk factors, 2001, *JAMA,* 289:76–79, 2003.
22. Field AE, Coakley EH, and Must A et al., Impact of overweight on the risk of developing common chronic diseases during a 10-year period, *Arch Intern Med,* 161:1581–1586, 2001.

23. Mokdad AH, Bowman BA, and Ford ES et al., The continuing epidemics of obesity and diabetes in the United States, *JAMA,* 286:1195–1200, 2001.
24. Maggio CA and Pi-Sunyer FX, Obesity and type-2 diabetes, *Endocrinol Metab Clin North Am,* 32:805–822, 2003.
25. van Dam RM, The epidemiology of lifestyle and risk for type-2 diabetes, *Europ J Epidemiol,* 18:1115–1125, 2003.
26. Wadden TA, Treatment of obesity by moderate and severe caloric restriction: Results of clinical research trials, *Ann Intern Med,* 119:688–693, 1993.
27. Lindstrom J, Louheranta A, and Mannelin M et al., Finnish Diabetes Prevention Study Group, The Finnish Diabetes Prevention Study (DPS): Lifestyle intervention and 3-year results on diet and physical activity, *Diabetes Care,* 26:3230–3236, 2003.
28. Knowler WC, Barrett-Connor E, and Fowler SE et al., Reduction in the incidence of type-2 diabetes with lifestyle intervention or metformin, *N Engl J Med,* 346:393–403, 2002.
29. Eriksson KF and Lindgarde F, Prevention of type-2 (non-insulin-dependent) diabetes mellitus by diet and physical exercise: The 6-year Malmo feasibility study, *Diabetologia,* 34:891–898, 1991.
30. Pan XR, Li GW, and Hu YH et al., Effects of diet and exercise in preventing NIDDM in people with impaired glucose tolerance: The Da Qing IGT and diabetes study, *Diabetes Care,* 20:537–544, 1997.
31. Palmer AJ, Roze S, and Valentine WJ et al., Intensive lifestyle changes or metformin in patients with impaired glucose tolerance: Modeling the long-term health economic implications of the diabetes prevention program in Australia, France, Germany, Switzerland, and the United Kingdom, *Clin Ther,* 26:304–321, 2004.
32. Parillo M and Riccardi G, Diet composition and the risk of type-2 diabetes: Epidemiological and clinical evidence, *Br J Nutr,* 92:7–19, 2004.
33. Hu FB, van Dam RM, and Liu S, Diet and risk of type II diabetes: The role of types of fat and carbohydrate, *Diabetologia,* 44:805–817, 2001.
34. Vessby B, Unsitupa M, and Hermansen K et al., KANWU Study, Substituting dietary saturated for monounsaturated fat impairs insulin sensitivity in healthy men and women: The KANWU study, *Diabetologia,* 44:312–319, 2001.
35. van Dam RM, Willett WC, and Rimm EB et al., Dietary fat and meat intake in relation to risk of type-2 diabetes in men, *Diabetes Care,* 25:417–424, 2002.
36. Harding AH, Day NE, and Khaw KT et al., Dietary fat and the risk of clinical type-2 diabetes: The European prospective investigation of Cancer–Norfolk study, *Am J Epidemiol,* 159:73–82, 2004.
37. Costacou T and Mayer-Davis EJ, Nutrition and prevention of type-2 diabetes, *Annu Rev Nutr,* 23:147–170, 2003.
38. Kopp W, High-insulinogenic nutrition—an etiologic factor for obesity and the metabolic syndrome? *Metabolism,* 52:840–844, 2003.
39. Chen J, Campbell TC, Li JY, and Peto R, *Diet, Life-style, and Mortality in China,* Oxford: Oxford University Press, 1990.
40. Gross LS, Li L, and Ford ES et al., Increased consumption of refined carbohydrates and the epidemic of type-2 diabetes in the United States: An ecologic assessment, *Am J Clin Nutr,* 79:774–779, 2004.
41. Salmeron J, Ascherio A, and Rimm EB et al., Dietary fiber, glycemic load, and risk of NIDDM in men, *Diabetes Care,* 20:545–550, 1997.
42. Salmeron J, Manson JE, and Stampfer MJ, Dietary fiber, glycemic load, and risk of non-insulin-dependent diabetes mellitus in women, *JAMA,* 277:472–477, 1997.
43. Schulze MB, Liu S, and Rimm EB et al., Glycemic index, glycemic load, and dietary fiber intake and incidence of type-2 diabetes in younger and middle-aged women, *Am J Clin Nutr,* 80:348–356, 2004.
44. Ebbeling CB, Leidig MM, and Sinclair KB et al., A reduced-glycemic load diet in the treatment of adolescent obesity, *Arch Pediatr Adolesc Med,* 157:773–779, 2003.
45. Pi-Sunyer FX, Glycemic index and disease, *Am J Clin Nutr,* 76:290S–298S, 2002.
46. Williams DE, Wareham NJ, and Cox BD et al., Frequent salad consumption is associated with a reduction in the risk of diabetes mellitus, *J Clin Epidemiol,* 52:329–335, 1999.
47. Ford ES and Mokdad AH, Fruit and vegetable consumption and diabetes mellitus incidence among U.S. adults, *Prev Med,* 32:33–39, 2001.
48. Murtaugh MA, Jacobs DR, Jr, and Jacob B et al., Epidemiological support for the protection of whole grains against diabetes, *Proceed Nutr Soc,* 62:143–149, 2003.

49. Jiang R, Manson JE, and Stampfer MJ et al., Nut and peanut butter consumption and risk of type-2 diabetes in women, *JAMA,* 288:2554–2560, 2002.

50. Nkondjock A and Receveur O, Fish-seafood consumption, obesity, and risk of type-2 diabetes: An ecological study, *Diabetes Metab,* 29:635–642, 2003.

51. Salazar-Martinez E, Willett WC, and Ascherio A et al., Coffee consumption and risk for type-2 diabetes mellitus, *Ann Intern Med,* 140:1–8, 2004.

52. Montonen J, Knekt P, and Jarvinen R et al., Dietary antioxidant intake and risk of type-2 diabetes, *Diabetes Care,* 27:362–366, 2004.

53. Lopez-Ridaura R, Willett WC, and Rimm EB et al., Magnesium intake and risk of type-2 diabetes in men and women, *Diabetes Care,* 27:134–140, 2003.

54. Song Y, Manson ME, and Buring JE et al., Dietary magnesium intake in relation to plasma insulin levels and risk of type-2 diabetes in women, *Diabetes Care,* 27:59–65, 2003.

55. Nadler JL, A new dietary approach to reduce the risk of type-2 diabetes? *Diabetes Care,* 27:270–271, 2004.

56. Schulze MB and Hu FB, Dietary patterns and risk of hypertension, type-2 diabetes mellitus, and coronary heart disease, *Curr Atheroscler Rep,* 4:462–467, 2002.

57. Lieberman LS, Dietary, evolutionary, and modernizing influences on the prevalence of type-2 diabetes, *Annu Rev Nutr,* 23:345–377, 2003.

58. Eriksson JG, Forsen TJ, and Osmond C et al., Pathways of infant and childhood growth that lead to type-2 diabetes, *Diabetes Care,* 26:3006–3010, 2003.

59. McCance DR, Pettitt KJ, and Hanson RL et al., Birth weight and non-insulin dependent diabetes: Thrifty genotype, thrifty phenotype, or surviving small baby genotype? *BMJ,* 308:942–945, 1994.

60. Pettitt DJ, Forman MR, Hanson RL, Knowler WC, and Bennett PH, Breastfeeding and incidence of non-insulin-dependent diabetes mellitus in Pima Indians, *Lancet,* 350:166–168, 1997.

61. Young TK, Martens PJ, and Taback SP, et al., Type-2 diabetes mellitus in children: Prenatal and early infancy risk factors among native Canadians, *Arch Pediatric Adolesc Med,* 156:651–655, 2002.

62. Executive Summary of the Third Report of the National Cholesterol Education Program (NCEP) Expert Panel on Detection, Evaluation, and Treatment of High Blood Cholesterol in Adults (Adult Treatment Panel III), *JAMA,* 285:2486–2497, 2001.

63. Franz MJ, Bantle JP, and Beebe CA et al., American Diabetes Association, Nutrition principles and recommendations in diabetes, *Diabetes Care,* 27(Suppl 1):S36–46, 2004.

64. Sherwin RS, Anderson RM, and Buse JB et al., American Diabetes Association, National Institute of Diabetes and Digestive and Kidney Diseases, Prevention or delay of type-2 diabetes, *Diabetes Care,* 27(Suppl 1):S47–54, 2004.

65. Klein S, Sheard NF, and Pi-Sunyer X et al., American Diabetes Association, North American Association for the Study of Obesity, American Society for Clinical Nutrition, Weight management through lifestyle modification for the prevention and management of type-2 diabetes: Rationale and strategies, A statement of the American Diabetes Association, the North American Association for the Study of Obesity, and the American Society for Clinical Nutrition, *Am J Clin Nutr,* 80:257–263, 2004.

66. Byers T, Nestle M, and McTiernan A et al., American Cancer Society 2001 Nutrition and Physical Activity Guidelines Advisory Committee, American Cancer Society guidelines on nutrition and physical activity for cancer prevention: Reducing the risk of cancer with healthy food choices and physical activity, *CA Cancer J Clin,* 52:92–119, 2002.

67. U.S. Dietary Guidelines Advisory Committee Report, http://www.health.gov/dietaryguidelines/dga2005/report/, Accessed January 25, 2005.

68. Chobanian AV, Bakris GL, and Black HR et al., Joint National Committee on Prevention, Detection, Evaluation, and Treatment of High Blood Pressure, National Heart, Lung, and Blood Institute, National High Blood Pressure Education Program Coordinating Committee, Seventh Report of the Joint National Committee on Prevention, Detection, Evaluation, and Treatment of High Blood Pressure, *Hypertension,* 42:1206–1252, 2003.

4 Nutritional Strategies for Patients with Obesity and the Metabolic Syndrome

Robert F. Kushner and Julie L. Roth

CONTENTS

The rising prevalence of obesity among children and adults is one of the most significant threats to our nation's health in the twenty-first century. According to the Surgeon General's Call to Action [1], obesity resulting from an unhealthy diet and physical inactivity is a major cause of preventable death which now accounts for approximately 400,000 deaths per year [2]. Among a multitude of disorders associated with obesity is the rising prevalence of type-2 diabetes mellitus (T2DM) and other cardiovascular risk factors. Although the correlation between obesity and cardiovascular risk has been known for decades, recent clinical observation and basic research studies have helped to further explain this association. Emerging from this research is the central role of abdominal adipose tissue and the adipocyte.

DEFINING THE METABOLIC SYNDROME

Although it has been nearly 50 years since the original observation was made that an android (trunk or abdominal) body fat distribution was associated with more metabolic abnormalities than a gynoid (hips, buttock, or thigh) body fat distribution [3], this association has only recently emerged as a major cardiovascular risk factor. In 1988, Reaven proposed the name "Syndrome X" to describe the clustering of hypertension, hyperglycemia, glucose intolerance, elevated triglycerides, and low HDL cholesterol with insulin resistance [4]. Since then, this constellation of abnormalities has been given many names including the "Deadly Quartet," the "Insulin Resistance Syndrome," the "Dysmetabolic Syndrome," and the "Metabolic Syndrome." Although the specific pathogenic mechanisms that link the various metabolic derangements are still being defined, insulin resistance with compensatory hyperinsulinemia appears to play a central role. The primary outcome of the metabolic syndrome is an increased risk for T2DM [5] and cardiovascular disease (CVD) [6].

In 1999 the World Health Organization (WHO) provided a working definition for the metabolic syndrome that included insulin resistance as a required component [7]. Although this view is scientifically sound, a potential disadvantage of this criterion is the need for special testing of a 2-hour postprandial glucose or measurement of insulin resistance by the glucose clamp technique or homeostasis-model assessed (HOMA) calculation. The National Cholesterol Education Program's Adult Treatment Panel III report (ATP III), released in 2002, identified the metabolic syndrome as a multiplex risk factor for CVD [8]. In contrast to the WHO criteria, explicit demonstration of insulin resistance is not required for diagnosis. Instead, measurement of impaired fasting glucose and other metabolic abnormalities are used as surrogate indicators. The ATP III panel specifically chose criteria that could be more routinely obtained in clinical practice. A third set of clinical criteria for the metabolic syndrome is proposed by the American College of Endocrinology (ACE) Task Force on the Insulin Resistance Syndrome [9]. The ACE definition relies on identifying patients who present with risk factors for insulin resistance, e.g., family history of T2DM, polycystic ovary syndrome, sedentary lifestyle, and two or more specific abnormalities. Unlike the WHO and ATP III definitions, overweight, obesity, and abdominal obesity are considered risk factors rather than diagnostic features. A comparison of criteria used for defining the metabolic syndrome for the three organizations is shown in Table 4.1. The International Diabetes Federation has also provided a definition of the metabolic syndrome that incorporates many of the components listed in Table 4.1 [10]. The primary controversy regarding the current criteria used to define the metabolic syndrome is that all components are weighted equally for risk of CVD, the presumed uniformity of risk across ethnic groups, and the use of "cut points" for some of variables that are continuous, such as waist circumference.

Although the components and cutoff values selected to define the metabolic syndrome are useful for clinical practice, the constellation of abnormalities associated with insulin resistance are much broader. As shown in Table 4.2, these include increased biomarkers of chronic inflammation (C-reactive protein [CRP], tumor necrosis factor-α [TNF-α], and interleukin-6 [IL-6]), a prothrombotic state (increased plasma plasminogen activator inhibitor-1 [PAI-1], and fibrinogen), endothelial dysfunction (decreased endothelium-dependent vasodilatation), hemodynamic changes (increased sympathetic nervous activity and renal sodium retention), hyperuricemia, and nonalcoholic fatty liver disease (NAFLD) [9–14]. When viewed in this context, it is clear that the metabolic syndrome is more than the sum of its parts and may explain the diversity of conditions associated with abdominal obesity. This concept has been recently challenged by the American Diabetes Association and European Association for the Study of Diabetes and is currently the subject of debate [15].

THE SCOPE OF THE PROBLEM

The prevalence of the metabolic syndrome as defined by ATP III using data from the Third National Health and Nutrition Examination Survey (NHANES III, 1988–1994) was 23.7% [16]. The prev-

TABLE 4.1
Comparison Criteria for the Diagnosis of the Metabolic Syndrome

Risk Factor	ATP-III Defining Level (three or more of)	WHO-Defining Level (#3 and/or insulin resistance plus any two of the remaining)[a]	ACE-Defining Level (an individual with risk factors plus 2 or more of)[b]
1. Overweight/ obesity	Waist circumference > 102 cm (> 40 in) for men and > 88 cm (> 35 in) for women	BMI >30 kg/M^2 and/or waist-to-hip ratio of > 0.9 for men and > 0.8 for women	BMI >25 kg/M^2, or > 102 cm (> 40 in) for men and > 88 cm (> 35 in) for women
2. Blood pressure	>130/85 mm Hg	>140/90 mm Hg	>130/85 mm Hg
3. Glucose	Fasting >110 mg/dL	Fasting between 110–125 mg/dL, 2-hour plasma glucose 140–199 mg/dL, or diabetes (fasting glucose >126 mg/dL and/or 2-hour plasma glucose >200 mg/dL	Fasting between 110–126 mg/dL, 2-hour postglucose challenge > 140 mg/dL
4. Triglycerides	>150 mg/dL	>150 mg/dL	>150 mg/dL
5. HDL cholesterol	< 40 mg/dL for men, < 50 mg/dL for women	< 35 mg/dL for men, < 39 mg/dL for women	< 40 mg/dL for men, < 50 mg/dL for women
6. Microalbuminuria	Not used in diagnosis	Urinary albumin excretion rate >20 mg/minute or albumin/creatinine ratio >30 mg/g	Not used in diagnosis

[a] World Health Organization (WHO) criteria: insulin resistance = insulin clamp-assessed glucose uptake below the 25th percentile, or homeostasis-model assessed (HOMA; fasting insulin/fasting glucose $\times$ 22.5) insulin resistance above the 75th percentile, as measured among subjects with no metabolic abnormalities [7].

[b] American College of Endocrinology (ACE) criteria: risk factors = diagnosis of CVD, hypertension, polycystic ovarian syndrome (PCOS), non-alcoholic fatty liver disease (NAFLD), or acanthosis nigricans; family history of T2DM, hypertension, or CVD; history of gestational diabetes or glucose intolerance; non-caucasian ethnicity; sedentary lifestyle; body mass index (BMI) > 25.0 kg/M^2 (or waist circumference > 40 inches in men, > 35 inches in women; age > 40 years [9]. Although displayed in the table, ACE considers overweight, obesity, and abdominal obesity a risk factor rather than a diagnostic criteria for the metabolic syndrome. ACE uses the term insulin resistance syndrome instead of metabolic syndrome.

alence increased from 6.7% among people aged 20 through 29 years to ≥ 42.0% for those aged 60 years or greater. The condition was highest among Mexican Americans (31.9%) followed by whites (23.8%) and African-Americans (21.6%). Using 2000 census data, about 47 million U.S. residents have the metabolic syndrome. For the entire population, the prevalence of having ≥ 3, ≥ 4 or 5 metabolic abnormalities was 23.7%, 10.4% and 2.7%, respectively. Perhaps not surprisingly, the metabolic syndrome was present in 4.6%, 22.4%, and 59.6% of normal-weight, overweight, and obese men, respectively, and a similar distribution was observed in women [17]. In individuals over 50 years old, there is a stepwise increase in prevalence of metabolic syndrome with worsening glucose tolerance from 26% in those with normal fasting glucose rising to 86% in those with diabetes [18]. In contrast, diabetes without metabolic syndrome was uncommon, occurring in only 13% of participants. These observations highlight the need to screen for components of the metabolic syndrome in overweight and diabetic individuals.

Although ATP III and WHO use different criteria to define the metabolic syndrome, they identify similar people at risk. In comparison to ATP III, 25.1% of NHANES III participants were identified as having the metabolic syndrome using WHO criteria and over 85% were similarly classified under the two definitions [19]. The largest difference occurred among African-American

TABLE 4.2
Abnormalities Associated with the Metabolic Syndrome

The Core Cluster	
Central Obesity	
Dyslipidemia	Hypertriglyceridemia
	Low HDL cholesterol
	Small, dense LDL cholesterol
	Postprandial lipemia
Glucose intolerance	Impaired fasting glucose
	Impaired glucose tolerance
	T2DM
Insulin resistance	
Hypertension	
Other Associated Features	
Microalbuminuria	
Hyperuricemia and gout	
Impaired fibrinolysis and increased coagulability	Elevated PAI-1
	Elevated fibrinogen
Increased inflammatory markers	Elevated CRP
	Elevated TNF-α
	Elevated IL-6
Increased sympathetic activity	
Endothelial dysfunction	Impaired endothelium-dependent vasodilatation
Fatty liver disease	
Polycystic ovary syndrome	
Obstructive sleep apnea	

Abbreviations: HDL—high-density lipoprotein; LDL—low-density lipoprotein; PAI-1—plasminogen activator inhibitor-1; CRP—C-reactive protein; TNF-α—tumor-necrosis factor-α; IL-6—interleukin-6

Source: Adapted from References [12,13].

men, of whom 16.5% had the metabolic syndrome using ATP III criteria and 24.9% using WHO criteria. Prevalence figures for the metabolic syndrome in four ethnic communities in Canada ranged from 41.6% among Native Indians, 25.9% among South Asians, 22.0% among Europeans, to 11.0% among Chinese [20].

PATHOPHYSIOLOGY

Two factors appear to be intricately linked in the pathogenesis of the metabolic syndrome: insulin resistance and obesity. Multiple research studies have investigated the relationship between these two variables over the past decade. Key studies have demonstrated a positive curvilinear relationship between body mass index (BMI) and insulin resistance, which begins to plateau at more severe levels of obesity [21]. A 5-year follow up from the Insulin Resistance Atherosclerosis Study (IRAS) suggests that obesity, particularly abdominal obesity, precedes the development of other components of the metabolic syndrome [22]. In fact, the relationship between deteriorating glucose disposal and body fat is directly correlated with visceral adipose tissue [23,24]. Visceral adipose tissue refers to adipose tissue located within the abdominal cavity below abdominal muscles and comprised of omental and mesenteric adipose tissue, as well as adipose tissue of the retroperitoneal and peri-nephric regions. In addition to overall mass and distribution of fat, the size of adipocytes is a predictor of insulin resistance [25]. Visceral fat accumulation has also been shown to have a significant negative impact on glycemic control in patients with T2DM through decreased insulin sensitivity and an enhancement of gluconeogenesis [26].

Although the visceral fat depots represent approximately 20% and 6% of total body fat in men and women, respectively [27,28], the biological properties of this regional adipose tissue provide the basis for the multiple disturbances seen in the metabolic syndrome. Compared with adipose cells obtained from the gluteal and hip regions, visceral fat cells display more active lipolysis, have higher rates of catecholamine-induced lipolysis, express more $\beta1$ and $\beta2$ adrenergic receptors and glucocorticoid receptors, and have increased lipoprotein lipase responsiveness to glucocorticoids [29]. Since visceral fat drains into the portal venous system, free fatty acids and other secreted products act directly on the liver to stimulate hepatic triglyceride secretion [30]. In addition to the visceral compartment, other ectopic fat depots are important in determining insulin resistance. Obesity is accompanied by high-plasma nonesterified fatty acids that cause insulin resistance in skeletal muscle and overload the liver with lipid. A number of studies have found a correlation between the triglyceride content of skeletal muscle and hepatic tissue (hepatic steatosis) and the severity of insulin resistance [31]. Unger et al. [32–34] proposed that insulin resistance and the metabolic syndrome occur as a result of lipotoxicity due to the surplus of fat in the visceral depot and these other ectopic tissues.

Recent studies have linked the metabolic and inflammatory abnormalities seen in abdominal obesity to the secretion of adipocyte and adipose-connective tissue products, or adipokines. Secreted factors include leptin, IL-6, TNF-α, angiotensinogen, PAI-1, transforming growth factor-β (TGF-β), and adiponectin, among many others [35]. Secretion of these products results in endocrine, paracrine, and autocrine functions. For example, IL-6 leads to hypertriglyceridemia by stimulating lipolysis and hepatic triglyceride secretion, and TNF-α directly decreases insulin sensitivity and increases lipolysis in adipocytes. Adiposity is negatively correlated with production of adiponectin, a hormone that decreases gluconeogenesis and increases lipid oxidation in muscle. Hepatic production of CRP, stimulated by increased cytokine production, reflects the inflammatory response [36,37] and correlates with increased CVD risk [5,6]. Several research groups have identified macrophage accumulation in adipose tissue as the source of TNF-α expression [38–40]. Sonnenberg et al. [41] recently proposed that TNF-α-stimulated activation of nuclear transcription factor-κB (NF-κB) augments production of cytokines and oxidative stress, whereas adiponectin inhibits activation of NF-κB and thereby promotes a more protective metabolic profile. Although the mechanism is still unraveling whereby obesity increases insulin resistance and worsens components of the metabolic syndrome, identification and treatment of the high-risk obese patient is a practical matter.

OBESITY

Over the past three decades, the prevalence of obesity has increased sharply. Such increases cut across all ages, racial and ethnic groups, and both genders [42]. The combined prevalence of overweight and obesity (BMI > 25.0) for persons 20 years of age or older is about 67% for men and 57% for women. While overweight and obesity are common in both sexes and all age groups, differences in prevalence exist in many segments of the population—particularly among blacks and Mexican Americans. For example, 50% of adult African-American women and 40% of Hispanic women are obese compared with 30% of white women, and Mexican-American men have a higher prevalence of overweight and obesity (75%) than non-Hispanic white men (67%) and non-Hispanic black men (61%). Concurrent increases in overweight and obesity in the United States also are occurring in pediatric and adolescent populations. Today, there are nearly twice as many overweight children and almost three times as many overweight adolescents as there were in 1980 [43]. Using the 95th percentile as the cut point, 15% of children and adolescence are considered obese. Because obesity is the primary risk factor for the metabolic syndrome, increasing prevalence rates for this comorbid condition can be expected over the coming decade.

IDENTIFICATION AND EVALUATION OF THE OBESE PATIENT

According to the National Heart, Lung, and Blood Institute (NHLBI) [44], North American Association for the Study of Obesity (NAASO) [45], and American Medical Association (AMA) [46] guidelines, assessment of risk status due to overweight or obesity is based on the patient's BMI, waist circumference, and the presence of comorbid conditions. BMI is calculated as [weight (kg)/height $(M)^2$], or as [weight (lb)/height $(inches)^2 \times 703$]. A BMI table is more conveniently used for simple reference (see Table 4.3). A desirable or healthy BMI is 18.5–24.9 kg/M^2, over-weightkg/M^2), class II (35.0–39.9 kg/M^2), and class III ($\geq$40 kg/M^2) (see Table 4.4). Patients at very high absolute risk of death include those with a high BMI and the following: (1) established coronary heart disease; (2) presence of other atherosclerotic diseases such as peripheral arterial disease, abdominal aortic aneurysm, or symptomatic carotid artery disease; (3) T2DM; and/or (4) sleep apnea. The presence of the metabolic syndrome and insulin resistance should prompt urgent treatment due to increased cardiovascular risk [48,49]. Other symptoms and diseases that are directly or indirectly related to obesity are listed in Table 4.5.

BMI may not accurately predict increased risk in people who are highly muscular. Therefore, abdominal obesity may also be used as one of the criteria to define the metabolic syndrome. Measurement of waist circumference should be obtained in those individuals with a BMI $\leq$ 35 kg/M^2. Abdominal fat is clinically defined as a waist circumference $\geq$ 102 cm ($\geq$ 40 inches) in men and $\geq$ 88 cm ($\geq$ 35 inches) in women. Waist circumference is measured by first locating the upper hip bone and the top of the right iliac crest and then placing a measuring tape in a horizontal plane around the abdomen at the level of the iliac crest, ensuring that the tape is snug and parallel to the floor but not compressing the skin [45]. Then, the measurement is made at the end of a normal expiration [45]. Because visceral adipose tissue is often measured with a single computed tomography or magnetic resonance imaging slice at the L4–L5 level and because the iliac crest is closer to L4–L5 than other locations recommended for the waist circumference, measurement above the iliac crest is appropriate as a surrogate marker for visceral adipose tissue [50]. An increased waist circumference has been found to be predictive of the risk of having hypertension, diabetes, dyslipidemia, and the metabolic syndrome, compared to those with normal waist circumference among men and women in the healthy, overweight, and class I obese categories [51]. Waist circumference is also more closely linked to cardiovascular disease risk factors than is BMI [52,53]. In the Insulin Resistance Atherosclerosis Study, waist circumference was the single best predictor of incident metabolic syndrome in both men and women [22]. Several authors have suggested adding measurement of fasting serum triglyceride to the waist circumference as a convenient and practical means to identify the high-risk patient [54–56]. An increased waist circumference accompanied by hypertriglyceridemia predicts an increased risk of having traditional coronary heart disease biomarkers (low HDL cholesterol, elevated LDL cholesterol, fasting glucose, and blood pressure) and non-traditional coronary heart disease biomarkers (hyperinsulinemia, increased apolipoprotein B, and small LDL particles). In contrast, McLaughlin et al. [57] suggest that the most practical approach to identify overweight patients who are insulin resistant is to use either a triglyceride cut point of 130 mg/dL or a triglyceride-HDL concentration ratio of 3:1.

TREATMENT OF OBESITY

The primary goal of obesity treatment is to improve obesity-related comorbid conditions and reduce the risk of developing future comorbidities. The decision of how aggressively to treat the patient and which modalities to use is determined by the patient's risk status, level of motivation, and the availability of various resources. Therapy for obesity always begins with lifestyle management and may include pharmacotherapy or surgery. Setting an initial weight loss goal of about 10% over 6 months is reasonable and clinically significant. Lifestyle management incorporates the three essential components of obesity care: dietary therapy, physical activity, and behavior therapy. The NHLBI

TABLE 4.3
Body Mass Index (BMI) Table

BMI	19	20	21	22	23	24	25	26	27	28	29	30	31	32	33	34	35
Height (inches)							Body Weight (pounds)										
58	91	96	100	105	110	115	119	124	129	134	138	143	148	153	158	162	167
59	94	99	104	109	114	119	124	128	133	138	143	148	153	158	163	168	173
60	97	102	107	112	118	123	128	133	138	143	148	153	158	163	168	174	179
61	100	106	111	116	122	127	132	137	143	148	153	158	164	169	174	180	185
62	104	109	115	120	126	131	136	142	147	153	158	164	169	175	180	186	191
63	107	113	118	124	130	135	141	146	152	158	163	169	175	180	186	191	197
64	110	116	122	128	134	140	145	151	157	163	169	174	180	186	192	197	204
65	114	120	126	132	138	144	150	156	162	168	174	180	186	192	198	204	210
66	118	124	130	136	142	148	155	161	167	173	179	186	192	198	204	210	216
67	121	127	134	140	146	153	159	166	172	178	185	191	198	204	211	217	223
68	125	131	138	144	151	158	164	171	177	184	190	197	203	210	216	223	230
69	128	135	142	149	155	162	169	176	182	189	196	203	209	216	223	230	236
70	132	139	146	153	160	167	174	181	188	195	202	209	216	222	229	236	243
71	136	143	150	157	165	172	179	186	193	200	208	215	222	229	236	243	250
72	140	147	154	162	169	177	184	191	199	206	213	221	228	235	242	250	258
73	144	151	159	166	174	182	189	197	204	212	219	227	235	242	250	257	265
74	148	155	163	171	179	186	194	202	210	218	225	233	241	249	256	264	272
75	152	160	168	176	184	192	200	208	216	224	232	240	248	256	264	272	279
76	156	164	172	180	189	197	205	213	221	230	238	246	254	263	271	279	287

BMI	36	37	38	39	40	41	42	43	44	45	46	47	48	49	50	51	52	53	54
58	172	177	181	186	191	196	201	205	210	215	220	224	229	234	239	244	248	253	258
59	178	183	188	193	198	203	208	212	217	222	227	232	237	242	247	252	257	262	267
60	184	189	194	199	204	209	215	220	225	230	235	240	245	250	255	261	266	271	276
61	190	195	201	206	211	217	222	227	232	238	243	248	254	259	264	269	275	280	285
62	196	202	207	213	218	224	229	235	240	246	251	256	262	267	273	278	284	289	295
63	203	208	214	220	225	231	237	242	248	254	259	265	270	278	282	287	293	299	304
64	209	215	221	227	232	238	244	250	256	262	267	273	279	285	291	296	302	308	314
65	216	222	228	234	240	246	252	258	264	270	276	282	288	294	300	306	312	318	324
66	223	229	235	241	247	253	260	266	272	278	284	291	297	303	309	315	322	328	334
67	230	236	242	249	255	261	268	274	280	287	293	299	306	312	319	325	331	338	344
68	236	243	249	256	262	269	276	282	289	295	302	308	315	322	328	335	341	348	354
69	243	250	257	263	270	277	284	291	297	304	311	318	324	331	338	345	351	358	365
70	250	257	264	271	278	285	292	299	306	313	320	327	334	341	348	355	362	369	376
71	257	265	272	279	286	293	301	308	315	322	329	338	343	351	358	365	372	379	386
72	265	272	279	287	294	302	309	316	324	331	338	346	353	361	368	375	383	390	397
73	272	280	288	295	302	310	318	325	333	340	348	355	363	371	378	386	393	401	408
74	280	287	295	303	311	319	326	334	342	350	358	365	373	381	389	396	404	412	420
75	287	295	303	311	319	327	335	343	351	359	367	375	383	391	399	407	415	423	431
76	295	304	312	320	328	336	344	353	361	369	377	385	394	402	410	418	426	435	443

Guidelines [44] recommend initiating treatment with a low-calorie Step 1 diet producing a calorie deficit of 500–1000 kcal/day. In general, this translates into prescribing diets containing 1000–1200 kcal/day for most women and between 1200 kcal/day and 1600 kcal/day for men. However, in practice there is little value in calculating the patient's current dietary caloric intake since dietary records and the recall method are typically inaccurate and underestimate actual intake [58]. Rather, the focus should be on where and how the patient will reduce daily calories. Because portion control is one of the most difficult strategies for patients to manage, patients should be taught to read food labels and measure food servings. The use of food models and visual aids can teach patients to estimate appropriate portion sizes. The use of pre-prepared products, called meal replacements, is another strategy that eliminates the need for patients to make food choices. Meal replacements are foods that are designed to take the place of a meal while at the same time providing nutrients and good taste within a known caloric limit [59]. Examples include frozen entrees, canned beverages, and bars. In a meta-analysis of six studies with a study duration ranging from 3–51 months, use of partial meal replacements resulted in a 7–8% weight loss [60].

Although exercise alone is only moderately effective for weight loss, the combination of dietary modification and exercise is the most effective behavioral approach for treatment of obesity. Additionally, physical activity is beneficial for improved cardiorespiratory fitness, cardiovascular

TABLE 4.4
Classification of Weight Status and Risk of Disease

		Risk of Disease (relative to having a healthy weight and waist size)	
		Waist circumference:[a] 35″ or less (women) 40″ or less (men)	Waist circumference:[a] More than 35″ (women) More than 40″ (men)
Underweight	BMI below 18.5		
Healthy weight	BMI 18.5–24.9		
Overweight	BMI 25.0–29.9	Increased	High
Obesity Class I	BMI 30.0–34.9	High	Very high
Obesity Class II	BMI 35.0–39.9	Very high	Very high
Obesity Class III	BMI 40 or more	Extremely high	Extremely high

[a] Note: If patient is 18 years or older, use the BMI and waist circumference to estimate weight status and relative risk for diabetes, high blood pressure, or heart disease. An increased waist circumference may indicate increased disease risk even at a normal weight.

Source: Adapted from Reference [44].

disease, cancer risk reduction, and improved mood and self-esteem. Currently, the public health recommendation for physical activity is a minimum of 30 minutes of moderate intensity physical activity on most, preferably all, days of the week [61]. A useful first step in counseling is to focus on simple ways to add physical activity into the normal daily routine, such as walking, using the stairs, doing home and yard work, and increasing recreational activity. Studies have demonstrated that lifestyle activities are as effective as structured exercise programs in improving cardiorespiratory fitness [62] and weight loss [63]. The most important role of exercise appears to be the maintenance of weight loss at a level higher than generally recommended for public health [64]. The American College of Sports Medicine (ACSM) recommends that overweight and obese individuals progressively increase to a minimum of 150 minutes of moderate intensity physical activity per week as a first goal [65]. However, for long-term weight loss, higher amounts of exercise (e.g., 200–300 minutes/week or ≥ 2000 kcal/week) are needed [65]. The ACSM also recommends a resistance exercise program in addition to an endurance exercise program [65]. Many patients would benefit from consultation with an exercise physiologist or personal trainer.

Adjuvant pharmacological treatments should be considered for patients with a BMI > 30 kg/M^2 or with a BMI > 27 kg/M^2 who also have concomitant obesity-related risk factors or diseases and for whom dietary and physical activity therapy have not been successful. Patients meeting criteria of the metabolic syndrome should be considered for pharmacotherapy on an individual basis. There are currently only two medications approved by the FDA for both weight loss and maintenance of weight loss supported by at least 2-year clinical outcome data. Sibutramine functions both as a serotonin and norepinephrine re-uptake inhibitor (SNRI). It produces a dose-dependent weight loss over a range of 5–20 mg daily, with an average loss of about 8–10% of initial body weight at 6 months [66]. Several studies have demonstrated the effect of sibutramine in improving glycemic control in patients with T2DM [67–70] and improvement in cardiovascular risk factors [71–73]. The most commonly reported adverse effects of sibutramine are headache, dry mouth, insomnia, and constipation. These are generally mild and well-tolerated. The principal concern is a dose-related increase in blood pressure and heart rate that may require discontinuation of the medication. A dose of 10–15 mg causes an average increase in systolic and diastolic blood pressure of 2–4 mm Hg and an increase in heart rate of 4–6 beats/minute. For this reason, all patients should be monitored closely and re-evaluated within one month after initiating therapy. Contraindications to sibutramine use include uncontrolled hypertension, congestive heart failure, symptomatic coronary heart disease, arrhythmias, or history of stroke. Caution is needed when using sibutramine in

TABLE 4.5
Obesity-Related Organ Systems Review

Cardiovascular	Respiratory
Hypertension	Dyspnea
Congestive heart failure	Obstructive sleep apnea
Cor pulmonale	Hypoventilation syndrome
Varicose veins	Pickwickian syndrome
Pulmonary embolism	Asthma
Coronary artery disease	
Endocrine	**Gastrointestinal**
Metabolic syndrome	Gastroesophageal reflux disease (GERD)
T2DM	Non-alcoholic fatty liver disease (NAFLD)
Dyslipidemia	Cholelithiasis
Polycystic ovarian syndrome (PCOS)	Hernias
Hyperandrogenism	Colon cancer
Infertility/menstrual disorders	
Musculoskeletal	**Genitourinary**
Hyperuricemia and gout	Urinary stress incontinence
Immobility	Obesity-related glomerulopathy
Osteoarthritis (knees and hips)	Hypogonadism (male)
Low back pain	Breast and uterine cancer
	Pregnancy complications
Psychological	**Neurologic**
Depression/low self esteem	Stroke
Body image disturbance	Idiopathic intracranial hypertension
Social stigmatization	Meralgia paresthetica
Integument	**Integument**
Striae distensae (stretch marks)	Cellulitis
Stasis pigmentation of legs	Intertrigo, carbuncles
Lymphedema	Acanthosis nigricans/skin tags

Source: From Reference [47] with permission.

conjunction with selective serotonin re-uptake inhibitors (SSRI). Similar to other anti-obesity medications, weight reduction is enhanced when the drug is used along with behavioral therapy and body weight increases once the medication is discontinued [74].

Orlistat is a synthetic hydrogenated derivative of a naturally occurring lipase inhibitor, lipostatin, produced by the mold Streptomyces toxytricini. Orlistat is a potent, slowly reversible inhibitor of intestinal lipases that are required for the hydrolysis of dietary fat in the gastrointestinal tract into fatty acids and monoacylglycerols. The drug's activity takes place in the lumen of the stomach and small intestine by forming a covalent bond with the active serine residue site of these lipases. A therapeutic oral dose of 120 mg TID blocks the digestion and absorption of about 30% of dietary fat. On a diet containing 30% fat, this effect typically results in a caloric deficit of approximately 200 kcal daily. When orlistat therapy is discontinued, fecal fat usually returns to normal concentrations within 48–72 hours [75]. Multiple randomized, 1- to 2-year double-blind placebo-controlled studies have shown that after 1 year, orlistat produces a weight loss of about 9–10% compared with a 4–6% weight loss in the placebo-treated groups [76,77]. Orlistat has been demonstrated to improve diabetic control and insulin sensitivity [78–80], reduce cardiovascular risk factors [81,82], and reduce the incidence of T2DM [83,84]. Since orlistat is minimally (< 1%) absorbed from the gastrointestinal tract, it has no systemic side effects. Tolerability to the drug is related to the malabsorption of dietary fat and subsequent passage of fat in the feces. Six gastrointestinal tract adverse effects have been reported to occur in at least 10% of orlistat-treated patients: oily spotting, flatus with discharge, fecal urgency, fatty/oily stool, oily evacuation, and increased defecation. The events are generally experienced early, diminish as patients control their dietary fat intake, and infrequently cause patients to withdraw from clinical trials. In fact, avoidance behavior (decreasing dietary fat to diminish orlistat-induced steatorrhea) contributes to weight loss. It has recently been shown that psyllium mucilloid is helpful in controlling the orlistat-induced glycemic index (GI) side effects when taken concomitantly with the medication [85]. Serum concentrations of the fat-soluble vitamins D and E and β–carotene have been found to be significantly lower in some of the trials, although they generally remain within normal ranges. The manufacturer's package insert for orlistat recommends that patients using orlistat take a vitamin supplement at bedtime to prevent potential deficiencies.

Metformin and the thiazolidinediones (TZD) are not approved for treatment of the metabolic syndrome. Studies utilizing metformin have demonstrated improved insulin sensitivity in individuals with impaired glucose tolerance [86] and decreased food consumption with associated weight loss [87]. A hypocaloric, carbohydrate-modified (low glycemic index) diet combined with metformin led to long-term (2–4 years) weight reduction in addition to improved fasting insulin levels [88].

Surgical intervention is an option for carefully selected patients with a BMI > 35 kg/M^2 and the metabolic syndrome. For these patients, the benefits of an invasive intervention should outweigh the risks. Although there are no defined criteria for a specified length of time or description of what constitutes an eligible 'less invasive' treatment, many consider this to be formal participation in a medically supervised diet and exercise program for 6 months or longer. Several bariatric procedures are available that either alter the amount of food a patient can eat (restrictive operations) or the amount of calories and nutrients absorbed (malabsorptive operations). Mean weight loss following the restrictive Roux-en-Y gastric bypass procedure (RGB) is approximately 35% of the pre-operative weight and is reached between 12 and 18 months postoperatively. Weight loss following the mal-absorptive procedures is reported to be greater than gastric restrictive procedures, but with a greater incidence of metabolic complications. Multiple studies have demonstrated complete resolution or improvement of obesity-related comorbid conditions following surgery, notably, T2DM, obstructive sleep apnea, obesity hypoventilation, gastroesophageal reflux disease (GERD), and peripheral edema [89,90]. Although there is an immediate reduction in the prevalence of hypertension, these benefits may diminish after 8 years of followup [91].

Often, medications for T2DM and CVD may be reduced or eliminated entirely following bariatric surgical procedures. As far back as 1984, gastric bariatric procedures were associated with post-operative improvements in mean hemoglobin A1C (A1C) levels (11.8% preoperative to 7.9% post-operative), fasting BG, and glucose tolerance [92]. In insulin-resistant obese patients undergoing biliopancreatic diversion (BPD) procedures, ideal body weight is re-established with normalized glucose tolerance [93]. This physiologic adaptation may result from reduced muscle gene expression of TNF-α, pyruvate dehydrogenase kinase isoform 4 (PDK4), uncoupling proteins 2 and 3 (UCP2, UCP3), and increased glucose transporter 4 (GLUT4) [94–96]. In addition, sterol regulatory element-binding protein 1c (SREBP1c) gene expression declines and there is decreased intramyocytic lipid accumulation [97]. Many of these events, as well as increased insulin receptor number, are mediated by the reduction of adiponectin with calorie restriction [98]. Furthermore, after Roux-en-Y gastric bypass or BPD surgery to induce weight loss, enteroinsular axis (GIP, GLP-1) defects are restored, leading to resolution of T2DM [99]. Each of these events may act in concert to reduce inflammation, endothelial dysfunction, and overall cardiovascular risk after bariatric surgery [100].

WEIGHT LOSS AND DIETARY APPROACHES TO THE METABOLIC SYNDROME

As discussed above, the metabolic syndrome is a constellation of several cardiovascular risk factors. Although prescription of a diet that meets the major tenets of several US organizations is reasonable

TABLE 4.6
Recommendations for Addressing Components of the Metabolic Syndrome

Component	Dietary Guidelines	Lifestyle Modification	Practical Advice	Evidence Level
Abdominal obesity	Clinical Guidelines on the Identification, Evaluation, and Treatment of Overweight and Obesity in Adults [44]	Weight loss	Decrease calories by 500 calories/day (1 lb/week weight loss); aim for a 5–10% reduction over 6 months	4
		Increase daily physical activity	30 minutes of moderate activity 5 out of 7 days/week	
Elevated blood pressure	Dietary Approaches to Stop Hypertension (DASH) Diet [137–139]	Weight loss	Aim for 5–10% reduction over 6 months	1
		Modest salt restriction	No salt shaker at the table; no added salt when cooking	
		Increase number of servings of fruits and vegetables	Get at least 5 servings/day of fruits and vegetables	
		Incorporate low-fat dairy products	Two servings/day skim milk or low-fat yogurt or cheese	
Suppressed HDL cholesterol level	Therapeutic Lifestyle Changes (TLC) Diet [109]	Get help to stop smoking	—	1
		Weight loss	Aim for 5–10% weight reduction over 6 months	
		Increase physical activity	Exercise 30 minutes 5 out of 7 days/week	
		Replace carbohydrates in diet with modest amounts of monounsaturated fats	Use small amounts of unsalted almonds, walnuts, and peanuts to replace cookies, candy, cake as snacks	
Elevated fasting triglyceride level	Therapeutic Lifestyle Changes (TLC) Diet [109]	Weight loss	Aim for 5–10% weight reduction over 6 months	1
		Reduce intake of simple carbohydrates	Reduce amount of soft drinks and juices; switch to seltzer, water, or diet sodas	
		Limit alcohol intake	Limit to one alcoholic beverage/day with a meal	
		Increase omega-3 fatty acids in diet	Eat fresh or canned fish at least 2 times/week	
Impaired fasting glucose level	Diabetes Prevention Program Diet [124]	Weight loss	Aim for 5–10% weight reduction over 6 months	1
		Increase soluble fiber intake	Eat more whole wheat grains and cereals; switch from white to brown grains	

Source: Adapted from Szapary PO, Hark LA, and Burke FM, The metabolic syndrome: A new focus for lifestyle modification, *Patient Care,* 75–88, 2002.

(e.g., consumption of a variety of foods, decreased intake of fat, saturated fat, and cholesterol, increased consumption of fruits, vegetables, and whole grains, and maintenance of a healthy body weight) [101], specific treatment recommendations will vary depending on which components are present. While the NHLBI Guidelines [44] recommend a Step 1 diet that is composed of 55% carbohydrate, ≤ 30% fat, and 15% protein, it primarily targets patients with hypercholesterolemia and may not be appropriate for patients with the metabolic syndrome. Table 4.6 highlights the specific dietary guidelines and lifestyle modifications needed to target individual components of the metabolic syndrome.

When the BMI is greater than 25 kg/M^2, calorie restriction along with increased physical activity should be prescribed. Intervention studies have repeatedly shown that a weight loss of 5–10% is clinically significant and leads to improvements in glycemic [102], lipemic [103], and hypertensive control [44]. Greater than 10% weight loss is associated with improvements in insulin resistance and in markers of vascular inflammation (decrease in serum concentrations of IL-6, IL-18, and CRP with an increase in adiponectin levels) [104]. Glycemic control is improved within 24 hours of calorie restriction before any weight loss occurs [105], whereas dyslipidemia requires moderate weight loss for improvement [106]. Observational studies have shown lower fasting insulin concentrations in association with decreased body weight and waist-to-hip ratio in individuals reporting higher dietary fiber intake (> 10.5 g/1000 kcal/day intake) [107]. Some studies evaluating the effect of fiber-rich carbohydrates on insulin sensitivity have demonstrated beneficial results [108,109], while others have been inconclusive [110]. At least one study comparing an *ad libitum* low-fat, high-carbohydrate diet (63% carbohydrates/26 g fiber per 1000 kcal) vs. a control diet (45% carbohydrates/7 g fiber per 1000 kcal) found a greater decrease in body weight and a higher percentage of body fat loss in the high-carbohydrate diet [111]. The addition of aerobic exercise training to the high-carbohydrate diet did not change the results. A current area of intense controversy is the use of low-carbohydrate diets for weight loss. Although the public and media tend to lump all of the low-carbohydrate popular diets into one category, they actually represent a continuum of carbohydrate percentage levels and differ slightly in theory. Figure 4.1 displays the currently used popular diets for treatment of obesity ranked by carbohydrate percentage. The Unified Diet [101] consisting of 55% carbohydrate, 30% fat, and 15% protein is a reasonable anchor to separate higher-carbohydrate diets (Ornish) from lower-carbohydrate diets (Atkins Diet®, South Beach Diet®, Zone Diet®, and Sugar Busters!™). As seen, all of the lower-carbohydrate diets except Atkins recommend a carbohydrate level of approximately 40–46%. In contrast, the Atkins diet contains 5–15% carbohydrate depending on the phase of the diet. Whereas Atkins believes that all carbohydrates are the primary cause of obesity and insulin resistance, the other lower carbohydrate diets place a greater emphasis on choosing low-glycemic index foods to reduce dietary insulin response.

Until recently, the theories and arguments of popular lower-carbohydrate diet books have relied on poorly controlled, non-peer-reviewed studies and anecdotes [112]. Over the past year, four randomized, controlled trials have demonstrated greater weight loss at 6 months with improvement in coronary heart disease risk factors, including an increase in HDL cholesterol and a decrease in triglyceride levels [113–117]. However, weight loss between groups did not remain statistically significant at one year [113]. The one study that enrolled patients with diabetes and the metabolic syndrome showed relative improvements in glycemic control, insulin sensitivity and dyslipidemia in those subjects randomized to the lower carbohydrate diet [116,117].

Because lower carbohydrate diets are just now being scrutinized with greater scientific vigor, it is premature to make definitive conclusions regarding their role in the treatment of obesity and/or metabolic syndrome. However, conclusions from two recent reviews are pertinent. The Executive Summary of a United States Drug Administration (USDA) conference on popular diets concluded that diets reducing calorie intake result in weight loss regardless of macronutrient composition (Evidence Level I) [118]. A systemic review by Bravata et al. [119] concluded that there is insufficient evidence to make recommendations for or against the use of low-carbohydrate diets and that participant weight loss was principally associated with decreased calorie intake and increased diet duration, but not with reduced carbohydrate content.

Physical activity appears to have an additional impact on the metabolic syndrome independent of weight loss. An increased clustering of metabolic syndrome parameters and higher cardiovascular and all-cause mortality occur with decreased cardiovascular fitness [6,120]. In contrast, there is a decreased incidence of "high-risk" parameters with increased cardiovascular fitness [121,122]. The Harvard Nurses' studies [123,124] reported a 30% reduction in the incidences of T2DM and

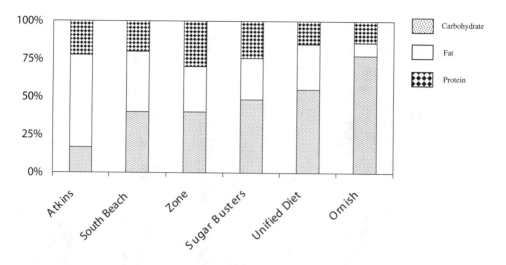

FIGURE 4.1 Comparison of popular diet books for treatment of obesity ranked by percent macronutrients.

coronary heart disease (CHD) by engaging in brisk walking for at least 3 hours/week. The Physicians' Health Study [125] showed a significantly decreased risk of developing T2DM with exercise greater than once per week. Ross et al. [126] found that weight loss induced by daily physical activity without calorie restriction is more effective than calorie reduction-induced weight loss in decreasing truncal obesity and insulin resistance in men.

Pharmacotherapy such as orlistat has been shown to be effective not only for weight loss but also for improving lipid profiles, fasting insulin, and glucose levels [127,128]. Metformin has also been shown to improve the components of the metabolic syndrome, but it is not currently approved in the clinical treatment of the disorder [129–131].

THE DYSLIPIDEMIA COMPONENT

PREVALENCE

The prevalence of the two dyslipidemic components of the metabolic syndrome, low HDL cholesterol, and hypertriglyceridemia vary by gender and race [17] and are shown in Figure 4.2. According to NHANES III, the prevalence of a low HDL cholesterol is 35.2% and 39.3% in men and women, respectively, with the highest levels among Mexican-Americans (39.6%). The prevalence of hypertriglyceridemia is 35.1% and 24.7% in men and women, respectively, with the lowest levels among African-Americans (17.7%) and highest among Mexican-Americans (37.7%).

PATHOPHYSIOLOGY

As previously stated, abdominal obesity is not only a component of the metabolic syndrome but also linked to the pathogenesis of the metabolic syndrome. Although still under speculation, the dyslipidemia component of the metabolic syndrome is thought to be due to insulin resistance driving an increased flow of free fatty acids from adipose tissue to the liver [132]. This increased availability of free fatty acids leads to triglyceride formation and increased hepatic secretion of triglyceride-rich lipoproteins—leading secondarily to low HDL cholesterol levels. Although patients with the metabolic syndrome usually have normal LDL cholesterol levels, their LDL particles are often small, dense, and oxidized, leading to a higher atherogenic potential.

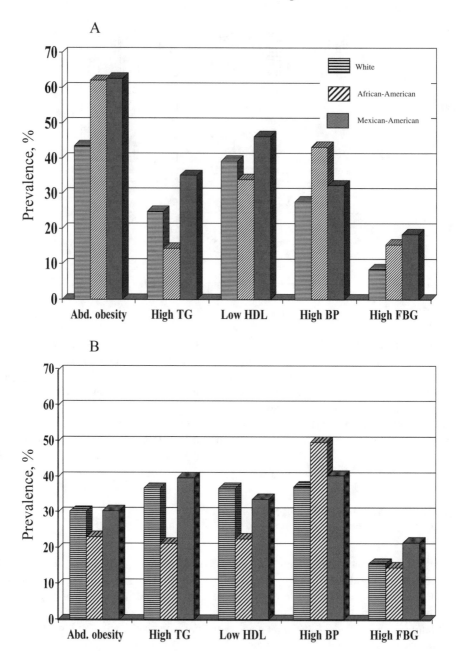

FIGURE 4.2 Metabolic syndrome criteria in women (A) and men (B). Data from the Third National Health and Nutrition Examination Survey (NHANES III) [16].

LIFESTYLE MANAGEMENT

The Third Report of the Expert Panel on Detection, Evaluation, and Treatment of High Blood Cholesterol [133] is the most current clinical guideline for blood lipid testing and management recommended by the National Cholesterol Education Program (NCEP). The fundamental approaches of therapy in ATP III are similar to the previous ATP II guidelines. ATP III continues

TABLE 4.7
Nutrient Composition of the Therapeutic Lifestyle Changes (TLC) Diet

Nutrient	Recommended Intake
Saturated fat[a]	<7% of total calories
Polyunsaturated fat	Up to 10% of total calories
Monounsaturated fat	Up to 20% of total calories
Total fat	25–35% of total calories
Carbohydrate[b]	50–60% of total calories
Fiber	20–30 g/day
Protein	Approximately 15% of total calories
Cholesterol	< 200 mg/day
Total calories[c]	Balance energy intake and expenditure to maintain desirable body weight/prevent weight gain

[a] Trans-fatty acids are another LDL-raising fat that should be kept at low intake.

[b] Carbohydrates should be derived predominantly from foods rich in complex carbohydrates including grains (especially whole grains), fruits, and vegetables.

[c] Daily energy expenditure should indicate at least moderate physical activity (contributing approximately 200 kcal/day).

Source: Adapted from Expert Panel on Detection, Evaluation, and treatment of high blood cholesterol in adults, Third report of the National Cholesterol Education Program, *JAMA*, 285:2486–2497, 2001 [125].

to identify risks for CHD by focusing on low-density lipoprotein-cholesterol (LDL cholesterol) of <100 mg/dL as a primary treatment target for all patients with CHD or its equivalent, T2DM. However, ATP III guidelines change the definition of low HDL cholesterol levels to < 40 mg/dL from < 35 mg/dL and mandate more stringent goals for triglycerides to < 150 mg/dL. More importantly, ATP III shifts the focus from dietary "steps" to "therapeutic lifestyle changes" (TLC), reinforcing both dietary intake and physical activity as essential components of weight control. The nutrient composition of the TLC diet is listed in Table 4.7. Another change of ATP III is a focus on high-risk populations, with multiple risk factors (metabolic syndrome), who are candidates for intensified therapeutic lifestyle changes. ATP III identifies metabolic syndrome as a secondary target for risk-reduction therapy after achieving the primary target of optimal LDL cholesterol. Since first-line therapy for metabolic syndrome is weight control, early referral to a registered dietitian for medical nutrition therapy is strongly encouraged.

ATP III identifies lifestyle intervention as the preferred approach to long-term prevention and treatment of CHD risk factors, primarily LDL cholesterol and the metabolic syndrome. When treating low HDL cholesterol levels accompanied by hypertriglyceridemia, total fat intake should consist of 25–35% of total calories. Unsaturated fats, such as olive oil, canola oil, nuts, and seeds, should be included in the diet—as opposed to saturated fats such as fried and fatty foods and commercially baked goods—to decrease the risk of CHD [134,135]. It is important to note that these foods can be calorically dense and restriction must still be applied for control of body weight. A high carbohydrate (53%)/high-fiber diet (54 g), compared with a low carbohydrate (42%)/low-fiber (20 g) or high-carbohydrate (53%)/low-fiber (16 g) diet, improves LDL cholesterol levels and glycemic control in type-1 diabetes mellitus (T1DM) and T2DM [136].

A major concern of the TLC diet in treating patients with the metabolic syndrome is that the 50–60% carbohydrate content of the diet may be too high for patients with hypertriglyceridemia [137,138]. The Institute of Medicine (IOM) Report, published in 2002 [139], recommends a broader range of macronutrient levels that may be more suitable for targeted treatment. Specifically, the

IOM Report recommends that adults should consume 45–65% of their total calories from carbohydrates, 20–35% of total calories from fat, and 10–35% of total calories from protein.

The final component of lifestyle interventions aimed at raising low HDL cholesterol and lowering triglyceride levels is physical activity. Lipid improvements are seen when diet therapy is combined with structured physical activity (working toward a goal of 45 minutes of activity three times per week in fitness classes) or combined with lifestyle activity (moderate-intensity physical activity for 30 minutes per day on most days of the week) [63]. The latter recommendation is important as many patients mention lack of membership or ability for membership to a health club as a reason for not increasing physical activity.

If patients require medication to achieve their LDL cholesterol goal, the 3-hydroxyl-3-methyl-glutaryl coenzyme A (HMG-CoA) reductase inhibitors ("statins") are recommended as first-line therapy. However, patients with the metabolic syndrome will be unlikely to achieve HDL cholesterol and triglyceride goals with statin therapy alone. Consideration should then be given to adding a second lipid-lowering drug such as nicotinic acid or fibric acid, with close attention to the risk for myopathy. Beneficial effects are seen in patients with dyslipidemia treated with rosuvastatin [140], fibrates [141,142], and sibutramine (as a result of weight loss) [72,143].

THE IMPAIRED FASTING GLUCOSE COMPONENT

PREVALENCE

The prevalence of impaired fasting glucose (IFG) from the NHANES III sample is the lowest of the five components of the metabolic syndrome (see Figure 4.2). The overall prevalence is 12.6%, higher among men (15.6%) than women (10.0%). IFG is highest among Mexican-Americans (overall [20.0%], in men [21.4%] and women [18.5%]) [16]. 25–50% of hypertensive patients demonstrate insulin resistance and hyperinsulinemia [144,145].

PATHOPHYSIOLOGY

Abdominal obesity is considered a causative factor in the pathogenesis of insulin resistance. Free fatty acids produced by the adipocyte promote gluconeogenesis by the liver, impair glucose utilization by the skeletal muscle, and may impair β-cell function directly. Each component plays an important role in the development of insulin resistance.

Early in insulin resistance, glucose tolerance remains normal due to pancreatic β-cell compensation, which increases insulin output. Over time, the β-cells are unable to sustain the hyperinsulinemic state and postprandial hyperglycemia ensues. A further decline in insulin output, in addition to an increase in hepatic gluconeogenesis, leads to impaired fasting hyperglycemia. Islet cell function is impaired by both chronic hyperglycemia (glucose toxicity) and by elevations of free fatty acid levels (lipotoxicity) [146,147].

LIFESTYLE MANAGEMENT

Lifestyle interventions have proven useful in preventing the development of T2DM in at-risk individuals and lowering the blood glucose in patients with T2DM. The primary lifestyle interventions for an overweight or obese individual with insulin resistance are weight loss by calorie restriction and increased physical activity. Physical activity—either structured or through increased activities of daily living of 30 minutes duration on most days of the week—should be recommended to all patients.

The Diabetes Prevention Program [148] evaluated the prevention of T2DM in 3,234 nondiabetic, overweight, insulin-resistant individuals. This study compared metformin with both placebo and lifestyle intervention. The lifestyle intervention, achieving at least 7% weight loss by calorie restriction, modification of dietary fat to < 25%, and at least 150 minutes of physical activity per

TABLE 4.8
Composition of the Diabetes Prevention Program (DPP) Diet

Component	Recommended Goal
Body weight	7% loss of body weight with maintenance
Total fat	< 25% of total calories
Total calories	1200–1800 kcal/day
Physical activity	> 150 minutes/week physical activity

Source: Diabetes Prevention Program Research Group, Reduction in the incidence of T2DM with lifestyle intervention or metformin, *N Engl J Med,* 346:393–403, 2002 [140].

week, resulted in a 58% decrease in the development of T2DM. The lifestyle intervention plan is summarized in Table 4.8. Although less successful than lifestyle intervention, metformin decreased the incidence of T2DM by 31%. In individuals older than 60 years, metformin had less effect but diet and exercise had a clinical outcome similar to the other age groups. The Finnish Diabetes Prevention Study [149], which evaluated the effect of reducing total and saturated fat and increasing fiber intake and physical activity in subjects with impaired glucose tolerance, showed similar decreases in the development of T2DM. Subjects in this study also demonstrated significant weight loss, decreased triglyceride levels, increased HDL cholesterol levels, and decreased blood pressure.

In a previously-mentioned study of obese subjects of which 43% had the metabolic syndrome and 39% had T2DM, a low-carbohydrate diet (< 30 g/day) was compared to a calorie restricted and low-fat diet (500 calories/day deficit, < 30% total calories from fat) [116,117]. The low-carbohydrate diet led to greater weight loss, greater decreases in triglyceride levels, and improved insulin sensitivity. Improvements in obesity and insulin resistance have also been shown with weight loss induced by physical activity without calorie restriction [102].

In obese subjects, orlistat has been shown to decrease the rate of progression to impaired glucose tolerance and T2DM [81,83] and to improve insulin sensitivity [81] and lipid profiles, including LDL cholesterol levels [128,150]. At 8 years, surgically induced weight loss significantly decreases the incidence of T2DM with no effect on the incidence of hypertension [91].

PCOS is characterized by hyperandrogenism and is often associated with features of the metabolic syndrome. Approximately 50% of women with PCOS are overweight or obese [151] and 20–49% demonstrate impaired glucose tolerance [152]. Hypocaloric diets alone and in combination with medication have shown an HDL cholesterol level increase of 6% and triglyceride level improvements to within ATP III guidelines in 34% of women with PCOS [129,153]. Clinical and biochemical improvements are seen in PCOS subjects with the addition of the insulin-sensitizing agents metformin [129,130,153] and troglitazone [154].

THE HYPERTENSIVE COMPONENT

PREVALENCE

The prevalence of high blood pressure or medication use for blood pressure control in the U.S. population is 34%, as shown in Figure 4.2. Prevalence levels for men and women are 38.2% and 29.3%, respectively, with the highest values seen among African-American men (49.6%) and women (43.3%) and Mexican-American men (40.2%) [16].

PATHOPHYSIOLOGY

The exact mechanism by which insulin resistance leads to elevated blood pressure is unclear. Proposed mechanisms include impaired endothelial function with impaired vasodilation as the result of dyslipidemia; increased renal sodium reabsorption, leading to increased plasma volume; and

TABLE 4.9
Nutrient Composition of the DASH Diet

Nutrient	Recommended Intake
Grains & Grain Products	7–8 servings/day
Vegetables	4–5 servings/day
Fruits	4–5 servings/day
Low-fat/Fat-free Dairy	2–3 servings/day
Meats, Poultry, Fish	≤ 2 servings/day
Nuts, Seeds, Dry Beans	4–5 servings/week
Fats and Oils	2–3 servings/day
Sweets	5 servings/week
Sodium	1500 mg/day

Source: Adapted from DASH (Dietary Approaches to Stop Hypertension-Sodium) eating plan, http: //www.nhlbi.nih.gov/hbp/prevent/h_eating/h_eating.htm. Accessed March 30, 2004 [152].

increased sympathetic nervous system activation due to hyperinsulinemia, leading to renal vaso-constriction with increased sodium retention [155]. It has also been theorized that the normal vasodilatory effect of insulin may be blocked with insulin resistance. Another theory involves hyperinsulinemia, leading to blood vessel wall hypertrophy resulting from enhanced growth factor activity (via increased flux through the mitogen-activating protein kinase (MAPK) insulin-signaling pathway), leading to a decreased lumen of the vessels [156].

LIFESTYLE MANAGEMENT

Lifestyle approaches recommended to reduce blood pressure include: weight reduction; decreasing sodium intake; increasing potassium intake; increasing consumption of fruits, vegetables, and low-fat dairy products; moderating of alcohol intake; and increasing physical activity. These measures serve as initial therapy for blood pressure control and may also prevent the development of hypertension [157]. Older individuals [158] and African-Americans are especially sensitive to the effects of diet on blood pressure. Studies have also found adding exercise to weight reduction to be an effective means of decreasing diastolic blood pressure in individuals with the metabolic syndrome [159].

The Dietary Approaches to Stop Hypertension (DASH) diet [160–162] emphasizes fruits, vegetables, and low-fat dairy products—all intended to enrich the diet in calcium, magnesium, and potassium. The DASH Eating Plan is outlined in Table 4.9. Without sodium restriction, the DASH diet vs. a control diet led to significant reductions in systolic and diastolic blood pressure of 5.5 mm Hg and 3.3 mm Hg, respectively, in normotensive individuals [157]. In hypertensive individuals, the DASH diet reduced systolic and diastolic blood pressure more than the control diet by 11.4 mm Hg and 5.5 mm Hg, respectively. When combined with low salt intake (1500 mg/day), the DASH diet led to a mean reduction in systolic blood pressure of 7.1 mm Hg in subjects without hypertension and 11.5 mm Hg in subjects with hypertension [158].

CONCLUSIONS AND RECOMMENDATIONS

The metabolic syndrome is a constellation of cardiovascular risk factors including: abdominal obesity, low HDL cholesterol levels, high triglyceride levels, high blood pressure, and impaired fasting glucose. The syndrome is associated with an increased risk of cardiovascular disease and T2DM that is linked to insulin resistance and abdominal obesity.

To achieve improved metabolic control, dietary treatment recommendations must be individu-alized to the metabolic profile of the patient. Individuals presenting with abdominal obesity associated with one or more components of the metabolic syndrome will benefit from weight loss as a key treatment recommendation. Lifestyle changes, including calorie restriction and physical activity, should aim for 5–10% weight reduction over 6 months. A calorie restriction of 500–1000 kcal/day should be combined with at least 30 minutes of physical activity on most, preferably all, days of the week. Physical activity has the added benefits of decreased risk of cardiovascular disease and improved quality of life. Specific recommendations for other components are listed in Table 4.6. If low HDL cholesterol levels and hypertriglyceridemia are present, moderation of dietary carbohydrates and liberation of dietary fats may be helpful to improve the dyslipidemia. A diet consistent with ATP III's therapeutic lifestyle change should be recommended. If elevated blood pressure is the predominant presenting component of the syndrome, then the DASH diet—with emphasis on fruits, vegetables, and low-fat dairy products—should be prescribed. Following the dietary guidelines of the Diabetes Prevention Program will be useful when treating patients with impaired glucose tolerance. It must be kept in mind, however, that regardless of the metabolic profile of the patient, dietary counseling must always take the patient's personal food preferences, lifestyle, and cultural norms into consideration. Failure to do so will lead to nonadherence and poor metabolic outcomes.

REFERENCES

1. U.S. Department of Health and Human Services, The surgeon general's call to action to prevent and decrease overweight and obesity, (Rockville, MD): U.S. Department of Health and Human Services, Public Health Services, Office of the Surgeon General, 2001.
2. Makdad AH, Marks JS, and Stroup DF et al., Actual causes of death in the United States, 2000, *JAMA,* 291:1238–1245, 2004.
3. Vague J, The degree of masculine differentiation of obesities: A factor determining predisposition to diabetes, atherosclerosis, gout, and uric calculous disease, *Am J Clin Nutr,* 4:20–34, 1956.
4. Reaven GM, Banting lecture 1988, Role of insulin resistance in human disease (review), *Diabetes,* 37:1595–1607, 1988.
5. Sattar N, Gaw A, and Scherbakova O et al., Metabolic syndrome with and without C-reactive protein as a predictor of coronary heart disease and diabetes in the west of Scotland coronary prevention study, *Circulation,* 108:414–419, 2003.
6. Lakka HM, Laaksonen DE, and Lakka TA et al., The metabolic syndrome and total and cardiovascular disease mortality in middle-aged men, *JAMA,* 288:2709–2716, 2002.
7. World Health Organization, Definition, diagnosis, and classification of diabetes mellitus and its complications: Report of the WHO consultation, Part 1: Diagnosis and classification of diabetes mellitus, Geneva, Switzerland: World Health Organization 1999, Available at: http://whqlibdoc.who.int/hq/1999/WHO_NCD_NCS_99.2.pdf, Accessed February 29, 2004.
8. Third Report of the National Cholesterol Education Program (NCEP) Expert Panel on Detection, Evaluation, and Treatment of High Blood Cholesterol in Adults (Adult treatment panel III), Final report, National Heart, Lung, and Blood Institute, National Institutes of Health, NIH publication No, 02-5215, September, 2002.
9. Einhorn D, Reaven GM, and Cobin RH et al., American College of Endocrinology position statement on the insulin resistance syndrome, *Endocr Pract,* 9:237–252, 2003.
10.) International Diabetes Federation. The IDF consensus worldwide definition of the metabolic syndrome, Available at: http://www.idf.org/webdata/docs/IDF Metasyndrome definition.pdf, Accessed October 19, 2005.
11. Reilly MP and Rader DJ, The metabolic syndrome, More than the sum of its parts? *Circulation,* 108:1546–1551, 2003.
12. Isomaa B, A major health hazard: The metabolic syndrome, *Life Sciences,* 73:2395–2411, 2003.
13. Reaven G, Metabolic syndrome, Pathophysiology and implications for management of cardiovascular disease, *Circulation,* 106:286–288, 2002.
14. Grundy SM, Brewer B, and Cleeman JI et al., Definition of metabolic syndrome, Report of the National Heart, Lung, and Blood Institute/American Heart Association conference on scientific issues related to definition, *Circulation,* 109:433–438, 2004.

15.) Kahn, R, Buse J, Ferrannini E, Stern M. The metabolic syndrome: time for a critical appraisal. *Diabetes Care*, 28:2289-2304, 2005.

16. Ford ES, Giles WH, and Dietz WH, Prevalence of the metabolic syndrome among U.S. adults, Findings from the third national health and nutrition examination survey, *JAMA*, 287:356–359, 2002.

17. Park YW, Zhu S, and Palaniappan L et al., The metabolic syndrome, Prevalence and associated risk factor findings in the U.S. population from the Third National Health and Nutrition Examination Survey, 1988–1994, *Arch Intern Med*, 163:427–436, 2003.

18. Alexander CM, Landsman PB, and Teutsch SM et al., NCEP-defined metabolic syndrome, diabetes, and prevalence of coronary heart disease among NHANES III participants age 50 years and older, *Diabetes*, 52:1210–1214, 2003.

19. Ford ES and Giles WH, A comparison of the prevalence of the metabolic syndrome using two proposed definitions, *Diabetes Care*, 26:575–581, 2003.

20. Anand SS, Yi Q, and Gerstein H et al., Relationship of metabolic syndrome and fibrinolytic dysfunction to cardiovascular disease, *Circulation*, 108:420–425, 2003.

21. Cnop M, Landchild M, and Vidal J et al., The concurrent accumulation of intra-abdominal and subcutaneous fat explains the association between insulin resistance and plasma leptin concentrations: Distinct metabolic effects of two fat compartments, *Diabetes*, 52:1005–1015, 2002.

22. Palaniappan L, Carnethon MR, and Wang Y et al., Predictors of the incident metabolic syndrome in adults, *Diabetes Care*, 27:788–793, 2004.

23. Banerji MA, Lebowitz J, and Chaiken RL et al., Relationship of visceral adipose tissue and glucose disposal is independent of sex in black NIDDM subjects, *Am J Physiol*, 273:E425–E432, 1997.

24. Wagenknech LE, Langefeld CD, and Scherzinger AL et al., Insulin sensitivity, insulin secretion, and abdominal fat, The Insulin Resistance Atherosclerosis Study (IRAS) family study, *Diabetes*, 52:2490–2496, 2003.

25. Weyer C, Foley JE, and Bogardus C et al., Enlarged subcutaneous abdominal adipocyte size, but not obesity itself, predicts T2DM independent of insulin resistance, *Diabetologia*, 43:1498–1506, 2000.

26. Gastaldelli A, Miyazaki Y, and Pettiti M et al., Metabolic effects of visceral fat accumulation in T2DM, *J Clin Endocrinol Metab*, 87:5098–5103, 2002.

27. Ross R, Leger L, and Morris D et al., Quantification of adipose tissue by MRI: Relationship with anthropometric variables, *J Appl Physiol*, 72:787–95, 1992.

28. Ross R, Rissanen J, and Martel Y et al., Adipose tissue distribution measured by magnetic imaging in obese women, *Am J Clin Nutr*, 57(Suppl 4):470–475, 1993.

29. Montague CT and O'Rahilly S, The perils of portliness, Causes and consequences of visceral adiposity, *Diabetes*, 49:883–888, 2000.

30. Zammit VA, Waterman D, and Tpooing D et al., Insulin stimulation of hepatic triacylglyceride secretion and the etiology of insulin resistance, *J Nutr*, 131:2074–2077, 2001.

31. Kelly DE, Goodpaster BH, and Storlien L, Muscle triglyceride and insulin resistance, *Annu Rev Nutr*, 22:325–346, 2002.

32. Unger RH, Lipotoxic diseases, *Annu Rev Med*, 53:319–336, 2002.

33. Unger RH, The physiology of cellular liporegulation, *Annu Rev Physiol*, 63:333–347, 2003.

34. Unger RH, Minireview: Weapons of lean body mass destruction: The role of ectopic lipids in the metabolic syndrome, *Endocrinology*, 144:5159–5165, 2003.

35. Fruhbeck G, Gomez-Ambrosi J, and Muruzabal FJ et al., The adipocyte: A model for integration of endocrine and metabolic signaling in energy metabolism regulation, *Am J Endocrinol Metab*, 280:E827–E847, 2001.

36. Grundy SM, Inflammation, metabolic syndrome, and diet responsiveness, *Circulation*, 108:126–128, 2003.

37. Grundy SM, Inflammation, hypertension, and the metabolic syndrome, *JAMA*, 290:3000–3002, 2003.

38. Weisberg SP, McCann D, and Desai M et al., Obesity is associated with macrophage accumulation in adipose tissue, *J Clin Invest*, 112:1796–1808, 2003.

39. Xu H, Barnes GT, and Yang Q et al., Chronic inflammation in fat plays a crucial role in the development of obesity-related insulin resistance, *J Clin Invest*, 112:1821–1830, 2003.

40. Wellen KE and Hotamisligil GS, Obesity-induced inflammatory changes in adipose tissue, *J Clin Invest*, 112:1785–1788, 2003.

41. Sonnenberg GE, Krakower GR, and Kissebah AH, A novel pathway to the manifestations of metabolic syndrome, *Obes Res,* 12:180–186, 2004.
42. Flegal KM, Carroll MD, and Ogden CL et al., Prevalence and trends in obesity among U.S. adults, 1999–2000, *JAMA,* 288:1723–1727, 2002.
43. Jolliffe D, Extent of overweight among U.S. children and adolescents from 1971 to 2000, *Int J Obesity,* 28:4–9, 2004
44. National Heart, Lung, and Blood Institute (NHLBI) and National Institute for Diabetes and Digestive and Kidney Diseases (NIDDKD), Clinical guidelines on the identification, evaluation, and treatment of overweight and obesity in adults, The Evidence Report, *Obes Res,* 6(Suppl 2):51S–210S, 1998.
45. National Heart, Lung, and Blood Institute (NHLBI) and North American Association for the Study of Obesity (NAASO), *Practical Guide on the Identification, Evaluation, and Treatment of Overweight and Obesity in Adults,* Bethesda, MD: National Institutes of Health; 2000, NIH Publication number 00-4084, October, 2000.
46. Kushner RF, *Roadmaps for Clinical Practice: Case Studies in Disease Prevention and Health Promotion—Assessment and Management of Adult Obesity: A Primer for Physicians,* Chicago, Illinois: American Medical Association; 2003, Available at: www.ama-assn.org/ama/pub/category/10931.html.
47. Kushner RF and Roth JL, Assessment of the obese patient, *Endocrinol Metab Clin N Am,* 32(4):915–934, 2003.
48. Reaven GM, Importance of identifying the overweight patient who will benefit the most by losing weight, *Ann Intern Med,* 138:420–423, 2003.
49. Wilson PWF and Grundy SM, The metabolic syndrome: Practical guide to origins and treatment: Part 1, *Circulation,* 108:1422–1425, 2003.
50. Wang J, Thornton JC, and Bari S et al., Comparisons of waist circumferences measured at four sites, *Am J Clin Nutr,* 77:379–384, 2003.
51. Janssen I, Katzmarzyk PT, and Ross R, Body mass index, waist circumference, and health risk: Evidence in support of current national institutes of health guidelines, *Arch Intern Med,* 162:2074–2079, 2002.
52. Zhu SK, Wang ZM, and Heshka S et al., Waist circumference and obesity-associated risk factors among whites in the third national health and nutrition examination survey: Clinical action thresholds, *Am J Clin Nutr,* 76:743–749, 2002.
53. Janssen I, Katzmarzyk PT, and Ross R, Waist circumference and not body mass index explains obesity-related health risk, *Am J Clin Nutr,* 79:379–384, 2004.
54. Lemieux I, Pascot A, and Couillard C et al., Hypertriglyceridemic waist: A marker of the atherogenic metabolic triad (hyperinsulinemia; hyperapolipoprotein B; small, dense LDL) in men? *Circulation,* 102:179–184, 2000.
55. Depres JP, Lemieux I, and Prud'homme D, Treatment of obesity: Need to focus on high-risk abdominally obese patients, *BMJ,* 322:716–720, 2001.
56. Kahn HS and Valdez R, Metabolic risks identified by the combination of enlarged waist and elevated triacylglycerol concentration, *Am J Clin Nutr,* 78:928–934, 2003.
57. McLaughlin T, Abbasi F, and Cheal K et al., Use of metabolic markers to identify overweight individuals who are insulin resistant, *Ann Intern Med,* 139:802–809, 2003.
58. Black AE, Prentice AM, and Goldberg GR et al., Measurements of total energy expenditure provide insights into validity of dietary measurements of energy intake, *J Am Diet Assoc,* 93:572–579, 1993.
59. Bowerman S, The role of meal replacements in weight control, In: Bessesen DH and Kushner R, Eds., *Evaluation & Management of Obesity,* Philadelphia, PA: Hanley & Belfus, Inc., 53–58, 2002.
60. Heymsfield SB, van Mierlo CAJ, and van der Knaap HCM et al., Weight management using meal replacement strategy: Meta and pooling analysis from six studies, *Int J Obes,* 27:537–549, 2003.
61. Pate RR, Pratt M, and Blair SN et al., Physical activity and public health: A recommendation from the Centers for Disease Control and Prevention and the American College of Sports Medicine, *JAMA,* 273:402–407, 1995.
62. Dunn AL, Marcus BH, and Kampert JB et al., Comparison of lifestyle an structured interventions to increase physical activity and cardiorespiratory fitness, A randomized trial, *JAMA,* 281:327–334, 1999.
63. Anderson RE, Wadden TA, and Bartlett SJ et al., Effects of lifestyle activity vs. structured aerobic exercise in obese women, A randomized trial, *JAMA,* 281:335–340, 1999.

64. Votrubo SB, Horvitz MA, and Schoeller DA, The role of exercise in the treatment of obesity, *Nutrition,* 16:179–188, 2000.
65. Jakacic JM, Clark K, and Coleman E, et al., Appropriate intervention strategies for weight loss and prevention of weight regain for adults, *Med Sci Sports Exerc,* 33:2145–2156, 2001.
66. Bray GA, Blackburn GL, and Ferguson JA et al., Sibutramine produces dose-related weight loss, *Obes Res,* 7:189–198, 1999.
67. Finer N, Bloom SR, and Frost GS, et al., Sibutramine is effective for weight loss and diabetic control in obesity with T2DM, A randomized, double-blind, placebo-controlled study, *Diabetes Obes Metab,* 2:105–112, 2000.
68. Fujioka K, Seaton TB, and Rowe E et al., Weight loss with sibutramine improves glycaemic control and other metabolic parameters in obese patients with T2DM mellitus, *Diabetes Obes Metab,* 2:175–187, 2000.
69. Gokcel A, Karakose H, and Ertorer EM et al., Effects of sibutramine in obese female subjects with T2DM and poor blood glucose control, *Diabetes Care,* 24:1957–1960, 2001.
70. McNulty SJ, Ur E, and Williams G, A randomized trial of sibutramine in the management of obese type-2 diabetic patients treated with metformin, *Diabetes Care,* 26:125–131, 2003.
71. James WPT, Astrup A, and Finer N et al., Effect of sibutramine on weight maintenance after weight loss, A randomized trial, *Lancet,* 356:2119–2125, 2000.
72. Dujovne CA, Zavoral JH, and Rowe E et al., Effects of sibutramine on body weight and serum lipids, A double-blind, randomized, placebo-controlled study in 322 overweight and obese patients with dyslipidemia, *Am Heart J,* 142:489–497, 2001.
73. Krijs GJ, Metabolic benefits associated with sibutramine therapy, *Int J Obes,* 26:S34–37, 2002.
74. Fanghanel G, Cortinas L, and Sachez-Reyes L et al., Second phase of a double-blind study clinical trial on sibutramine for the treatment of patients suffering essential obesity: 6 months after treatment cross-over, *Int J Obes,* 25:741–747, 2001.
75. Lucas KH and Kaplan-Machlis B, Orlistat—a novel weight loss therapy, *Ann Pharmacother,* 35:314–328, 2001.
76. Sjostrom L, Rissanen A, and Anderson T et al., Randomized placebo-controlled trial of orlistat for weight loss and prevention of weight regain in obese patients, *Lancet,* 352:167–173, 1998.
77. Davidson MH, Hauptman J, and DiGirolamo M et al., Weight control and risk factor reduction in obese subjects treated for 2 years with orlistat, A randomized trial *JAMA,* 281:235–242, 1999.
78. Hollander PA, Elbein SC, and Hirsch IB et al., Role of orlistat in the treatment of obese patients with T2DM, *Diabetes Care,* 21:1288–1294, 1998.
79. Miles JM, Leitter L, and Hollander P et al., Effect of orlistat in overweight and obese patients with T2DM treated with metformin, *Diabetes Care,* 25:1123–1128, 2002.
80. Kelley DE, Kuller LH, and McKolanis TM et al., Effects of moderate weight loss and orlistat on insulin resistance, regional adiposity, and fatty acids in T2DM, *Diabetes Care,* 27:33–40, 2004.
81. Tong PCY, Lee ZS, and Sea MM et al., The effect of orlistat-induced weight loss, without concomitant hypocaloric diet, on cardiovascular risk factors and insulin sensitivity in young obese Chinese subjects with or without T2DM, *Arch Intern Med,* 162:2428–2435, 2002.
82. Lindgarde F, The effect of orlistat on body weight and coronary heart disease risk profile in obese patient, The Swedish multimorbidity study, *J Intern Med,* 248:245–254, 2000.
83. Heymsfield SB, Segal KR, and Hauptman J et al., Effects of weight loss with orlistat on glucose tolerance and progression to T2DM in obese adults, *Arch Intern Med,* 160:1321–1326, 2000.
84. Torgerson JS, Hauptman J, and Boldrin MN et al., Xenical in the prevention of diabetes in obese subjects (XENDOS) study, A randomized study of orlistat as an adjunct to lifestyle changes for the prevention of T2DM in obese patients, *Diabetes Care,* 27:155–161, 2004.
85. Cavaliere H, Floriano I, and Medeiros-Neto G, Gastrointestinal side effects of orlistat may be prevented by concomitant prescription of natural fibers (psyllium mucilloid), *Int J Obes,* 25:1095–1099, 2001.
86. Lehtovirta M, Forsen B, and Gullstrom M et al., Metabolic effects of metformin in patients with impaired glucose tolerance, *Diabetic Med,* 18:578–583, 2001.
87. Lee A and Morley JE, Metformin decreases food consumption and induces weight loss in subjects with obesity with type II non-insulin-dependent diabetes, *Obes Res,* 6:47–53, 1998.

88. Mogul HR, Peterson SJ, and Weinstein BI et al., Long-term (2–4 year) weight reduction with metformin plus carbohydrate-modified diet in euglycemic, hyperinsulinemic, midlife women (Syndrome W), *Heart Dis,* 5(6):384–392, 2003.

89. Sjostrom CD, Lissner L, and Wedel H et al., Reduction in incidence of diabetes, hypertension and lipid disturbances after intentional weight loss induced by bariatric surgery, The SOS Intervention study, *Obes Res,* 7:477–484, 1999.

90. Schauer PR, Ikramuddin S, and Gourash W et al., Outcomes after laparoscopic Roux-en-Y gastric bypass for morbid obesity, *Ann Surg,* 232:515–529, 2000.

91. Sjostrom CD, Peltonen M, and Wedel H, Differentiated long-term effects of intentional weight loss on diabetes and hypertension, *Hypertension,* 36:20–5, 2000.

92. Herbst CA, Hughes TA, and Gwynne JT et al., Gastric bariatric operation in insulin-treated adults, *Surgery,* 95:209–214, 1984.

93. Castagneto M, De Gaetano A, and Mingrone G et al., Normalization of insulin sensitivity in the obese patient after stable weight reduction with biliopancreatic diversion, *Obes Surg,* 4:161–168, 1994.

94. Mingrone G, Rosa G, and Di Rocco P, et al., Skeletal muscle triglycerides lowering is associated with net improvement of insulin sensitivity, TNF-α reduction and GLUT4 expression enhancement, *Int J Obes,* 26:1165–1172, 2002.

95. Rosa G, Di Rocco P, and Manco M et al., Reduced PDK4 expression associates with increased insulin sensitivity in postobese patients, *Obes Res,* 11:176–182, 2003.

96. Mingrone G, Rosa G, and Greco AV et al., Decreased uncoupling protein expression and intramyocytic triglyceride depletion in formerly obese subjects, *Obes Res,* 11:632–640, 2003.

97. Mingrone G, Rosa G, and Greco AV et al., Intramyocitic lipid accumulation and SREBP-1c expression are related to insulin resistance and cardiovascular risk in morbid obesity, *Atherosclerosis,* 170:155–161, 2003.

98. Pender C, Goldfine ID, and Tanner CJ et al., Muscle insulin receptor concentrations in obese patients post bariatric surgery: Relationship to hyperinsulinemia, *Int J Obes Relat Metab Disord,* 28:363–369, 2004.

99. Patriti A, Facchiano E, and Sanna A et al., The enteroinsular axis and the recovery from type-2 diabetes after bariatric surgery, *Obes Surg,* 14:840–848, 2004.

100. Vazquez LA, Pazos F, and Berrazueta JR et al., Effects of changes in body weight and insulin resistance on inflammation and endothelial function in morbid obesity after bariatric surgery, *J Clin Endocrinol Metab,* 90:316–322, 2005.

101. Deckelbaum RJ, Fisher EA, and Winston M et al., Summary of a scientific conference on preventive nutrition, Pediatrics to geriatrics, *Circulation,* 100:450–456, 1999.

102. Ross R, Dagnone D, and Jones PJH et al., Reduction in obesity and related comorbid conditions after diet-induced weight loss or exercise-induced weight loss in men, A randomized, controlled trial, *Ann Intern Med,* 133:92–103, 2000.

103. Janssen I, Fortier A, and Hudson R et al., Effects of an energy-restrictive diet with or without exercise on abdominal fat, intermuscular fat, and metabolic risk factors in obese women, *Diabetes Care,* 25:431–438, 2002.

104. Esposito K, Pontillo A, and Di Palo C et al., Effect of weight loss and lifestyle changes on vascular inflammatory markers in obese women, *JAMA,* 289:1799–1804, 2003.

105. Kelley DE, Wing R, and Buonocore C et al., Relative effects of calorie restriction and weight loss in non-insulin-dependent diabetes mellitus, *J Clin Endocrinol Metab,* 77:1287–1293, 1993.

106. Markovic TP, Campbell LV, and Balasubramanian S et al., Beneficial effect on average lipid levels from energy restriction and fat loss in obese individuals with or without T2DM, *Diabetes Care,* 21:695–700, 1998.

107. Ludwig DS, Pereira MA, Kroenke CH, and Hilner JE et al., Dietary fiber, weight gain, and cardiovascular disease risk factors in young adults, *JAMA,* 282:1539–1546, 1999.

108. Lovejoy J and DiGirolamo M, Habitual dietary intake and insulin sensitivity in lean and obese adults, *Am J Clin Nutr,* 55:1174–1179, 1992.

109. Strazinsky N, O'Callaghan C, and Barrington V et al., Hypotensive effect of a low-fat, high-carbohydrate diet can be independent of changes in plasma insulin concentrations, *Hypertension,* 34:580–585, 1999.

110. Jenkins DJA, Axelson M, and Kendall CWC et al., Dietary fiber, lente carbohydrates, and the insulin-resistant diseases, *Br J Nutr*, 83(Suppl 1):S157–163, 2000.

111. Hays NP, Starling RD, and Liu X et al., Effects of an ad libitum low-fat, high-carbohdyrate diet on body weight, body composition, and fat distribution in older men and women, *Arch Intern Med*, 164:210–217, 2004.

112. Cheuvront SN, The Zone Diet phenomenon: A closer look at the science behind the claims, *J Am Coll Nutr*, 22:9–17, 2003.

113. Foster GD, Wyatt HR, and Hill JO et al., A randomized trial of a low-carbohydrate diet for obesity, *New Engl J Med*, 348:2082–2090, 2003.

114. Yancy WS, Olsen MK, and Guyton JR et al., A low-carbohydrate, ketogenic diet versus a low-fat diet to treat obesity and hyperlipidemia, *Ann Intern Med*, 140:769–777, 2004.

115. Brehm BJ, Seeley RJ, and Daniels SR et al., A randomized trial comparing a very low-carbohydrate diet and a calorie-restricted low-fat diet on body weight and cardiovascular risk factors in healthy women, *J Clin Endocrinol Metab*, 88:1617–1623, 2003.

116. Samaha FF, Iqbal N, and Seshadri P et al., A low-carbohydrate as compared with a low-fat diet in severe obesity, *N Engl J Med*, 348:2074–2081, 2003.

117. Stern L, Iqbal N, and Seshadri P et al., The effects of low-carbohydrate versus conventional weight loss diets in severely obese adults, One-year follow-up of a randomized trial, *Ann Intern Med*, 140:778–785, 2004.

118. Freedman MR, King J, and Kennedy E, Popular diets: A scientific review, *Obes Res*, 9(Suppl 1):1S–40S, 2001.

119. Bravata DM, Sanders L, and Huang J et al., Efficacy and safety of low-carbohydrate diets, A scientific review, *JAMA*, 289:1837–1850, 2003.

120. Whaley MH, Kampert JB, and Kohl HW et al., Physical fitness and clustering of risk factors associated with the metabolic syndrome, *Med & Sci Sports Exerc*, 31:287–293, 1999.

121. Irwin ML, Ainsworth BE, and Mayer-Davis EJ et al., Physical activity and the metabolic syndrome in a tri-ethnic sample of women, *Obes Res*, 10:1030–1037, 2002.

122. Rennie KL, McCarthy N, and Yazdgerdi S et al., Association of the metabolic syndrome with both vigorous and moderate physical activity, *Int J Epidemiol*, 32:600–606, 2003.

123. Hu FB, Sigal RJ, and Rich-Edwards JW et al., Walking compared with vigorous physical activity and risk of T2DM in women, A prospective study, *JAMA*, 282:1433–1439, 1999.

124. Manson JE, Hu FB, and Rich-Edwards JW et al., A prospective study of walking as compared with vigorous exercise in the prevention of coronary heart disease in women, *N Engl J Med*, 341:650–650, 1999.

125. Manson JE, Nathan DM, and Krolewski AS et al., A prospective study of exercise and incidence of diabetes among U.S. male physicians, *JAMA*, 268:63–67, 1992.

126. Ross R, Dagnone D, and Jones PJ et al., Reduction in obesity and related comorbid conditions after diet-induced weight loss or exercise-induced weight loss in men, A randomized, controlled trial, *Ann Intern Med*, 133:92–103, 2000.

127. Heymsfield SB, Segal KR, and Hauptman J et al., Effects of weight loss with orlistat on glucose tolerance and progression to T2DM in obese adults, *Arch Intern Med*, 160:1321–1326, 2000.

128. Muls E, Kolanowski J, and Scheen A et al., ObelHyx Study Group, The effects of orlistat on weight and on serum lipids in obese patients with hypercholesterolemia, A randomized, double-blind, placebo-controlled, multicenter study, *Int J Obes Relat Metab Disord*, 25:1713–1721, 2001.

129. Pasquali R, Gambineri A, and Biscotti D et al., Effect of long-term treatment with metformin added to hypocaloric diet on body composition, fat distribution, and androgen and insulin levels in abdominally obese women with and without the polycystic ovary syndrome, *J Clin Endocrinol Metab*, 85:2767–2774, 2000.

130. Moghetti P, Castello R, and Negri C et al., Metformin effects on clinical features, endocrine and metabolic profiles, and insulin sensitivity in polycystic ovary syndrome, A randomized, double-blind, placebo-controlled, 6-month trial, followed by open, long-term clinical evaluation, *J Clin Endocrinol Metabolism*, 85:139–146, 2000.

131. DeFronzo RA, Pharmacologic therapy for T2DM mellitus, *Ann Intern Med*, 131:281–303, 1999.

132. Ginsberg HN and Goldberg IJ, Disorders of lipoprotein metabolism, In: *Harrison's Principles of Internal Medicine*, 15th ed., New York: McGraw-Hill, 2245–2257, 2001.

133. Executive summary of the third reports of the National Cholesterol Education Program (NCEP) Expert Panel on Detection, Evaluation, and Treatment of High Blood Cholesterol in Adults (Adult treatment panel III), *JAMA,* 285:2486–2497, 2001, Available at: http://www.nhlbi.nih.gov/guidelines/cholesterol/atp3xsum.pdf, Accessed March 30, 2004.

134. Gordon DJ, Cholesterol and mortality: What can meta-analysis tell us? In: Gallo LL, Ed., *Cardiovascular Disease 2: Cellular and Molecular Mechanisms, Prevention, and Treatment,* New York: Plenum Press, 333–40, 1995.

135. Gordon DJ, Cholesterol lowering and total mortality, In: Rifkind BM, Ed., *Lowering Cholesterol in High-risk Individuals and Populations,* New York: Marcel Dekker, Inc., 333–348, 1995.

136. Riccardi G, Rivellese A, and Pacioni D et al., Separate influence of dietary carbohydrates and fiber on the metabolic control in diabetes, *Diabetologia,* 26:116–121, 1984.

137. Garg A, Grundy SM, and Unger RH, Comparison of effects of high- and low-carbohydrate diets on plasma lipoproteins and insulin sensitivity in patients with mild NIDDM, *Diabetes,* 41:1278–1285, 1992.

138. Bonanome A, Visona A, and Lusiani L et al., Carbohydrate and lipid metabolism in patients with non-insulin-dependent diabetes mellitus: Effects of a low-fat, high-carbohydrate diet vs. a diet high in monounsaturated fatty acids, *Am J Clin Nutr,* 54:586–590, 1991.

139. National Research Council, *Dietary Reference Intakes for Energy, Carbohydrate, Fiber, Fat, Fatty Acids, Cholesterol, Protein, and Amino Acids,* Washington, D.C.: National Academy Press, 2002, 936 pages.

140. Ballantyne CM, Stein EA, and Paoletti R et al., Efficacy of rosuvastatin 10 mg in patients with the metabolic syndrome, *Am J Cardiol,* 91(Suppl):25C–28C, 2003.

141. Watts GF, Barrett HR, and Ji J et al., Differential regulation of lipoprotein kinetics by atorvastatin and fenofibrate in subjects with the metabolic syndrome, *Diabetes,* 52:803–811, 2003.

142. Robins SJ, Rubins HB, and Faas FH et al., VA-HIT Study Group, Insulin resistance and cardiovascular events with low-HDL cholesterol, *Diabetes Care,* 26:1513–1517, 2003.

143. McMahon FG, Fujioka K, and Singh BN et al., Efficacy and safety of sibutramine in obese white and African American patients with hypertension, A 1-year, double-blind, placebo-controlled, multicenter trial, *Arch Intern Med,* 160:2185–2191, 2000.

144. Zavaroni I, Mazza S, and Dall'Aglio E et al., Prevalence of hyperinsulinaemia in patients with high blood pressure, *J Intern Med,* 231:235–240, 1992.

145. Lind L, Berne C, and Lithell H, Prevalence of insulin resistance in essential hypertension, *J Hypertens,* 13:1457–1462, 1995.

146. Powers AC, Diabetes mellitus, In: *Harrison's Principles of Internal Medicine,* 15th ed., New York: McGraw-Hill, 2109–2137, 2001.

147. Boden G, Lebed B, and Schatz M et al., Effects of acute changes of plasma free fatty acids on intramyocellular fat content and insulin resistance in healthy subjects, *Diabetes,* 50:1612–1617, 2001.

148. Diabetes Prevention Program Research Group, Reduction in the incidence of T2DM with lifestyle intervention or metformin, *N Engl J Med,* 346:393–403, 2002.

149. Tuomilehto J, Lindstrom J, and Eriksson JG et al., Finnish Diabetes Prevention Study Group, Prevention of T2DM mellitus by changes in lifestyle among subjects with impaired glucose tolerance, *N Engl J Med,* 344:1343–1350, 2001.

150. Reaven G, Segal K, and Hauptman J et al., Effect of orlistat-assisted weight loss in decreasing coronary heart disease risk in patients with syndrome X, *Am J Cardiol,* 87:827–831, 2001.

151. Pasquali R and Casimirri F, The impact of obesity on hyperandrogenism and polycystic ovary syndrome in premenopausal women, *Clin Endocrinol,* 39:1–16, 1993.

152. Dunaif A, Insulin resistance and the polycystic ovary syndrome: Mechanism and implications for pathogenesis, *Endocr Rev,* 18:774–800, 1997.

153. Glueck CJ, Papanna R, and Wang P et al., Incidence and treatment of metabolic syndrome in newly referred women with confirmed polycystic ovarian syndrome, *Metabolism,* 52:908–915, 2003.

154. Ehrmann DA, Schneider DJ, and Sobel BE et al., Troglitazone improves defects in insulin action, insulin secretion, ovarian steroidogenesis, and fibrinolysis in women with polycystic ovary syndrome, *J Clin Endocrinol Metab,* 82:2108–2116, 1997.

155. Reaven GM, Diet and syndrome X, *Curr Atheroscler Rep,* 2:503–507, 2000.

156. Mediratta S, Fozailoff A, and Frishman W, Insulin resistance in systemic hypertension: Pharmaco-therapeutic implications, *J Clin Pharmacol*, 35:943–956, 1995.

157. The Trials of Hypertension Prevention Collaborative Research Group, Effects of weight loss and sodium reduction intervention on blood pressure and hypertension incidence in overweight people with high-normal blood pressure, The trials of hypertension prevention, phase II, *Arch Intern Med*, 157:657–667, 1997.

158. Whelton PK, Appel LJ, and Espeland MA et al., TONE Collaborative Research Group, Efficacy of sodium reduction and weight loss in the treatment of hypertension in older persons, Main results of the randomized, controlled trial of nonpharmacologic interventions in the elderly (TONE), *JAMA*, 279:839–846, 1998.

159. Watkins LL, Sherwood A, and Feinglos M et al., Effects of exercise and weight loss on cardiac risk factors associated with syndrome X, *Arch Intern Med*, 163:1889–1895, 2003.

160. Appel LJ, Moore TJ, and Obarzanek E et al., DASH Collaborative Research Group, A clinical trial of the effects of dietary patterns on blood pressure, *N Engl J Med*, 336:1117–1124, 1997.

161. Sacks FM, Svetkey LP, and Vollmer WM et al., DASH-Sodium Collaborative Research Group, Effects on blood pressure of reduced dietary sodium and the dietary approaches to stop hypertension (DASH) diet, *N Engl J Med*, 344:3–10, 2001.

162. Windhauser MM, Ernst DB, and Karanja NM et al., DASH Collaborative Research Group, Translating the dietary approaches to stop hypertension diet from research to practice: Dietary and behavior change techniques, *J Am Diet Assoc*, 99:S90–95, 1999.

5 Medical Nutrition Therapy for Patients with Type-2 Diabetes

Bantwal Suresh Baliga, Zachary Bloomgarden, and Cathy Nonas

CONTENTS

GOALS AND COMPONENTS OF MEDICAL NUTRITION THERAPY

An essential component of effective diabetes management is medical nutrition therapy (MNT). Nutritional recommendations for diabetes, as recommended by the American Diabetes Association (ADA), should be based on scientific knowledge, taking into account individual, cultural, and ethnic circumstances and preferences. Goals for nutrition are broad:

- Attain and maintain optimal metabolic outcomes.
- Modify nutrient intake and lifestyle to prevent and treat:
    - Obesity
    - Dyslipidemia

- Cardiovascular disease
- Hypertension
- Nephropathy
- Improve health through healthy food choices and physical activity [1]

Typically, the largest percentage of calories should be derived from carbohydrates, with at least 15–20% from protein, and the rest from fat. However, within those parameters, there is evidence for choosing foods wisely, including high-fiber carbohydrates, low-fat protein, and fats that are relatively low in saturated fatty acids, trans-fatty acids, and dietary cholesterol [1]. The actual distribution of macronutrients may change according to individual needs. For example, persons with elevated low-density lipoprotein cholesterol (LDL-c) are given fewer calories from fats (20–30%), while those with hypertriglyceridemia are given fewer calories from carbohydrates (40–45%).

The ADA recommends avoiding dietary prescriptions that specifically refer to the terms "simple sugars," "complex carbohydrates," and "fast-acting carbohydrates." Quantitatively, the carbohydrate content of food predicts post prandial increases in blood glucose and, therefore, all carbohydrates in foods should be carefully considered. Types and examples of carbohydrates are given in Table 5.1.

DIETARY COMPONENTS OF MEDICAL NUTRITION THERAPY FOR TYPE-2 DIABETES MELLITUS

CALORIE RESTRICTION—WEIGHT LOSS

Short-term studies of weight loss with calorie restriction in subjects with type-2 diabetes mellitus (T2DM) are associated with improvement in many indices including insulin sensitivity, glucose control, lipids, and blood pressure—independent of the distribution of calories. The most effective diet for the obese patient with T2DM in the short-term is a very low-calorie diet (VLCD), which is defined as < 800 calories/day. VLCDs improve glycemic control, despite a relatively high carbohydrate content [2–6]. This is independent of weight loss and due to the severity of the calorie restriction which reduces fasting glucose by 30–50% within the first 7–10 days [3,7,8]. In one study, subjects were randomized to either a VLCD of 400 calories/day or a low-calorie diet (LCD) of 1000 calories/day, and glucose control was compared after both groups lost 11% of their weight [9]. Results showed that the 400 calories/day VLCD group had better glycemic control [9]. Both groups were restudied 15 weeks later, when the 400 calories/day group was increased to 1000 calories/day [9]. The 400 to 1000 calories/day group showed a slight worsening of glycemic control despite continued weight loss while the constant LCD group showed continued weight loss and improved glycemic control [9].

LCDs consist of 800–1500 calories/day, or a 500–1000 calorie deficit per day, resulting in 1–2 lb of weight loss per week [10]. LCDs are recommended by the ADA [1]. However, for some people, adherence with a LCD is difficult due to psychological factors and logistical issues in food selection and preparation. This has led to the recently increased popularity of meal replacements. Meal replacements provide a defined amount of macronutrients and have been marketed as formula products. They are used on a regular basis to replace 1–3 meals per day and can result in significant weight loss [10]. Although some clinicians are concerned with the amount of sugar in some of the liquid meal replacements, subjects randomized to either a meal replacement containing lactose, fructose and sucrose, or a meal replacement containing oligosaccharides have similar reductions in fasting glucose levels [11]. Furthermore, serum glucose was lower in both of these meal replacement groups when compared to the conventional diet group [11]. Again, this is due to calorie restriction since most meal replacements contain < 300 calories. In another study of meal replacements and T2DM [12], subjects were randomized to a standardized LCD weight loss program or

TABLE 5.1
Dietary Carbohydrates

Starches
Rice
Pasta
Bread
Cereals
Starchy vegetables

Sugars
Lactose in milk and many other dairy products
Fructose, in fruits and fruit juices
Sucrose in table sugars and in many desserts

Fibers found in fruits, vegetables, whole grains, and beans
Cellulose
Hemicellulose
Lignin
Gums
Pectins

---

a meal replacement plus sibutramine for one year. There was a significant reduction of diabetes medications due to improved glycemic control in the intervention group, compared with the control group in the standard program [12].

There is a paucity of studies on the long-term success of calorie-restricted diets in people with or without T2DM. The Diabetes Prevention Study [13] showed long-term success in preventing diabetes in people with impaired glucose tolerance (IGT). By adherence to a low-fat, LCD, and 150 minutes/week of physical activity resulting in 5–7% weight loss, development of frank diabetes was reduced by 58% [13]. In a study comparing the meal-replacement product Slim-Fast® twice daily to a self-selected isocaloric diet, the former group lost more weight and maintained that weight to a greater extent with 4-year follow-up [14]. The National Weight Control Registry, an ongoing study of people who have lost at least 30 lb and kept it off for a year or longer, found that the majority of members consume a LCD (1400 kcal/day) that is low in fat (24% of total daily calories) and eat a regular breakfast [15]. These persons are physically active, expending 2800 calories of physical activity per week, and weigh themselves at least weekly [15]. This study indicates that structured, intensive lifestyle changes, incorporating regular physical activity in conjunction with fat and calorie restriction, are necessary for long-term weight losses of 5–7%. The existing evidence also shows that, although exercise has only a modest effect on weight loss, it is necessary for long-term maintenance of weight loss [13–17]. Exercise also improves insulin sensitivity and lowers blood pressure [1].

Behavioral therapy (helping individuals to modify lifestyles to improve outcomes) is also important as an adjunct therapy for weight loss success [18,19]. Maintenance of weight loss is often unsuccessful: within the first year, most people gain one third to one half of the weight initially lost, so that weight loss from baseline rarely exceeds 5 kg at 1 year [20]. However, maintenance of weight loss is improved with regular contact with a clinician [12,21]. Clinicians have balked at the potential cost of such an intensive program though even less intense programs may still show metabolic improvement. In a Dutch study of people with IGT, physical activity and nutrition information was given to participants every 3 months for 2 years, resulting in a statistically significant reduction of 2-hour glucose levels [22].

CALORIE RESTRICTION—BEYOND WEIGHT LOSS

Calorie restriction of 10–30% below usual intake for prolonged periods drastically reduces the risk of developing diabetes and atherosclerosis [23]. In a study, a calorie restriction group consuming between 1100 and 1950 calories/day (depending upon height, weight, and gender) with 26% protein, 28% fat, and 46% complex carbohydrates, was compared to a control group consuming between 1975 and 3550 calories/day with 18% protein, 32% fat, and 50% carbohydrates, including refined and processed starches. The calorie restricted group had lower LDL-c comparable to the lowest 10% of the population in their respective age groups; higher high-density lipoprotein cholesterol (HDL-c) levels in the 85–90th percentile for middle-aged men, and significantly lower triglycerides than 95% of Americans [23]. The calorie restricted group also had much lower blood pressure, the average being 100/60 mm Hg, compared to an average blood pressure of 130/80 mm Hg in the control group [23]. As expected, the calorie restricted group also showed much lower fasting glucose and insulin levels as well [23].

DIETARY CARBOHYDRATE

Studies of postprandial glycemia in persons with T2DM have shown that the amount of carbohydrates in meals is more important than the source or type of carbohydrates [1,24]. However, the glycemic response is affected by myriad factors [25,26], including:

- The type of sugar (glucose, fructose, sucrose, or lactose)
- The nature of the starch (whether it is a straight chain carbohydrate such as amylose)
- The presence of rapidly digestible branched chain carbohydrates (such as amylopectin)
- The presence of a resistant starch (which enters the colon and acts as a slowly digested carbohydrate in the small intestine)
- The cooking and food-processing method (which results in varying degrees of starch gelatinization, particle size, and cellular form)
- The additional food components that slow digestion (including lectins, phytates, tannins, fats, other lipid components, and proteins)

Some research has shown that both sucrose and fructose may increase serum triglycerides and total cholesterol compared with starch intake, although naturally occurring fructose in fruits and vegetables is unlikely to cause metabolic problems [27]. The use of high-fructose corn syrup (HFCS) as the predominant sweetener in foods and beverages has made the idea of ranking carbohydrate foods, according to their "glycemic index" (GI) very attractive, since the type and amount of carbohydrate influences postprandial glucose levels and, therefore, insulin sensitivity [28].

The GI has become a popular way to quantify the varying glycemic responses to foods of similar carbohydrate content [29,30]. The GI system numerically ranks carbohydrate-containing foods according to the degree to which they raise blood sugar immediately after eating them, and compares them to one of two reference foods (white bread or glucose). The GI is defined as the incremental positive area under the blood glucose curve of 50 g of carbohydrate from a test food divided by the incremental area of 50 g of reference food [31]. A high GI is > 70, medium GI 56–69, and low GI < 55. Certain foods, such as potatoes and many types of bread, increase blood glucose levels more than equivalent caloric quantities of glucose and are therefore considered to have a high GI [26,32]. Other foods, such as pasta and beans, raise blood sugars to a lower extent and are considered to have a low GI [26,32]. Typically, low-GI foods contain starch made up of the less rapidly digested amyloses while high-glycemic foods contain starches made up of the more rapidly digested amylopectins [33]. A food with low GI is more desirable because the absorption of glucose into the blood stream is slower, thereby reducing insulin secretory requirements. Indeed, in a meta-analysis of the GI, A1C was significantly reduced in people with T2DM following a low-GI diet when compared to those who adhered to a high-GI diet [34]. Studies done in T2DM have not shown consistent improvements in A1C, fructosamine, or insulin levels with low-GI diets [35–37]. Furthermore, there is controversy as to the effects of low-GI foods on lipids [34,38]. In a meta-analysis of people who had T2DM, low-GI diets resulted in a decrease in LDL-c as compared with high-GI diets, but there was no change in HDL-c or serum triglycerides.

Although individual carbohydrates have differing glycemic responses, the existing data show weak outcome benefits when adjustments are made for body mass index (BMI) and waist circumference [39]. Furthermore, research has not been carried out on the long-term effects of low-GI diets on glycemic control and lipids. What does seem clear is that a diet can be both high in carbohydrates and low in GI and that such a diet may be beneficial.

A related concept that is gaining recognition is the glycemic load (GL) of foods. The GL is calculated by multiplying the GI of a food by the number of grams of available carbohydrate in that food. [40]. A high GL is > 20, medium 11–19, and low < 10. The GI requires both the portions of the reference food and test foods to contain the same grams of carbohydrates and ignores usual serving size. The GL defines the glycemic effect of a typical serving size of the food and has more practical applicability. Some foods that have a high GI may, in actuality, have a low GL due to the small amount of carbohydrate per serving of food. An example of this is the carrot. In order to reach the standard 50 g of carbohydrate found in carrots, which have a high GI ranging from 95–131, a person would have to eat 1½ lb of carrots. In fact, a single serving of carrots has only 8 available grams of carbohydrate and therefore has a low GL [41].

Diets that adhere to the principles of GI or GL can be difficult to follow because only about 750 different foods have been tested for their GI [33]. Furthermore, one person's glycemic response to a food may be markedly different from another's [31]. In addition, combining foods with different GI numbers, such as baked potatoes with sour cream, results in a different GI number from that of eating each food separately [42]. These drawbacks are consistent with the controversy of whether dietary prescriptions for people with diabetes should incorporate recommendations based on GI and/or GL (see Table 5.2).

Dietary Fiber

The use of foods high in dietary fiber gained popularity when a series of studies were reported indicating the efficacy of fiber in preventing a variety of malignancies, including colon [43] and breast cancers [44], as well as a number of other conditions including diverticular disease [52], cardiovascular disease, [46–49] and diabetes [50–54]. In a review of international recommendations on fiber and diabetes, Anderson et al. [55] compared high-fiber/moderate carbohydrate intakes to low-fiber/moderate carbohydrate intakes, and found higher-fiber diets were associated with reductions in: fasting, postprandial and average plasma glucose, LDL-c, and triglycerides levels. In light of extensive evidence that a high-fiber diet was associated with significant reduction in disease, the Food and Nutrition Board of the Institute of Medicine (IOM) recently recommended dietary fiber intakes of approximately 14 g for every 1000 calories consumed [56]. For adults, this translates to a total daily intake of 38 g for men and 25 g for women < 50 years of age, and 30 g for men and 21 g for women > 50 years of age [56]. To put this in context, the usual American diet contains an estimated 12–18 g/day of fiber, or half of what is recommended by the IOM and others [56–60].

Dietary fiber refers to the edible but indigestible cell walls of plants and is only found in plant-based foods. Dietary fiber resists the acids in the stomach and other digestive enzymes in the intestine and ultimately reaches the large intestine intact. There are two types of dietary fibers: soluble and insoluble. Soluble fiber readily dissolves in water and is fermented by bacteria in the large bowel. Such fiber is found in oat bran, oatmeal, ground flax seeds, beans, and the pulps of certain fruits such as apples. Soluble fiber has been shown to lower blood glucose, presumably by delaying absorption. In a study of patients with T2DM randomized to a high-fiber diet (50 g total, 50% soluble fiber) vs. a low-fiber diet (24 g total, 33% soluble fiber), there was a significant

TABLE 5.2
Glycemic Index (GI) and Glycemic Load (GL) Values for Various Foods[a]

| Food | GI based on | | GL based on | |
	Glucose = 100	Bread = 100	Reference Serving	GL
Coca-Cola®	63	90	250 mL	16
Gatorade®	78	111	250 mL	12
Bagel, frozen, Lender's®	72	103	70 g	25
100% Whole-grain bread	51	73	30 g	7
Cornflakes	92	130	30 g	24
Raisin Bran®	61	87	30 g	12
White rice	52	74	150 g	19
Brown rice	50	72	150 g	16
Apple juice	40	57	250 mL	12
Apple	40	57	120 g	6
Banana, ripe, all yellow	51	73	120 g	13
Grapefruit, raw	25	36	120 g	3
Kidney beans	23	33	150 g	6
Glucerna®, vanilla	31	44	237 mL	7
Spaghetti	58	83	180 g	28
Milk chocolate	49	70	50 g	14
Corn chips	42	60	50 g	11
Cashew nuts	22	31	50 g	3
Carrots (Romania)	16	23	80 g	1
Baked potato	85	121	150 g	26

[a] GI are based on either glucose as a reference or bread as a reference; see Reference [33] for a more extensive list of foods.

decrease in 24-hour plasma glucose, a 12% reduction in plasma insulin, and a decreased urinary glucose excretion in the high-fiber/high-soluble fiber group [61]. In contrast, insoluble fiber does not dissolve in water and is not easily fermented by colonic bacteria. It increases gastrointestinal transit time and contributes to stool bulk. This kind of fiber is found in garden vegetables such as broccoli, turnip greens, collard greens, celery, and squash, as well as in fruit peels and wheat bran. The ADA clinical practice guidelines call for an increased amount of total fiber containing two thirds to three quarters insoluble fiber [62]. However, due to the difficulty in accurately assessing the physiological and chemical effects between soluble and insoluble fiber, the National Academy of Sciences Panel has recommended that the terms "soluble fibers" and "insoluble fibers" gradually be eliminated and replaced by specific beneficial physiological effects of a fiber [63].

There is an inverse relationship between fiber intake and coronary heart disease (CHD) rates [64]. A study that looked prospectively at the relationship between dietary fiber and risk of CHD in 43,757 American male health professionals, 40–75 years of age and free from diagnosed cardiovascular disease and diabetes, showed that each 10-g increment in dietary fiber was associated with a 19% reduction in CHD risk [65]. Another study looking at the effects of fiber on vascular outcomes suggested that cereal fiber is most strongly associated with reduced risk of myocardial infarction and that fruit and vegetable intake significantly correlate with decreased stroke risk [66]. In an analysis of 10 prospective cohort studies from the United States and Europe on dietary fiber intake and coronary heart disease with 6–10 years follow-up, it was found that a high-fiber intake, particularly from cereals and fruit, was inversely associated with risk of CHD [67].

A prospective cohort study showed an inverse association between dietary fiber and cardiovascular disease risk (CVD) and myocardial infarction (MI) [68]. Even though this was not significant after adjusting for cardiovascular risk factors [68], increasing consumption of fiber-rich whole grains, fruits, and vegetables represents a primary preventive strategy against CVD. High-fiber foods also contain higher levels of antioxidant vitamins, folate, phytonutrients, potassium, and lower fat content. These are all characteristic of a "heart-healthy diet" that may reduce cardiovascular disease risk [69].

In summary, there is some evidence that dietary fiber should be part of all diets, for the general population as well as for persons with diabetes. Individuals should be encouraged to incorporate a variety of fiber-containing foods (whole grains, fruits, and vegetables) in their diets. Higher fiber intakes improve glycemic control, lower serum cholesterol, and LDL-c levels [70] and may reduce serum triglyceride values [80]. Fiber intake also reduces risk for CHD [72] and assists in weight management [73].

DIETARY PROTEIN

For persons with diabetes, insulin deficiency and insulin resistance do not affect protein metabolism as severely as they affect carbohydrate metabolism. However, there is mounting evidence that persons exhibiting all ranges of hyperglycemia have increased protein turnover. In one study of 48 subjects, inflammatory cytokines that may regulate production of acute-phase proteins were increased with severe hyperglycemia [74]. Even moderate hyperglycemia can contribute to increased protein turnover [75]. The average daily protein intake in the U.S. is well above levels which might lead to borderline degrees of protein malnutrition. Unfortunately, diabetes may produce a protein-deficient state in populations with lower dietary protein intake. Studies in healthy subjects and persons with well-controlled T2DM have shown that glucose derived from dietary proteins does not appear in the circulation and hence is unlikely to contribute to hyperglycemia. Furthermore, the peak plasma glucose concentration in response to a carbohydrate meal is similar to that of a meal consisting of an equal quantity of carbohydrates with additional protein, suggesting that protein does not alter the absorption or disposition of glucose derived from dietary carbohydrates [1].

DIETARY FATS

A diet high in dietary fat may increase calories, thereby increasing the risk of weight gain, insulin resistance, and worsening glucose control [76,77]. Furthermore, because people with diabetes are at increased risk for CVD, the type of fat consumed will affect risk. Dietary saturated fat is an important determinant of plasma LDL-c, with a 2.7 mg/dL increase in cholesterol per 1% increase in saturated fat content of the diet [78]. Saturated fats (derived from meat and dairy products), and trans-fats, such as vegetable oils treated with hydrogen to increase solidity for food preservation, comprise approximately 11 and 3%, respectively, of the typical diet. These fats raise LDL-c levels, with trans-fats also lowering HDL-c levels [79]. In the Nurses Health Study [80], higher consumption of trans-fats and, to a lesser extent, saturated fats increased the risk of diabetes.

Recent United States Department of Agriculture (USDA) guidelines recommend consumption of less than 10% of calories from saturated fatty acids and less than 300 mg/day of cholesterol, and minimal consumption of trans-fatty acid [81]. Replacement of saturated fats with monounsaturated fatty acids (MUFA) decrease LDL-c and increase HDL-c as well as improve insulin sensitivity [82].

Metabolic studies have shown that when isocaloric, weight-maintaining diets low in saturated fats and enriched with cis-MUFA are employed, LDL-c is consistently lowered [82]. This could be a useful approach for some persons with diabetes [82]. Furthermore, results from the Dietary Approaches to Hypertension (DASH) Trial suggest that a high-fiber, high-carbohydrate, high-cis-MUFA diet has a variety of benefits [83]. The DASH dietary pattern is high in fruits (~5 servings/day), vegetables (~4 servings/day), grains (~8 servings/day), and low-fat dairy products (~2 servings/day) [83]. It emphasizes fish and chicken rather than red meat and is low in total fat (~26%), saturated fat (~7%), cholesterol (~150 mg), sugar, and refined carbohydrates. Sodium intake is also low (3000 mg/day) and body weight is kept constant [83]. The fiber content of the diet is approximately 30 g/day [83]. After 8 weeks, the DASH diet significantly reduces resting systolic and diastolic blood pressure and total LDL-c, compared with a control (typical American) diet [83]. There was also a small but significant decrease in HDL-c concentration (0.09 mmol/L) [83]. Despite the fact that the DASH diet is roughly 55–60% carbohydrate, blood triglyceride concentrations did not increase in weight-stable subjects and were reduced in those who lost weight [83].

Plant stanols (found in some margarines) have fewer calories than fat and consumption of 2–3 g/day reduces LDL-c by about 10% [84]. Fish oils containing omega-3 unsaturated fatty acids (n-3 FA) and plant oils found in soy, canola, and a variety of nuts, decrease triglycerides and increase insulin sensitivity [85], while plant n-3 fatty acids, such as linoleic acid, may lack these beneficial lipid effects [86,87]. However, these effects may disappear if the fat intake increases to > 38% of total calories [88].

ALCOHOL INTAKE

Epidemiological studies indicate that light-to-moderate alcohol ingestion (5–15 g/day) in healthy adults is associated with increased insulin sensitivity and decreased risk of developing T2DM, coronary artery disease, and stroke [89–91]. This level of alcohol intake in adults with diabetes has been shown to decrease the risk for developing coronary artery disease [89,91,92]. The beneficial effect of alcohol may be related to its ability to raise HDL-c [90,92].

Chronic excessive alcohol ingestion is associated with adverse effects including higher blood pressure, both in men and women [89–91]. The ADA recommends that patients with diabetes observe the same precautions as the general public if they choose to drink alcohol. This includes ingestion of not more than two alcohol-containing drinks per day for men and no more than one drink per day for women. One alcohol drink is defined as 12 oz of beer, 5 oz of wine, or 1.5 oz of distilled spirits, each of which contains approximately 15 g of alcohol (7.1 kcal/g). Alcohol use is not recommended for women who are pregnant, patients with history of pancreatitis, or patients with evidence of liver disease, alcohol abuse, depression, or other psychiatric disease, advanced neuropathy, or severe hypertriglyceridemia [89]. Furthermore, alcohol may cause either hyper- or hypoglycemia in persons with diabetes depending upon the amount of alcohol consumed, whether it is consumed with or without food and the medications taken, so that persons with diabetes must exhibit caution [89]. All potential adverse interactions with other medications should be investigated. Perhaps the greatest argument fueling the controversy of whether or not the medical profession should be recommending, or condoning, routine light-to-moderate alcohol intake for health promotion, is the association of alcohol intake with motor vehicle accidents. Clearly, physicians must exercise discretion, on an individualized basis, when broaching this topic with patients.

MICRONUTRIENT INTAKE

It is important for all persons with or without diabetes to consume adequate amounts of vitamins and minerals from natural whole food sources as much as possible [81]. Since diabetes represents a state of increased oxidative stress, and observational studies demonstrate beneficial effects of dietary consumption of antioxidants, there has been considerable interest in using antioxidants in persons with diabetes. However, at present, trials of dietary antioxidants such as vitamin C, vitamin E, selenium, and beta-carotenes have not shown evidence of benefit in the prevention of cardiovascular disease, diabetes, or cancer [93,94]. Furthermore, some studies have suggested adverse effects of antioxidant vitamins [95]. The role of folate supplementation to reduce hyperhomocysteinemia and to reduce cardiovascular events is not clear, with a recent study suggesting that this approach may actually increase the likelihood of restenosis following coronary artery stenting [96]. In another study, homocysteine levels were correlated with the incidence of neuropathy [97]. Okada et al. [98] compared vitamin B12 and vitamin B6 supplementation in dialysis patients with peripheral neuropathy and found vitamin B6 to be effective in reducing symptoms. In another study, vitamin B1 (thiamin) was shown to be effective in reducing the proliferation of arterial smooth muscle cells induced by high glucose and insulin [99]. Deficiencies of minerals such as magnesium, zinc, and chromium may result in carbohydrate intolerance. The interest in chromium as a nutritional enhancement to glucose metabolism can be traced back to the 1950s, when it was suggested that brewer's yeast contained a glucose tolerance factor that prevented diabetes in experimental animals. In a meta-analysis of randomized controlled trials of chromium supplementation in healthy persons and those with diabetes, data showed no effect of chromium on glucose or insulin concentrations in nondiabetic subjects, and inconclusive results in subjects with diabetes [100].

NON-SUCROSE SWEETENERS

Fructose is associated with a lower postprandial rise in blood sugar than sucrose, but may affect lipids adversely [101–103]. Sugar alcohols produce lower glycemic responses compared to sucrose, fructose, and glucose, but can cause diarrhea [27]. Saccharin, aspartame, acesulfame potassium, and sucralose are the four Food and Drug Administration (FDA)-approved nonnutritive artificial sweeteners [104]. Aspartame (NutraSweet®) consists of two amino acids (aspartic acid and pheny-lalanine) and is 180 times as sweet as sucrose. It cannot be used in baking or cooking as it is heat-labile. Saccharin is a nonnutritive sweetener which is still being used despite an FDA warning about its potential for bladder carcinogenicity with long-term use [103]. Sucralose (Splenda®) is 600 times sweeter than sucrose and is heat-stable for cooking and baking. The FDA approved its use in 1998 and concluded that this sweetener did not pose carcinogenic, reproductive, or neuro-logical risk to humans [104].

THE FOOD PYRAMID

A potential meal plan would be one based on the 1996 Food Guide Pyramid of the USDA guidelines for healthy Americans (see Figure 5.1) [105]. This guideline is based on "seven healthy principles" of good nutrition:

1. Eat a variety of foods for energy, protein, vitamins, minerals, and fiber.
2. Balance food intake with physical activity to maintain or improve weight.
3. Choose a diet moderate in salt to reduce the risk of high blood pressure.
4. Eat more grain products, vegetables, and fruits that provide needed phytonutrients, vita-mins, minerals, fiber, and complex carbohydrates.
5. Choose a diet low in fats and cholesterol which would reduce the risk of CVD and certain malignancies and help maintain health weight.
6. Choose a diet moderate in sugars to reduce calories as well as to increase micronutrient intake and decrease the likelihood of dental caries.
7. If you choose to drink alcohol, do so in moderation as alcoholic beverages provide little or no nutritional value and can lead to health problems, accidents, or addiction.

The food pyramid is divided into four levels of foods. The highest and least desirable is that of fats, oils, and sweets, as found in salad dressings, oils, cream, butter, margarine, sugars, soft drinks, candies, and sweet desserts. These foods provide calories with little nutritional value and should be used sparingly. At the next level are (1) products largely derived from animal sources, including milk and dairy, meat, poultry, fish, and eggs, and (2) dry beans and nuts, foods high in protein, calcium, iron, and zinc, but also relatively high in calories and fats. The next level includes vegetables and fruits, while the lowest level, with the highest intake advised, includes a variety of starches. It is clear that although widely used and available [106], there may be problems in following these dietary recommendations for the person with T2DM. For instance, the majority of this diet consists of high glycemic load carbohydrate foods.

The new 2005 dietary guidelines from the Department of Health and Human Services and the Department of Agriculture [81] emphasize weight reduction and healthy weight maintenance, provide

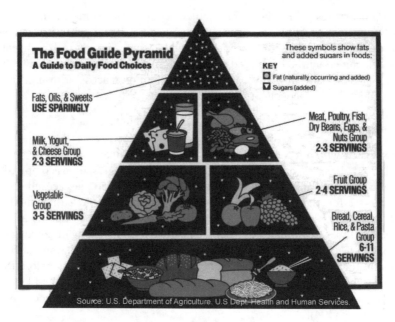

FIGURE 5.1 The Food Pyramid [105].

more precise, unambiguous quantities of recommended foods, set specific limits on fat and salt, and encourage plenty of physical activity. Some of the new dietary recommendations are given below:

- Food groups to encourage:
  - Consume a sufficient amount of fruits and vegetables while staying within energy needs. Two cups of fruit and 2½ cups of vegetables per day are recommended for a reference 2000-calorie intake, with higher or lower amounts depending on the calorie level.
  - Choose a variety of fruits and vegetables each day. In particular, select from all five vegetable subgroups (dark green, orange, legumes, starchy vegetables, and other vegetables) several times a week.
  - Consume three or more ounce-equivalents of whole-grain products per day, with the rest of the recommended grains coming from enriched or whole-grain products. In general, at least half the grains should come from whole grains.
  - Consume 3 cups/day of fat-free or low-fat milk or equivalent milk products.
- Fats: Limit the total fat intake to 20–35% of total daily caloric intake and also keep consumption of trans-fats to a minimum.
- Carbohydrates: Choose fiber-rich fruits, vegetables, and whole grains often.
- Sodium: It is recommended to keep daily salt intake to no more than 1 tsp (approximately 2300 mg).

THE EXCHANGE LIST

There are many approaches, which have been designed to specifically address meal planning for persons with diabetes. A popular method involves teaching persons with diabetes the use of exchange lists. Each exchange is considered in terms of the three different food components, carbohydrates, proteins, and fats, as well as in terms of caloric content (see Table 5.3). All foods

TABLE 5.3
Carbohydrate, Fat, and Protein Exchanges

Food	Carbohydrate (g)	Protein (g)	Fat (g)	Calories
Starch/bread	15	3	trace	80
Meat				
Very lean	—	7	0–1	35
Lean	—	7	3	55
Medium fat	—	7	5	75
High-fat	—	7	8	100
Vegetable	5	2	—	25
Fruit	15	—	—	60
Milk				
Skim	12	8	0–3	90
Low-fat	12	8	5	120
Whole	12	8	8	150
Fat	—	—	5	45

Source: From Reference [113].

in a given exchange have roughly the same amount of these components [107]. The six exchanges are starch/bread, meat, vegetable, fruit, milk, and fat, with sublists of meat and milk products based on fat content. This is an approach that helps persons with diabetes to select from the low-fat groups to whatever extent possible.

DIET AND DIABETES PREVENTION TRIALS

Lifestyle interventions have been shown to significantly reduce the incidence of diabetes. In the Da Qing [108] study of 577 persons with IGT, followed for 6 years with programs of diet, exercise, and combined lifestyle intervention, the likelihood of progression to T2DM was reduced by 42%. Participants in the Finnish Diabetes Prevention Study [109] of 531 persons with IGT followed a diet including whole grains, vegetables, fruit, low-fat milk, and lean meats, and had a 58% reduction in development of T2DM. Similarly, in the U.S., the Diabetes Prevention Program [13] of 3324 persons, including a group receiving a lifestyle intervention, also demonstrated reduced development of T2DM by 58%. In the Nurses Health Study [106], follow-up was available for approximately 95% of the large cohort (85,000 nurses) regarding nutrition, physical activity, and health status. Trans-fats and, to a lesser extent, saturated fats increased the risk of diabetes, while polyunsaturated and monounsaturated fats reduced this risk, with total fat not influencing the risk of developing diabetes at all [110].

The Iowa Women's Health Study [111] analyzed responses to a dietary questionnaire in approximately 40,000 women, suggesting that greater ingestion of whole grains was strongly associated with other lifestyle characteristics and was also associated with lower body weight. When correcting for body weight, there remained a 20% reduction in diabetes risk with whole-grain ingestion [111]. The Health Professional's Study [112] similarly showed that cereal fiber was associated with decreased diabetes risk. Fasting insulin levels and body weight decreased with increasing whole-grain intake in these and other studies [112]. A summary of evidence-based conclusions linking various dietary components with clinical parameters in T2DM is given in Table 5.4.

Specific Diets

Various commercialized diets have been advocated and publicized in medical literature and the general media targeting patients with obesity and T2DM. These diets vary according to macronutrient composition and fad selection strategies for whole foods and dietary supplements. Of these,

TABLE 5.4
Summary of Evidence-Based Conclusions Linking Nutrition and T2DM

Carbohydrates

Recommendation Grade A

Foods containing carbohydrate from whole grains, fruits, vegetables, and low-fat milk should be included in a healthy diet.
With regard to the glycemic effects of carbohydrates, the total amount of carbohydrate in meals or snacks is more
  important than the source or type.
As sucrose does not increase glycemia to a greater extent than isocaloric amounts of starch, sucrose and sucrose-
  containing foods do not need to be restricted by people with diabetes; however, they should be substituted for other
  carbohydrate sources or, if added, covered with insulin or other glucose-lowering medication.
Non-nutritive sweeteners are safe when consumed within the acceptable daily intake levels established by the Food and
  Drug Administration.

Recommendation Grade B

Individuals receiving intensive insulin therapy should adjust their premeal insulin doses based on the carbohydrate
  content of meals.
Although the use of low-glycemic index foods may reduce postprandial hyperglycemia, there is not sufficient evidence
  of long-term benefit to recommend use of low-glycemic index diets as a primary strategy in food/meal planning.
As with the general public, consumption of dietary fiber is to be encouraged; however, there is no reason to recommend
  that people with diabetes consume a greater amount of fiber than other Americans.

Proteins

B-level Evidence

In persons with controlled type-2 diabetes, ingested protein does not increase plasma glucose concentrations, although
  protein is just as potent a stimulant of insulin secretion as carbohydrate.
For persons with diabetes, especially those not in optimal glucose control, the protein requirement may be greater than
  the Recommended Dietary Allowance, but not greater than usual intake.

Fats

A-level Evidence

Less than 10% of energy intake should be derived from saturated fats. Some individuals (i.e., persons with LDL-c
  > 100 mg/dL) may benefit from lowering saturated fat intake to < 7% of energy intake.
Dietary cholesterol intake should be <300 mg/day. Some individuals (i.e., persons with LDL-c > 100 mg/dL) may benefit
  from lowering dietary cholesterol to < 200 mg/day.

B-level Evidence

To lower LDL cholesterol, energy derived from saturated fat can be reduced if weight loss is desirable or replaced with
  either carbohydrate or monounsaturated fat when weight loss is not a goal.
Intake of trans-fatty acids should be minimized.
Reduced-fat diets when maintained long-term contribute to modest loss of weight and improvement in dyslipidemia.
Two to three servings of fish per week provide dietary n-3 polyunsaturated fat and can be recommended.

Source: From Reference [1].

low-carbohydrate diets have become the most popular among patients with T2DM since they claim to address not only glycemic control, but also obesity and lipid metabolism. In a study by Dansinger et al. [113], four different popular diets achieved similar weight loss results, and both cardiac risk reduction and greater weight loss success were attributed more to adherence than to any specific diet. This variability is consistent with the lack of proven efficacy of many fad diets over the long-term [114,115]. A summary of several popular commercial diets used in T2DM is given in Table 5.5 and more detailed discussions are given below.

TABLE 5.5
Some Commercialized Diets and Their Effects on Patients with T2DM

Diet	Premise	Benefit	Risk	Evidence	Grade
Atkins	↑Insulin sensitivity	↓ Weight ↓ Sugars ↓ Lipids	Calciuresis Nephropathy Renal stones	3 (short term) 4 (long term)	D
South Beach	↑ Complex carbs beneficial	↓ Weight	Renal stones	4	
GI Diet	↑ Complex carbs beneficial	↓ Weight	—	4	C
Zone	Optimal insulin production ↑ Protein beneficial	↓ Weight	Calciuresis Nephropathy Renal stones	4	D
Low-fat/ high complex carbohydrate	↓ Fat beneficial for CVD ↑ Complex carbs beneficial	CHD regression ↓ LDL-c ↓ Insulin ↓ Glucose ↓ Weight (short term)	Poor adherence	2	B

See text for abbreviations.

Atkins Diet

Low-carbohydrate diets, like the Atkins Nutritional Approach™, have received a great deal of publicity. The IOM recommends no less than 100 g of carbohydrates per day, per person, while the Atkins Nutritional Approach recommends 20–90 g, depending upon the individual's "metabolic resistance" [116]. The original rationale for the very low carbohydrate approach is that carbohydrate deprivation and the resulting mild ketosis force the body to utilize more stored fat for energy needs, causing greater weight loss. Thus far, however, this does not appear to be valid [114] though there are some data to conclude that low-carbohydrate diets may be more effective in reducing serum triglycerides [117]. The decreased appetite claimed to be due to ketosis is probably more due to the high-protein content [118] as well as orectic peptide signals, including insulin itself.

The Atkins Nutritional Approach also refers to "Atkins Carbohydrate Equilibrium" instead of directly encouraging ketosis. This diet asserts that a high content of refined carbohydrates, typically found in conventional diets, leads to hyperinsulinemia and eventually obesity and T2DM. However, the clinical evidence indicates that regardless of the type of diet, weight loss of only 5–10% is associated with increased insulin sensitivity, decreased fasting blood glucose, improved A1C levels, and decreased medication requirements [119,120].

As originally proposed, the diet consists of a four-step program. Phase 1, or the "induction" phase, typically lasts a minimum of 2 weeks. During this phase, the dieter is expected to severely restrict carbohydrates to less than 20 g/day and take a multivitamin and potassium citrate. All breads, pastas, sugars, fruit, milk, and most vegetables are eliminated from the diet, and carbohydrates are primarily from salads and other nonstarchy vegetables. Trans-fats are avoided and exercise is encouraged. "Healthy proteins" and "natural fats" are eaten ad lib. Phase 2, the "ongoing weight loss" (OWL) phase, allows reintroduction of certain nutrient-dense fiber-rich, low-GI foods. Carbohydrates are adjusted by 5 g/day every week until weight loss is reduced and a moderate rate sustained. This usually occurs with consumption of 40–60 g of carbohydrate per day and is not stopped until the patient is within 5–10 lb of their goal weight. In phase 3, or the "maintenance" phase, carbohydrates are increased by 10 g increments. If the dieter starts gaining weight, the diet's total carbohydrate intake is dropped by 10 g increments until very slight weight loss resumes. During this phase the dieter is encouraged to start planning long-term carbohydrate consumption based on activities and exercise. Finally, in phase 4, which is referred to as the "lifetime maintenance" phase, there is reintegration of a variety of carbohydrates.

The majority of persons who start the Atkins Diet lose a significant amount of weight in the first few weeks primarily due to fluid loss and secondarily due to calorie restriction, since carbohydrates account for the bulk of calories in a normal diet. However, this effect is short-lived, as evidenced by a study comparing the Atkins Diet with a conventional diet over a year [110]. In this study of 63 obese, nondiabetic subjects, there was a 7% loss of body weight by 3–6 months in the low-carbohydrate, high-protein, high-fat (treatment) group, compared with 3% in the conventional diet group—but only 4% loss of body weight by 1 year in the treatment group compared with 3% in the conventional diet group [110]. There was a greater decrease in triglycerides and increase in HDL cholesterol in the Atkins group at 3 months, which was sustained at 1 year [114]. There were no differences in LDL-c at 6 or 12 months [114]. Both groups showed evidence of sustained improvement in insulin sensitivity [114]. Urinary ketones were increased with the Atkins Diet through 3 months, but showed no subsequent significant difference compared with the conventional diet group [114]. In a similar study of 132 persons comparing low-fat and low-carbohydrate diets, of which 39% of participants had T2DM, there was a greater fall in fasting glucose in those randomized to the low-carbohydrate diet. [121]. Since many patients were lost to follow-up in these studies, compromising "intention-to-treat" analyses, the subtle benefits gleaned from the data, particularly early benefits, are weakly substantiated [122].

A synthesis of 107 studies of low-carbohydrate diet with 3268 participants suggests that weight loss with these approaches is principally due to decreased total calorie intake and increased duration of diet adherence, rather than the reduction in carbohydrate content per se [123]. In a study by Johnston et al. [118], energy restricted, isocaloric low-fat diets with varying amounts of protein (15 or 30% total daily calories) promoted weight loss over a 6-week period with the high-protein group experiencing less hunger. In a study by Hertzler et al. [124], reduced-carbohydrate energy bars decreased postprandial glycemia, but not insulin levels, compared with moderate- and high-carbohydrate bars. In sum, the data argue against the premise that low-carbohydrate diets induce greater long-term (12 months) weight loss due to the composition of the diet purported to lower insulin levels. If there is weight loss with low-carbohydrate diets, it is simply due to [1] early depletion of glycogen stores and increased excretion of bound water and [2] decreased total caloric intake. In addition, there are still no short- or long-term data indicating that low-carbohydrate diets are associated with regression of CHD.

Various risks are intrinsic to low-carbohydrate diets though proponents of the Atkins Diet debate the extent of clinical proof for each of these risks. The potential risks include: (1) high protein can induce or contribute to renal hyperfiltration, hyperammonemia, renal stones, calcium loss, osteoporosis, and dehydration; (2) low-carbohydrate intake deprives subjects of recommended amounts of phytonutrients, especially fiber and antioxidants, and can lead to severe ketosis and cardiomyopathy; last, (3) high-fat content can increase LDL-c [125]. Additionally, high-protein diets have the potential to exacerbate nephropathy [126], though in one study this adverse effect was not observed [121].

The lack of fiber in traditional low-carbohydrate diets has prompted the marketing of diets advertising "net carbohydrates" that only include carbohydrates significantly affecting the blood glucose level and do not generally include nonabsorbable carbohydrates, which could now be freely consumed. Fiber, glycerin, and sugar alcohols are not included in net carbohydrate counts since they only minimally affect blood sugar. The subject of low-carbohydrate diets is currently being studied in many centers and, in patients who need the psychological motivation from immediate success, these diets play a role as an "induction" phase to more balanced caloric-restrictive diets. However, the medical profession should not promulgate generalized "carbophobia" since clinical data do not support the preferred use of low-carbohydrate diets over high-fiber high-carbohydrate diets which incorporate balanced reduction in total daily calories and an emphasis on fresh fruit and vegetable intake [127–129].

South Beach Diet

This diet is also marketed as a low-carbohydrate diet, though it contains 40–45% carbohydrates after the first phase [130]. The South Beach Diet consists of three phases and focuses on eliminating highly refined carbohydrates as the predominant source of food [130]. In phase 1, cravings for carbohydrates are supposed to be eliminated via carbohydrate limitation. This phase lasts for about 2 weeks. This is followed by gradual resumption of low-GI, high-fiber foods. Weight loss generally occurs in phase 2 and lasts until ideal weight is achieved. There should be a gradual loss of weight at a rate of 1–2 lb/week. Normal foods with normal portions, avoiding high-carbohydrate, refined, or heavily processed foods, are used in phase 3. The diet menu consists of proteins from low-fat sources, MUFA, green vegetables, berries, and nuts. Low-fat milk products and fat-free yogurt have recently been added to phase 1, and bananas, a low-GI food, have recently been added to phase 2. Clinical data are lacking to support the use of this diet for weight loss or improved glycemic control in T2DM, compared with a general strategy of balanced caloric restriction that incorporates fresh fruit and vegetables.

Glycemic Index (GI) Diet: The Easy Healthy Way to Permanent Weight Loss

This diet streamlines the idea of low vs. high glycemic foods by categorizing them into columns of green, yellow, and red [131]. Similar to Epstein & Squire's pediatric obesity "StopLight Diet" [132], all high-glycemic foods are in the red column, indicating that they are off the diet, no matter what the circumstances. Although this diet does not count calories per se, any weight loss diet that recommends eating low-calorie, low-GI foods such as vegetables and fresh fruit may increase satiety and improve weight loss [133].

One must be careful in selecting low-GI foods. High-fat, high-protein foods such as red meat and whole milk, although having a low GI index, can adversely affect cardiovascular health. This diet recommends low-fat, high-protein foods such as skinless chicken, low-fat dairy and seafood, as well as high-fiber, low-carbohydrate foods. The GI Diet contains a revised food pyramid that indicates approximate serving sizes. This diet plan consists of two phases. In phase 1, which is associated with weight loss, dieters are instructed to limit their food intake to lean meat, no-fat dairy, whole-wheat products, and certain low-GI fruits. Dieters avoid high-GI foods such as high-sugar drinks, high-carbohydrate foods, high-fat dairy and high-fat meat. This diet also recommends that fruits and vegetables replace grains as the most abundant source in the food pyramid, suggesting that half of each meal should consist of fruits and vegetables with low-GI grains and fats kept to a minimum. Phase 2 starts after the dieter reaches target BMI. During this phase the dieter gradually increases calorie consumption by selecting foods such as nuts, low-fat dairy, higher-GI fruits, and vegetables [131]. No scientific studies have been conducted on the GI Diet.

Zone Diet

Barry Sears, Ph.D., created the Zone Diet [134] and claims it is safe for patients with type-1 diabetes mellitus (T1DM) or T2DM. The rationale behind this diet is that by eating the proper ratio of low-density carbohydrates, dietary fat, and protein, the dieter can keep the body's insulin production within a therapeutic zone, making it possible to burn excess body fat (and keep the fat off permanently). He describes the "Zone" as a state of homeostasis that allows a person's body and mind to work together at their ultimate best. In order to get to the "Zone," the diet has to consist of a ratio of macronutrients made up of less total carbohydrates and more protein (40% carbohydrate:30% protein:30% fat) than is usually prescribed by conventional dietary guidelines (55% carbohydrates:15% protein:30% fat). The 0.75 protein:carbohydrate ratio (three times the ratio found in conventional diets) is thought to reduce the insulin:glucagon ratio and eicosanoid metabolism. There are no level 1–3 clinical scientific data to support these claims. It turns out that this ratio may actually increase the area under the insulin curve and, in general, much of the scientific literature at hand contradicts many of the claims advanced by Zone Diet enthusiasts [135]. Furthermore, claims that a Zone composition of sports drinks (i.e., not having the traditionally high-carbohydrate load) is beneficial on performance have not been scientifically substantiated and may even be detrimental [136,137] A similar ratio of protein:carbohydrate is used in the Sugar Busters!™ diet.

From a pragmatic standpoint, each meal or snack in The Zone Diet should contain the following rough portion sizes: protein—size and thickness of your palm; favorable (complex) carbohydrate—two fists; unfavorable (simple) carbohydrate—one fist; fat added (if not in the protein)—a few nuts, some olive oil, or a couple of olives. Patients are instructed to eat five times a day (three meals and two snacks) without more than 5 hours between meals or snacks.

The diet is planned such a way that it provides adequate amounts of protein, essential fat, and micronutrients. The Zone recommends limiting high-density and high-GI carbohydrates such as grains, breads, pasta, rice, and starches. It recommends limiting protein sources that are rich in arachidonic acid, such as egg yolks, fatty red meat, and organ meat. The Zone also recommends regular exercise to promote health. Dr. Sears posits that our diet should mimic the dietary habits of our Neolithic ancestors, which included lean meats, fruits, and vegetables. He notes that human genetics have not changed substantially throughout history and the current western diet is not really suited to our digestive tract. Furthermore, the harmony of the Neolithic people was disrupted 10,000 years ago by the development of agriculture with the introduction of grains and dairy products.

The applicability of hunter-gatherer diets to scientifically-based, health-promoting, and disease-preventing nutritional strategies remains contested. In fact, since dietary intake was not regular throughout the day 10,000 years ago, and consisted of long periods of relative undernutrition punctuated by periods of binging after a kill, one might argue that regular consumption of food altogether is unnatural for humans. Suffice it to say, no conclusive clinical studies have been conducted on the Zone Diet [134] and, at present, it remains a fad diet without any scientific merit.

Very Low-Fat/High-Carbohydrate Diet

Defined usually as 10% or less of total energy from fat and greater than 55% of energy from carbohydrate [138], low-fat and very low-fat diets were originally developed for individuals with heart disease. Low-fat and very low-fat diets that are high in complex carbohydrates, fruits, and vegetables are naturally high in fiber and low in energy density. The original low-fat diets were high in refined carbohydrates and this approach should be avoided in diabetics. Programs such as Dr. Dean Ornish's Program for Reversing Heart Disease [139] and Dr. Nathan Pritikin's Program [140] fall into this category.

There are more data on low-fat diets than high-fat diets. As with all diets for weight loss, low-fat, high-carbohydrate diets reduce LDL cholesterol, blood pressure, insulin levels, and serum glucose, but their effect on serum triglycerides is equivocal. As with most diets, they produce weight loss in the range of 6–10% of baseline weight over a 3–6 month period [151]. Ornish et al. [152] have reported regression of coronary atherosclerosis [153] and successful 1- and 5-year follow-up data for individuals eating a very low-fat diet. Unfortunately, these low-fat diets are extremely difficult to adhere to, especially for a long time.

SYNCHRONIZATION OF DIET WITH MEDICATIONS IN TYPE-2 DIABETES MELLITUS

A common misconception among patients with T2DM and their families is that they must eat at specified times throughout the day to avoid hypoglycemia. In the past, this was true as patients were treated primarily with sulfonylureas and neutral pH–protamine–Hagedorn insulin (NPH).

However, with modern-day diabetes management, more flexible eating patterns are possible depending on the treatment regimen. Sulfonylureas act for up to 24 hours and a patient taking one of these medications must have regular carbohydrate-containing meals to avoid hypoglycemia. The shorter-acting meglitinides can be taken only at mealtimes and meals can be skipped. In addition, repaglinide doses can be adjusted for variability in carbohydrate intake from meal to meal, or day to day. Patients taking only an insulin sensitizer, metformin, or a thiazolidinedione are not at risk for hypoglycemia if a meal is missed, as these medications do not stimulate insulin secretion. Likewise, the α-glucosidase inhibitors do not pose any risk of hypoglycemia and are only taken with a carbohydrate-containing meal.

Various insulin regimens are used to treat patients with T2DM. When a "basal-bolus regimen" is used (i.e., rapid-acting analog pre-meals and long-acting insulin once or twice daily), the flexibility in meal times is greatest as there is only minimal basal insulin acting between meals. Patients have even been able to fast for religious purposes on such a regimen with careful monitoring. Furthermore, patients can adjust the premeal insulin dose based on the carbohydrate content of the meal. Often, to limit the number of injections a patient takes, NPH or a premixed insulin (i.e., 70/30 or 75/25) will be used at breakfast. The purpose is for the intermediate-acting insulin to cover the lunchtime carbohydrates. However, if lunch is delayed or if the patient has a noncarbohydrate lunch, hypoglycemia will occur. Such regimens allow little flexibility for day-to-day variation in carbohydrate intake.

It is essential for the physician to make sure that a T2DM patient who needs to lose weight is not being forced to eat more to avoid hypoglycemia as a result of medications. Medication doses can be lowered or regimens changed to allow for dieting. A patient who has been controlled on a regimen including a sulfonylurea, a meglitinide, or insulin who then begins a low-carbohydrate diet for weight loss is at substantial risk of hypoglycemia and must consult with a physician for medication adjustment prior to starting the diet.

CONCLUSION

The ideal components of a diet for the person with T2DM are no different than the current USDA dietary guidelines [90] for all Americans: primarily, maintain or attain a healthy weight and increase physical activity to 30–90 minutes/day; consume a total of 9 servings of fresh fruit and vegetables (with an emphasis on vegetables); consume approximately 6–9 servings of grains, half of which must be whole grains; and limit saturated fats and eliminate trans-fats. Given the evidence on vitamins, it may be useful to take a multivitamin and, depending upon the age, a calcium supplement may also be warranted, but more studies need to be done before additional supplements can be recommended.

REFERENCES

1. Franz MJ, Bantle JP, and Beebe CA et al., American Diabetes Association. Nutrition principles and recommendations in diabetes, *Diabetes Care*, 27:S36–46, 2004.
2. Henry RR, Wiest-Kent TA, and Scheaffer L et al., Metabolic consequences of very-low-calorie diet therapy in obese non-insulin-dependent diabetic and nondiabetic subjects. *Diabetes* 35:155–164, 1986.
3. Amatruda JM, Richeson JF, and Welle SL et al., The safety and efficacy of a controlled low-energy ('very-low-calorie') diet in the treatment of non-insulin-dependent diabetes and obesity. *Arch Intern Med*, 148:873–877, 1986.
4. Weck M, Hanefeld M, and Schollberg K, Effects of VLCD in obese NIDDM (non-insulin-dependent diabetes) on glucose, insulin, and C-peptide dynamics. *Int J Obes Relat Metab Disord*, 13:159–160, 1989.

5. Anderson JW, Brinkman-Kaplan V, and Hamilton CC et al., Food-containing hypocaloric diets are as effective as liquid-supplement diets for obese individuals with NIDDM, *Diabetes Care,* 17:602–604, 1994.

6. Capstick F, Brooks BA, and Burns CM et al., Very low calorie diet (VLCD): A useful alternative in the treatment of the obese NIDDM patient, *Diabetes Res Clin Pract,* 36:105–111, 1997.

7. Christiansen MP, Linfoot PA, and Neese RA et al., Effect of dietary energy restriction on glucose production and substrate utilization in type-2 diabetes, *Diabetes,* 49:1691–1699, 2000.

8. Kelley DE, Wing R, and Buonocore C et al., Relative effects of calorie restriction and weight loss in noninsulin-dependent diabetes mellitus, *J Clin Endocrinol Metab,* 77 (Suppl 5):1287–1293, 1993.

9. Wing RR, Blair EH, and Bononi P et al., Caloric restriction per se is a significant factor in improvements in glycemic control and insulin sensitivity during weight loss in obese NIDDM patients. *Diabetes Care,* 17:30–36, 1994.

9. National Institutes of Health, National Heart, Lung, and Blood Institute, *Clinical Guidelines on the Identification, Evaluation, and Treatment of Overweight and Obesity in Adults,* Bethesda, MD: National Institutes of Health, 2002, NIH Publication No. 02-4084.

10. Ashley, JM, St. Jeor ST, and Perumean-Chaney SP et al., Meal replacements in weight intervention, *Obes Res,* 9:312S–320S, 2001.

11. Yip I, Go VL, and DeShields S et al., Liquid meal replacements and glycemic control in obese type-2 diabetes patients, *Obes Res,* 9:341S–347S, 2001.

12. Redmon JB, Raatz SK, and Reck KP et al., One-year outcome of a combination of weight loss therapies for subjects with type-2 diabetes, A randomized trial. *Diabetes Care,* 26:2505–2511, 2003.

13. Knowler WC, Barrett-Conner E, and Fowler SE et al., Reduction in the incidence of type-2 diabetes with lifestyle intervention or metformin. *N Engl J Med,* 346:393–403, 2002.

14. Fletchner-Mors M, Ditschuneit HH, and Johnson TD et al., Metabolic and weight loss effects of long-term dietary intervention in obese patients, Four-year results, *Obes Res,* 8:399–402, 2000.

15. Wing RR and Hill JO, Successful weight loss maintenance, *Ann Rev Nutr,* 21:323–341, 2001.

16. Ewbank PP, Darga LL, and Lucas CP, Physical activity as a predictor of weight maintenance in previously obese subjects, *Obes Res,* 3:257–263, 1995.

17. Wing RR, Venditti E, and Jakicic JM et al., Lifestyle intervention in overweight individuals with a family history of diabetes, *Diabetes Care,* 21:350–359, 1998.

18. Wadden TA, Brownell KD, and Foster GD, Obesity: Responding to the global epidemic, *J Consult Clin Psychol,* 70:510–525, 2002.

19. Wadden TA, Behavioral treatment, In: Foster GD and Nonas CA, Eds., *Managing Obesity: A Clinical Guide,* American Diabetes Association, 65–75, 2004.

20. Hensrud DD, Dietary treatment and long-term maintenance in type-2 diabetes, *Obes Res,* (Suppl 4):348S–353S, 2001.

21. Perri MG, McAllister DA, and Gange JJ et al., Effects of four maintenance programs on the long-term management of obesity, *Clin Psychol,* 56:529–534, 1988.

22. Mensink M, Blaak E, and Corpeleijn E et al., Lifestyle intervention according to general recommendations improves glucose tolerance, *Obes Res,* 11:1588–1596, 2003.

23. Fontana L, Meyer TE, and Klein S et al., Long-term calorie restriction is highly effective in reducing the risk for atherosclerosis in humans, *Proc Natl Acad Sci USA,* 101:6659–63, 2004.

24. Bantle JP, Sawnson JE, and Thomas W et al., Metabolic effects of dietary sucrose in type-II diabetic subjects, *Diabetes Care,* 16:1301–1305, 1993.

25. Jenkins DJ, Wolever TM, and Taylor RH et al., Exceptionally low blood glucose response to dried beans: Comparison with other carbohydrate foods, *Br Med J,* 281:578–80, 1980.

26. Jenkins DJ, Wolever TM, and Jenkins AL, et al., Low glycemic response to traditionally processed wheat and rye products: Bulgur and pumpernickel bread, *Am J Clin Nutr,* 43:516–20, 1986.

27. Barnett JP and Garg M, Preventing cardiovascular complications in diabetes, In: Carson JS, Burke FM, and Hark LA, Eds., *Cardiovascular Nutrition,* American Dietetic Association, 89–212, 2004.

28. Ludwig DS, The glycemic index: Physiological mechanisms relating to obesity, diabetes, and cardiovascular disease, *JAMA,* 287:2414–2432, 2002.

29. John L, Sievenpiper MS, and Vuksan V, Commentary, Glycemic index in the treatment of diabetes: The debate continues, *J Am Coll Nutr,* 23:1–4, 2004.

30. Jenkins DJ, Wolever TM, and Taylor RH et al., Glycemic index of foods: A physiological basis for carbohydrate exchange, *Am J Clin Nutr,* 34:362–366, 1981.

31. Coulston, AM, Hollenbeck CB, and Swislocki AL et al., Effect of source of dietary carbohydrate on plasma glucose and insulin responses to mixed meals in subjects with NIDDM, *Diabetes Care,* 10:395–400, 1987.

32. Jenkins DJ, Wolever TM, and Taylor RH et al., Exceptionally low blood glucose response to dried beans: Comparison with other carbohydrate foods, *Br Med J,* 281:578–580, 1980.

33. Foster-Powell K, Holt SHA, and Brand-Miller JC, International table of glycemic index and glycemic load values, *Am J Clin Nutr,* 76:5–56, 2002.

34. Opperman AM, Venter CS, and Oosthuizen W et al., Meta-analysis of the health effects of using the glycaemic index in meal-planning, *Br J Nutr,* 92:367–381, 2004.

35. Franz MJ, Carbohydrate and diabetes: Is the source or the amount of more importance? *Curr Diab Rep,* 1:177–86, 2001.

36. Jenkins DJ, Kendall CW, and Augustin LS et al., High-complex carbohydrate or lente carbohydrate foods? *Am J Med,* 13 (Suppl 9B):30S–37S, 2002.

37. Heilbronn LK, Noakes M, and Clifton PM, The effect of high- and low-glycemic index energy restricted diets on plasma lipid and glucose profiles in type-2 diabetic subjects with varying glycemic control, *J Am Coll Nutr,* 21:120–7, 2002.

38. Sloth B, Krog-Mikkelsen I, and Flint A et al., No difference in body weight decrease between a low-glycemic-index and a high-glycemic-index diet but reduced LDL cholesterol after 10-wk ad libitum intake of the low-glycemic-index diet, *Am J Clin Nutr,* 80:337–47, 2004.

39. Hodge AM, English DR, and O'Dea K et al., Glycemic index and dietary fiber and the risk of type-2 diabetes, *Diabetes Care,* 27:2701–2706, 2004.

40. Liu S, Manson JE, and Stampfer MJ et al., Dietary glycemic load assessed by food-frequency questionnaire in relation to plasma high-density-lipoprotein cholesterol and fasting plasma triacylglycerols in postmenopausal women, *Am J Clin Nutr,* 73:560–566, 2001.

41. Brody JE, Personal health: Fear not that carrot, potato, or ear of corn, *New York Times,* June 11, 2002.

42. Pi-Sunyer FX, Glycemic index and disease, *Am J Clin Nutr,* 76:290S–298S, 2002.

43. Kim YI, AGA technical review: Impact of dietary fiber on colon cancer occurrence, *Gastroenterology,* 2000;118:35–57, 2002.

44. Gerber M, Fibre & breast cancer, *Eur J Cancer Prev,* 7:S63–S67, 1998.

45. West AB and Losada M, The pathology of diverticulosis coli, *J Clin Gastroenterol,* 38(5 Suppl):S11–16, 2004.

46. Anderson JW, Chen WJ, and Sieling B, Hypolipidemic effects of high-carbohydrate, high-fiber diets, *Metabolism,* 29:551–558, 1980.

47. Anderson JW, Zeigler JA, and Deakins DA, et al., Metabolic effects of high-carbohydrate, high-fiber diets for insulin-dependent diabetic individuals, *Am J Clin Nutr,* 4:936–943, 1991.

48. Anderson JW, Garrity TF, and Wood CL et al., Prospective, randomized, controlled comparison of the effects of low-fat and low-fat plus high-fiber diets on serum lipid concentrations, *Am J Clin Nutr,* 56:887–894, 1992.

49. Rimm EB, Ascherio A, and Giovannucci E et al., Vegetable, fruit and cereal fiber intake and risk of coronary heart disease among men, *JAMA,* 275:447–451, 1996.

50. Salmeron J, Manson JE, and Stampfer MJ et al., Dietary fiber, glycemic load and risk of non-insulin-dependent diabetes mellitus in women, *JAMA,* 277:472–477, 1997.

51. Salmeron J, Ascherio A, and Rimm EB et al., Dietary fiber, glycemic load, and risk of NIDDM in men, *Diabetes Care,* 20:545–550, 1997.

52. Meyer KA, Kushi LH, and Jacobs DR et al., Carbohydrates, dietary fiber, and incident type-2 diabetes in older women, *Am J Clin Nutr,* 71:921–930, 2000.

53. Fung TT, Hu FB, and Pereira MA, et al., Whole-grain intake and the risk of type-2 diabetes, A prospective study in men, *Am J Clin Nutr,* 76:535–40, 2002.

54. Ludwig DS, The glycemic index physiological mechanisms relating to obesity, diabetes, and cardiovascular disease, *JAMA,* 287:2414–2423, 2002.

55. Anderson JW, Randles KM, and Kendall CWC et al., Carbohydrate and fiber recommendations for individuals with diabetes, A quantitative assessment and meta-analysis of the evidence, *J Am Coll Nutr,* 23:5–17, 2004.

56. Institute of Medicine, Dietary, Functional, and Total Fiber, Dietary Reference Intakes for Energy, Carbohydrate, Fiber, Fat, Fatty Acids, Cholesterol, Protein, and Amino Acids, Washington, D.C.: National Academies Press, 265–334, 2002.
57. American Diabetes Association: Nutrition recommendations and principles for people with diabetes mellitus, *Diabetes Care,* 24(Suppl 1):S44–46, 2001.
58. Krauss RM, Eckel RH, and Howard B, et al., AHA dietary guidelines, revision 2000: A statement for healthcare professionals from the nutrition committee of the American Heart Association, *Circulation,* 102:2296–2311, 2000.
59. U.S. Department of Agriculture and U.S. Department of Health and Human Services, Dietary Guidelines for Americans, 5th ed., Home and Garden Bulletin, No. 232, Washington, D.C., 2000.
60. Food and Nutrition Board and the Institute of Medicine, Dietary Reference Intakes for Energy, Carbohydrate, Fiber, Fat, Fatty Acids, Cholesterol, Protein, and Amino Acids (Macronutrients), National Academies Press, Washington, D.C., 2002.
61. Chandalia M, Garg A, and Lutjohann D et al., Beneficial effects of high dietary fiber intake in patients with type-2 diabetes mellitus, *N Engl J Med,* 342:1392–1398, 2000.
62. American Dietetic Association Position Statement, Health implications of dietary fiber, *J Am Diet Assoc,* 102:993–1000, 2002.
63. Panel on the Definition of Dietary Fiber, Standing Committee on the Scientific Evaluation of Dietary Reference Intakes, Food and Nutrition Board, Dietary Reference Intakes Proposed Definition of Dietary Fiber, National Academies Press, 1–64, 2001.
64. Khaw KT and Barrett-Connor E, Dietary fiber and reduced ischemic heart disease mortality rates in men and women, A 12-year prospective study, *Am J Epidemiol,* 126:1093–1102, 1987.
65. Rimm EB, Ascherio A and Giovannucci E et al., Vegetable, fruit, and cereal fiber intake and risk of coronary heart disease among men, *JAMA,* 275:447–451, 1996.
66. Gillman MW, Cupples LA, and Gagnon D et al., Protective effect of fruits and vegetables on development of stroke in men, *JAMA,* 273:1113–1117, 1996.
67. Pereira MA, O'Reilly E, and Augustsson K et al., Dietary fiber and risk of coronary heart disease, A pooled analysis of cohort studies, *Arch Intern Med,* 164:370–376, 2004.
68. Liu S, Burning J, and Sesso H et al., A prospective study of dietary fiber intake and risk of cardiovascular disease among women, *J Am Coll Cardiol,* 39:49–56, 2002.
69. Bazzano LA, Dietary intakes of fruits and vegetables and risk of cardiovascular disease, *Curr Atheroscler Rep,* 5:492–499, 2003.
70. Brown L, Rosner B, and Willett WW et al., Cholesterol-lowering effects of dietary fiber, A meta-analysis, *Am J Clin Nutr,* 69:30–42, 1999.
71. Anderson JW, Dietary fiber prevents carbohydrate-induced hypertriglyceridemia, *Curr Artheroscler Rep,* 2:536–541, 2000.
72. Anderson JW, Hanna TJ, and Peng X et al., Whole grain foods and heart disease risk, *J Am Coll Nutr,* 19:291S–9S, 2000.
73. Food and Drug Administration, Wholegrain Foods Authoritative Statement Claim Notification docket, Washington, DC, 99P-2209P, 1999.
74. Stentz FB, Umpierrez GE, and Cuervo R et al., Proinflammatory cytokines, markers of cardiovascular risks, oxidative stress, and lipid peroxidation in patients with hyperglycemic crises, *Diabetes,* 43:2079–2086, 2004.
75. Franz MJ, Protein and diabetes: Much advice, little research, *Curr Diabetes Rep,* 2:457–464, 2002.
76. Riccardi G, Giacco R, and Rivellese AA, Dietary fat, insulin sensitivity, and the metabolic syndrome, *Am J Clin Nutr,* 23:447–456, 2004.
77. Tremblay A, Dietary fat and body weight set point, *Nut Rev,* 62:S75–77, 2005.
78. Fetcher ES, Foster N, and Anderson JT et al., Quantitative estimation of diets to control serum cholesterol, *Am J Clin Nutr,* 20:475–492, 1967.
79. de Roos NM, Bots ML, and Katan MB, Replacement of dietary saturated fatty acids by trans fatty acids lowers serum HDL cholesterol and impairs endothelial function in healthy men and women, *Arterioscler Thromb Vasc Biol,* 21:1233–1237, 2001.
80. Mozaffarian D, Pischon T, and Hankinson SE et al., Dietary intake of trans fatty acids and systemic inflammation in women, *Am J Clin Nutr,* 79:606–12, 2004.

81. U.S. Department of Agriculture, 2005 Dietary Guidelines Advisory Committee, Nutrition and your health: Dietary guidelines for Americans, http://www.health.gov/dietaryguidelines/dga2005/report/, Accessed on February 26, 2005.
82. Garg A, Bonanome A, and Grundy SM et al., Comparison of a high-carbohydrate diet with a high-monounsaturated-fat diet in patients with non-insulin-dependent-diabetes mellitus, *New Engl J Med,* 319:829–834, 1988.
83. Harsha DW, Sacks FM, and Obarzanek E et al., Effect of dietary sodium intake on blood lipids, Results from the DASH-sodium trial, *Hypertension,* 43:393–398, 2004.
84. Law M, Plant sterol and stanol margarines and health, *BMJ,* 320:861–864, 2000.
85. Kris-Etherton PM, Zhao G, and Binkoski AE et al., The effects of nuts on coronary heart disease risk, *Nutr Rev,* 59:103–111, 2001.
86. Hu FB, Bronner L, and Willett WC et al., Fish and omega-3 fatty acid intake and risk of coronary heart disease in women, *JAMA,* 287:1815–1821, 2002.
87. Zambon D, Sabate J, and Munoz S et al., Substituting walnut for monounsaturated fat improves the serum lipid profile of hypercholeterolemic men and women, A randomized crossover trial, *Ann Intern Med,* 132:538–546, 2000.
88. Riccardi G and Rivellese AA, Dietary treatment of the metabolic syndrome—the optimal diet, *Br J Nutr,* 83(Suppl 1):S143–148, 2000.
89. van de Wiel A, Diabetes mellitus and alcohol, *Diabetes Metab Res Rev,* 20:263–267, 2004.
90. Pownall HJ, Alcohol: Lipid metabolism and cardioprotection, *Curr Atheroscler Rep,* 4:107–112, 2002.
91. Shai I, Rimm EB, and Schulze MB et al., Moderate alcohol intake and markers of inflammation and endothelial dysfunction among diabetic men, *Diabetologia,* 47:1760–1767, 2004.
92. Avogaro A, Watanabe RM, and Dall'Arche A et al., Acute alcohol consumption improves insulin action without affecting insulin secretion in type-2 diabetic subjects, *Diabetes Care,* 27:1369–1374, 2004.
93. Dagenais GR, Marchioli R, and Yusuf S et al., Beta-carotene, vitamin C, and vitamin E and cardiovascular diseases, *Curr Cardiol Rep,* 4:293–299, 2000.
94. Yusuf S, Dagenais G, and Pogue J et al., Vitamin E supplementation and cardiovascular events in high-risk patients, The Heart Outcomes Prevention Evaluation Study Investigators, *N Engl J Med,* 342:154–160, 2000.
95. Miller ER, Pastor-Barriuso P, and Dlal D et al., Meta-analysis of high-dosage vitamin E supplement may increase all-cause mortality, *Ann Int Med,* 142:37–46, 2005.
96. Lange H, Suryapranata H, and De Luca G et al., Folate therapy and in-stent restenosis after coronary stenting, *N Engl J Med,* 350:2673–2681, 2004.
97. Ambrosch A, Dierkes J, and Lobmann R et al., Relation between homocysteinaemia and diabetic neuropathy in patients with type-2 diabetes mellitus, *Diabetic Med,* 18:185–192, 2001.
98. Okada H, Moriwaki K, and Kanno Y et al., Vitamin B6 supplementation can improve peripheral polyneuropathy in patients with chronic renal failure on high-flux haemodialysis and human recombinant erythropoietin, *Nephrol Dial Transplant,* 15:1410–1413, 2000.
99. Avena R, Arora S, and Carmody BJ et al., Thiamine (Vitamin B1) protects against glucose- and insulin-mediated proliferation of human infragenicular arterial smooth muscle cells, *Ann Vasc Surg,* 14:37–43, 2000.
100. Althuis MD, Jordan NE, and Ludington EA et al., Glucose and insulin responses to dietary chromium supplements, A meta-analysis, *Am J Clin Nutr,* 76:148–155, 2002.
101. Malerbi DA, Paiva ESA, and Duarte AL et al., Metabolic effects of dietary sucrose and fructose in type II diabetic subjects, *Diabetes Care,* 19:1249–1256, 1996.
102. Fried SK and Rao SP, Sugars, hypertriglyceridemia and cardiovascular disease, *Am J Clin Nutr,* 78:873S–880S, 2003.
103. Bantle JP, Raatz SK, and Thomas W et al., Effects of dietary fructose on plasma lipids in healthy subjects, *Am J Clin Nutr,* 72:1128–1134, 2000.
104. American Dietetic Association, Position of the American Dietetic Association: Use of nutritive and nonnutritive sweeteners, *J Am Dietet Assoc,* 104:355–375, 2004.
105. U.S. Department of Agriculture Center for Nutrition Policy and Promotion, The food guide pyramid, Home and Garden Bulletin, No. 252, October 1996, http://www.usda.gov/cnpp/pyrabklt.pdf, Accessed on February 27, 2005.

106. Davis CA, Britten P, and Myers EF, Past, present, and future of the Food Guide Pyramid, *J Am Diet Assoc,* 101:881–885, 2001.

107. Bowes SK, Diabetes and nutrition, http://www.nursingceu.com/NCEU/courses/dmdiet/, Accessed on February 27, 2005.

108. Pan XR, Li GW, and Hu YH et al., Effects of diet and exercise in preventing NIDDM in people with impaired glucose tolerance, The Da Qing IGT and Diabetes Study, *Diabetes Care,* 20:537–544, 1997.

109. Lindstrom J, Louheranta A, and Mannelin M et al., Finnish Diabetes Prevention Study Group, The Finnish Diabetes Prevention Study (DPS): Lifestyle intervention and 3-year results on diet and physical activity, *Diabetes Care,* 26:3230–3236, 2003.

110. Hu FB, Manson JE, and Stampfer MJ et al., Diet, lifestyle, and the risk of type-2 diabetes mellitus in women, *N Engl J Med,* 345:790–797, 2001.

111. Meyer KA, Kushi LH, and Jacobs DR et al., Carbohydrates, dietary fiber, and incident type-2 diabetes in older women, *Am J Clin Nutr,* 71:921–930, 2000.

112. McCullough M, Feskanich D, and Rimm E et al., Adherence to the Dietary Guidelines for Americans and risk of major chronic disease in men, *Am J Clin Nutr,* 72:122–131, 2000.

113. Dansinger ML, Gleason JA, and Griffith JL et al., Comparison of the Atkins, Ornish, Weight Watchers, and Zone diets for weight loss and heart disease risk reduction, *JAMA* 293:43–53, 2005.

114. Foster GD, Wyatt HR, and Hill JO, et al., A randomized trial of a low-carbohydrate diet for obesity, *N Engl J Med,* 348:2082–2090, 2003.

115. Nonas CA and Foster GD, Popular diets in the management of obesity, In: Carson JH, Burke FM, and Hark L, Eds., *Cardiovascular Nutrition,* American Diabetes Association, 265–280, 2004.

116. Atkins RC, *Dr. Atkins' New Diet Revolution,* New York: HarperCollins, 2002.

117. Layman DK, Boileau RA, and Erickson DJ, et al., A reduced ratio of dietary carbohydrate to protein improves body composition and blood lipid profiles during weight loss in adult women, *J Nutr,* 133:411–417, 2003.

118. Johnston CS, Tjonn SL, and Swan PD, High-protein, low-fat diets are effective for weight loss and favorably alter biomarkers in healthy adults, *Nutrition,* 134:586–591, 2004.

119. Wing RR, Koeske R, and Epstein LH et al., Long-term effects of modest weight loss in type-II diabetic patients, *Arch Int Med,* 147:1749–1753, 1987.

120. McLaughlin T, Abbasi F, and Kim HS et al., Relationship between insulin resistance, weight loss, and coronary heart disease in healthy, obese women, *Metabolism,* 50:795–800, 2001.

121. Samaha FF, Iqbal N, and Seshadri P et al., A low-carbohydrate as compared with a low-fat diet in severe obesity, *N Engl J Med,* 348:2074–2081, 2003.

122. Ware JH, Interpreting incomplete data in studies of diet and weight loss, *N Engl J Med,* 348:2136–2137, 2003.

123. Bravata DM, Sanders L, and Huang J et al., Efficacy and safety of low-carbohydrate diets: A systematic review, *JAMA,* 289:1837–1850, 2003.

124. Hertzler SR and Kim Y, Glycemic and insulinemic responses to energy bars of differing macronutrient composition in healthy adults, *Med Sci Monit,* 9:CR84–90, 2003.

125. Larosa JC, Fry AG, and Muesing R et al., Effects of high-protein, low-carbohydrate dieting on plasma lipoproteins and body weight, *J Am Diet Assoc,* 77:264–270, 1980.

126. Gannon MC, Nuttall FQ, and Saeed A et al., An increase in dietary protein improves the blood glucose response in persons with type-2 diabetes, *Am J Clin Nutr,* 78:734–741, 2003.

127. Bonow RO and Eckel RH, Diet, obesity, and cardiovascular risk, *N Engl J Med,* 348:2057–2058, 2003.

128. Lara-Castro C and Garvey WT, Diet, insulin resistance, and obesity: Zoning in on data for Atkins dieters living in South Beach, *J Clin Endocrinol Metab,* 89:4197–4205, 2004.

129. Stephenson J, Low-carb, low-fat diet gurus face off, *JAMA,* 289:1772–1771, 2003.

130. Agaston A, *The South Beach Diet,* New York: Rodale Press, 2003.

131. Gallop R, *The GI Diet: The Easy Healthy Way to Permanent Weight Loss,* New York: Workman, 2003.

132. Epstein L and Squires S, *The Stoplight Diet,* New York: Little, Brown & Co., 1988.

133. Rolls BJ, Ello-Martin JA, and Tohill BC, What can intervention studies tell us about the relationship between fruit and vegetable consumption and weight management? *Nutr Rev,* 62:1–17, 2004.

134. Sears B and Lawren B, *The Zone: A Dietary Road Map to Lose Weight Permanently: Reset Your Genetic Code: Prevent Disease: Achieve Maximum Physical Performance,* New York: Regan Books, 1995.

135. Cheuvront SN, The Zone Diet phenomenon: A closer look at the science behind the claims, *J Am Coll Nutr,* 22:9–17, 2003.
136. Jarvis M, McNaughton L, and Seddon A et al., The acute 1-week effects of the Zone diet on body composition, blood lipid levels, and performance in recreational athletes, *J Strength Cond Res,* 16:50–57, 2002.
137. Cheuvront SN, The Zone diet and athletic performance, *Sports Med,* 27:213–228, 1999.
138. Freedman MR, King J, and Kennedy E, Popular diets, A scientific review, *Obes Res,* 9:1S–40S, 2001.
139. Ornish D, *Eat More, Weigh Less: Dr, Dean Ornish's Life Choice Program for Losing Weight Safely While Eating Abundantly,* New York: Perennial Currents, 2001.
140. Pritikin, N, *Pritikin Permanent Weight Loss Manual,* New York: Bantam, 1982.
141. Kennedy E, Dietary approaches: Overview, In: Foster GD and Nonas CA, Eds., *Managing Obesity: A Clinical Guide,* American Diabetes Association, Chicago, 91–97, 2004.
142. Ornish D, Brown SE, and Scherwitz LW et al., Can lifestyle changes reverse coronary heart disease? The Lifestyle Heart Trial, *Lancet,* 336:129–133, 1990.
143. Ornish D, Scherwitz LW, and Billings JH et al., Intensive lifestyle changes for reversal of coronary heart disease, *JAMA,* 280:2001–2007, 1998.

6 Nutrition and Type-1 Diabetes Mellitus

Stuart Weiss

CONTENTS

Type-1 diabetes mellitus (T1DM) is a complex disorder characterized by the autoimmune destruction of the insulin producing β-cells of the pancreas. With the loss of insulin production, the transport of glucose into cells is impaired and hyperglycemia results. Over time, this can lead to microvascular and macrovascular complications. For many years, several dietary factors have been thought to trigger or suppress the autoimmune mechanisms, which result in T1DM. These include cow's milk [1], the timing of cereal exposure to the immature gut [2], nitrates or nitrites [3], and vitamin D deficiency [4]. Also, population studies show a link between vegetables infested with Streptomyces and an increased incidence of T1DM [5]. Gastrointestinal immunologic mechanisms have been proposed as possibly causative in the autoimmune destruction of the β-cells of the pancreas. No conclusive data is yet available but population studies continue to perpetuate theoretical arguments for dietary causality in T1DM.

The variability in the rate of progression of T1DM and development of complications calls into question the relationship between environment and genetics. This relationship is complex and poorly understood. There are type-1 diabetics with good glycemic control who develop complications as well as those with poor control who, for a long period of time, remain complication-free. It was not until publication of the Diabetes Control and Complications Trial (DCCT) [6] that the relationship between glucose control and the incidence of diabetes complications was clearly established. Some researchers have postulated that the composition of a patient's diet may influence the development of microvascular complications. For example, diets rich in foods containing high levels of advanced glycation endproducts (AGE), implicated in the development of microvascular complications, are associated with high blood levels of AGE in people with diabetes [7].

The scientific literature related to the nutritional approach to T1DM, and the role of nutrients other than carbohydrates in the natural history of T1DM, is sparse. There is also limited evidence-based consensus on managing dietary protein in patients with diabetic nephropathy. Likewise, dietary lipids and their cardiovascular impact are not clearly defined. Even the most basic questions about diet and glucose management are subject to controversy. As the scientific community continues to address basic questions about the etiology of disorders associated with T1DM, we are left with the pragmatic challenge of glycemic control. Patients must be taught to balance the glucose derived from foods they eat with the exogenous insulin they administer. This chapter will use the limited extant scientific data and clinical experience to establish nutritional strategies for controlling glucose levels in patients with T1DM.

INSULIN REGIMENS

The control of blood glucose levels in T1DM is best understood as an attempt to synchronize the peak of the derived glucose load from a meal to the peak of the insulin used to meet that glucose challenge. In the past, coordinating the timing of wide peaks in insulin action of available animal and human preparations was difficult. With newer synthetic insulin preparations, the more rapid and shorter duration peaks in insulin action more easily synchronize with meal-derived glucose. The rapid-acting insulin analogs aspart, lispro, and glulisine provide better glucose control and less hypoglycemia compared to regular insulin, and are recommended for most patients [8,9]. These insulin analogs are used in combination with basal insulin preparations ("basal-bolus regimen"). Small and steady amounts of basal insulin cover non-food-related insulin requirements due to glycogenolysis and gluconeogenesis in the fasting and postabsorptive states. The basal insulin analogs glargine and possibly detemir fulfill this role reasonably well. With the introduction of these long-acting, peakless insulins, it is easier to separate basal and prandial insulin requirements. Previously, when intermediate-acting insulins were used as a basal, they also covered some carbohydrates because of peaks in their action. Thus, the technique of carbohydrate counting, often previously reserved for patients on insulin pumps, is now the standard of care for most patients with T1DM. Furthermore, as compared with NPH, the insulin analogs glargine [8] and detemir [9] lower the risk of nocturnal hypoglycemia in patients with T1DM on a basal-bolus regimen. Insulin pump therapy is an acceptable and often preferred alternative to multiple daily injections for patients with T1DM.

MODERN DIABETES MANAGEMENT

While the newer insulins facilitate glycemic control, the American diet has become much more varied and complex. We are presented with food choices from all over the world as well as new chemically altered foods that can be digested either more slowly or more rapidly than unaltered foods. The glycemic index (GI) and glycemic load (GL), measures of the potential for a particular food to raise blood glucose levels, are only recently becoming part of an acceptable approach to understanding how quickly a food will be converted into glucose in the circulation. There are an enormous variety of foods for which carbohydrate amounts and GI are not readily available. We are often faced with food combinations that give rapid or, more commonly, slowed absorption of carbohydrates. This, along with gastrointestinal factors such as diabetic gastroparesis, can alter the time course of absorption and conversion of a meal's carbohydrates to glucose. Ultimately, this makes a purely scientific attempt at glucose control difficult.

Technological advances in home glucose monitoring systems have empowered patients to have greater control over their glucose levels throughout the day. Glucometers are faster, more precise, and easier to use than ever before. Continuous glucose monitoring systems currently are imperfect but available and highly useful. Numerous software programs are available that allow patients to track carbohydrate intake, insulin doses, and downloadable glucometer results. Thus, in very general terms, complete normalization of glucose is not possible but reasonable goals are more easily achieved than in past years.

CARBOHYDRATE COUNTING

Most clinicians who treat patients with T1DM accept carbohydrate counting as a preferred method for calculating an insulin dose prior to a meal. Carbohydrate counting is an approach to glycemic control which focuses on the carbohydrate ingestion as the primary determinant of blood glucose. The patient is taught to match insulin doses to carbohydrate amounts consumed. This method provides the greatest flexibility in terms of food choices, portion size, and timing of meals. Increasing the carbohydrate amount of a meal does not result in deterioration of control as long as the pre-meal insulin dose is adjusted accordingly [10]. An alternate approach is to give patients a meal plan based on carbohydrate servings or "exchanges" along with a fixed pre-meal insulin dose. This approach to glucose control can be a limited technique unless patients maintain a consistent carbohydrate intake from day to day. The standard diet 30 years ago was fairly constant in its nutritional composition: the carbohydrate, protein, and fat intake did not vary much from day to day. Now with readily available cheap, flavorful, high-carbohydrate "fast foods," a standing pre-meal insulin dosing approach is antiquated. In one study, this simpler option was least preferred by patients, compared to carbohydrate counting, meal plans based on food exchanges, and the use of qualitative adjustments of insulin for exercise and stress [11]. Prescribing standing pre-meal rapid-acting insulin doses remains a good launching pad from which carbohydrate counting techniques can be introduced. For patients with T1DM who are unable or unwilling to count carbohydrates and inject insulin four times daily, meal planning with day-to-day consistency in the amount and source of carbohydrate is associated with improved control on a regimen of two injections per day [12].

For the vast majority of patients, the first task is to teach them to recognize the carbohydrates in their diet. Newer mandatory food labels have made carbohydrate counting much easier. It is essential to teach patients that when reading food labels they must add up the total carbohydrates and not just the sugars. The carbohydrate content of some common foods is listed in Table 6.1. With the expanding variety of foods available in our diet, the carbohydrate content is not always easily recognizable. Often, the only way a patient finds out about the carbohydrates in the food is when their monitored glucose is elevated. By monitoring postprandial glucose levels, patients can learn which foods are likely to raise their blood sugars. With adjustments in the dose and timing of the insulin injection(s), a strategy to improve their glucose control is developed.

The next step necessitates characterizing a patient's insulin and carbohydrate sensitivity. In practice, a typical patient with T1DM will require 1 unit of insulin to cover between 5-15 g of carbohydrate. Carbohydrate sensitivity can vary dramatically from patient to patient. The ratio is tested by having the patient eat several meals of known carbohydrate content and testing the glucose 2 hours postprandially. These test meals are taken when the pre-meal glucose is within the target range. Total daily prandial insulin requirements are typically in the range of 50–60% of the total daily insulin dose but vary depending on the carbohydrate content of the diet.

One also needs to determine how much insulin is required to correct an elevated glucose. A typical patient with T1DM will drop their blood glucose by 20–80 mg/dL for every unit of insulin given subcutaneously. This number is referred to as the "correction factor." Several different formulas have been proposed to calculate a correction factor for a patient whose insulin sensitivity is not known. These take a number ranging from 1500–1800 divided by the total daily dose of insulin [13]. Bear in mind that these numbers are highly variable and influenced by many factors, including weight, age, sex, renal function, stress level, gastric emptying, physical activity, degree of hyperglycemia, length of the meal, composition of the food consumed, and time of day. For example, insulin sensitivity is often lowest and insulin requirements highest with the morning meal. Therefore, carbohydrate:insulin ratios can vary at different times of the day [10,14]. To further

TABLE 6.1
Carbohydrate Amounts of Some Common Foods

Food Name	Amount	Unit	Grams Carbohydrate
Apple	1	Medium	21
Apple juice	8	Oz	26
Apricots, dried	¼	Cup	20
Banana	1	Medium	27
Beans, black, cooked	½	Cup	20
Beer, regular	12	Fl oz	13
Blueberries	½	Cup	10
Bread, white	1	Slice	15
Cake, angel-food	1	Slice	16
Carrots, fresh	1	Medium	6
Cereal, Cheerios®	1	Cup	16
Cereal, cooked oatmeal	1	Cup	25
Cola	12	Fl oz	38
Crackers, Ritz®	1	Cracker	2
Croissant	1	Medium	26
Doughnuts, jelly	1	Each	31
Doughnuts, plain	1	Each	23
Ice cream, vanilla	½	Cup	15
Milk	8	Oz	12
Peanut butter	2	Tbsp	7
Peanuts, dry roasted	½	Cup	16
Peas, green, cooked	½	Cup	13
Popcorn, oil popped	1	Cup	6
Potato chips	1	Oz	15
Potatoes, mashed	½	Cup	18
Pretzels	1	Oz	20
Raisins	1½	Oz	33
Rice, white, cooked	½	Cup	22
Soup, chicken noodle	1	Cup	19
Soup, minestrone	1	Cup	19
Soup, split pea	1	Cup	28
Spaghetti	2	Oz	41
Spaghetti sauce	½	Cup	20
Sugar	1	Tsp	4
Syrup, maple	¼	Cup	53
Waffles	1	Each	15
Yogurt, fruit on bottom	6	Oz	29
Yogurt, plain	6	Oz	14

complicate management, the same patient can often respond differently to the same regimen of insulin, diet, and activity.

THE GLYCEMIC INDEX

The GI is a system of classification in which the glycemic response of various foods are indexed against a standard; either 50 g of dextrose or white bread (depending on the laboratory used) over a standard 120-minutes time course [15]. The glucose response is expressed as the area under a curve and is measured from an isolated carbohydrate food that is given to 6–10 individuals; the results are expressed as the group's mean value. This technique helps to scientifically demonstrate the differences in the observed glycemic response to different carbohydrates when served by weight alone. It also allows sugar to be seen as a carbohydrate that is less glycemic than a whole variety of carbohydrate-based foods. Fructose [16], but not high-fructose corn syrup [17], has a lower GI than sucrose or glucose due to hepatic uptake of fructose. Most fruits are less glycemic than white bread [18]. Cooked foods generally have higher GI than raw foods, which have more resistant starch (a starch that is not digested by the small intestine) [19]. Legumes have the lowest GI, followed by dairy products [20]. In patients with T1DM treated with insulin lispro, the GI predicts the glycemic response to dietary carbohydrates [21]. Foods that have high GIs will raise the blood glucose level more rapidly and may require adjustments in the timing or dosing of insulin therapy. These foods must be consumed closer to the peak in insulin action. Foods with lower GIs can be less difficult to match to the insulin peak and will be less likely to cause wide swings in blood glucose values. With these low-GI foods there can be early postprandial hypoglycemia followed by later hyperglycemia as the insulin peak can occur before all the carbohydrates in the meal are converted to glucose. The use of this index in patients with T1DM is best thought of as a method to help assess the timing of the conversion of a food to glucose in the blood. This would enable coordination of the peak in blood glucose with the peak in the exogenous insulin that the patient takes.

The GI is accurate when a food is eaten by itself but loses validity in mixed meals composed of fats [22], protein [22], and fiber [23] that alter gastrointestinal food processing. In addition, GI can vary with food preparation. There can also be substantial within-subject variability in the glycemic response to a particular food [24]. Moreover, the glycemic response to a meal can be altered by the GI of the prior meal [25]. The glycemic response to foods may differ among non-diabetic, type-2 diabetic, and type-1 diabetic patients [26]. This tool is also not well-accepted or developed and is to be used with caution by patients who do not do use frequent glucose monitoring while attempting to obtain tight glucose control.

GLYCEMIC LOAD

Because the GI is a qualitative measurement of a carbohydrate, and not a quantitative measure, the GL is an approach to look at the GI per gram of carbohydrate consumed. The GL takes into account the amount of carbohydrates in a food serving. For example, certain vegetables have a high GI but a low GL. This calculation is not a scientifically well-established method for glucose control but has clinical merit for insulin dosing. The total carbohydrate intake determines the number of units needed to cover a meal. The GI and GL of some common foods are listed in Table 6.2.

PROTEIN

Although amino acids can be converted into glucose via gluconeogenesis, ingestion of protein by normal subjects does not increase blood glucose levels [27]. Several theories have been proposed to explain this phenomenon [28]. The same is not true in the presence of insulin deficiency. Peters

TABLE 6.2
Glycemic Index and Glycemic Load of Some Common Foods

Food	Glycemic Index	Carbohydrates (g)	Serving Size	Glycemic Load
Cake, angel-food	67	29	50 g	19
Croissant	42	26	57 g	17
Doughnut	76	23	47 g	17
Cola	63	26	250 mL	16
Orange juice	50	26	250 mL	13
Bagel, Lenders®	72	35	70 g	25
Baguette	95	15	30 g	15
Multigrain bread	51	30	30 g	7
Cornflakes	92	26	30 g	24
Raisin Bran®	61	19	30 g	12
Shredded Wheat®	83	20	30 g	17
White rice	52	37	150 g	19
Brown rice	50	33	150 g	16
Ice cream	27	12	250 g	3
Apple	40	16	120 g	6
Banana	51	25	120 g	13
Grapes	46	18	120 g	8
Mango	41	20	120 g	8
Orange	42	11	120 g	5
Pineapple	59	13	120 g	7
Baked beans	48	15	150 g	7
Chick peas	28	30	150 g	8
Kidney beans	23	25	150 g	6
Lentils	30	18	150 g	6
Pizza	80	27	100 g	16
Sushi, salmon	48	36	100 g	17
Macaroni and cheese®	64	51	180 g	32
Capellini	45	45	180 g	20
Chocolate milk	42	31	50 g	13
Peanut M&M®	33	17	30 g	6
Jelly beans	78	28	30 g	22
Cashews	22	13	50 g	3
Popcorn	55	11	20 g	6
Corn	60	18	80 g	11
Carrots (Canada)	47	6	80 g	3
Baked potato	85	30	150 g	26
French fries	75	29	150 g	22
Mashed potato	85	20	150 g	17
Sweet potato	48	34	150 g	16

Source: Foster-Powell K, Holt SH, and Brand-Miller JC, International table of glycemic index and glycemic load values, *Am J Clin Nutr*, 76:5-56, 2002.

and Davidson [29] demonstrated that in patients with T1DM, the glucose response and insulin requirements were greater when protein was added to a standard meal. Low doses of insulin may be required to cover a very high-protein meal. In another study, a high-protein, low-fat evening meal increased plasma glucagon concentrations and increased plasma glucose concentrations later in the night, as compared with a low-protein, high-fat meal with equivalent carbohydrate amounts [30]. This has led to the common recommendation of including protein with a bedtime snack when glucose is low.

FIBER

The inclusion of soluble fiber in a mixed meal reduces the expected rise in blood glucose [31]. A high-fiber diet was shown to improve glycemic control and reduce the incidence of hypoglycemia as compared to a low-fiber diet with similar macronutrient content in type-1 diabetic patients receiving their usual treatment regimen [32]. It is a common practice recommendation that if a meal contains more than 5 g of fiber to subtract out the number of grams of fiber from the amount of carbohydrate in the meal [33]. A meta-analysis of randomized controlled trials supports that ingestion of dietary fiber, primarily from fruits, vegetables, and whole grains, is recommended in amounts 25–50 g/day or 15–25 g/1000 kcal to facilitate glycemic control [34].

SUGAR

It is a common misconception that elevated blood sugars are the result of consumption of sugar and that sugar should therefore be avoided by patients with diabetes. It was demonstrated in 1986 that the substitution of sucrose for complex carbohydrate does not result in deterioration of glycemic control [35]. Despite this knowledge, the American Diabetes Association has only recently taken the position that sucrose and other sugars can be incorporated into the diet of patients with diabetes as long as it is substituted for other carbohydrates [36]. In fact, terms like "simple sugars," "complex carbohydrates," and "fast-acting sugars" are now discouraged from use [37]. One exception is the use of sugar-based beverages which have a high GL and are deficient in micronutrients. The recommended overall intake of carbohydrate is 45–55% of total calories. Low-carbohydrate diets are not recommended for people with diabetes because carbohydrate-containing foods are an important source of vitamins, minerals, fiber, and energy [38].

FAT

The incorporation of fat into a carbohydrate meal delays gastric emptying and lowers postprandial glucose and insulin responses in normal subjects [39]. The rate of gastric emptying does not vary with different types of fat [40]. The slower absorption of carbohydrates may necessitate a change in insulin dosing. For high-carbohydrate meals, lispro is best given before the meal, but for meals with high-fat content, lispro may best be given postprandially [41]. Administering lispro after a high-fat meal may decrease the risk for hypoglycemia [42]. Another strategy is to use a mix of rapid-acting and regular insulin for a high-fat meal.

The majority of studies related to the health effects of fat intake in patients with diabetes have been performed in subjects with type-2 diabetes mellitus (T2DM). In one study involving patients with T1DM, lipid profiles improved (lower low-density lipoprotein [LDL], lower very low-density lipoprotein [VLDL]) following a diet high in monounsaturated fatty acids (MUFA) (43–46% carbohydrate, 37–40% fat, 17–20% MUFA) compared with a high-carbohydrate, low-fat diet (54–57% carbohydrate, 27–30% fat, 10–13% MUFA) [43]. An earlier study showed higher circulating postprandial atherogenic lipoproteins after a high-MUFA (40% fat, 45% carbohydrate) vs. a high-carbohydrate diet (24% fat vs. 61% carbohydrate) [44]. Omega-3 fatty acids have been shown to decrease cholesterol ester transfer protein, and therefore the potential atherogenicity of LDL particles, in patients with T1DM [45]. The American Diabetes Association (ADA) recommends that patients with diabetes limit their intake of saturated fats to < 10% of energy and limit dietary intake of cholesterol to 300 mg/day [46]. Further restrictions to < 7% saturated fat and 200 mg/day of cholesterol are recommended if the patient's LDL is >100 mg/dL [46]. Trans-fatty acids should also be minimized to avoid increases in LDL and decreases in high-density lipoprotein (HDL). Current recommendations for fat intake do not distinguish between patients with T1DM vs. T2DM.

GETTING STARTED

With a newly-diagnosed patient with T1DM, it is best to initiate carbohydrate counting once a basic insulin and diet regimen has been established. Once a patient can return to a regular lifestyle, the diet and insulin adjustments can begin. For a week the patient is told to eat a reasonable diet and record all the food that was eaten, noting the time it was consumed (see patient handout in Appendix 4). The insulin dose is also noted with the time it was given. Glucose values are measured before the insulin is given and again 2 hours postprandially. Records should include at least an approximation of the number of grams of carbohydrate, protein, and fat ingested. Any significant physical activity should also be recorded. There are many patients who are reluctant to keep detailed records, but once patients are motivated, all the details can be helpful. More often than not, the best information you can get is the foods eaten and an approximation of the total amount of food (i.e., a big bowl of oatmeal). Given the complexity of the human system, it is safest to initially start with treatment goals designed to prevent hypoglycemia. This is done by underestimating both carbohydrate content and insulin sensitivity. Once the patient presents recordings of their diet, insulin dosing, and glucose response, the fine tuning of the insulin/diet interaction can begin. The erratic nature of "real life" can make this simple plan very complicated.

Once the record is made available, the details can be reviewed and food patterns can be discovered. Breakfast is usually high in simple carbohydrates and can result in dramatic rises in post-meal glucose values. Many foods that are labeled as sugar-free contain significant amounts of carbohydrate; for breakfast people usually eat sugar-free jellies and cereals without counting the naturally occurring sugars and total carbohydrates. For lunch, fast food is often eaten, containing foods that are rich in carbohydrates and fats. The portion sizes are difficult, and even those patients who usually can readily approximate carbohydrate portions can easily under- or overestimate the proper insulin dose. In these situations, a 2-hour postprandial glucose check will be helpful as an evaluation of the delivered insulin dose or as a guide for repeated meals at the same restaurant. For supper, the situation can be easier for carbohydrate counting. At home, portions can be weighed and insulin doses readily calculated. When eating at restaurants, the dosing of insulin can be complicated by unexpected carbohydrates served with a meal. Often the best approach to this scenario is to give supplemental rapid-acting insulin either during or after the meal. If the patient is only willing to take a single injection, it is best to take the rapid-acting insulin prior to the meal based on anticipated intake than after the meal adjusted for actual meal size consumed [47]. There are many foods that have greater impact on blood glucose than their carbohydrate content reveals. For example, pizza results in significant and prolonged hyperglycemia greater than a control meal composed of high-GI foods with similar macronutrient content [48]. Often, there are hidden starches or sugars in restaurant foods, such as certain sauces or sushi rice. In addition, there are combinations of foods which, for unknown or unrealized reasons, impact on a patient's blood glucose.

There is some variability in the time to the peak of the insulin as well as the duration of the action of the subcutaneous administration. In old parlance, there are "early peakers" and there are "late peakers." The trick is to identify them. This is best done with a continuous glucose monitor. Otherwise, frequent glucose monitoring throughout the day with minimal between-meal insulin coverage and snacks can often identify an individual's tendency for early or late peaks in insulin action. As noted above, the optimal time of the prandial insulin injection may vary with the content of the meal.

Gastroparesis is a common neuropathic complication of long-standing diabetes. Acute hyperglycemia also slows gastric emptying [49]. Patients with gastroparesis may have lower prandial insulin requirements [50]. Although it has not been studied, the time action of regular insulin may better match the absorption of carbohydrate in the patient with gastroparesis, as compared with rapid-acting insulins.

The lessons learned over years of reviewing these records seem to be as many as the number of records seen. Several of the more important lessons are:

- Never assume that the records are complete.
- All carbohydrates are not created the same.
- All patients are not created the same.
- People can vary from day to day.
- Some patients can do the same routine and have vastly different glucose responses to the same food and activity.
- Portion size is not always easy to deduce from the label.
- Portion size varies from one restaurant or bakery to the next.
- Patients rarely eat a precise portion size.
- Mixed meals change the glycemic response to foods but foods with a high GI will still raise the blood glucose quickly.
- The GI helps but does not give the whole story.
- Large protein portions will contribute to the glycemic load of a meal.
- Soups are loaded with carbohydrates that are often missed.
- Thick sauces, especially those with cornstarch, will raise blood glucose values.
- Split insulin doses will cover multi-course meals well.
- Cornstarch can raise and keep blood glucose high for a surprisingly long time. In the past, nocturnal hypoglycemia on low doses of intermediate-acting insulin was treated with cornstarch.

EXPERIENCE OVER TIME

Over time, patients develop better carbohydrate counting techniques. Experience is usually the best teacher, yet it is still helpful to set up a few basic ground rules to follow. One slice of bread had traditionally been attributed to have 15 g of carbohydrates. The range for bread can be from 8–20 g. Now, with carbohydrate-modified breads some sliced breads can have as few as 4 g per slice. Patients are taught to take equivalent portions of other carbohydrates to correspond to one slice of bread as was done with the old American Diabetes Association exchange system. This conceptual model helps as a first look approach. With monitoring and dietary record keeping, individuals can expand their knowledge of foods, and how they can use insulin to control their blood glucose levels.

Sometimes it is helpful for a particular patient who is having difficulty with glucose control to eat a diet that contains the same foods on each day of the week or the same diet everyday. On each day the portion sizes are nearly constant and the insulin dose is adjusted to better cover the 2-hour post-meal glucose value. This can be one of the more frustrating as well as most rewarding approaches to controlling glycemia in diabetics.

CONSEQUENCES OF IMPROVED METABOLIC CONTROL

Weight gain is often the first sign of improved glucose control. The patient that learns to control their blood glucose will better incorporate the glucose derived from carbohydrates into body fat.

There will be less glucose spilled into the urine and less glucose available to upset metabolism via cross-linking proteins and formation of AGE.

Hypoglycemia is a problematic result of tight glucose control. Often patients will temper their attempts to get good blood glucose values for fear of having a repeat severe hypoglycemic episode. These episodes can be limited by having patients use as little insulin as possible for each change made in the insulin to carbohydrate ratio as well as only gradually adjusting the insulin correction ratio. Hypoglycemia frequently occurs when an insulin bolus is given too close to the previous bolus. Exercise can always complicate the matter in a variety of ways and glucose tabs or gel need to be on hand to correct hypoglycemia during or after exercise.

CONTINUOUS GLUCOSE MONITORING SYSTEMS AS A TOOL FOR EVALUATING DIETARY MANAGEMENT

Continuous glucose monitoring is the best way to understand the relationship between an individual's diet, insulin, and exercise lifestyle. The tracings obtained, along with the patient's diet, insulin, and activity records can identify gaps in the records and help to characterize a patient's response to different foods as well as the insulin used. It can be particularly useful to identify periods of hypoglycemia and adjust therapy [51].

The current technology for continuous glucose monitoring is not yet adequate for a closed-loop glucose-sensing and insulin-administering system, but it can often be quite accurate. As the technology continues to improve and the cost goes down, this tool promises to be a very rewarding way to help a type-1 diabetic learn how to match his diet and insulin to best limit the expected glucose excursions.

REFERENCES

1. Wasmuth HE and Kolb H, Cow's milk and immune-mediated diabetes, *Proc Nutr Soc*, 59:573–579, 2000.
2. Norris JM, Barriga K, and Klingensmith G et al., Timing of initial cereal exposure in infancy and risk of islet autoimmunity, *JAMA*, 290:1713–1720, 2003.
3. Virtanen SM, Jaakkola L, and Rasanen L et al., Nitrate and nitrite intake and the risk for type-1 diabetes in Finnish children, Childhood Diabetes in Finland Study Group, *Diabetic Med*, 11:656–662, 1994.
4. Giulietti A, Gysemans C, and Stoffels K et al., Vitamin D deficiency in early life accelerates type-1 diabetes in non-obese diabetic mice, *Diabetologia*, 47:451–462, 2004.
5. Myers MA, Hettiarachchi KD, and Ludeman JP et al., Dietary microbial toxins and type-1 diabetes, *Ann NY Acad Sci*, 1005:418–422, 2003.
6. The effect of intensive insulin treatment of diabetes on the development and progression of long-term complications in insulin-dependent diabetes mellitus. The Diabetes Control and Complications Trial Research Group, *N Engl J Med*, 329:977–986, 1993.
7. Uribarri J, Peppa M, and Cai W et al., Dietary glycotoxins correlate with circulating advanced glycation end product levels in renal failure patients, *Am J Kidney Dis*, 42:532–538, 2003.
8. Murphy NP, Keane SM, and Ong KK et al., Randomized cross-over trial of insulin glargine plus lispro or NPH insulin plus regular human insulin in adolescents with type-1 diabetes on intensive insulin regimens, *Diabetes Care*, 26:799–804, 2003.
9. Russell-Jones D, Simpson R, and Hylleberg B et al., Effects of QD insulin detemir or neutral protamine Hagedorn on blood glucose control in patients with type-1 diabetes mellitus using a basal-bolus regimen, *Clin Ther*, 26:724–736, 2004.
10. Rabasa-Lhoret R, Garon J, and Langelier H et al., Effects of meal carbohydrate content on insulin requirements in type-1 diabetic patients treated intensively with the basal-bolus (ultralente-regular) insulin regimen, *Diabetes Care*, 22:667–673, 1999.

11. Kalergis M, Pacaud D, and Strychar I et al., Optimizing insulin delivery: Assessment of three strategies in intensive diabetes management, *Diabetes Obes Metab,* 2:299–305, 2000.

12. Wolever TM, Hamad S, and Chiasson JL et al., Day-to-day consistency in amount and source of carbohydrate associated with improved blood glucose control in type-1 diabetics, *J Am Coll Nutr,* 18:242–247, 1999.

13. Stoller WA, Individualizing insulin management: Three practical cases, rules for regimen adjustment, *Postgrad Med,* 111:51–54, 59–60, 63–66, 2002.

14. Vlachokosta FV, Piper CM, and Gleason R et al., Dietary carbohydrate, a Big Mac, and insulin requirements in type-I diabetes, *Diabetes Care,* 11:330–336, 1988.

15. Wolever TM, The GI, *World Rev Nutr Diet,* 62:120–85, 1990.

16. Lee BM and Wolever TM, Effect of glucose, sucrose, and fructose on plasma glucose and insulin responses in normal humans: Comparison with white bread, *Eur J Clin Nutr,* 52:924–928, 1998.

17. Hung CT, Effects of high-fructose (90%) corn syrup on plasma glucose, insulin, and C-peptide in non-insulin-dependent diabetes mellitus and normal subjects, *Taiwan Yi Xue Za Zhi,* 88:883–885, 1989.

18. Gregersen S, Rasmussen O, and Larsen S et al., Glycaemic and insulinaemic responses to orange and apple compared with white bread in non-insulin-dependent diabetic subjects, *Eur J Clin Nutr,* 46:301–303, 1992.

19. Garcia-Alonso A and Goni I, Effect of processing on potato starch: In vitro availability and glycaemic index, *Nahrung,* 44:19–22, 2000.

20. Jenkins DJ, Wolever TM, and Taylor RH et al., Glycemic index of foods: A physiological basis for carbohydrate exchange, *Am J Clin Nutr,* 34:362–366, 1981.

21. Mohammed NH and Wolever TM, Effect of carbohydrate source on postprandial blood glucose in subjects with type-1 diabetes treated with insulin lispro, *Diabetes Res Clin Pract,* 65:29–35, 2004.

22. Guillford MC, Bicknell EJ, and Scarpello JH, Differential effect of protein and fat ingestion on blood glucose responses to high- and low-glycemic-index carbohydrates in noninsulin-dependent diabetic subjects, *Am J Clin Nutr,* 50:773–777, 1989.

23. Behme MT and Dupre J, All bran vs. corn flakes: Plasma glucose and insulin responses in young females, *Am J Clin Nutr,* 50:1240–1243, 1989.

24. Wolever TM, Csima A, and Jenkins DJ et al., The GI: Variation between subjects and predictive response, *J Am Coll Nutr,* 8:235–247, 1989.

25. Wolever TM, Jenkins DJ, and Ocana AM et al., Second-meal effect: Low-glycemic-index foods eaten at dinner improve subsequent breakfast response, *Am J Clin Nutr,* 48:1041–1047, 1988.

26. Simpson RW, McDonald J, and Wahlqvist ML et al., Macronutrients have different metabolic effects in nondiabetics and diabetics, *Am J Clin Nutr,* 42:449–453, 1985.

27. Westphal SA, Gannon MC, and Nuttall FQ, Metabolic response to glucose ingested with various amounts of protein, *Am J Clin Nutr,* 52:267–272, 1990.

28. Franz MJ, Protein: Metabolism and effect on blood glucose levels, *Diabetes Educ,* 23:643–646, 648, 650–651, 1997.

29. Peters AL and Davidson MB, Protein and fat effects on glucose responses and insulin requirements in subjects with insulin-dependent diabetes mellitus, *Am J Clin Nutr,* 58:555–560, 1993.

30. Winiger G, Keller U, and Laager R et al., Protein content of the evening meal and nocturnal plasma glucose regulation in type-I diabetic subjects, *Horm Res,* 44:101–104, 1995.

31. Nuttal FQ, Dietary fiber in the management of diabetes, *Diabetes,* 42:503–508, 1993.

32. Giacco R, Parillo M, and Rivellese AA et al., Long-term dietary treatment with increased amounts of fiber-rich low-glycemic index natural foods improves blood glucose control and reduces the number of hypoglycemic events in type-1 diabetic patients, *Diabetes Care,* 23:1461–1466, 2000.

33. Bazel Geil P, Carbohydrate counting: Part 2, *Diabetes Self-Management,* November/December 1998.

34. Anderson JW, Randles KM, and Kendall CWC et al., Carbohydrate and fiber recommendations for individuals with diabetes: A quantitative assessment and meta-analysis of the evidence, *J Am Coll Nutr,* 23:5–17, 2004.

35. Peterson DB, Lambert J, and Gerring S et al., Sucrose in the diet of diabetic patients—just another carbohydrate? *Diabetologia,* 29:216–20, 1986.

35. American Diabetes Association, Evidence-based nutrition principles and recommendations for the treatment and prevention of diabetes and related complications, *Diabetes Care,* 25:S50–60, 2002.

36. Kelley DE, Sugars and starch in the nutritional management of diabetes mellitus, *Am J Clin Nutr*, 78:858S–864S, 2003.
37. American Diabetes Association, *Standards of Medical Care in Diabetes*, 28:S4–36, 2005.
38. Cunningham KM and Read NW, The effect of incorporating fat into different compounds of a meal on gastric emptying and postprandial blood glucose and insulin responses, *Br J Nutr*, 61:285–290, 1989.
39. Porsgaard T, Swtraarup EM, and Hoy CE, Gastric emptying in rats following administration of a range of different fats measured as acetaminophen concentrations in plasma, *Ann Nutr Metab*, 47:13208, 2003.
40. Strachan MW and Frier BM, Optimal time of administration of insulin lispro. Importance of meal composition, *Diabetes Care*, 1:26–31, 1998.
41. McAulay V, Ferguson SC, and Frier BM, Postprandial administration of insulin lispro with a high-fat meal minimizes the risk of hypoglycemia in type-1 diabetes, *Diabetic Med*, 21:953–954, 2004.
42. Strychar I, Ishac A, and Rivard M et al., Impact of a high-monounsaturated-fat diet on lipid profile in subjects with type-1 diabetes, *J Am Diet Assoc*, 103:467–474, 2003.
43. Georgopoulos A, Bantle JP, and Noutsou M et al., Differences in the metabolism of postprandial lipoproteins after a high-monounsaturated fat versus a high-carbohydrate diet in patients with type-1 diabetes mellitus, *Arterioscler Throm Vasc Biol*, 18:773–782, 1998.
44. Bagdade JD, Ritter M, and Subbaiah PV, Marine lipids normalize cholesteryl ester transfer in IDDM, *Diabetologia*, 39:487–491, 1996.
45. American Diabetes Association, Evidence-based nutrition principles and recommendations for the treatment and prevention of diabetes and related complications, *Diabetes Care*, 26;S51–61, 2003.
46. Jovanovic L, Giammattei J, and Acquistapace M et al., Efficacy comparison between preprandial and postprandial insulin aspart administration with dose adjustment for unpredictable meal size, *Clin Ther*, 26:1492–1497, 2004.
47. Ahern JA, Gatcomb PM, and Held NA et al., *Diabetes Care*, 16:578–580, 1993.
48. Kong MF, Macdonald IA, and Tattersall RB, Gastric emptying in diabetes, *Diabetic Med*, 13:112–129, 1996.
49. Ishii M, Nakamura T, and Kasai F et al., Altered postprandial insulin requirements in IDDM patients with gastroparesis, *Diabetes Care,* 17:901–903, 1994.
50. Tanenberg R, Bode B, and Lane W et al., Use of a continuous glucose monitoring system to guide therapy in patients with insulin-treated diabetes, A randomized clinical trial, *Mayo Clin Proc*, 79:1521–1526, 2004.

7 Carbohydrate Counting: Description and Resources

Hope S. Warshaw

CONTENTS

Carbohydrate counting is one of several meal planning approaches that can be taught to and used by patients with diabetes. Carbohydrate counting has gained popularity in the U.S. in the last decade. It was used effectively in the intensively managed group in the Diabetes Control and Complications Trial (DCCT) to achieve glycemic control while allowing patients lifestyle flexibility [1]. It is also based on the principle that carbohydrate is the main nutrient that impacts postprandial blood glucose levels, and therefore the focus of the teaching is on the impact of only one nutrient [2,3].

Carbohydrate counting encompasses two meal planning approaches with different levels of complexity: basic carbohydrate counting and advanced carbohydrate counting [4]. This meal planning approach can also be thought of as a continuum because patients who are taught to use advanced carbohydrate counting need to master the concepts of basic carbohydrate counting before advancing their skills and knowledge.

BASIC CARBOHYDRATE COUNTING

The goal of basic carbohydrate counting is to teach patients to identify the foods that contain carbohydrates and to encourage them to eat consistent amounts of carbohydrates at meals and, if necessary or desired, snacks at similar times each day. Basic carbohydrate counting is most appropriate for patients with type-2 diabetes mellitus (T2DM) whose glucose is controlled with a healthy eating and a physical activity plan, with or without the addition of oral diabetes medications.

To count carbohydrates, patients can use either the averaged carbohydrate counts of the exchange system, e.g., one slice of bread equals 15 g of carbohydrate, or they can be taught how to count more accurately with grams of carbohydrates. If the averaged carbohydrate counts are used, they can utilize the resources based on the Exchanges Lists for Meal Planning published by American Diabetes Association and American Dietetic Association [5].

ADVANCED CARBOHYDRATE COUNTING

The goal of advanced carbohydrate counting is to teach patients to match the amount of rapid-acting insulin they take with the amount of carbohydrate they consume. Patients are taught to use an individualized insulin sensitivity factor (ISF) (see Table 7.1) and insulin-to-carbohydrate ratio (ICR) to achieve blood glucose control. Advanced carbohydrate counting is most appropriate for patients with type-1 diabetes mellitus (T1DM) or T2DM who use a multiple daily injections (MDI) regimen or continuous subcutaneous insulin infusion (CSII). The availability of the newer insulin analogs has allowed easier separation of basal and prandial insulin requirements, making this approach more precise and practical for many more individuals.

Patients using advanced carbohydrate counting should be taught to count their carbohydrate intake by grams. They should be discouraged from averaging with exchange or "choice" carbohydrate values. These values are not precise enough to guide bolus insulin dosing.

PROCESS OF BUILDING A PERSONAL FOOD DATABASE

The key to how well a patient uses carbohydrate counting is how well the individual is able and willing, over the long term, to estimate the amount of carbohydrate in the foods and meals. Patients trained in advanced carbohydrate counting using an insulin pump should be encouraged to make accurate decisions about their bolus doses based on the carbohydrate count of meals and snacks as well as their pre-set "insulin-on-board," ISFs, and target blood glucose values. These concepts are described in Table 7.1. Although today's insulin pumps can deliver precise bolus doses calculated out to two decimal points, if the carbohydrate count is not estimated accurately, the bolus dose will be wrong. In addition, if the bolus dose is not synchronized with the rise of blood glucose from the carbohydrate, blood glucose control will not be achieved [6]. Thus, carbohydrate counting remains critical to achieving good blood glucose control. Patients must have adequate and quality training in carbohydrate counting to implement it well. They also must be provided with educational resources and references.

In the beginning, individuals should be encouraged to build their personal food databases with carbohydrate counts. Although at first this seems like a difficult task, it generally requires minimal time because most patients eat a narrow list of foods and meals (combinations of foods) from day to day. Once they have built their personal food databases, it will decrease the time-intensive and arduous nature of constantly searching for the carbohydrate counts of foods and meals.

The following step-by-step process used in conjunction with the sample charts in Table 7.2 and Table 7.3 will help build a personal food database:

1. Brainstorm a list of the 50 to 100 foods regularly eaten. Observe foods in the refrigerator, pantry, and freezer. Think about the combination of foods used in common meals.
2. Write the amount of these foods usually eaten next to each food item, for example, ½ cup, two slices, or 3 oz. Weigh and measure the common amounts of these foods eaten to get precise carbohydrate counts. For example, fresh fruits or bagels can be weighed using a food scale. Portion sizes of foods such as mashed potatoes, rice, and corn can be determined easily using measuring cups.

3. Find the carbohydrate counts of these foods in the amounts recorded. Use the Nutrition Facts labels if available, books, online resources, searchable databases, and restaurant nutrition information to determine the carbohydrate counts. A list of these resources follows beneath the "Educational Resources" heading.
4. Determine the total carbohydrate count for common meals by adding up the carbohydrate counts for the combination of foods that make up common meals. Several insulin pumps allow one to enter the carbohydrate counts for commonly eaten meals.
5. Over a period of time, add new foods, meals, and their carbohydrate counts. Learn about unlabeled foods from experience, like a slice of pizza from the local pizza parlor. If you are uncertain about the carbohydrate amount of a particular food, then test your glucose level 2 hours after the meal to determine if the pre-meal insulin dose was correct.
6. Develop the personal food database in a portable format, for instance, a small notebook, laminated index cards, or PDA.

RESOURCES FOR CARBOHYDRATE AND NUTRITION INFORMATION

It is essential for patients with diabetes to be able to find the carbohydrate counts of the foods they eat. The Nutrition Facts label found on the packaging of many foods should be used as a primary reference. Patients should be taught to focus on two pieces of information from the Nutrition Facts label—the serving size and the total carbohydrates. One must consider the serving size that will be eaten and calculate the amount of carbohydrates for the serving. It is not necessary to consider the "sugars" on the Nutrition Facts label separately because these are factored into the total carbohydrate count. These sugars are not simply added sugars, they are, according to Food and Drug Administration (FDA) food labeling guidelines, all mono- and disaccharides. Therefore, sugars are both naturally occurring sugars, such as lactose or sucrose, and added sugars, such as dextrose or high-fructose corn syrup. For more precise insulin dosing, the number of grams of fiber to be consumed can be subtracted from the total carbohydrates, if patients are going to consume a high-fiber (> 5 g) food or meal. At present, many commonly eaten foods, such as fresh produce, meats, and restaurant foods, do not require a Nutrition Facts label. Several educational resources can be used to obtain the carbohydrate counts of foods that do not have a Nutrition Facts label.

TABLE 7.1
Insulin Pump Features to Factor into Bolus Dosing Decisions

Feature	Concept
Insulin-on-board (IOB)	Amount of active bolus insulin remaining in the body from previous bolus doses within the past few hours. Patients set a duration of hours on their IOB feature of most pumps in consultation with their pump trainer and health care provider. Generally patients are advised to set the duration for insulin-on-board some point between 3–5 hours.
Insulin sensitivity factor (ISF)	Number of mg/dL that one unit of rapid-acting insulin lowers blood glucose (on average). The ISF is used to correct blood glucose results above the pre- and post-meal blood glucose targets. Patients can set most of today's pumps with several ISFs for various time periods of the day.
Target blood glucose values	Target numbers or ranges for blood glucose to factor in to the decision for bolus doses. Patients can have a variety of targets for pre-meal, post-meal, and bedtime, for instance. Today's insulin pumps allow the setup of several target goals and several pumps also allow patients to set these up as ranges.

Source: Sansum, W.D., *The Normal Diet*, 2nd ed., St. Louis: C.V. Mosby, 1928. With permission.

TABLE 7.2
Sample Personal Food Database

Food	Amount I Eat	Carbohydrate Count (g)
Bran flakes	¾ cup	23
Honey Nut Cheerios®	¾ cup	17
Milk, fat-free	1 ¼ cups	15
Banana	1 small	21
Apple, Granny Smith	1 small/6 oz	23
Whole wheat bread—Arnold®	1 slice	18
American cheese slices—2% milk	1 slice	2
Tomato soup—Campbell's®	1 can/8 oz, prepared with one container of fat-free milk	31

TABLE 7.3
Sample Carbohydrate Counts of Common Meals

Meals	Amount I Eat		Carbohydrate Count (g)
Breakfast #1			
Bran flakes	¾ cup		23
Honey Nut Cheerios®	¾ cup		17
Milk, fat-free	1 ¼ cups		15
Banana	1 small		21
		Total	76
Breakfast #2			
Whole wheat bread – Arnold®	2 slices		36
American cheese slices	2 slices		2
Apple	1 medium		23
		Total	61

EDUCATIONAL RESOURCES

BOOKS

1. *Bowes and Church Food Values of Portions Commonly Used,* 17th ed., by Janet Pennington, et al., Lippincott Williams & Wilkins, 1998, 481 pages.
2. *Calories and Carbohydrates*, 14th ed., by Barbara Kraus, Signet Book, 2001, 476 pages.
3. *Corinne T. Netzer Carbohydrate Counter*, 7th ed., by Corinne T. Netzer, Dell, 2002, 496 pages.
4. *The Diabetes Carbohydrate and Fat Gram Guide: Quick, Easy Meal Planning Using Carbohydrate and Fat Gram Counts*, 1st ed., by Lea Ann Holzmeister, American Diabetes Association, 2000, 422 pages.
5. *The Doctor's Pocket Calorie, Fat, & Carbohydrates Counter 2004: Plus 170 Fast-Food Chains & Restaurants*, by Allan Borushek, Family Health Publications, 2004, 304 pages.

RESTAURANT FOODS

1. *The Complete Guide to Healthy Restaurant Eating*, 1st ed., by Hope Warshaw, American Diabetes Association, 2006, 650 pages.
2. *Nutrition in the Fast Lane*, Dennis Jones, Ed., Franklin Publishing Inc., 2000, 113 pages.

ONLINE INFORMATION FROM WEB SITES

1. www.nal.usda.gov/fnic/foodcomp: These are the federal government's nutrient databases of about 6000 foods. It is searchable and can be downloaded at no charge.
2. www.calorieking.com.
3. www.nutritiondata.com.
4. www.dietfacts.com.
5. Restaurant carbohydrate information: Some of the web sites of the large chain restaurants provide nutrition information. This is more common for "walk up and order" restaurants than for the "sit down and order" restaurants. Much of this information is available in a portable format in the 1st edition of the book noted above: *The Complete Guide to Healthy Restaurant Eating*.

DOWNLOADABLE DATA FOR PERSONAL DIGITAL ASSISTANCE

1. EZManager Plus® from Animas (www.animascorp.com).
2. Several products: GlucoPilot®, BalanceLog®, PX Nutrition info.
3. www.calorieking.com.

COOKBOOKS USING CARBOHYDRATE COUNTING

1. *Carb Counter's Diabetic Cookbook*, by Hope Warshaw, Better Homes and Gardens, 2002, 256 pages.
2. *The Carbohydrate Counting Cookbook*, 1st ed., by Tami Ross and Patti Bazel Geil, Wiley, 1998, 108 pages.

The above cookbooks provide basic information about carbohydrate counting as well as recipes with carbohydrate counts. However, patients do not need to purchase carbohydrate counting cookbooks because the majority of cookbooks as well as recipes in diabetes and healthy eating magazines provide the carbohydrate counts.

PROFESSIONAL RESOURCES FOR TEACHING CARBOHYDRATE COUNTING

1. *Practical Carbohydrate Counting: A How-to-Teach Guide for Health Professionals*, 1st ed., by Hope S. Warshaw and Karen M. Bolderman, American Diabetes Association, 2003, 64 pages.

CONSUMER BOOKS FOR LEARNING CARBOHYDRATE COUNTING

1. *ADA Complete Guide to Carb Counting*, 2nd ed., by Hope S. Warshaw, et al., American Diabetes Association, 2004, 256 pages.
2. American Diabetes Association: Basic carbohydrate counting, 2003. This is a pamphlet that opens into a larger poster.

3. American Diabetes Association: Advanced carbohydrate counting, 2003. This is a 30-page pamphlet that covers the basics of this meal planning approach.
4. International Diabetes Center: Carbohydrate counting for patients with diabetes, 2002. This is a 16-page pamphlet.

CONSUMER MATERIALS ON THE EXCHANGE SYSTEM

1. American Diabetes Association and American Dietetic Association, Exchanges Lists for Meal Planning, 2003.
2. American Diabetes Association and American Dietetic Association, Official Pocket Guide to Diabetic Exchanges, 2003.

Manufacturers of diabetes-related products make available various materials on the topic of carbohydrate counting. Talk to the sales representatives from these companies to determine what resources they have and their availability.

MAKING REFERRALS FOR CARBOHYDRATE COUNTING TRAINING

Patients must be taught how to count carbohydrates if they are to be successful in applying this knowledge to their lifestyle and diabetes management. Physicians should refer patients who want to be trained in carbohydrate counting to a dietitian specialized in diabetes. Generally, it requires a minimum of two 1-hour sessions to learn basic and advanced carbohydrate counting. A written referral should be made for this training as a referral for "Medical Nutrition Therapy" (MNT). Many patients are able to get reimbursed through their health plan for MNT. Today Medicare Part B provides coverage for MNT, both for initial training and annually for patients who meet the diagnostic criteria for diabetes.

Many dietitians are able to provide patients with the skills and resources to do basic carbohydrate counting. Training patients to use advanced carbohydrate counting for MDI or CSII requires advanced level skills and competencies [7]. Dietitians who provide this training should be able to feel comfortable providing ISFs and ICRs, and in teaching patients how to use insulin pump features such as insulin-on-board, temporary basal, and extended bolus.

Registered dietitians who are certified diabetes educators (CDE) or are board-certified in advanced diabetes management (BC-ADM) can be found by locating American Diabetes Association Education Recognition Programs in the area at: www.diabetes.org/education/eduprogram.asp or by calling 1-800-DIABETES (1-(800) 342-2383).

REFERENCES

1. The DCCT Research Group, Nutrition interventions for intensive therapy in the DCCT, *J Am Diet Assoc,* 93(Suppl 7):768–772, 1993.
2. American Diabetes Association, Nutrition principles and recommendations in diabetes, *Diabetes Care,* 27:S36, 2004.
3. Sheard NF, Clark NG, and Brand-Miller JC et al., Dietary carbohydrate (amount and type) in the prevention and management of diabetes: A statement by the American Diabetes Association, *Diabetes Care,* 27:2266–2271, 2004.
4. Warshaw HS and Bolderman KM, *Practical Carbohydrate Counting: A How-to-Teach Guide for Health Professionals,* American Diabetes Association, 2001.
5. American Diabetes Association and American Dietetic Association, Exchanges Lists for Meal Planning, 2003.

6. Warshaw HS, *Rapid-Acting Insulin: Action Curve Update with Practical Tips, On the Cutting Edge*, Diabetes Care and Education Dietetic Practice Group and the American Dietetic Association, Summer 2005, (In press).

7. Kulkarni K, Boucher JL, and Daly A et al., American Dietetic Association, Standards of practice and standards of professional performance for registered dietitians (generalist, specialist, and advanced) in diabetes care, *J Am Diet Assoc*, 105(Suppl 5):819–824, 2005.

8 Continuous Insulin Infusion Therapy and Nutrition

Andrew Jay Drexler and Carolyn Robertson

CONTENTS

RATIONALE FOR INSULIN PUMP THERAPY

Insulin pump therapy or continuous subcutaneous insulin infusion (CSII) was first introduced in the late 1970s. However, it has been only in the past 5–10 years that there has been a dramatic increase in its use. In part, this is a consequence of its increased use among pediatricians. Smaller, more sophisticated pumps and the availability of insulin analogs have also contributed to its increased use. Insulin pumps are mechanical devices that deliver very small amounts of short-acting insulin, such as regular human insulin (RHI), or a rapid-acting analog such as lispro, aspart, or glulisine, via a catheter into the subcutaneous space for eventual absorption into the circulation. The pump is programmed to deliver a small amount of insulin called the "basal rate" at all times. This rate, determined by the patient or health professional, can vary at different times of the day. Once established, the basal program is delivered without further action on the part of the patient. Basal rates are usually expressed as "units of insulin per hour," with a typical range of 0.5 units/hour –1.5 units/hour, but this can be more or less in individual cases. At meal times, the patient must interact with the pump to activate delivery of insulin, known as a "bolus," which is issued to cover the expected rise in blood sugar from the meal. This bolus is expressed as units of insulin for a reference amount of food (usually carbohydrate) and therefore provides for flexibility in the amount of food that is ingested.

Insulin pump therapy has been shown to result in improvement of hemoglobin A1C (A1C) levels with reduced frequency of severe hypoglycemia in individuals with type-1 diabetes mellitus (T1DM) [1], often with a reduction in total daily insulin dose [2]. There are many reasons for a particular patient to utilize CSII, including increased flexibility of lifestyle, avoidance of injections, ease of meal dosing, and the potential for improved control. The strongest indication for CSII is in the patient with a major manifestation of the "dawn phenomenon." The dawn phenomenon is a rise in plasma glucose or insulin requirements in the early morning hours before rising in the absence of antecedent hypoglycemia [3]. For these patients, the only alternative is to awaken in the middle of the night and take an insulin injection. In one recent study, the use of insulin aspart in the pump resulted in lower glycemic exposure—as determined by a continuous glucose monitoring system (CGMS)—as compared with multiple daily injections (MDI) therapy using aspart

125

and glargine, without increased risk of hypoglycemia [4]. This was attributed to the ability to control the dawn phenomenon with adjustment of nighttime basal rates and the flexibility in mealtime dosing.

BASAL-BOLUS INSULIN THERAPY

With the current understanding of T1DM, the optimal management strategy is thought to be that which most closely mimics insulin secretion in the non-diabetic or "basal-bolus therapy." While basal-bolus therapy can be equally successful with either MDI or CSII, many people assume that CSII always implies basal-bolus therapy. This is not true and depends on the actual distribution of insulin between basal and bolus doses.

The definition of basal-bolus therapy implies a complete separation between the insulin given to meet the body's non-food-related insulin requirements (basal) and the insulin given to cover meals (bolus). In general, the 24-hour basal dose of insulin will be 40–50% of the total daily dose. Under normal circumstances, insulin's role in carbohydrate metabolism is to adjust for the changes from fasting, eating, and the post-absorptive state. During meal ingestion, a small amount of food is utilized for energy but the majority is stored for future use. The ingested carbohydrates are predominantly converted to glycogen for storage in the liver. During fasting, this glycogen is broken down into glucose most importantly to meet the needs of the brain. The interaction between glucose in the circulation and the liver can be in either of two different states: glycogen synthesis or glycogenolysis. The status of glycogen utilization depends on the relative levels of insulin and glucagon in the blood. Eating in the non-diabetic individual results in up to a tenfold increase in insulin levels in the portal vein [5]. This high insulin level induces the enzymes of glycogen synthesis and inhibits glucose release by the liver. However, insulin levels never reach zero even when fasting. In the non-absorptive state, the lower levels of insulin in the circulation allow the release of glucose by the liver either by glycogenolysis or gluconeogenesis. This lower level of insulin also allows preferential uptake of glucose from the circulation by non-insulin-requiring tissues such as the brain. It also allows the maintenance of normal protein and lipid metabolism. This lower level of serum insulin is called the basal insulin requirement and is regulated so that glucose release by the liver matches glucose utilization by the brain, muscles, and other organs. The correctness of the basal dose can be measured by glucose monitoring devices during an extended period of fasting to confirm that the blood glucose level neither rises nor falls.

One of the first defects noted in type-2 diabetes mellitus (T2DM) is a loss of first-phase insulin secretion [6]. No currently available insulin pump is able to reproduce the biphasic nature of endogenous meal-stimulated insulin secretion. In the non-diabetic, the first phase corresponds to a rapid initial response to food. This is followed by a larger second phase which accounts for the majority of the insulin response to food. In theory, first-phase insulin secretion, along with the incretin response, may allow the pancreas to sense how much total insulin will be required. This biphasic nature of endogenous insulin secretion (see Figure 8.1) should not be confused with the dual bolus feature of insulin pumps described later. Another critical factor in understanding insulin physiology is the rapid clearance of the high levels of insulin from the blood stream. This is achieved because of the short half-life of insulin in the blood, estimated at 5–10 minutes [7,8]. The ability to rapidly adjust serum insulin levels is what allows for the exquisite degree of glycemic control while eating either complex or simple carbohydrates.

It is very important to recognize the difference in kinetics between rapid-acting insulin analogs used in a subcutaneous insulin pump and endogenous insulin secretion. All current commercially available insulin pumps deliver the insulin into the subcutaneous space. Since the insulin only becomes effective when it is in the systemic circulation, the kinetics of action require time for absorption from the subcutaneous space. Endogenous insulin on the other hand is secreted directly into the portal vein circulation. Approximately half the insulin that passes through the liver is metabolized there and hence does not reach the systemic circulation. Portal vein insulin levels are

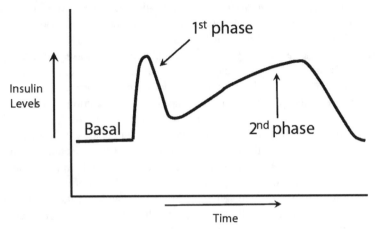

FIGURE 8.1 The biphasic insulin response to glucose.

therefore twice the levels of the systemic circulation. Since the portal insulin concentration influences the enzymatic actions of the liver, resulting in either glycogen synthesis or glycogenolysis, insulin from an insulin pump programmed to achieve the required levels must produce systemic hyperinsulinemia. Because subcutaneous insulin depots act as a reservoir, no insulin delivery program, either by CSII or by injection, can match the rate of change of insulin levels seen in the non-diabetic individual. Rapid-acting insulin analogs have improved these problems but not solved them.

Extracellular glucose in the body is distributed in four compartments: the blood, interstitial fluid, liver glycogen, and muscle glycogen. The smallest component is in the blood stream. Assuming a blood sugar of 100 mg/dL and a blood volume of 5 L, there are only 5 g of glucose in the blood. The body's total amount of exchangeable glucose accounts for about 300 g and muscle glycogen 400–500 g. In total then, stored glycogen is sufficient for only a short period of fasting and the body soon turns to gluconeogenesis to meet the brain's requirement for glucose. Since the brain uses approximately 150 g of glucose/day, or 6.25 g/hour, and the blood stream contains only an approximate 5 g of glucose, it is clear that while the serum glucose level remains relatively constant, it does so by maintaining a large flux between the various compartments. It is important to note that while the liver, using alanine as a substrate, is the main organ of gluconeogenesis, the kidney, using primarily glutamine as substrate, is also important in gluconeogenesis. This latter fact has important consequences for patients on CSII with renal failure. The basal insulin dose then primarily controls hepatic glucose metabolism. It does not provide any glucose lowering nor does it contribute to disposing of meal-ingested carbohydrates. Ensuring the physiological distribution of ingested nutrients, primarily carbohydrates, is the function of the bolus insulin dose.

It has been know for many years that the insulin output is greater when the same amount of carbohydrate is given orally rather than intravenously. This is now thought to be due to the action of hormones in the intestine, primarily GIP (glucose-dependent insulinotropic polypeptide) and GLP-1 (glucagon-like peptide 1). In the non-diabetic individual, these hormones are secreted upon ingestion of food and augment the insulin response, presumably based on the amount and type of carbohydrate ingested. Neither CSII nor any current insulin therapy in the treatment of T1DM replaces this function. Drugs to augment this function are now available for the treatment of T2DM but are unlikely to be useful in T1DM since they act on pancreatic β-cells to augment insulin secretion.

Historically, nutrition therapy for the individual with T1DM has been dictated by the rate of absorption of the insulin used to cover the meal-induced rise in blood sugar. Because regular human insulin (RHI) has such a delayed onset of action, late peak, and prolonged duration of action, it was necessary to limit carbohydrates to those that best matched this action. Rapidly absorbed carbohydrates had to be avoided because of the delayed onset of the insulin; the late peak required slowly absorbed carbohydrates, and the prolonged duration of action required a snack several hours after the meal even with a meal of complex carbohydrates. Essentially, the diet had to be made to fit the kinetics of the RHI. With rapid-acting insulin analogs and insulin pumps, it is possible to deliver insulin to more closely match the food. The rapid-acting insulin analogs allow the intake of more rapidly absorbed carbohydrates. Rapid-acting insulins also have a shorter duration of action, eliminating the need for planned snacks. However, even rapid-acting insulin analogs cannot produce the very rapid rise and peak levels in portal vein insulin seen with endogenous insulin secretion. Therefore, there is still a restriction on the use of very rapid-acting carbohydrates such as fruit juices.

The distinction between different types of carbohydrates concerns the influence of the rate of their absorption into the blood and the rate of the absorption of the injected insulin. The inclusion of fats and fiber in a meal also influences the kinetics of the carbohydrate absorption. However, there is a belief that this distinction does not adequately define the difference in carbohydrates. Data from patients performing blood glucose self-monitoring indicated that the quality of carbohydrate had as great an effect as the quantity of carbohydrate. That is, not all carbohydrates had the same rate of absorption from the gastrointestinal tract. The glycemic index (GI) was developed as a way of solving this problem and determining the amount of insulin needed for different carbohydrates. The GI is developed by comparing the area under the curve of 100 g of the food being tested compared to the area under the glucose curve of a comparator, initially glucose and then white bread. An American Diabetes Association position statement concluded that use of the GI can provide an additional benefit over that observed when total carbohydrate is considered alone [9].

In summary, most patients using CSII must consider several factors before taking a bolus: (1) how many grams of carbohydrates will be eaten; (2) is a supplemental dose required to correct an elevated premeal glucose; (3) is the content of the meal such that an extended bolus or dual bolus is preferable; and (4) has some preceding event such as exercise necessitated a change in their insulin-to-carbohydrate ratio. While there are guidelines, there are no guaranteed rules and patients must assess the success of their decisions based on pre- and post-meal blood sugar testing. With CSII it is also important to remember that an unexpectedly high blood sugar reading may result from a technical problem such as a dislodged catheter and not be related to the food at all.

SOME TECHNICAL ASPECTS OF CSII USE

The currently available short-acting insulins that are used in insulin pumps are given in Table 8.1. Today most individuals use one of the three rapid-acting analogs, but there are still patients using RHI. While the long duration of action of RHI often necessitates snacks between meals, the rapid-acting analogs may not last long enough for some foods and meals. With the ingestion of slowly-absorbed carbohydrates and fats, it is possible that the duration of the action of the insulin to be less than the time for absorption of the meal. This is also true of meals eaten over an extended period of time. There are significant differences in the duration variation of the post-absorptive state at different times of the day and for meals of different quantities [10]. For individuals using injected insulin, this often means taking repeated injections for some meals or the use of mixtures of rapid-acting insulin analog and RHI.

Insulin pumps can address this problem through the use of a dual (combination) and/or extended (square wave) bolus feature. Under usual circumstances, the insulin pump delivers a bolus of insulin over a very short period of time, roughly comparable to the time it would take to inject the insulin with a syringe (though some pumps will allow the user to alter the speed of delivery). If a meal consists of both rapidly and slowly absorbed carbohydrate-containing foods, the dual bolus feature can be used. The pump would then be programmed to deliver a quantity of insulin immediately with the remainder delivered over an extended period of time. Alternatively, the pump can also be instructed to modify the delivery of the bolus over an extended period of time. This time of action can be up to 8 hours although the more common value is 2–4 hours. This square wave bolus is functionally similar to using a higher temporary basal rate. The onset of action will then be the

TABLE 8.1
Insulins Used in Insulin Pumps

Brand Name	Onset	Peak	Duration
Humulin R	½ hour	2–4 hours	6–8 hours
Novolin R	½ hour	2–4 hours	6–8 hours
Humalog	¼–½ hour	½–1½ hours	4–6 hours
Novolog	< ½ hour	1–3 hours	3–5 hours
Apidra	¼ hour	½–1½ hours	3–5 hours

same as with an injection by a syringe but the duration of action will be increased. This extended bolus feature will produce a lower initial dose of insulin, which differs more than usual from the normal pattern of first-phase insulin secretion.

This capability to provide an extended bolus and a dual bolus is unique to insulin pumps and is not easily duplicated by subcutaneous insulin injections unless the patient is willing to mix rapid- and short-acting insulins. For these features to be used, the patient must have a good understanding of the types and amounts of foods in the meal. General guidelines suggest that the square wave bolus is used for extended meals such as a buffet or a high-fat, high-protein, low-carbohydrate meal. The dual, or combination bolus, is used when the meal is both high in carbohydrate and high in fat [11,12]. In studies evaluating these features, patients used a 50% ratio between the initial bolus and the 2-hour extended bolus. Clearly, additional comparison studies with different types of meals are needed to establish firm guidelines for the use of a dual or combination bolus. Compared with the extended bolus feature, the dual bolus feature requires a greater understanding of the nutritional content of the meal. In the absence of a consensus, it is still best for patients to develop their own individual guidelines based on careful trial and error with frequent postprandial glucose tests.

The newer insulin pumps may have two other unique features. The first allows the patient or health care provider to input their previously calculated insulin-to-carbohydrate ratio for specific meals or times. Once the patient inputs the amount of carbohydrate to be eaten, the math processor will calculate the recommended bolus using the formula that was previously entered and display the expected dosage. This feature functions as a simple calculator and is not a "closed loop" feature that would independently determine the appropriate dosage of insulin to deliver. The math processor can also be set to provide a supplemental dose of insulin for an elevated blood sugar, which is entered by the patient or transmitted directly from the meter—again, according to a formula provided by the patient or health care provider. A second recent feature added to some insulin pumps is known as the "insulin on board." This feature tells the patient how much insulin activity remains from the last bolus. This feature must be individualized by the patient but operates without any feedback from blood sugar testing. Since the duration of action of a particular insulin can vary among patients the duration of action is specifically programmed for the individual. For patients who take frequent supplemental boluses to correct for a high blood sugar, this feature is designed to remind the patient that insulin does not work immediately. It is also necessary for the patient to override this feature when extra insulin dosing is required to cover unanticipated carbohydrate ingested after the bolus was delivered.

MEDICAL NUTRITION THERAPY

While there are many approaches to teaching diet therapy to patients with diabetes, the two most common today are the "Diabetic Exchange Lists" and "Carbohydrate Counting." The first comment to be made is that these are not different diets but different ways of presenting dietary information to patients. Once a diet has been developed it can be described by either of these methods. The choice of method is made based on individual patient needs and not the form of insulin therapy used. The Diabetic Exchange List approach is simpler and defines all foods as belonging to seven categories with each category having a defined amount of carbohydrate, fat, and protein. Patients do not need to know the nutritional content of each category, only that they must have so many servings from each category. This approach is the easiest for the patient to follow, but it provides little flexibility for dietary changes by the patient.

On the other hand, the practice of carbohydrate counting involves estimating mealtime insulin requirements based only on the amount of carbohydrate in the meal and ignores the protein and fat content. Hence, a formula can be developed for each meal so that a patient takes a certain number of units of insulin for a certain number of grams of carbohydrate. This requires the patient to learn the amount of carbohydrate in each food he or she eats but allows for much greater flexibility in the amount of food eaten at the meal. For example, a patient may be instructed to take 2 units of insulin for each 15 g of carbohydrate ingested. The patient can then eat however much he wants so long as he calculates how many grams of carbohydrate will be eaten and multiplies that by the appropriate factor. Some patients will also adjust this figure for the GI of the carbohydrates eaten as well as the starting glucose. Today, most patients on CSII are taught carbohydrate counting. Of note, some of the newer pumps currently contain a carbohydrate reference database.

By definition, the basal rate settings of an insulin pump should be unaffected by nutritional intake, since insulin to match the absorption of carbohydrate is the role of the bolus secretion by the pump. However, there are select situations when the basal rate is altered by the nutritional status of the patient. This occurs when either there are no glycogen stores in the liver or the body's ability to produce glucose via gluconeogenesis is impaired. When this occurs, the basal rate must be decreased, especially the overnight rates. In addition, patients on very low carbohydrate diets or after prolonged fasting may need an increase in the basal rate because of an increased rate of gluconeogenesis. In either case, insulin pumps have a distinct advantage over injected basal insulins such as glargine or detemir, due to their ability to adjust the basal rates for different times of the day.

The impact of nutrients other than carbohydrates is much less important with CSII. With the exception of the glycerol moiety of triglycerides, fats cannot be converted to glucose, and therefore do not need to be taken into consideration in calculating the necessary bolus dose in a meal. However, fat in a mixed meal delays gastric emptying and may slow the rate of absorption of all nutrients including carbohydrates. Depending on the composition of the meal, the extended bolus feature may become important. Proteins, specifically some amino acids, can be converted into glucose—but this is slow process and is usually covered by the basal insulin. However, if the protein content in a meal is very high, an extended bolus or dual bolus feature may be required.

Alcohol is not metabolized like other carbohydrates and cannot be converted into glucose. Nevertheless, the amount of alcohol ingested is very important because the metabolism of large amounts of alcohol interferes with the liver's ability to release glucose. The metabolism of ethanol increases the ratio of nicotinamide adenine dinucleotide, reduced form (NADH) to nicotinamide adenine dinucleotide (NAD), which leads to a reduction in hepatic gluconeogenesis from lactate [13]. Glucose-6-phosphate levels are decreased, thereby activating glycogenolysis to maintain blood glucose. After alcohol is metabolized, glucose-6-phosphate levels increase, activating glycogen synthase; glycogen stores are repleted. This leads to a reduction in blood glucose if insulin levels are unchanged. Thus, patients using an insulin pump have the advantage of being able to decrease their overnight basal rates after alcohol ingestion to avoid hypoglycemia.

WEIGHT GAIN

The question often arises as to the impact of CSII therapy on weight. Data from the Diabetes Control and Complications Trial (DCCT) showed that patients receiving intensive insulin therapy had greater weight gain than patients receiving conventional therapy [14]. However, there was no difference between subjects in the intensive group on CSII versus those receiving insulin injections. As described above, all forms of subcutaneous insulin therapy lead to systemic insulin levels greater than portal levels and hence systemic hyperinsulinemia. The weight gain from this is not unique or different with CSII. Unless there is a decrease in caloric intake as glycemic control improves with insulinization and glycosuria decreases, weight gain is the expected outcome. It is also important to note that in patients enjoying the new ease of taking small boluses via CSII, they respond by the addition of multiple snacks. This results in weight gain related to the increased calories. On the other hand, many patients experience a decrease in their insulin requirement when transferring to CSII and may note some weight loss as compared to MDI. In fact, CSII has been shown to allow weight loss without deterioration in glucose control in adolescents with T1DM [15].

SPECIAL SITUATIONS

A number of special situations can occur that alter CSII management. These include illness in general, illnesses that produce nausea and vomiting, gastroparesis, lipodystrophy, pregnancy, and young children who may or may not eat a meal placed before them. With the exception of lipodystrophy, these are situations where the amount of food ingested is uncertain until after the meal. Thus, a small amount of the bolus, or none at all, can be taken at the start of the meal and then the remainder at the end of the meal. At that time, it is easier to estimate how much of the meal was eaten and absorbed.

The rate of carbohydrate absorption can also be altered by the presence of gastroparesis, a form of diabetic autonomic neuropathy that slows the transit of food from the stomach to the small intestine. When the delay in absorption is known, the use of the extended bolus feature is an important advantage of an insulin pump.

Lipodystrophy refers to skin changes associated with insulin injection. Most often these changes produce fibrosis which can delay insulin absorption. Insulin antibodies can also alter the kinetics of insulin absorption. In both these cases, the change prolongs the action of the insulin and decreases the benefits of rapid-acting insulin analogs in individual patients. Patients for whom this condition is a problem need to use a dietary program similar to those for patients on RHI.

Exercise is a situation where there is a high risk of hypoglycemia. To prevent this, patients using an insulin pump have the option of stopping or reducing the insulin delivery, or increasing carbohydrate intake. In the former case, extra glucose will be provided by hepatic glycogenolysis. Caution needs to be exercised so that insulin is not reduced too much or hyperglycemia and ketosis can result. The more advisable strategy is to increase carbohydrate intake since glucose is the most efficient energy source for muscle activity and depleting glycogen stores may have negative consequences hours later. However, patients who desire weight loss may prefer to reduce the basal rate to avoid taking in the extra calories. Note that the pump should never be stopped for more than an hour to ensure that the basal level of insulin does not drop too low.

The role of CSII in T2DM is still evolving. CSII has been shown to be safe and as effective as MDI therapy in T2DM patients [16]. Early in the course of the disease, it is primarily the prandial secretion of insulin that is decreased and basal insulin secretion is less affected. However, by the time most people with T2DM start insulin therapy, there is a decrease in both manifestations of insulin secretion. One difference between patients with T1DM and T2DM is that the ratio of bolus-to-basal insulin requirements may be greater for type-2 patients. Currently, Medicare will not pay for insulin pumps in patients with T2DM.

REFERENCES

1. Rudolph JW and Hirsch IB, Assessment of therapy with continuous, subcutaneous insulin infusion in an academic diabetes clinic, *Endocr Pract,* 8:401–405, 2002.

2. Hissa MN, Hissa AS, and Bruin VM et al., Comparison between continuous subcutaneous insulin infusion and multiple injection insulin therapy in type-1 diabetes mellitus, 18-month follow-up, *Endocr Pract,* 8:411–416, 2002.
3. Bolli GB and Gerich JE, The "dawn phenomenon"—a common occurrence in both non-insulin-dependent and insulin-dependent diabetes mellitus, *N Engl J Med,* 310:746–750, 1984.
4. Hirsch IB, Bode BW, and Garg S, et al., Insulin aspart CSII/MDI comparison study group, *Diabetes Care,* 28:533–538, 2005.
5. Nuttall FQ, Gannon MC, and Wald JL et al., Plasma glucose and insulin profiles in normal subjects ingesting diets of varying carbohydrate, fat, and protein content, *J Am Coll Nutr,* 4:437–450, 1985.
6. Del Prato S, Marchetti P, and Bonadonna RC, Phasic insulin release and metabolic regulation in type-2 diabetes, *Diabetes* 52:S109–116, 2002.
7. Rasio EA, Hampers CL, and Soeldner JS et al., Diffusion of glucose, insulin, inulin, and Evans blue protein into thoracic duct lymph of man, *J Clin Invest,* 46:903–910, 1967.
8. Sherwin RS, Kramer KJ, and Tobin JD et al., A model of the kinetics of insulin in man, *J Clin Invest,* 53:1481–1492, 1974.
9. Sheard NF, Clark NC, and Brand-Miller JC et al., Dietary carbohydrate (amount and type) in the prevention and management of diabetes, *Diabetes Care,* 27:2266–2271, 2004.
10. Polonsky KS, Given BD, and Hirsch LJ et al., Abnormal patterns of insulin secretion in non-insulin-dependent diabetes mellitus, *N Engl J Med,* 318:1231–1239, 1988.
11. Chase HP, Saib SZ, and MacKenzie T et al., Post-prandial glucose excursions following four methods of bolus insulin administration in subjects with type-1 diabetes, *Diabetic Med,* 19:317, 2002.
12. Lee SW, Cao M, and Sajid S et al., The dual-wave bolus feature in continuous subcutaneous insulin infusion pumps ctonrtrols prolonged post-prandial hyperglycemia better than standard bolus in type-1 diabetes, *Diabetes Nutr Metab,* 17:211–216, 2004.
13. Plougmann S, Hejlesen O, and Turner B et al., The effect of alcohol on blood glucose in type-1 diabetes—metabolic modeling and integration in a decision support system, *Int J Med Inform,* 70:337–344, 2003.
14. Adverse events and their association with treatment regimens in the diabetes control and complications trial, *Diabetes Care,* 18:1415–1427, 1995.
15. Raile K, Noelle V, and Landgraf R et al., Weight in adolescents with type-1 diabetes mellitus during continuous subcutaneous insulin infusion (CSII) therapy, *J Pediatr Endocrinol Metab,* 15:607–612, 2002.
16. Raskin P, Bode BW, and Marks JB et al., Continuous subcutaneous insulin infusion and multiple daily injection therapy are equally effective in type-2 diabetes, A randomized, parallel-group, 24-week study, *Diabetes Care,* 26:2598–2603, 2003.

9 Nutritional Strategies in Pregestational, Gestational, and Postpartum Diabetic Patients

Zohair Hussain and Lois Jovanovic

CONTENTS

INTRODUCTION

In the "pre-insulin" days, diabetes was virtually incompatible with successful pregnancy [1]. The prevailing notion that diabetes was "inconsistent with conception" eventually gave way, but for many years, pregnancies complicated by diabetes were very different from non-diabetic pregnancies. Pregnancies in diabetic women, whether the diabetes was pregestational or diagnosed during gestation, were still associated with significant maternal and fetal morbidity, mortality, and increased risks for complications [2].

Nutrition has always been an integral component of diabetes treatment and diet has always been the mainstay of treatment for diabetes in pregnancy. Even such pioneering figures as Dr. William D. Sansum, the first physician in the United States to administer insulin to a human being afflicted by diabetes, noted that "diet errors are very common, and such errors are undoubtedly responsible for many ailments" [3].

With the discovery of insulin in 1921, a marked improvement in the outcome of pregnancies complicated with diabetes was seen. At the Joslin Clinic, during the early years of insulin therapy, Dr. Priscilla White devoted her life to the study of type-1 diabetes mellitus (T1DM) [4]. By 1949, Dr. White still reported rates of spontaneous abortions as high as 25% and fetal loss rates as high as 18% [5,6]. Dr. White concluded early on that "good treatment of diabetes" clearly improved the outcome of pregnancies complicated by diabetes [5].

By the 1950s, several other American centers confirmed her impression that the "good treatment of diabetes" led to a more normalized pregnancy outcome [7]. Long et al. were the first to state that "excellent diabetic control was needed to carry the pregnancy safely to term" [8]. By the late 1960s and early 1970s it became clear that the higher the maternal blood glucose, the greater the risk for fetal or neonatal loss [9–11]. Even now, the American Diabetes Association states that the goal of therapy for pregnant diabetic women should be to achieve and maintain as near normal glycemia as is feasible [12].

Achieving normal glucose levels is crucial and diet is one of the most important tools in achieving this goal. As our knowledge about diabetes in pregnancy has advanced over time, the diets prescribed for diabetes have undergone an evolution. Though the original diets at the time of Dr. Sansum are not as specific or as scientifically calculated as they are now, there are several trends over time. In Table 9.1 there are two sample diets prescribed by Dr. Sansum. There is a "normal diet" for those individuals with no ailments and a "safe reducing diet" for those individuals that are overweight or suffering from conditions related to weight, including diabetes. The importance of these two diets is not the step-by-step prescription they entail, as these specifics have changed, but to see that even in the beginning of the inquiries into nutrition and diabetes, there was a consensus that a "reduced" diet is needed. Even in these early diets, we see a sharp cut in the allowed carbohydrate intake as well as decreased total caloric intake. Nevertheless, the original dietary recommendations by the American Diabetes Association (ADA) were varied and often resulted in excessive weight gain as well as severe postprandial hyperglycemia [12].

Medical nutritional therapy is now focused on providing adequate calories, nutrients, minerals, and vitamins to maintain a healthy pregnancy while keeping glucose levels as close to normal as possible. This strategy in diet and nutrition has been dubbed the "Euglycemic Diet" and attempts to normalize maternal glucose levels through carbohydrate restriction. Though controversy still exists regarding ideal macronutrient composition, it is clear that carbohydrate restriction is necessary [13].

PREGESTATIONAL DIABETES AND PRE-PREGNANCY PLANNING

Pregestational DM encompasses both T1DM, a state of absolute insulin deficiency caused by the autoimmune destruction of the pancreatic β-cells, and type-2 diabetes mellitus (T2DM), a state of relative insulin deficiency typically associated with insulin resistance and secretory defects [2]. In women with pregestational DM, it is essential that glucose control be optimized prior to conception to reduce the risk for congenital malformations and perinatal loss [13]. The fetus is affected by maternal blood glucose even in the first few weeks post-conception before a home pregnancy test will be positive. If excellent glucose control is not established until after the onset of pregnancy, these women are at increased risk of bearing a malformed fetus since organogenesis is complete by the eighth gestational week. Thus, in order to minimize the losses due to congenital anomalies, programs to normalize maternal blood glucose must begin before conception. Reproductive-aged women with diabetes must be taught early on the importance of avoiding an unplanned pregnancy.

Ideally, preconception care should be handled by a team approach in which the physician, registered dietitian, certified diabetes nurse educator, and patient are all actively involved in planning the pregnancy [2]. The initial evaluation should include an A1C level, which reflects approximately the past two to three months of glycemic control. Ideally, A1C levels should be 5–6% prior to conception. Women who enter pregnancy in poor metabolic control, as reflected by an elevated hemoglobin A1C (A1C) (greater than 2–3 standard deviations above the mean of a normal population of pregnant women), are at greater risk for spontaneous abortion and major malformations of the fetus as seen in Figure 9.1 [2]. The most common congenital malformations in infants of diabetic women are summarized in Table 9.2 [2]. Fortunately, normalizing blood glucose before and early in pregnancy can reduce the risk of spontaneous abortion and malformations to nearly

TABLE 9.1
"Normal Diet" and "Safe Reducing Diet" from 1928

	Normal Diet	**Safe Reducing Diet**
Breakfast		
	melon	1 grapefruit
	shredded wheat with milk and sugar	—
	scrambled eggs	2 eggs
	toast and butter	thin slice of toast with 1/2 square butter
	coffee with cream and sugar	coffee or tea (clear)
	orange juice	skim milk (2/3 glass)
Dinner		
	tomato bisque	—
	roast chicken with dressing	tenderloin steak—small serving
	mashed potato and gravy	mushrooms—3 tablespoons
	baked squash and buttered celery	stewed tomato/celery—4 tablespoons
	pineapple and marshmallow salad with whipped cream	asparagus salad
	bread and butter	—
	chocolate sundae and cake	watermelon—medium slice
	tea with cream and sugar	tea (clear)
Supper		
	creamed macaroni	baked potato—medium
	spinach on toast with poached egg	black bass—small serving
	baked tomato	cabbage salad
	bread and butter	—
	assorted fresh fruits	sliced orange—1 medium
	milk	tea (clear)
Composition		
Carbohydrate (g)	300	115
Fat (g)	80	68
Protein (g)	100	30
Bulk (g)	800	900
Calories (kcal)	2420	1002

Source: From Reference [3].

the occurrence rate of the general population [14]. It is recommended that all women, with or without diabetes, who plan to become pregnant, increase their daily intake of folic acid to 400 mcg/day to prevent neural tube defects in the fetus. However, folic acid supplementation does not decrease the risk of anencephaly and caudal agenesis, the two diabetes-specific neural tube defects related to poor glycemic control.

ORAL MEDICATIONS AND INSULIN

For most women with T2DM, medical nutritional therapy alone will not be enough to maintain normal glycemic levels. Even if glucose is well-controlled with diet alone prior to pregnancy, by the 5th–6th gestational week most women with T2DM require insulin therapy despite minimizing carbohydrate ingestion to 30–35% of total calories. None of the oral hypoglycemic agents are currently approved for use in pregnancy. While there are limited data demonstrating safety and

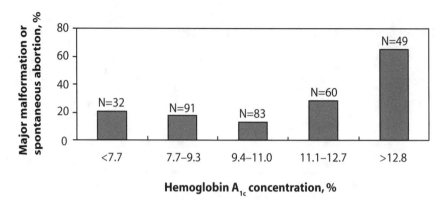

FIGURE 9.1 Deleterious effect of poor glycemic control on fetal outcome. Combined incidence of major malformation and spontaneous abortion according to hemoglobin A1C concentration during the first trimester of pregnancy in 315 women with insulin-dependent diabetes mellitus. The risk rises markedly at A1C concentrations above 11% [2].

TABLE 9.2
Congenital Malformations in Infants of Diabetic Mothers

	Ratios of Incidence Compared with:
Anomaly	**Control Population**
Caudal regression	252
Spina bifida, hydrocephalus, or other CNS defect	2
Anencephalus	3
Heart anomalies (include VSD, ASD, and transposition of the great vessels)	4
Anal/rectal atresia	3
Renal anomalies	5
Agenesis	6
Cystic kidney	4
Ureter duplex	23
Situs inversus	84

Abbreviations: CNS—central nervous system; VSD—ventricular septal defects; ASD—atrial septal defects

Source: From Reference [2].

efficacy of glyburide during pregnancy, the evidence is not conclusive and the safety of currently available oral antidiabetic agents has not been established [15]. Although no adverse effects of metformin have been reported, it too has not been adequately studied during pregnancy. Therefore, if a pregnant woman is taking any form of an oral antidiabetic agent, it should be stopped immediately, blood glucose concentrations monitored, and insulin therapy initiated at the moment that the blood glucose concentrations drift outside the target range.

PREPREGNANCY ASSESSMENT OF DIABETES-RELATED MEDICAL CONDITIONS

Retinopathy

Diabetic retinopathy often progresses during pregnancy, although it is unlikely to appear *de novo* in women without preexisting retinopathy [16]. Preexisting cases of diabetic retinopathy are associated with longer duration of diabetes and worse glycemic control. In women with diabetes for longer than 15 years duration, approximately 98% demonstrate retinopathy with 20–25% displaying severe proliferative changes [17]. Unfortunately, rapid normalization of glucose in pregnancy has been associated with deterioration of the retinal status [18]. Since the degree to which this occurs is related to the degree of hyperglycemia at conception, a woman planning pregnancy should be evaluated by a ophthalmologist prior to conception and laser treatment used as needed for proliferative disease. If a woman is already pregnant and has evidence of retinopathy, the ophthalmologist should be informed that her retinopathy might deteriorate as the blood glucose levels are improved in an attempt to improve the outcome for the fetus. Treatment of severe, proliferative retinopathy with laser therapy diminishes the risk of worsening neovascularization, hemorrhage, detachment, and macular edema. For women who are planning pregnancy but have uncontrolled DM and diabetic retinopathy, glycemic control preceding pregnancy should be best attained gradually over 3–6 months. Studies have not shown any correlation between the improvement of retinopathy and intake of vitamin C or E [19,20].

Renal Function

As part of the pre-pregnancy evaluation in diabetic women, renal function must be assessed with a 24-hour urinary collection for creatinine clearance and total protein. Hypertension and preeclampsia are frequently associated with nephropathy and can result in additional serious complications for the fetus, including growth retardation, fetal distress, premature labor, and intrauterine demise [7]. Pregnancy itself has not been shown to increase the risk for future diabetic nephropathy and it is not associated with permanent worsening of renal function in the majority of diabetic patients [21]. However, the physiological changes accompanying pregnancy, such as hyperfiltration and increased protein excretion, may aggravate preexisting diabetic nephropathy. In those women with preexisting T1DM or T2DM and uncontrolled hypertension or a baseline creatinine value higher than 1.5 mg/dL, worsening of renal disease can be expected in roughly one third of the patients [2].

Pregnant women with diabetic nephropathy should maintain 1 g/kg/day protein to ensure proper nutrition for the developing fetus. Although protein restriction is often recommended to preserve renal function, decreased protein content in a woman's diet during pregnancy can have detrimental effects on the developing fetus. One recent study has shown evidence that soy protein in particular has several beneficial effects that help improve renal function as well as serum lipid levels. The study suggests that consumption of soy protein may improve several markers that can be beneficial for a patient with nephropathy [22]. In addition, the restriction of dietary sodium to 2–2.4 g/day may help control hypertension [23].

Heart Disease

While debate has existed over the use of high-fat/low-carbohydrate diets, and in particular over which type of fat to prescribe in a diet, current evidence shows fat content of a diet is not a factor of great concern for the pregnant woman with diabetes. Dietary fat is perfectly safe for both the woman and fetus and that the main focus of diet should be normalizing blood glucose as opposed to fat reduction. The purpose of the ADA recommendations for lower fat intake in pregnant women is to limit weight gain.

GESTATIONAL DIABETES MELLITUS

Gestational diabetes mellitus (GDM) is defined as any degree of glucose intolerance with its onset or first recognition during pregnancy. GDM affects up to 14% of pregnant women, or approximately 135,000 women/year in the United States [24]. GDM prevalence rates are highest in African-Americans, Hispanics, Native Americans, and Asians [25]. Factors that put women at the greatest risk for developing GDM include a family history of diabetes, pre-pregnancy obesity, age older than 25 years, nonwhite ethnicity, abnormal glucose metabolism, or a prior poor obstetric outcome [25].

To varying degrees, insulin resistance occurs in all pregnancies as a result of increased caloric intake, decreased exercise, increased adiposity, and increased anti-insulin placental hormones. This leads to free fatty acid elevation, intramyocellular accumulation of diacylglycerol, protein kinase-b-II and d-isoform activation, reduction of tyrosine phosphorylation of insulin receptor substrate-1 (IRS-1), inhibition of activation of phosphatidylinositol-3-kinase (PI-3), and ultimately glucose uptake [26]. Women who are unable to compensate for pregnancy-induced insulin resistance with a normal pattern of insulin secretion develop GDM. The first-phase insulin response to a meal acutely inhibits hepatic gluconeogenesis and glycogenolysis. The second phase of insulin secretion is functionally coupled to the first-phase response and has an extended secretion pattern that disposes the ingested carbohydrate [27] (see Figure 9.2a). When the first phase is lost, the second-phase response can be exaggerated due to rapidly appearing carbohydrates from the meal plus uninhibited hepatic glucose production (see Figure 9.2b). The rapid fall of blood glucose 2–3 hours later triggers food-seeking behavior, further perpetuating a vicious cycle between hyperglycemia and hypoglycemia (see Figure 9.2c). In lean women developing GDM during late gestation, there is a decline in first-phase insulin response [28,29]. However, in obese women developing GDM, the first-phase response is unaltered and the second-phase response is enhanced [30]. In African-American women with a parental history of GDM, there are defects in first-phase insulin responses consistent with a genetic defect differing from the defect that confers the T2DM phenotype [31]. In a study of Finnish women with GDM or T2DM, functional variants of the sulfonylurea receptor 1 (SUR1) gene were identified [32]. Thus the physiological and molecular similarities between T2DM and GDM reinforce the use of carbohydrate-restricted diet in women with GDM.

In GDM, similar to pregestational diabetes, even slight degrees of maternal hyperglycemia can result in fetal abnormalities. However, unlike pregestational diabetes mellitus, GDM does not appear until the second or third trimester, when organogenesis has already been completed in a euglycemic environment, making major congenital abnormalities uncommon.

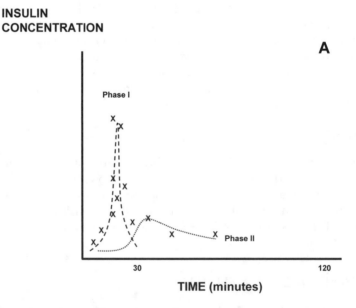

FIGURE 9.2A Normal insulin secretion over time in response to food stimulus. "x" denotes sampling points reflecting both phase I and phase II insulin secretion.

**INSULIN
CONCENTRATION**

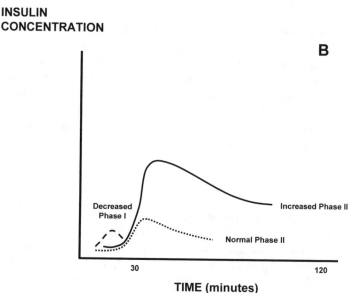

B

Decreased
Phase I

Increased Phase II

Normal Phase II

30   120

TIME (minutes)

FIGURE 9.2B Insulin secretion in women with GDM in response to food stimulus. The overworked pancreas fails to secrete the initial insulin spike in response to food ingestion that occurs in normal individuals. To compensate for the lack of a 1st-phase response, the pancreas exaggerates the 2nd gradual phase of insulin secretion.

**GLUCOSE
CONCENTRATION**

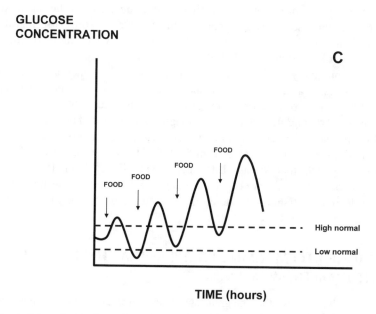

C

FOOD

FOOD

FOOD

FOOD

High normal

Low normal

TIME (hours)

FIGURE 9.2C Blood glucose levels for women with gestational diabetes as food is consumed. This follows the rise and fall of glucose levels in response in accordance with phase I and phase II of insulin secretion.

RISKS OF GESTATIONAL DIABETES MELLITUS

Women with GDM do not have the vasculopathy that often accompanies those with pregestational diabetes mellitus, and so surveillance for retinopathy, nephropathy, and neuropathy is generally not needed [2]. The greatest risk of GDM is fetal macrosomia related to maternal hyperglycemia. The Diabetes in Early Pregnancy Study identified 28.5% of infants from diabetic mothers weighed more than the 90th percentile infant birth weight [33]. Other studies have documented that nearly 40% of infants are greater than the 90th percentile for gestational age and sex [2]. Fetal macrosomia increases the risk of birth injuries such as shoulder dystocia and metabolic derangements, including neonatal hypoglycemia. These are the main dangers of GDM and provide the rationale for intensive glycemic control.

SCREENING FOR GESTATIONAL DIABETES MELLITUS

The assessment of expectant mothers falls into three risk categories: low-, medium-, and high-risk. Low risk is characterized by age < 25 years, normal weight before pregnancy, ethnicity with a low prevalence of GDM, no known diabetes in first degree relatives, no history of abnormal glucose tolerance, and no history of poor obstetric outcome. High risk is characterized by marked obesity, past history of GDM, a family history of diabetes, and the presence of glucosuria. Medium risk falls between high- and low-risk categories. Various organizations have espoused different criteria for the screening of GDM (see Table 9.3). According to ADA Guidelines, pregnant women of low-risk status require no testing. Women with average- or high-risk status can be screened by a one-step or a two-step method.

Screening for GDM is performed between 24–28 weeks of gestation. The one-step approach consists of a diagnostic oral glucose tolerance test (OGTT) using a 75 g oral glucose load and measuring plasma glucose at fasting, at 1 and 2 hours. The test should be done after an overnight fast of 8–14 hours with normal physical activity and an unrestricted diet in the days prior to the test. If the plasma glucose levels are greater than 95 mg/dL fasting, 180 mg/dL at 1 hour, and 155 mg/dL at 2 hours, the diagnosis of GDM is made. Two or more of the plasma glucose concentrations must be met or exceeded for a positive diagnosis.

In the more commonly used two-step approach, high-risk women are screened early in pregnancy and then retested at 24–48 weeks if the initial screen was normal. The initial screening is performed by measuring plasma or serum glucose 1 hour after a 50 g oral glucose load. If the glucose value is > 140 mg/dL at 1 hour, the diagnosis of GDM should be confirmed by using a 100 g OGTT with plasma glucose measurements at 1, 2, and 3 hours. If a cutoff of > 130 mg/dL at 1 hour is used, the yield is increased from 80–90%. The diagnosis of GDM is confirmed if the plasma glucose is greater than 95 mg/dL fasting, 180 mg/dL at 1 hour, 155 mg/dL at 2 hours, and 140 mg/dL at 3 hours. Two or more of the plasma glucose concentrations must be met or exceeded for a positive diagnosis. It should be noted that the one-step approach is cost-effective and more efficient in high-risk patients.

DIETS DESIGNED TO MINIMIZE POSTPRANDIAL HYPERGLYCEMIA FOR THE PREGNANT DIABETIC WOMAN

Numerous studies have shown that the greatest indicator of infant birth weight and fetal macrosomia is the 1-hour postprandial glucose level [38]. It does not matter whether the women has pregestational or gestational diabetes; an elevated 1-hour postprandial glucose level translates to an increased risk for macrosomia, a risk for all infants of both the pregestational and the gestational diabetic woman.

Postprandial hyperglycemia is a result of both peripheral insulin resistance and decreased pancreatic insulin secretion. Postprandial glucose is dependent on the carbohydrate content of the

TABLE 9.3
Criteria for the Diagnosis of Gestational Diabetes Mellitus

	NDDG [34]	ADA [35,36]	ADA [35,36]	WHO [37]
Glucose load or OGTT (g)	100	100	75	75
FBG (mg/dL)	105	95	95	140
1 hr BG (mg/dL)	190	180	180	n/p
2 hr BG (mg/dL)	165	155	155	200 (140)[a]
3 hr BG (mg/dL)	145	140	n/p	n/p

Abbreviations: NDDG—National Diabetes Data Group (need two or more abnormally high values for diagnosis), ADA—American Diabetes Association (need two or more abnormally high values for diagnosis; the test should be performed in the morning after an overnight fast of between 8–14 hours and after 3 days of consuming at least 150 g carbohydrate per day), WHO—World Health Organization (need one or more abnormally high values for diagnosis); n/p—not performed.

[a] GDM if over 200 mg/dL; gestational impaired glucose tolerance if over 140 mg/dL.

Source: From Reference [25]; divide value in mg/dL by 18 to compute value in nmol/L.

meal plan and the efficiency of glucose clearance as the carbohydrates are metabolized [39]. Thus, the peak postprandial response is minimized when carbohydrates are restricted in the meal plan. A normal fasting blood glucose level in pregnancy is 55–65 mg/dL and there should be no blood glucose level greater than 105 mg/dL one hour after a meal. The risk of macrosomia increases rapidly when the maternal glucose concentrations are greater than a fasting of 90 mg/dL and the 1-hour postprandial glucose concentrations are greater than 120 mg/dL [38]. Goals for glycemic control during pregnancy are below these targets. Thus, if the dietary prescription fails to maintain the glucose concentrations in the target ranges, then insulin therapy is initiated.

The search for a "euglycemic diet" began when it was recognized that the American Diabetes Association's original recommendation of 35 kcal/kg pregnant weight, composed of 50–60% carbohydrates in the meal plan, not only caused excessive weight gain, but also resulted in severe postprandial hyperglycemia [12]. Carbohydrates and total calories must be reduced while maintaining adequate protein intake. Studies have shown that diabetic women may be more vulnerable to protein malnutrition than non-diabetic women during gestation. In addition, animal studies have shown that pup growth was stunted, maternal glucose tolerance was impaired, and insulin secretory response was absent in those pups of female rats that faced severe protein-energy malnutrition from a limited diet [25]. From a few preliminary studies it has been shown that an obese sedentary woman, who does not expend as many calories as a lean woman who is participating in a cardiovascular program, would need fewer carbohydrate calories during pregnancy [12].

A study designed to evaluate calorie restriction for obese patients with GDM, compared groups consuming 2400 kcal/day diet to those consuming 1200 kcal/day diet. After 6 weeks the low-calorie group had lower average glucose levels and fasting insulin levels, but fasting glucose levels and post-glucose challenge levels were not significantly different [40]. However, after just 1 week, the 50% calorie restricted group developed ketonemia and ketonuria. Upon this discovery investigators concluded that the 1200-kcal diet is too restrictive, may have negative impact on the developing fetus, and should not be recommended. In another trial with a 33% restricted diet, glycemia improved (fasting and mean 24-hour glucose) in the restricted group and ketonemia did not develop [41]. This indicates that a mild restriction of calories for obese diabetics is both safe and effective. While the effect of ketones in pregnancies complicated with diabetes remains controversial, some data suggest that those offspring may have lower IQ scores [42]. However, since the methodology used in this study was controversial, it is unclear whether chorioamnionitis may have caused the impairment [25]. It has also been shown that pregnant women after a 6-hour fast will have lower levels of plasma glucose, plasma alanine, and plasma insulin levels with coincident rises in plasma FFA and beta-hydroxybutyrate, as compared to non-pregnant women. The studies indicate that "accelerated starvation" ketosis will be noted even with the minor dietary deprivation common in routine clinical circumstances. To help avoid ketonaemia during pregnancy, it is recommended that pregnant women avoid skipping breakfast [33,43]. To further fuel the controversy regarding ketones, there may be a difference between the ketonemia produced from starvation and the ketonemia produced from poorly controlled diabetes. Studies showed that neonatal complications were tied to maternal ketones only in those mothers with ketonemia from hyperglycemia and not from starvation [44,45].

Nutritional counseling by a dietitian trained in maternal nutrition is essential for management of pregestational and gestational diabetes mellitus. An effective diet should provide the necessary nutrients, prevent ketosis, normalize glucose, and allow for appropriate weight gain. The caloric intake per day is based upon ideal body weight. For women, the recommended caloric intake is roughly [46]:

- 40 kcal per present pregnant weight in kilograms per day in underweight women (< 80% of ideal body weight)
- 30 kcal per present pregnant weight in kilograms per day in normal-weight women (80–120% of ideal body weight)
- 24 kcal per present pregnant weight in kilograms per day in overweight women (120–150% of ideal body weight)
- 12–15 kcal per present pregnant weight in kilograms per day in obese women (> 150% of ideal body weight)

The overall carbohydrate content of the diet is 40% of the total calories and is distributed as described in Table 9.4. Though there are no randomized control trials focusing on an optimal diet for patients with GDM, a study was conducted that looked at carbohydrate content by meal. In the study, 14 subjects were enrolled at 32–36 weeks gestation and all were > 130% ideal body weight and did not require insulin. The patients consumed a 24-kcal/kg/day diet with 12.5% of the total caloric requirement for breakfast and 28% for both lunch and dinner, and the rest of the calories split between three snacks [12]. The study found that the 1-hour postprandial glucose levels correlated with the percentage of carbohydrate in the meal. The study further showed that the relationship was most significant at dinner and more variable at breakfast and lunch. The study proposed to maintain ideal control of postprandial glucose < 120 mg/dL and required 10% of the daily carbohydrates allowed at breakfast, 30% at lunch, and 30% at dinner, not including snacks [12]. This caloric and percentage carbohydrate prescription serves to guide the initial dietary prescription, and can be modified by the patient's food preferences and activities. Some general dietary food suggestions are summarized in Table 9.5. In particular, high-fiber foods are recommended. Non-absorbable fibers are a good option for women with diabetes since they confer the sensation of being full; in fact, these fibers go right through the digestive tract with very little actual absorption, thus reducing appetite without affecting blood glucose. Absorbable fibers contain slow-releasing sugars, which are fine for consumption since the delayed release times often match up to the bodies own insulin.

In addition to carbohydrate restriction one must ensure adequate intake of vitamins and minerals during pregnancy. A balanced diet usually provides adequate amounts of all the vitamins and minerals that are required, with the exception of folate. Prior to conception and during the first 12 weeks of pregnancy, the folate intake should be increased to minimize the risk of neural tube defects [47]. Dietary supplements containing 400 μg of folic acid daily in addition to a balanced diet should provide the necessary amount of folate. In general, women taking prenatal multivitamins get all the necessary vitamins and minerals. Though data exist on the salutary effects of magnesium [48], chromium [48,49], and zinc [48] on maternal insulin sensitivity and glucose homeostasis, the routine use of these dietary supplements in pregnancy is not evidence-based and therefore not recommended (grade D).

TABLE 9.4
The "Euglycemic Diet" for GDM Women: Calorie Distribution to Maintain Normoglycemia and 80–120% of Ideal Body Weight

Time	Meal	Fractional kcal	% Daily Carbohydrate Allowed
0800	breakfast	2/18	10
1030	snack	1/18	5
1200	lunch	5/18	30
1500	snack	2/18	10
1700	dinner	5/18	30
2000	snack	2/18	10
2300	snack	1/18	5

Source: From References [12,38].

PROPER WEIGHT GAIN

Optimal weight gain during pregnancy is related to pre-pregnancy weight. The weight gain should be gradual with only 2–5 lb gained during the first trimester and a 0.5–1-lb/week gain during the second and third trimester [2]. Women who are 80–120% ideal body weight should expect weight gains between 25–35 lb. Those women who are obese would benefit from a more modest weight gain of less than 15 lb. The National Academy of Sciences concluded that healthy obese pregnant women (> 150% of ideal body weight) would benefit from this most if weight gain were limited to 6.5 lb or less.

While the common myth holds that larger women give birth to big babies, this is simply not true. If maternal weight gain is properly adjusted for pre-pregnancy weight, fetal abnormalities of growth and development can be avoided. Studies have shown that for women who were underweight prior to pregnancy, the greater the gestational weight gain, the lower the perinatal mortality [50]. It was also seen for women with desirable pre-pregnancy weights that perinatal mortality rates increased with excessive weight gain. This might be explained by the correlation between high birth weights and the rise in rates of shoulder dystocia and other complications of labor [50]. Women who began pregnancy already above the desired weight range had the highest levels of perinatal mortality when weight gain in pregnancy was not controlled.

EXERCISE

Exercise helps decrease peripheral insulin resistance in women with T2DM or GDM. Occasionally, exercise may make insulin therapy unnecessary. The safest form of exercise for both mother and fetus is one that does not cause fetal distress, low birth weight, uterine contractions, or maternal hypertension [51]. The best exercises for pregnant women are ones that use the upper body muscles, placing little stress on the trunk region, such as the arm ergometry and the recumbent bicycle [12]. When excessive weight bearing by the lower body is avoided, workload can be increased safely, leading to an effective cardiovascular workout without fear of fetal distress [12]. Prior to beginning an exercise regimen, women should be taught how to palpate their own uterus for contractions. Exercise should be stopped immediately if contractions begin. Most experts agree that women who were exercising prior to pregnancy can continue their usual activity.

TABLE 9.5
Dietary Guidelines for Women with GDM or at Risk for GDM

Avoid sugar and concentrated sweets

No cookies, cakes, pies, sugared soft drinks, chocolate, table sugar, fruit juices, fruit drinks, Kool-Aid®, Hi-C®, nectars, jams, or jellies

Read labels: avoid foods containing sucrose, fructose, corn syrup, dextrose, honey, molasses, natural sweeteners, cornstarch, and concentrated fruit juices

Avoid convenience foods

No instant noodles, canned soups, instant potatoes, frozen meals, or packaged stuffing

Eat small frequent meals

Eat about every 3 hours

Include a good source of protein at every meal and snack

High-protein foods are low-fat meats, chicken, fish, low-fat cheese, peanut butter, cottage cheese, eggs, and turkey

Eat a very small breakfast

No more than one starch/bread exchange

Choose high-fiber foods

Whole-grain breads and cereals

Fresh and frozen vegetables

Beans and legumes

Fresh fruits (except at breakfast)

Lower fat intake

Buy lean protein foods: chicken, roast beef, turkey, ham, and fish

Limit lunch meat, bacon, sausage, and hot dogs

Remove/trim all visible fat and skin of poultry

Bake, broil, steam, boil, or barbecue foods (no frying)

Use nonstick vegetable oil spray or small amounts (1–2 tsp) of oil for cooking

Use skim or low-fat (1%) milk and dairy products

Eat boiled (not refried) beans

Reduce added fat in the diet, such as butter, margarine, sour cream, mayonnaise, nuts, avocados, cream cheese, or salad dressings

Free foods—eat as desired

Cabbage, cucumbers, green onions, mushrooms, zucchini, spinach, celery, green beans, radishes, and lettuce

Source: From Reference [1].

INSULIN THERAPY

If diet and exercise are not successful in achieving normal glycemia in women with T2DM or GDM, insulin therapy needs to be initiated. For women with T1DM, the insulin requirement rises progressively throughout pregnancy, with insulin rates rising as high as > 1.0 unit/kg by the 3rd trimester [25]. The key to insulin dosages for pregnant women with T1DM is matching the food and insulin dosage [2]. One method of estimating insulin requirements for pregnancy is found in Table 9.6.

The type of insulin prescribed in T2DM or GDM should be based on the specific blood glucose levels. A diet-controlled gestational diabetic should check her blood glucose at least four times a day (fasting and 1 hour post-meal), whereas the preexisting diabetic women should check blood glucose levels at least six times (before and 1 hour after meals) [25]. In the case of a woman with gestational diabetes treated with diet only, if the fasting glucose is elevated above 90 mg/dL, then

TABLE 9.6
Algorithm for Calculating Insulin Dosage Regimen during Pregnancy

STEP 1	**Calculate total daily dose (TDD) of insulin which includes basal and bolus doses**	
	a. Gestational week 0–12	k = 0.7
	b. Gestational week 13–28	k = 0.8
	c. Gestational week 29–34	k = 0.9
	d. Gestational week > 34	k = 1.0
	TDD = [k times weight (in kg)]/24 hours	
	BASAL INSULIN = ½ TDD	
	BOLUS INSULIN = ½ TDD	
STEP 2	**Calculate basal insulin dose with intermediate-acting insulin (NPH)**	
	Before breakfast	= 1/6 TDD
	Before dinner	= 1/6 TDD
	Before bedtime	= 1/6 TDD
STEP 3	**Calculate bolus insulin dose with rapid-acting insulin (lispro or aspart)**	
	Before breakfast	= 1/6 TDD
	Before lunch	= 1/6 TDD
	Before dinner	= 1/6 TDD

See text for abbreviations.

intermediate-acting insulin (NPH) should be given before bed, starting with doses of 0.2 units/kg/day and monitoring the results. If the 1-hour postprandial glucose levels are elevated above 120 mg/dL, then rapid-acting insulin should be prescribed starting with a dose of 1 unit per 10 g of carbohydrates in the meal [2,12]. Recent studies have shown that the rapid-acting insulin analogs, lispro and aspart, are safe and efficacious during pregnancy [52,53].

If both fasting and postprandial glucose levels are elevated, a four-injections-per-day regimen should be prescribed similar to a protocol for women with T1DM. To help mimic the normal pancreas, mealtime boluses using a combination of neutral pH-protamine-Hagedorn insulin (NPH) and rapid-acting insulin analog are used [25]. The total dose of insulin per day is dependent on body weight and gestational week. In the first trimester, the insulin requirement for type-1 diabetic women is 0.7 units/kg/day in the first trimester, 0.8 units/kg/day in the second trimester, and up to 0.9–1.0 units/kg/day in the third trimester. To date, the use of the long-acting insulin analogs, glargine and detemir, have not been studied in human pregnancies and therefore should be avoided.

POSTPARTUM CARE

A woman with GDM should be able to resume a regular diet after pregnancy. However, she should continue to measure blood glucose at home for a few weeks after discharge from the hospital and report any high values to her physician, especially if she was diagnosed early in gestation or required insulin during the pregnancy. As long as postpartum glucose levels are well-controlled, women with diabetes recover at the same rate as normal women. While breastfeeding is encouraged, if maternal glucose levels remain elevated postpartum, this increase will be passed along to the infant through the milk. Therefore, if planning to breastfeed, maternal glucose levels must be monitored and kept as normal as possible. When returning to a regular diet, if one wishes to breastfeed, it must be noted that roughly an additional 640 kcal/day is needed above the normal prepregnancy caloric intake to lactate. Women should also be encouraged to resume an exercise program as early as 2 weeks after a vaginal delivery and 4–6 weeks after a cesarean delivery.

The 15-year prevalence of T2DM in women with a history of GDM is roughly 60%, if obese during pregnancy, and 30%, if lean during pregnancy [54], with overall rates reported in the literature ranging from 17–63% [55]. Risk factors for developing T2DM include early gestational age at GDM diagnosis, obesity, and the need for insulin [56]. Recurrence rates for GDM are 35–80% and depend on parity, body mass index (BMI), early diagnosis of GDM, insulin requirements, weight gain, and the interval between pregnancies [56].

Approximately 6–8 weeks after delivery, or shortly after cessation of breastfeeding, all women with previous GDM should undergo an oral glucose tolerance test. A 2-hour 75-g oral glucose tolerance test is recommended by the American Diabetes Association and the Third International Workshop-Conference on gestational diabetes mellitus. The diagnosis of T2DM is made if the fasting blood glucose concentration is > 126 mg/dL (7 mmol/L) and if any value at or after 2 hours is higher than 200 mg/dL (11.1 mmol/L) [57]. Although women with GDM who develop diabetes after pregnancy usually develop T2DM, a small subset may develop T1DM [2]. For these women with T2DM, lifestyle changes including exercise, diet, and maintenance of ideal body weight is essential. A postpartum woman with normal glucose tolerance should be counseled regarding her risk for developing GDM in subsequent pregnancies and possible T2DM in the future.

REFERENCES

1. Hadden D, History of diabetic pregnancy, In: Hod M, Jovanovic L, Di Renzo GC, de Leiva A, and Langr O, Eds., *Textbook of Diabetes and Pregnancy*, London: Martin Dunitz, 1–12, 2003.
2. Hugo K and Jovanovic L, Diabetes in Pregnancy, In: Leahy J, Clark N, and Cefalu W, Eds., *Medical Management of Diabetes Mellitus*, New York: Marcel Dekker, Inc., 183–200, 2000.
3. Sansum W.D., *The Normal Diet*, 2nd ed., St. Louis: The C.V. Mosby Co., 1928.
4. Jovanovic L, Medical nutritional therapy in pregnant women with pregestational diabetes mellitus, *J Maternal-Fetal Med,* 9:21–28, 2000.
5. White P, Pregnancy complicating diabetes, *JAMA,* 128:181–182, 1945.
6. White P, Pregnancy complicating diabetes, *Am J Med,* 7:609–616, 1949.
7. White P, Gillespie L, and Sexton L, Use of female sex hormone therapy in pregnant diabetic patients, *Am J Med,* 71:57–69, 1956.
8. Long NW, Hartmann WL, and Futcher PH et al., Diabetes mellitus and pregnancy, *Obstet Gynecol,* 3:160–168, 1954.
9. Harley JMG and Montgomery DAD, Management of pregnancy complicated by diabetes, *Br Med J,* 1:14–18, 1965.
10. Delany JJ and Ptacek J, Three decades of experience with diabetic pregnancies, *Am J Obstet Gynecol,* 106:550–556, 197.
11. Karlsson K, Kjellmer I, The outcome of diabetic pregnancies in relation to the mother's blood sugar level, *Am J Obstet Gynecol,* 112:213–220, 1972.
12. Jovanovic L, American Diabetes Association's Fourth International Workshop-Conference on Gestational Diabetes Mellitus: Summary and discussion, *Diabetes Care,* 21(Suppl 2):B131–137, 1998.
13. Jovanovic, Lois, Medical nutritional therapy in pregnant women with pregestational diabetes mellitus, *J Maternal-Fetal Med,* 9:21–28, 2000.
14. Greene MF, Hare JW, and Clohert JP, First trimester hemoglobin A1 and risk for major malformation and spontaneous abortion in diabetic pregnancy, *Teratology,* 39; 225–231, 1989.
15. Langer O, Conway DL, and Berkus MD et al., A comparison of glyburide and insulin in women with gestational diabetes mellitus, *N Engl J Med,* 343(16):1134–1138, 2000.
16. Elman KD, Welch RA, and Frank RN, Diabetic retinopathy in pregnancy, A review, *Obstet Gynecol,* 75:119, 1990.
17. Klein R, Klein BEK, and Moss S, The Wisconsin epidemiologic study of diabetic retinopathy: Prevalence and risks of diabetic retinopathy when age at diagnosis is less than 30 years, *Arch Ophthalmol,* 102:520, 1984.
18. Chew EY, Mills JL, and Metzger BE, Metabolic control and progression of retionopathy, The diabetes in early pregnancy study, *Diabetes Care,* 18:631, 1995.

19. Millen AE, Klein R, and Folsom AR et al., Relation between intake of vitamins C and E and risk of diabetic retinopathy in the Atherosclerosis Risk in Communities Study, *Am J Clin Nutr*, 79(5):865–873, 2004.
20. Mayer-Davis EJ, Bell RA, and Reboussin BA et al., Antioxidant nutrient intake and diabetic retinopathy: The San Luis Valley Diabetes Study, *Ophthalmology*, 105(12):2264–2270, 1998.
21. Miodovnik M, Rosenn BM, and Khoury JC, Does pregnancy increase the risk for development and progression of diabetic nephropathy? *Am J Obstet Gynecol,* 174:1180, 1996.
22. Teixeira SR, Tappenden KA, and Carson L et al., Isolated soy protein consumption reduces urinary albumin excretion and improves the serum lipid profile in men with type-2 diabetes mellitus and nephropathy, *J Nutr*, 134(8):1874–1880, 2004.
23. Franz MJ and Wheeler ML, Nutrition therapy for diabetic nephropathy, *Curr Diab Rep*, 3(5):412–417, 2003.
24. Coustan DR, Gestational diabetes, In: Harris MI, Cowie CC, Stern MP, and Boyko EJ et al., Eds., *Diabetes in America*, 2nd ed., Baltimore, MD: National Institutes of Health, 703–717, 1995:
25. Jovanovic L, Pettitt DJ, Gestational diabetes mellitus, *JAMA,* 286:20, 2516–2518, 2001.
26. Sivan E and Boden G, Free fatty acids, insulin resistance, and pregnancy, *Curr Diab Rep*, 3:319–322, 2003.
27. van Haeften TW, Early disturbances in insulin secretion in the development of type-2 diabetes mellitus, *Mol Cell Endocrinol,* 197:197–204, 2002.
28. Catalano PM, Tyzbir ED, and Wolfe RR, et al., Carbohydrate metabolism during pregnancy in control subjects and women with gestational diabetes, *Am J Physiol,* 264:E60–70, 1993.
29. Kuhl C, Etiology and pathogenesis of gestational diabetes, *Diabetes Care,* 21(Suppl 2):B19–26, 1998.
30. Catalano PM, Huston L, and Amini SB et al., Longitudinal changes in glucose metabolism during pregnancy in obese women with normal glucose tolerance and gestational diabetes, *Am J Obstet Gynecol,* 180:903–916, 1999.
31. Osei K, Gaillard TR, and Schuster DP, History of gestational diabetes leads to distinct metabolic alterations in nondiabetic African-American women with a parental history of type-2 diabetes, *Diabetes Care,* 21:1250–1257, 1998.
32. Rissanen J, Markkanen A, and Karkkainen P et al., Sulfonylurea receptor 1 gene variants are associated with gestational diabetes and type-2 diabetes but not with altered secretion of insulin, *Diabetes Care,* 23:70–73, 2000.
33. Jovanovic-Peterson L, Peterson CM, and Reed GF et al., The National Institute of Child Health and Human Development—The Diabetes in Early Pregnancy Study, Maternal postprandial glucose levels and infant birth weight, The diabetes in early pregnancy study, *Am J Obstet Gynecol,* 164:103–111, 1991.
34. National Diabetes Data Group, Classification and diagnosis of diabetes mellitus and other categories of glucose intolerance, *Diabetes*, 28:1039–1057, 1979.
35. Metzger BE and Coustan DR, Summary and recommendations of the Fourth International Workshop-Conference on Gestational Diabetes Mellitus, *Diabetes Care,* 21(Suppl 2):B161–167, 1998.
36. American Diabetes Association, Gestational diabetes mellitus, *Diabetes Care,* 27(Suppl 1):S88–93, 2004.
37. WHO Study Group, *Prevention of Diabetes Mellitus*, Geneva, Switzerland: World Health Organization, 1994, WHO Technical Report Series, No. 844.
38. Jovanovic L, Role of diet and insulin treatment of diabetes in pregnancy, *Clinical Obstet Gynecol,* 43:1, 46–55, 2000.
39. Peterson CM and Jovanovic-Peterson L, Percentage of carbohydrate and glycemic response to breakfast, lunch, and dinner in women with gestational diabetes, *Diabetes*, 40(Suppl 2):172–174, 1990.
40. Magee MS, Knopp RH, and Benedetti TJ, Metabolic effects of 1200-kcal diet in obese pregnant women with gestational diabetes, *Diabetes,* 39:234–240, 1990.
41. Knopp RH, Magee MS, and Raisys V, Hypocaloric diets and ketogenesis in the management of obese gestational diabetic women, *J AM Coll Nutr,* 10:649–667, 1991.
42. Churchill JA, Berrendes HW, and Nemore J, Neuropsychological deficits in children of diabetic mothers, A report from the Collaborative Study of Cerebral Palsy, *Am J Obstet Gynecol*, 105:257–268, 1969.

43. Metzger BE, Ravnikar V, and Vileisis RA et al., "Accelerated starvation" and the skipped breakfast in late normal pregnancy, *Lancet*, 1(8272):588–592, 1982.

44. Rizza T, Metzger BE, and Urns WJ et al., Correlations between antepartum maternal metabolism and intelligence of offspring, *N Engl J Med*, 343:1134–1138, 2000.

45. Jovanovic L, Metzger B, and Knopp RH, Beta-hydroxybutyrate levels in type-1 diabetic pregnancy compared with normal pregnancy, *Diabetes Care*, 21:1–5, 1998.

46. L Jovanovic and CM Peterson, Guest editorial: Nutritional management of the obese gestational diabetic woman, *J Am Coll Nutr,* 11:246, 1992.

47. Dormhorst A and Frost G, Nutritional management in diabetic pregnancy: A time for reason, not dogma, In: Moshe Hod, Lois Jovanovic, and Gian Carlo Di Renzo et al., Eds., *Textbook of Diabetes and Pregnancy*, London: Martin Dunitz, 340–358, 2003:

48. Catalano PM, Kirwan JP, and Haugel-de Mouzon S et al., Gestational diabetes and insulin resistance: Role in short- and long-term implications for mother and fetus, *J Nutr*, 133:1674S–1683S, 2003.

49. Jovanovic-Peterson L and Peterson CM, Vitamin and mineral deficiencies which may predispose to glucose intolerance of pregnancy, *J Am Coll Nutr,* 15:14–20, 1996.

50. *Nutrition During Pregnancy*, Washington, D.C.: National Academy Press, 1990.

51. Durak EP, Jovanovic L, and CM Peterson, Comparative evaluation of uterine response to exercise on five aerobic machines, *Am J Obstet Gynecol,* 162:754, 1990.

52. Jovanovic L, Ilic S, and Pettitt DJ et al., Metabolic and immunologic effects of insulin lispro in gestational diabetes, *Diabetes Care,* 22:1422–1427, 1999.

53. Pettitt DJ, Ospina P, and Kolaczynski JW et al., Comparison of an insulin analog, insulin aspart, and regular human insulin with no insulin in gestational diabetes mellitus, *Diabetes Care,* 26:183–186, 2003.

54. O'Sullivan JB, Body weight and subsequent diabetes mellitus, *JAMA,* 248:949–952, 1982.

55. Hanna FWF and Peters JR, Screening for gestational diabetes; past, present, and future, *Diabetic Med,* 19:351–358, 2002.

56. Ben-Haroush Y, Yogev Y, and Hod M, Epidemiology of gestational diabetes mellitus and its association with type-2 diabetes, *Diabetic Med,* 21:103–113, 2003.

57. Jovanovic L, Treatment and course of gestational diabetes mellitus, *Uptodate*, 2004.S

10 Nutritional Strategies for the Patient with Diabetic Nephropathy

Joseph A. Vassalotti

CONTENTS

Diabetes is the most common cause of chronic kidney disease (CKD) in the United States and accounts for 40% of end-stage renal disease (ESRD) patients requiring renal replacement therapy [1]. Compared with type-2 diabetes mellitus (T2DM), the duration of diabetes is better defined in type-1 diabetes mellitus (T1DM) where nephropathy rarely occurs before 5 years duration. The nephropathy incidence rises in T1DM after 5 years until a peak at 15–20 years [2]. There may even be a specifically susceptible population of T1DM patients, since the incidence of nephropathy declines after 20 years. African-Americans [3], Mexican-Americans [3], and Native Americans [4] have a higher prevalence of type-2 diabetic nephropathy than Caucasians.

Diabetic nephropathy is characterized by albuminuria in the absence of other clear etiologies, and is typically accompanied by hypertension and diabetic retinopathy. One study of T2DM patients with microalbuminuria demonstrated a close correlation between diabetic glomerular changes on renal biopsy and retinopathy [5]. An angiotensin-converting enzyme gene insertion/deletion polymorphism is associated with more rapid progression of diabetic nephropathy [6].

The classic histopathological lesion, first described by Kimmelsteil and Wilson in 1936 [7], is characterized by nodular mesangial sclerosis, thickened glomerular basement membranes, thickened tubular basement membranes, tubular atrophy, and interstitial fibrosis. Vascular morphologic changes include microaneurysms and hyaline arteriolosclerosis of both afferent and efferent arterioles. Renal biopsies in 30% of patients with T2DM and macroalbuminuria reveal other etiologies for kidney disease, while in patients with T1DM, there is nearly always classic diabetic nephropathy [8]. Important and potentially reversible diagnostic considerations are renal ischemia, secondary to renal artery stenosis, and drug-induced acute renal failure. Other etiologies for renal disease should be considered if there is active urinary sediment, less than 5-year duration of diabetes, absent diabetic retinopathy, or acute renal failure.

The most striking complication of diabetic kidney disease is the high risk of coexistent or subsequent cardiovascular disease. Diabetic nephropathy incidence, clinical presentation, and disease progression are remarkably similar in type-1 and type-2 patients [9]. Primary treatment aims of nutritional therapy are to attenuate kidney disease progression and to prevent cardiovascular events.

PATHOPHYSIOLOGY AND NATURAL HISTORY

The exact mechanism of diabetic nephropathy is poorly characterized, but putative factors include glomerular hyperfiltration, advanced glycation endproduct (AGE) accumulation [10], and growth factors including insulin-like growth factor (IGF)-1 and transforming growth factor (TGF)-β [10]. The course of diabetic renal disease follows five stages from hyperfiltration, to normal glomerular filtration rate (GFR) without microalbuminuria, to microalbuminuria, to overt albuminuria, and finally to ESRD. Glomerular hemodynamic alterations are thought to be related to renin-angiotensin-induced efferent arteriolar constriction and results in supra-normal GFR in the first stage. The long-term effects of increased GFR are detrimental. Serum creatinine, used to estimate GFR clinically, is not sensitive enough to detect hyperfiltration, so that most patients in this stage remain undiagnosed. Patients with hyperfiltration are at increased risk of progression, but not all patients who develop increased GFR experience advanced disease. The GFR then falls to the normal range in the absence of microalbuminuria in the second stage.

Microalbuminuria, characteristic of stage 3, is an important hallmark for increased risk of renal disease progression and cardiovascular events [11]. Traditionally, microalbuminuria was defined using a cumbersome 24-hour urine collection with albumin in the 30–300 mg/day range. Detection of microalbuminuria is now facilitated using a random urine albumin to creatinine ratio. The normal ratio is less than 17 mg albumin/g creatinine for men and less than 25 mg albumin per grams of creatinine for women. Microalbuminuria is defined as 17–250 mg albumin per grams of creatinine for men and 25–355 mg albumin per gram of creatinine for women (see Table 10.1) [12]. Stage 4 diabetic nephropathy is characterized by overt albuminuria and impaired GFR. Such patients are at high risk for progression to ESRD within a few years. In this fifth stage, when the GFR is markedly reduced, the proteinuria may attenuate. The five diabetic nephropathy stages should not be confused with the National Kidney Foundation's five CKD stages, which stratify patients ages 18–70 by GFR calculated using the simplified Modification of Diet in Renal Disease Study (MDRD) equation into stage 1: GFR > 90 mL/minute/1.73 M^2; stage 2: GFR 60–89 mL/minute/1.73 M^2; stage 3: GFR 30–59 mL/minute/1.73 M^2; stage 4: GFR 15–29 mL/minute/1.73 M^2; and stage 5: GFR < 15 mL/minute/1.73 M^2 or ESRD [12].

TABLE 10.1
Stages of Chronic Kidney Disease (CKD)

CKD Stage	GFR (cc/minute)	Description
1	> 90	Proteinuria
2	60–89	Proteinuria with mild decrease in GFR
3	30–59	Proteinuria with moderate decrease in GFR
4	15–29	Proteinuria with severe decrease in GFR
5	< 15	Renal failure

See text for abbreviations.

Source: http://www.kidney.org/atoz/atozItem.cfm?id=134#chart, Accessed on July 4, 2005.

TREATMENT OF DIABETIC NEPHROPATHY

HYPERTENSION

Hypertension contributes to the progression of diabetic nephropathy. Target blood pressure in diabetic kidney disease should be < 130/80 mm Hg to attenuate this progression [13]. Patients with diabetic kidney disease, with or without hypertension, should be treated with an angiotensin-converting enzyme inhibitor (ACE-I) or an angiotensin receptor blocker (ARB). For patients with normal or optimal blood pressure control, the target should be albuminuria attenuation. Clinical evidence supporting the use of ACE-I in T1DM is compelling, whereas the clinical evidence in T2DM is stronger for angiotensin receptor blocker (ARB) use.

ACE-Is are the best-studied drugs to treat established diabetic nephropathy in T1DM. There is a 50% reduction in renal disease progression using captopril, compared with placebo, in patients with more than 500 mg/day proteinuria and serum creatinine less than 2.5 mg/dL [14]. There are less data to support ARB therapy in this population, but ARB therapy is a reasonable alternative for patients who are unable to tolerate ACE-I due to cough.

In contrast, patients with T2DM and established nephropathy clearly benefit from ARB therapy based on two important studies. The Irbesartan Diabetic Nephropathy Trial [15] demonstrated significant reductions in the composite endpoint of doubling serum creatinine, ESRD, or death, with 20% reduction using irbesartan vs. placebo and 23% reduction using irbesartan vs. amlodipine. The blood pressure management was similar in the three groups. A similar Reduction of Endpoints in NIDDM with the Angiotensin II Antagonist (RENAAL) study of losartan revealed a 16% reduction in the same composite endpoint compared to placebo [16]. Both trials excluded patients with serum creatinine greater than 3.0 mg/dL. A recent trial of early nephropathy in T2DM demonstrated similar benefit in GFR slope at 5 years using high-dose ARB (telmisartan 80 mg daily) vs. medium-dose ACE-I (enalapril 20 mg daily) [17].

Concomitant ACE-I and ARB therapy may be more effective than treatment with either agent alone, but there are few studies comparing combination therapy to equivalent dose monotherapy. Patients with advanced CKD often require three or more agents to manage hypertension, including at the very least an ACE-I, ARB, and loop diuretic.

The hyperkalemia associated with ACE-I or ARB use leads to physician reluctance to employ these drugs and frequent drug interruption or discontinuation. The incidence of hyperkalemia secondary to ACE-I was 11% in one outpatient general medicine clinic [18], but an even higher incidence may be anticipated in high-risk diabetic nephropathy patients. Techniques for limiting hyperkalemia in such patients are prescribing a low potassium diet, avoidance of concomitant drugs that interfere with urinary potassium excretion, use of thiazide or loop diuretics that promote kaliuresis, and treatment of acidosis with sodium citrate or sodium bicarbonate [19].

An additional important cause of discontinuation of these drugs is a subsequent rise in serum creatinine. Physicians may choose to withhold therapy when the serum creatinine exceeds 3.0 mg/dL based on clinical trial designs that typically exclude such patients. This potentially precludes benefit for this population in which therapy could be critical. The clinician must be able to distinguish typical mild creatinine elevations, which result from drug-induced decreased glomerular filtration pressure, from more significant acute renal failure. For instance, the latter is an important sign of bilateral renal artery stenosis. A greater than 25% rise in serum creatinine during the first three months of ACE-I or ARB therapy should prompt magnetic resonance angiography to search for renal artery stenosis, and at least temporary discontinuation of drug therapy [13]. Increments in serum creatinine less than 25% over 3 months in serum creatinine should be anticipated. Well-informed patients who know and request serum creatinine data should be counseled regarding the anticipated short-term adverse effects of these drugs, as well as the long-term benefits, to avoid patient frustration, poor adherence, and self-discontinuation.

Clearly, ACE-I and/or ARB are crucial drugs to treat all patients with diabetic nephropathy. Moreover, both ACE-I [20] and ARB [21] reduce cardiovascular mortality in diabetes patients without established diabetic nephropathy. There is also speculation that these agents will actually prevent diabetes in the prediabetic patient at risk for subsequent diabetes. However, the universal application of these drugs to all diabetic and prediabetic patients carries a cost to society and side-effect risk to the individual patient. Overall, ACE-I or ARB therapy should be considered in each individual diabetic or prediabetic patient.

TOBACCO CESSATION

Tobacco smoking is an important and frequently overlooked contributing factor to both the onset and progression of diabetic nephropathy [22]. Prospective studies with near-optimal blood pressure control in both smokers and nonsmokers demonstrated more rapid progression of diabetic nephropathy in tobacco users for both T1DM [23] and T2DM [24]. One proposed mechanism of tobacco-associated renal injury involves acute hemodynamic alterations due to sympathetic activation, renin-angiotensin activation, increased endothelin production, and impaired endothelial cell-dependent vasodilatation [25]. Tobacco use is also associated with higher serum levels of AGE [26]. In practical terms, tobacco cessation delays the onset of diabetic nephropathy, attenuates the course of diabetic nephropathy, and reduces risk of cardiovascular events.

GLYCEMIC CONTROL

Intensive glycemic control reduced the development of diabetic nephropathy or microalbuminuria and attenuated the course of established diabetic nephropathy in three seminal studies, including the American Diabetes Control and Complications Trial [27] of patients with T1DM, the United Kingdom Prospective Diabetes Study [28] of patients with T2DM, and the Japanese Kumamoto Study [29] of patients with T2DM. The goal of therapy is an A1C less than 7% [27,28] or 6.5% [29]. It should be noted that in advanced diabetic nephropathy, a reduced erythrocyte survival occurs and can reduce A1C values. As a result of this "false-lowering" of the A1C, insulin therapy may be inappropriately delayed in patients with CKD. Metformin should be avoided in stages 2 to 5 CKD.

RENAL AND PANCREAS REPLACEMENT THERAPIES

Hemodialysis

Although the timing of dialysis initiation is challenging to anticipate clinically, patients with stage 5 CKD should be considered candidates for hemodialysis, peritoneal dialysis, and renal transplantation [12]. The major indications for emergent initiation of dialysis are metabolic acidosis, hyperkalemia, and volume overload. Uremic manifestations such as nutritional abnormalities, pericarditis, and encephalopathy are additional indications. Uremic manifestations that impact nutritional status are anorexia, dysgeusia, dyspepsia, early morning nausea, and vomiting. Uremic gastropathy can be difficult to distinguish from diabetic gastroparesis. Physicians must balance the nearly universal patient wish to forestall dialysis therapy with correction of the acute problems mentioned above. Stage 4 patients who are selected for hemodialysis should be prepared in advance with arteriovenous access creation [12], because hemodialysis therapy with catheters is associated with increased morbidity and mortality [30]. In addition, the patient with stage 4 CKD should be referred for renal transplantation evaluation immediately and not delayed unnecessarily until the diagnosis of ESRD is established. Patients with very limited life expectancy as a result of comorbidities, such as pancreatic carcinoma, should be offered the option of avoiding renal replacement after appropriate medical, palliative, and psychosocial assessments.

The high annual mortality of stage 5 CKD diabetic patients treated with hemodialysis in the U.S. is approximately 20% per year and is generally higher than the non-diabetic patient [1]. Myocardial infarction, cardiac arrhythmia, and cardiomyopathy account for more than 50% of the mortality [1].

Peritoneal Dialysis

The indications for therapy are as noted above. Peritoneal dialysis (PD) is probably underutilized in the U.S. for diabetic patients with ESRD. Selection bias limits morbidity and mortality comparisons between the dialysis modalities. Observational studies demonstrate mortality improvements in PD-treated patients, especially in the first few years of ERSD [31], reflecting improvements in this dialysis modality relative to hemodialysis or fewer comorbidities in PD patients at the time of dialysis initiation. Patients who are hemodynamically unstable as a result of cardiomyopathy or diabetic autonomic neuropathy may benefit from the more continuous nature of peritoneal dialysis, thus avoiding the frequent hypotensive episodes associated with intermittent hemodialysis. After 3 years of dialysis, the annual PD mortality is similar to hemodialysis, except that the increase in mortality in diabetic vs non-diabetic PD patients is more prominent [1]. Reluctance to offer PD in the U.S. is probably indicative of limited physician experience with this modality.

KIDNEY TRANSPLANTATION

A recent large observational study convincingly demonstrated that survival is enhanced for most diabetic patients, particularly the young, after kidney transplantation compared to continuing dialysis [33]. This therapy should be considered the optimal renal replacement modality for most T1DM and T2DM patients. Cardiovascular disease is the major limitation to transplantation in such patients. Selected T1DM patients should be referred for kidney–pancreas transplantation. Immunosuppressive therapy is associated with hyperglycemia, hypertension, and worsening of lipid metabolism, depending on the agents selected.

PANCREAS TRANSPLANTATION

The American Diabetes Association criteria for pancreas transplantation in patients with T1DM includes frequent acute and severe metabolic complications, clinical or emotional problems with insulin therapy, and consistent failure of insulin-based therapy to prevent secondary complications [34]. Pancreas transplantation is the only therapy capable of reversing the renal histopathologic alterations of diabetic nephropathy. One series of eight patients with T1DM who underwent renal biopsy before isolated pancreas transplant revealed significant improvement in both basement membrane thickness and mesangial sclerosis, but only after 10 years [35]. The pancreas may be transplanted alone, after kidney transplantation, or simultaneously at the time of kidney transplantation. Islet cell transplantation holds significant future promise, but at this time, should only be performed as part of a controlled clinical research trial [34].

NUTRITIONAL INTERVENTIONS IN DIABETIC NEPHROPATHY

Nutritional problems typically begin when the GFR is below 60 mL/minute/1.73 M^2 or with stages 3–5 CKD. Malnutrition is therefore common in CKD patients. Dietary counseling can impact the course of malnutrition, but is unfortunately underutilized, with only 1/3 of patients seeing a dietitian more than once in the year prior to initiating dialysis [1]. Medicare reimbursement for CKD nutritional care should improve access to dietary evaluation and therapy. Nutritional assessment in stages 3 and 4 CKD should include measurement of serum albumin and prealbumin, serum lipid profile, usual and actual edema-free body weights, percent ideal body weight, and body mass index (BMI; weight [kg]/height^2 [M^2]). Physicians or dietitians can perform a subjective global assessment [36], normalized protein nitrogen appearance (nPNA), and various anthropometric measurements, including bioelectrical impedance analysis. The nPNA calculations require multiple equations with different calculations for PD and HD [37].

SODIUM RESTRICTION

Patients with diabetes, particularly with hypertension also, have an increased pressor response to a dietary sodium load even in the setting of normal or supranormal GFR [38]. The mechanism may be over-activity of the renin-angiotensin system [38]. Furthermore, the pressor response to dietary sodium is usually exacerbated by decreased salt excretion in patients with impaired GFR [13]. Increased dietary sodium in diabetics also confers higher risks of albuminuria progression [38,39] and left ventricular hypertrophy [39]. High dietary sodium intake causes resistance to antihypertensive medicines, especially diuretics, ACE-I, and ARB. Sodium restriction is an essential nutritional measure to attain blood pressure in the target range and achieve edema-free body weight [12]. The spectrum of sodium restriction ranges from modest 2.4 g sodium to strict 1.5 g daily restriction and should be prescribed depending on a patient's CKD stage and ability to adhere to this dietary prescription [12]. This range of sodium intake is quite challenging for patients to achieve in the U.S., making flexibility for individual patients and ongoing nutritional intervention important features of care. The complete effect of blood pressure improvement with sodium restriction requires 5 weeks of intervention and adherence [39]. Moderate sodium restriction reduces systolic readings 5 mm Hg and diastolic blood pressure 2 mm Hg in hypertensive diabetics [40]. Assuming stable sodium intake in a steady state, the 24-hour urinary sodium can be used to estimate dietary salt intake. While the Dietary Approaches to Stop Hypertension (DASH) diet is an effective nutritional therapy for hypertension in the general population, the relatively high 1.4 g/kg/day protein intake and high potassium intake make it a poor choice for CKD patients [13]. Lastly, additional benefits of sodium restriction in diabetics include regression of left ventricular hypertrophy, decreased cerebrovascular events, albuminuria attenuation. and enhanced responses to antihypertensive medications [39].

LIPID MANAGEMENT

The principal reason to evaluate serum lipids in diabetic nephropathy is to detect abnormalities that may be treated to reduce the incidence of cardiovascular disease (CVD). Observational studies have conflicting results regarding the association of hyperlipidemia with kidney function deterioration in diabetic nephropathy, but lipid management may also improve or attenuate the course of kidney disease progression [41]. Inflammation in CKD is associated with increased low-density lipoprotein cholesterol (LDL-c), increased lipoprotein (a), and decreased high-density lipoprotein cholesterol (HDL-c) levels [42]. Heavy proteinuria in advanced diabetic nephropathy is associated with increased LDL-c levels secondary to decreased hepatic clearance. Also, advanced glycation endproducts (AGE) cross-linking to LDL-c may play a role in atherogenesis and observed increased cardiovascular mortality [42]. Typical lipid derangements found in patients with stage 5 CKD are increased triglycerides and low HDL-c [43].

Since CKD patients are at high risk for cardiovascular events [44], therapy with an 3-hydroxy-3-methylglutaryl coenzyme A (HMG-CoA) reductase inhibitor ("statin") should be considered for all patients with an LDL-c above 100 mg/dL (or above 70 mg/dL with diabetes and at high-risk for CVD) [31, 32]). Specific drug therapy for triglycerides above 500 mg/dL is also recommended [43]. Atorvastatin and simvastatin are the most efficacious in LDL-c reduction and have a reasonable safety profile. Once the LDL-c is at target levels, a fibrate may be used to treat the common hypertriglyceridemia of diabetic nephropathy [43]. Most fibrates (benzafibrate, clobibrate, and fenofibrate), except gemifbrozil, require dose adjustments for impaired GFR [43]. There are no safety data to support the use of ciprofibrate in CKD stages 2–5 [43]. Only gemfibrozil is recommended in stage 5 CKD patients because of insufficient data to support the use of other fibrates [43]. Combination therapy with a fibrate and statin must be prescribed cautiously because of the increased risk for rhabdomyolysis [43]. Immediate clinical evaluation and statin therapy interruption for patients with significant myalgia is probably more valuable than routine monitoring of serum CPK levels in asymptomatic individuals. Fish oil, containing omega-3 fatty acids, is an adjunctive therapy that requires close monitoring for LDL-c elevation. Nicotinic acid is also safe in CKD patients in the absence of liver disease [43].

Nutritional adjuvant therapies are an important component of lipid management. Low-fat diets are the primary therapy. For patients with an LDL-c above 70–100 mg/dL and adequate nutritional parameters, dietary content should be ≤ 7% saturated fat, ≤ 10% polyunsaturated fat, and ≤ 20% monounsaturated fat. Dietary fat restriction should be avoided in patients with protein energy malnutrition (PEM). Replacing saturated fat with carbohydrate in patients with diabetes has been shown by most, but not all, studies to result in LDL-c reduction with beneficial or neutral effects on plasma triglycerides [40]. The LDL-c reduction can also be enhanced by the addition of 2 g daily plant sterols and by 5–10 g soluble or viscous fiber [40]. Interestingly, the type of protein prescribed can increase the low HDL-c. A recent 8-week crossover trial of T2DM nephropathy revealed a mean 4.5% HDL-c rise with 0.5 g/kg soy protein, compared with 0.5 g/kg casein protein supplementation [45].

Weight reduction should be recommended for obese patients and an exercise program prescribed based on cardiovascular risks. Aerobic exercise modestly increases HDL-c and improves glycemic management. Although effective glycemic control usually reduces LDL-c and triglycerides in T1DM, obese patients with T1DM or T2DM usually require specific lipid-lowering therapy even when glycemic control is optimal [40].

PROTEIN–ENERGY REQUIREMENTS IN STAGE 1–4 CHRONIC KIDNEY DISEASE

The nutritional interventions in CKD patients must strike a balance in the spectrum between excessive protein-energy intake-induced deterioration in GFR and inadequate protein-energy intake contributing to PEM. The double-edged sword of protein energy dietary prescription in CKD contrasts with other nutritional interventions that are more in one direction only, i.e., increasing protein intake in the critically ill patient with PEM, or decreasing fat intake for the obese patient with hyperlipidemia [46]. Both the risks and benefits of protein energy dietary modification increase as CKD progresses, although there are little data to support this concept. In patients with CKD who do not require dialysis or transplant therapy, energy expenditure is similar to that of healthy patients without CKD [37]. The diet should therefore provide 35 kcal/kg/day to maintain neutral nitrogen balance and promote higher serum albumin concentrations [37]. In CKD patients 60 years of age or older, who tend to be less physically active, a reduced energy intake of 30–35 kcal/kg/day is recommended, although energy requirements for this age range have also been poorly investigated [37].

In a rat model of diabetic nephropathy, protein restriction reduces intraglomerular pressure, decreases glomerular hypertrophy, and decreases growth factor elaboration [47]. However, the precise mechanisms of these effects and their relevance to humans are unclear. Human studies of protein restriction in diabetic nephropathy are more promising than in other renal diseases in which intrarenal hemodynamic alterations are thought to play less of a prominent role [48]. The Modification of Diet in Renal Disease Study [49] is one of the largest trials showing the effects of different levels of protein restriction and blood pressure control on the progression of chronic renal failure. This study excluded insulin-treated diabetics and found that there was no statistically significant improvement in GFR with dietary protein restriction [49].

Prospective randomized controlled trials using diets with 0.3 g protein/kg/day with essential amino acid (L-lysine, L-threonine, L-tyrosine, and L-histidine) and keto-analogue (keto-leucine, keto-isoleucine, keto-valine, keto-phenylalanine, and hydroxyl-methionine) supplementation [50], 0.6 g protein/kg/day [51–54], 0.7 g protein/kg/day [55,56], and 0.8 g protein/kg/day [57,58] demonstrate attenuated declines in GFR compared to controls receiving higher intakes or unrestricted intakes of protein. When prescribing protein-restricted diets, at least 50–60% of the protein should be of high biological value to avoid negative nitrogen balance [59]. The concept of "biologic value" or "high quality" is subjective and based on how well the amino acid composition of the dietary protein matches the specific needs of the patient. In general, high biologic value is ascribed to animal protein like milk, eggs, and lean meats, followed by proteins from legumes (beans), cereals (rice, wheat, and corn), and roots. High biologic proteins are also highly digestible and absorbable with optimal proportions of the essential amino acids. The strategy in patients with diabetic nephropathy is to provide high-quality protein so that physiological needs are met with the least amount of nitrogen and deleterious fats.

Dietary protein modification trials in diabetic nephropathy have conflicting results. Most, but not all, of these trials demonstrate GFR benefit. Several randomized trials have also demonstrated a decrease in albuminuria with dietary protein restriction independent of blood pressure effects [50,52,53,55–58]. Two of these studies demonstrated improved glycemic control with protein restriction [50,57]. Interestingly one 4-year prospective randomized study revealed no significant change in GFR with 0.6 g protein/kg/day restriction, but revealed significant improvements in ESRD onset and mortality compared to the control group [60]. This suggests other beneficial effects that are independent of GFR. One important aspect of this well-designed trial was the concomitant ACE-I use in over 85% of patients in both treatment and control arms. In fact, optimal or nearly optimal blood pressure management is a prerequisite for any beneficial effect of dietary protein restriction [53]. In addition, adherence to low-protein diets is questionable even for selected patients in well-designed clinical research trials [54,57]. The National Kidney Foundation's clinical practice guidelines for nutrition in chronic kidney disease recommend consideration of 0.6–0.75 g/kg/day dietary protein restriction for stable patients with stage 4 CKD [37].

The primary risk of protein-restricted diets is PEM. One negative study of 0.6 g/kg/day dietary protein modification for 12 months in patients with diabetic nephropathy demonstrated significant reductions in both serum prealbumin at 9 months and albumin at 12 months, compared with controls [61]. However, similar trials of protein-restricted diets in diabetic nephropathy did not show significantly decreased serum albumin levels. Prealbumin levels not only reflect changes in visceral protein stores over a shorter time period, compared with albumin, but can also be confounded by GFR changes, dialysis, bleeding, and inflammation. Because the effects of PEM are potentially devastating, special care must be taken to ensure that protein-restricted diets do not yield a state of negative nitrogen balance. One helpful tool to estimate the actual protein intake or estimate dietary protein prescription adherence, assuming stable nitrogen balance, uses a 24-hour urine collection and the following formula [62]:

- Observed nitrogen intake = urinary nitrogen excretion
- Urinary nitrogen excretion = urine urea nitrogen (UUN) + nonurea nitrogen of 31 mg/kg

- Protein intake = 6.25 × urinary nitrogen excretion
- For example, an 80 kg man with 24-hour urine urea nitrogen of 8 g
- Protein intake = 6.25 (8 + 2.48) = 65.5 g or 0.82 g/kg/day

A more conventional method to estimate protein requirements is to estimate the protein catabolic rate: [24 hour UUN (g) + 4] × 6.25. Last, in acutely ill pre-dialysis CKD patients, protein intake should not be reduced [37].

PROTEIN–ENERGY REQUIREMENTS IN STAGE 5 CHRONIC KIDNEY DISEASE OR END-STAGE RENAL DISEASE

There is no single parameter that provides a comprehensive assessment of nutritional status in stage 5 CKD, making a combination of measurements optimal [37]. Such parameters include serum albumin, serum prealbumin, serum cholesterol, dietary interviews, dairies, nPNA, subjective global assessment, and edema-free body weight.

Energy requirements are identical to earlier stages of CKD, or 35 kcal/kg/day and a reduced intake of 30 to 35 kcal/kg/day for those 60 years of age or older [37]. The recommended protein intake for stable patients is 1.2 g/kg/day for hemodialysis and 1.2–1.3 g/kg/day for peritoneal dialysis with at least 50% high biological value [37,63]. Also similar to pre-dialysis CKD patients, protein intake should not be reduced in unstable or hospitalized stage 5 CKD patients [37]. Unfortunately, PEM is common in stage 5 CKD, occurring in up to 50% of patients [64,65]. The target serum albumin to prevent PEM is a minimum of 3.8 g/dL [37]. Low serum albumin is associated with increased risk of mortality in both hemodialysis- [66] and peritoneal dialysis-treated patients [67]. Important etiologies for inadequate nutrition in the diabetic dialysis patient include inadequate dialysis dose delivery [68], overly aggressive dietary restrictions, metabolic acidosis [69], and diabetic gastroparesis. Hemodialysis patients had lower protein and energy intakes on dialysis days than other days in two well-designed studies [70,71], but the etiology of this finding is unclear. In the first 1000 patients participating in a randomized trial of variations in hemodialysis dose (the HEMO study), the mean daily intake levels of energy were 24.1 and 21.8 kcal/kg, with dietary protein at 0.98 and 0.89 g/kg for men and women, respectively [64]. Compared to afore-mentioned National Kidney Foundation recommended intakes, these data indicate approximately 90% energy intake and 50% protein intake deficiency prevalence [65]. Peritoneal dialysis patients have additional etiologies: increased dialysate amino acid and protein losses [72] as well as impaired appetite due to abdominal fullness. Enhancements in suboptimal dialysis dose improve appetite and protein intake in hemodialysis- [68] and peritoneal dialysis-treated patients [73]. Unfortunately, increasing hemodialysis dose beyond the accepted minimum standard three times weekly did not improve nutritional parameters in the previously described HEMO study [74]. Underutilized home and in-center hemodialysis modalities that demonstrate the most promise to improve nutritional parameters in small observational studies include short frequent hemodialysis (five or more sessions per week) and long nocturnal hemodialysis [75].

The MIA syndrome, consisting of malnutrition, inflammation, and atherosclerosis, accounts for the excessively high mortality among ESRD patients and highlights the importance of nutritional therapy in CKD [76]. The first description came recently from Peter Stenvinkel. Proinflammatory cytokines, like tumor necrosis factor (TNF-α), can suppress appetite, induce muscle proteolysis, and promote atherosclerosis. Cardiac valvular calcification is enhanced by TNF-α, suggesting an additional link between MIA and deleterious calcium-phosphate metabolism [76]. Malnutrition increases mortality rates by aggravating established inflammation, which in turn worsens congestive heart failure, increases susceptibility to infection, and promotes atherogenesis [76]. Surprisingly, higher cholesterol levels, obesity, and relatively low homocysteine levels in ESRD confer favorable survival in hemodialysis patients in several studies [77]. This unexpected relationship is called the reverse epidemiology of ESRD by some authors [77]. The explanation may be related to the decreased prevalence of MIA syndrome in these patients. The reverse epidemiology relationship should not be interpreted as beneficial effects of obesity, dyslipidemia, and hyperhomocysteinemia, nor that these conditions should be untreated [77].

The MIA syndrome is an elegant concept [76] that is perhaps the most compelling non-traditional cardiovascular risk factor in CKD described to date. Although physicians can recall cases that clearly illustrate the MIA syndrome, how will this condition be definitively diagnosed–a triad of findings, such as serum albumin, C-reactive protein, and cardiac calcification on imaging? Future research should answer these questions, more precisely define diagnostic criteria, and provide specific nutritional and pharmacological therapies to improve the high cardiovascular CKD mortality associated with this syndrome.

ORAL AND ENTERAL PROTEIN–ENERGY SUPPLEMENTATION

If dietary modifications fail to improve nutritional status, oral protein supplementation is effective in improving nutritional parameters [65,78]. Protein supplements used in this setting should be low potassium, phosphate, and magnesium. Most protein supplements come in 8-oz cans or cartons. Nepro® (formulated for stage 5 CKD) and Suplena® (formulated for stages 3 and 4 CKD) are high in carbohydrate content and may require therapy for hyperglycemia. The lower amounts of carbohydrate provided by diabetes formulations Glucerna® and ReSource® Diabetic cause less hyperglycemia, but contain more potassium and phosphate [79]. Enteral feedings are underutilized in CKD because of lack of convenience and physician inexperience.

PERITONEAL DIALYSATE INSULIN AND AMINO ACID CONTENT

Conventional peritoneal dialysate solutions are composed of dextrose at concentrations of 1.5%, 2.5%, and 4.25%. Higher osmolarity concentrations increase ultrafiltrate removal. Since these solutions impact glycemic control, intraperitoneal insulin can be helpful. Peritoneal visceral absorption of intraperitoneal insulin into the portal circulation may be more rapid, consistent, and is associated with lower insulin levels in the systemic circulation than subcutaneous administration [80]. A potential disadvantage of intraperitoneal insulin administration is increased incidence of PD peritonitis [80]. Since the absorption benefits are at least in part counterbalanced by the infectious risks, there are no definitive data in the literature regarding the optimal use of intraperitoneal insulin. Additionally, icodextin is a recently Food and Drug Administration (FDA)-approved glucose-free peritoneal dialysis solution that has the potential advantage of improved glycemic control [81].

In patients with diabetic nephropathy treated with continuous ambulatory peritoneal dialysis (CAPD), in whom PEM and nitrogen balance remains impaired despite attempts to improve oral intake, one option is to add amino acids to one of the usual four daily peritoneal dialysis fluid (PDF) exchanges. Several studies, with treatment duration for at least 3 months, have demonstrated the beneficial effect of a 1.1% amino acid dialysis solution (e.g., Nutrineal®) on nitrogen balance, serum albumin, and serum amino acid concentrations, but at the expense of increased acidosis, need for antacid treatment, and decreased dialysis adequacy (evidence levels 2 and 3) [82–84]. In a PRCT involving 60 malnourished Chinese CAPD patients, there was no demonstrable benefit of amino acid-containing PDF [85]. There was no evidence of increased mortality or incidence of peritonitis with amino acid-containing PDF. Ohter effects of amino acid-containing PDF are improved peritoneal mesothelial cell physiology [86,87] and impairment of endothelial function [88]. Overall, there is insufficient conclusive evidence, especially in patients with diabetes, supporting the routine use of amino acid-containing PDF with respect to nutritional benefit (grade D). However, since this intervnetion is generally well-tolerated, it does offer the potential advantage to adult and pediatric patients with diabetes of introducing a lower glucose load, lower insulin requirement, improved glycemic control, and reduction in amino acid losses in the peritoneal effluent (evidence level 2) [89,90].

INTRADIALYTIC PARENTERAL NUTRITION

Intradialytic parenteral nutrition (IDPN), an admixture of amino acids, dextrose, lipid, and micro-nutrients, provides supplemental nutrition exclusively during the hemodialysis procedure via the patient's dialysis access. IDPN is a particularly convenient and attractive nutritional therapy for the hemodialysis patient in need of nutrition support. However, the time limitations of the hemodialysis sessions, typically 3–4 hours thrice weekly in the U.S., make this an inefficient treatment. There are no definitive data that demonstrate that IDPN improves morbidity and mortality. However, there are a number of small prospective IDPN series demonstrating improvements in nutritional parameters compared to controls in nondiabetic patients [91]. One retrospective IDPN study, including 33 diabetics of 81 studied, demonstrated a 12% increase in serum albumin, as well as a 12% improvement in survival over a mean 9-month follow up compared to controls [91]. A major flaw of IDPN trials is the absence of oral supplements or appetite stimulant use in the control groups [91,92].

There is insufficient clinical evidence for specific indications for IDPN, but it is reasonable to use IDPN in patients with (1) inadequate protein-calorie intake to meet their metabolic needs, (2) uncertain or nonfunctional GI function precluding sufficient enteral nutrition support and inadequate venous access for conventional peripheral or central parenteral nutrition, or (3) inability to meet nutritional needs with parenteral nutrition due to volume limitations (grade C). Another use of IDPN is in all malnourished dialysis patients, based on the sustained (> 3 months) presence of hypoalbuminemia, weight loss, decreased intake, and subjective global assessment [93]. It must be emphasized that IDPN is not a substitute for conventional parenteral nutrition since, by itself, it cannot provide sufficient nutrition with only three infusions per week. Specifically, IDPN only provides approximately 1100 kcal TIW (6 kcal/kg/day for a 70 kg patient) and 80 g protein TIW (0.5 g/kg/day for a 70 kg patient) [94]. Thus, total protein-calorie needs are only met when other sources of nutrition provide at least approximately 25–30 kcal/kg/day and 0.7 g/kg/day.

Diabetic patients receiving IDPN should receive insulin in the PN formula along with dextrose. Glucose determinations are made during and after the infusion, and the insulin dose is adjusted and optimized. Then, dextrose may be increased with commensurate increases in the insulin content. A typical IDPN formula contains 80 g of concentrated (15% solution; 4 kcal/g) amino acid (320 kcal), 100–150 g dextrose (as D70; 3.4 kcal/g; 340–510 kcal), 30 g lipid (as a 20% emulsion; 10 kcal/g; 300 kcal), 1 g calcium gluconate, trace elements, and multivitamins—with no sodium, potassium, phosphate, or magnesium—in a 1 L solution. Carnitine, 1–3 g, can also be added to the bag. Carnitine is particularly efficacious in treating refractory anemia, intradialytic hypotension, and myopathy [37]. One author recommends a minimum 4-hour hemodialysis treatment time to adequately address the volume infused and enhanced urea generation consequent to the fluid and amino acid content of IDPN respectively [65]. Future IDPN studies should address the morbidity and mortality outcomes and better characterize the target patient population [94].

ANABOLIC AGENTS AND APPETITE STIMULANTS

Anabolic agents studied in dialysis patients include recombinant human growth hormone (GH) and recombinant IGF-1 but these drugs have not been used outside of research protocols and can induce hyperglycemia [95]. Androgen therapy has been used to promote anabolism but there are no controlled studies in diabetics with nephropathy. Megestrol acetate, an appetite stimulant, has a role for treating malnutrition and anorexia in dialysis patients. An uncontrolled trial of 18 hypoalbuminemic (serum albumin < 3.5 g/dL) hemodialysis patients including 8 patients with diabetes treated with megestrol acetate, 400 mg twice daily, showed poor tolerance for this therapy with frequent hyperglycemia, diarrhea, confusion and headaches [96]. Other potential agents used to stimulate appetite include antidepressants, such as methylphenidate and mirtazapine. In general, as oral intake increases with appetite stimulation, diabetic medication will need to be adjusted.

Treatment of dysgeusia, common in stage 5 CKD patients [97], should improve appetite. Although studies published in the 1980s demonstrated evidence for reversibility of hypogeusia and dysgeusia with zinc supplementation [98,99], a more recent randomized placebo-controlled trial definitively showed no change in baseline taste disturbance with zinc supplementation [97].

PHOSPHATE RESTRICTION AND SECONDARY HYPERPARATHYROIDISM

Secondary hyperparathyroidism is generally evident with stages 3–5 CKD [100]. Phosphate retention is associated with a decline in GFR. Hyperphosphatemia directly stimulates post-translational parathyroid hormone (PTH) synthesis and indirectly inhibits renal vitamin D activation [101]. The combination of hyperphosphatemia and calcitriol deficiency promotes hypocalcemia and thus further increases PTH. Hyperphosphatemia and the increased calcium-phosphate cross-product are associated with increased mortality in hemodialysis patients [102], possibly through enhanced vascular calcification and atherosclerosis. The target phosphate level is 2.7–4.6 mg/dL, for stages 3 and 4 CKD patients, and 3.5–5.5 mg/dL, for stage 5 CKD [100]. The target PTH value is subject to debate, but is generally agreed to be 1.5x higher than the normal range, with a graded increase in target as CKD progresses from stage 3 to stage 5.

An important part of secondary hyperparathyroidism is dietary phosphate restriction. Dairy products, cereals, grains, and colored-sodas are rich sources of dietary phosphate. Most of the drug therapies that treat hyperphosphatemia and secondary hyperparathyroidism act independently. Phosphate binders include calcium carbonate, calcium acetate, lanthanum carbonate, and sevelamer, whereas vitamin D and its analogs include calcitriol, paricalcitol, and doxercalciferol. Calcitriol may induce hypercalcemia and increase the calcium-phosphate cross-product. Moreover, hyperphosphatemia blunts the effects of vitamin D and its analogs. Cinacalcet offers the advantage of both reducing phosphate and PTH [103]. This calcimimetic agent mimics the effect of calcium on the receptor in the parathyroid cell to limit secretion and gene transcription of PTH. In stage-5 CKD patients, hyperphosphatemia often occurs despite adequate dialysis dose delivery [102]. Therefore, since protein intake necessarily includes phosphorus intake, coordinating the intake of these dietary constituents is essential.

POTASSIUM AND MAGNESIUM RESTRICTION

Potassium restriction is important to prevent or limit hyperkalemia. This applies to at-risk diabetics with nephropathy and impaired GFR, type-IV renal tubular acidosis, and drug use such as ACE-I, ARB, and potassium-sparing diuretics. Frequently unrecognized sources of dietary potassium are salt substitutes, which are usually composed of potassium chloride. Common rich sources of dietary potassium include citrus fruits and their juices, bananas, and tomatoes. Patients without documented hyperkalemia do not need to restrict intake. Daily potassium intake is limited to 2–3 g in hemodialysis and 3–4 g in peritoneal dialysis treated patients.

Magnesium toxicity is essentially only observed in clinical medicine in CKD patients because of reduced renal clearance and in obstetrical patients with pre-eclampsia treated with exceptionally high doses of intravenous magnesium salts. Magnesium intake should be restricted to 200–300 mg daily [65]. Perhaps the most important practical aspect of magnesium restriction is avoidance of drugs containing magnesium salts such as antacids and laxatives.

VITAMINS, MINERALS, AND ANTIOXIDANTS

Dialysis population studies provide evidence of low blood concentrations of water-soluble vitamins and minerals because of inadequate intake, increased losses, and increased needs [104]. Of the water-soluble vitamins, folate deserves special mention. There has been much speculation that folate supplementation will correct the hyperhomocysteinemia of CKD, resulting in reduced cardiovascular morbidity and mortality. Unfortunately, no study has convincingly demonstrated improved outcomes in CKD with folate supplementation. Paradoxically, a recent study revealed increased morbidity and mortality in hemodialysis patients with lower homocysteine levels, perhaps as a reflection of PEM—as previously noted [105]. Overall, hemodialysis patients demonstrate hyperhomocysteinemia, yet relatively low levels may represent a nutritional marker [105].

Iron deficiency is common in hemodialysis patients by virtue of increased demands of erythropoietin and darbepoetin anemia therapies and the small amount of blood loss obligate with each treatment [106]. Hemodialysis patients should be treated with nondextran intravenous iron preparations, such as iron gluconate and iron sucrose. This avoids the side effects of poorly tolerated and generally ineffective oral iron [106]. The optimal mode of iron supplementation in patients with stages 1 to 4 CKD and those treated with PD is currently unknown. Such patients are usually treated with oral iron supplementation for convenience, but intravenous therapy should be considered for refractory iron deficiency.

Antioxidant properties of vitamins C and E make supplementation reasonable in CKD, but definitive studies demonstrating improved outcomes are lacking. In contrast, the reduced clearance of fat-soluble vitamin A metabolites by the normal kidney places stage-3 CKD patients at risk for hypervitaminosis A [104]. This is an important consideration when selecting a multivitamin that contains a combination of water- and fat-soluble vitamins. A number of vitamin preparations tailored to the special needs of stage-5 CKD patients are available including Nephrocaps®, Neph-Plex® Rx, NephroVite Rx®, Diatx™, Dialyvite, and Renax.

NUTRITIONAL ISSUES FOR THE KIDNEY- AND PANCREAS-TRANSPLANT DIABETIC PATIENT

KIDNEY TRANSPLANTATION

Certain immunosuppressive drugs, glucocorticoids, cyclosporine, and tacrolimus, are associated with hyperglycemia, new onset diabetes, or post-transplantation diabetes in approximately 10% of patients [107]. Glucocorticoids primarily induce postprandial hyperglycemia with less effect on fasting glucose levels. Although both calcineurin inhibitors cause reversible islet cell toxicity, tacrolimus is associated with more hyperglycemia than cyclosporine. Other immunosuppressive agents, azathioprine, mycophenolate mofetil, and sirolimus do not appear to have detrimental effects on glucose metabolism.

A different group of immunosuppressive agents, including prednisone, cyclosporine, and sirolimus, as well as graft dysfunction and genetic predisposition, are the major causes of dyslipidemia after renal transplantation [108]. The most common abnormality is LDL-c greater than 100 mg/dL observed in over 70% of patients 1 year after surgery in several observational studies [108]. Statin therapy has important drug interactions with immunosuppressive agents. Most statins are metabolized via the hepatic cytochrome p450 3A4 enzyme, such as atorvastatin or simvastatin. The calcineurin inhibitors cyclosporine and tacrolimus share this metabolism, resulting in increased statin levels during concomitant therapy [108]. Avoidance of rhabdomyolysis in this population requires a reduction in maximum statin dose and avoidance of other drugs that share similar metabolism, such as nicotinic acid and fibrates. Combination statin and fibrate therapy should be avoided in kidney-transplant patients [108]. Fluvastatin or pravastatin, the statins preferred by many transplant physicians, are metabolized differently from calcineurin inhibitors. Fibrate monotherapy may be considered for patients with triglycerides over 500 mg/dL who are not treated with a statin or unable to tolerate statin therapy [108].

Glucocorticoids, calcineurin inhibitors, and renal graft dysfunction contribute to hypertension. Systolic blood pressure (BP) greater than 140 mm Hg was found in 44% of patients at 1 year in one study, representing remarkably poor blood pressure management after renal transplantation [109]. Each 10 mm Hg increase in BP confers highly significant relative risks of 1.12 for graft failure and 1.18 for death [109]. Aggressive pharmacologic therapy and continued nutritional intervention particularly for sodium restriction should be emphasized.

Postoperative restoration of urine output allows for unrestricted fluid intake and increases in salt intake if blood pressure is well-managed. The anabolic effects of glucocorticoids and normal or improved urea clearance require increases in energy and protein intake. Overall nutritional status significantly improves in patients with diabetes 2 years after renal transplantation with 0.5 g/dL mean serum albumin increase, thicker midarm muscle circumference, and an approximate 10% body weight increase [110]. Nutritional benefits observed in patients with diabetes after renal transplantation are more pronounced than those found in nondiabetics [110]. Similar to CKD, hypoalbuminemia is associated with poorer outcomes [111], and cardiovascular mortality is the most common cause of death [112].

The course after transplantation has important nutritional implications in the diabetic patient. Uncomplicated courses result in dietary liberalization, better quality of life, enhanced appetite, improved nutritional parameters, and decreases in cardiovascular morbidity and mortality. Alternatively, postoperative episodes of rejection are treated with more intense immunosuppression, which in turn worsens hyperglycemia, hypertension, and hyperlipidemia. Acute rejection and infection impair appetite and are associated with hypoalbuminemia [111] and systemic inflammation. Such patients are more likely to suffer a cardiovascular event [112]. Course also impacts the prevalence of hypoalbuminemia. In one large series, the prevalence of hypoalbuminemia after renal transplanation revealed a 31% peak at 3 months, 12% nadir at 1 year, 14% prevalence at 4 years, and 20% prevalence at 8 years [111]. This bimodal or early peak and late gradual increase of hypoalbuminuria reflects a high incidence of acute complications in the first 3 months, followed by stabilization at 1 year, and culminating in gradual deterioration, perhaps secondary to hyperlipidemia and chronic rejection.

Obesity may limit renal transplant candidacy and was found in 15–20% of patients at the time of renal transplantation in one series [107]. Obesity carries important implications for post-transplant glycemic control. Sedentary lifestyle is a major risk factor for hyperglycemia and obesity post-transplant [107]. Intensive nutritional intervention including an exercise program tailored to the individual's capacity and cardiovascular risk is crucial for improved outcomes.

KIDNEY–PANCREAS TRANSPLANTATION

The balance of risks and benefits of dual-organ transplant compared to renal transplant alone on cardiovascular morbidity and mortality is unclear. Comparisons are complicated by selection bias and absence of randomized trials, which many consider unethical [113]. The simultaneous kidney–pancreas transplant requires a longer operation that confers higher short-term morbidity and mortality, which probably lasts 3 months compared to renal transplant alone. How much the long-term benefits of dual-transplant counterbalance the increased 3-month risk is an important consideration. Improved glucose control and freedom from insulin therapy results in elimination or marked reduction of dietary restrictions that contribute to enhanced quality of life [113]. Improvements or stabilization of other diabetic end-organ damage is observed in patients following kidney and pancreas transplantation [113]. Post-transplant hypoalbuminemia development is typically early, especially in patients with acute rejection. The long-term nutritional course may be better than the bimodal deterioration observed with renal transplantation alone. For example, hypoalbuminermia prevalence is 44% at 3 months, 15% at 1 year, and 8% at 3 years in one dual organ transplant series [114]. Persistent hypoalbuminemia is associated with increased risks of CMV infection and graft (pancreas and kidney) failure [114].

Interventions to treat and prevent PEM in transplant patients should be similar to CKD patients, except that post-transplant PEM carries different implications. Etiologies of transplant rejection and chronic infection such as CMV should be considered in PEM evaluation and therapy. Restrictions in potassium and phosphate are usually not required, depending on the GFR. The traditional

TABLE 10.2
Nutritional Therapy for Each CKD Stage

Nutrient	Stage 1	Stage 2	Stage 3	Stage 4	Stage 5
Sodium (g/day)	1.5–2.4	1.5–2.4	1.5–2.4	1.5–2 .4	1.5–2.4
Energy (kcal/kg/day)	(35 under age 60, and 30–35 age 60 and older for all stages)				
Fat	TLC[a]	TLC[a]	TLC[a]	TLC[a]	TLC[a]
Protein (g/kg/day)	0.8[a]	0.8[a]	0.6[a]	0.6[a]	1.2 (HD), 1.3 (PD)
Phosphate (mg/day)	none	none	800–1000	800–1000	800–1000
Potassium (g/day)	V[b]	V[b]	V[b]	V[b]	2–3 (HD), 3–4 (PD)

Abbreviations: TLC—therapeutic lifestyle changes; HD—hemodialysis; PD—peritoneal dialysis; V—variable.

Dietary fat restriction should be avoided for patients with protein-energy malnutrition. For patients with low-density lipoprotein cholesterol (LDL-c) 100 mg/dL and adequate nutritional parameters, dietary content should include < 7% saturated fat, 10% polyunsaturated fat, 20% monounsaturated fat, and 25–35% total fat content of all calories. Weight reduction for obese patients and exercise program graded to cardiovascular disease should be considered.

[a] The aim is to attenuate CKD progression in highly motivated patients with optimal (BP < 130/80 mm Hg) or nearly optimal BP management and adequate nutritional parameters. Close follow-up is critical to encourage and monitor compliance as well as prevent protein-energy malnutrition.

[b] Depending on the presence of preexisting hyperkalemia.

risk factors for CVD (tobacco smoking, dyslipidemia, hyperglycemia, and hypertension) play a more prominent role in transplant patients than in CKD patients [112]. Cardiovascular risks demand especially aggressive therapies to improve outcomes. Given the poor hypertension management in these patients [109], the importance of dietary sodium restriction should be emphasized. Although the MIA syndrome may not be applicable to patients post-transplant, inflammation may also be associated with cardiovascular mortality in this setting. CMV infection and acute rejection are examples of inflammatory modulation in kidney transplant recipients not observed in CKD without transplantation.

CONCLUSIONS AND RECOMMENDATIONS

Nutritional therapy of diabetic nephropathy can attenuate the course of CKD, reduce morbidity, and perhaps improve survival via reduction in cardiovascular mortality. Nutritional therapy should be individualized to the patient's level of renal function, composite CVD risk, glycemic control, nutritional status, ability to adhere to dietary modification, and motivation (see Table 10.2). The extraordinary complexity of these interventions—including sodium, fat, protein, potassium, and phosphate dietary modifications, above and beyond the diabetic carbohydrate limitations—make the complete nutritional prescription realistic only in a small minority of patients who are highly motivated. These patients will only achieve optimal care if the physician is appropriately informed of the indications, benefits, and risks of nutritional therapy.

The multidisciplinary approach to care, including a dietitian skilled in CKD management, is most likely to succeed in the highly motivated patient. At the other end of the spectrum are patients who are unable to comprehend or adhere to the complex dietary modifications. The focus for such patients should be early detection, treatment, and ideally prevention of hyperphosphatemia and PEM in a multidisciplinary fashion. The therapeutic armamentarium for PEM in diabetic nephropathy includes increasing high-biological-value dietary protein, oral protein supplementation tailored to CKD, enteral tube feedings, amino acid-containing PDF in select instances of hyperglycemia with PD, IDPN with hemodialysis, and total parenteral nutrition (TPN) (see Table 10.3). The grave mortality associations of hyperphosphatemia [102], high-calcium-phosphate cross-product [102], hypoalbuminemia [66,67],

TABLE 10.3
Evidence-Based Nutritional Interventions in CKD

Intervention	Evidence Level
High biological value protein	2
Oral protein supplements	2
Amino acid-containing peritoneal dialysis fluid	2-3
Intradialytic parenteral nutrition	3
Total parenteral nutrition	3
Multidiscipinary approach with dietitian	4
Enteral tube feedings	4

TABLE 10.4
Nutritional Therapy Goals to Potentially Limit PEM and Cardiac Calcification

Albumin 4.0 g/dL using the Bromcresol Green Assay
Phosphate 2.7–4.6 mg/dL for stages 3 & 4 CKD
Phosphate 3.5–5.5 mg/dL for stage 5 CKD
Calcium-phosphate cross-product < 55 mg^2/dL^2

See text for abbreviations.

Source: From References [37,100].

and the malnutrition, inflammation, and atherosclerosis syndrome (MIA) syndrome [76] in ESRD patients suggests that prevention and perhaps even improvement of established hyperphosphatemia and PEM will reduce mortality. Because hyperphosphatemia, malnutrition, and inflammation are common in stages 3 and 4 CKD [115], nutritional assessment and therapy are critical to the management of diabetic nephropathy. Prospective studies should be performed to address the benefit of improving nutritional status (see Table 10.4) on cardiovascular mortality in CKD.

REFERENCES

1. U.S. Renal Data System, USRDS 2004 Annual Report: Atlas of End-Stage Renal Disease in the United States, National Institutes of Health, National Institute of Diabetes and Digestive and Kidney Diseases, Bethesda, MD, 2004.
2. Krolewski AS, Warram JH, and Rand LI et al., Epidemiologic approach to the etiology of type-I diabetes mellitus and its complications, *N Engl J Med*, 317:1390–1398, 1987.
3. Cowie CC, Port FK, and Wolfe RA et al., Disparities in incidence of diabetic end-stage renal disease according to race and type of diabetes, *N Engl J Med*, 321:1074–1079, 1989.
4. Nelson RG, Bennett PH, and Beck GJ et al., Diabetic Renal Disease Study Group, Development and progression of renal disease in Pima Indians with non-insulin-dependent diabetes mellitus, *N Engl J Med*, 335:1636–1642, 1996.
5. Osterby R, Gall MA, and Schmitz A et al., Glomerular structure and function in proteinuric type-2 (non-insulin-dependent) diabetic patients, *Diabetologia*, 36:1064–1070, 1993.
6. Kennon B, Petrie JR, and Small M et al., Angiotensin-converting enzyme gene and diabetes mellitus, *Diabetic Med*, 16:448–458, 1999.
7. Kimmelsteil P and Wilson C, Intercapillary lesions in glomeruli of the kidney, *Am J Pathol*, 12:83, 1936.
8. Dalla Vestra M, Saller A, and Bortoloso E et al., Structural involvement in type-1 and type-2 diabetic nephropathy, *Diabetes Metab*, 26(Suppl 4):8–14, 2000.
9. Hasslacher C, Ritz E, and Wahl P et al., Similar risks of nephropathy in patients with type-I or type-II diabetes mellitus, *Nephrol Dial Transplant*, 4:859–863, 1989.

10. Brizzi MF, Dentelli P, and Rosso A et al., RAGE- and TGF-β receptor-mediated signals converge on STAT5 and p21waf to control cell-cycle progression of mesangial cells: A possible role in the development and progression of diabetic nephropathy, *FASEB J,* 18:1249–1251, 2004.
11. Deckert T, Kofoed-Enevoldsen A, and Norgaard K et al., Microalbuminuria: Implications for micro- and macrovascular disease, *Diabetes Care,* 15:1181–1191, 1992.
12. National Kidney Foundation, K/DOQI clinical practice guidelines for chronic kidney disease: Evaluation, classification, and stratification, *Am J Kidney Dis,* 39(Suppl 1):S1–245, 2002.
13. National Kidney Foundation, K/DOQI clinical practice guidelines on hypertension and antihypertensive agents in chronic kidney disease, *Am J Kidney Dis,* 43(5 Suppl 1):S1–290, 2004.
14. Lewis EJ, Hunsicker LG, and Bain RP et al., The Collaborative Study Group, The effect of angiotensin-converting-enzyme inhibition on diabetic nephropathy, *N Engl J Med,* 329:1456–1462, 1993.
15. Lewis EJ, Hunsicker LG, and Clarke WR et al., Renoprotective effect of the angiotensin-receptor antagonist irbesartan in patients with nephropathy due to type-2 diabetes, *N Engl J Med,* 345:851–860, 2001.
16. Brenner BM, Cooper ME, and de Zeeuw D et al., RENAAL Study Investigators, Effects of losartan on renal and cardiovascular outcomes in patients with type-2 diabetes and nephropathy, *N Engl J Med,* 345:861–869, 2001.
17. Barnett AH, Bain SC, and Bouter P et al., Diabetics Exposed to Telmisartan and Enalapril Study Group, Angiotensin-receptor blockade versus converting-enzyme inhibition in type-2 diabetes and nephropathy, *N Engl J Med,* 351:1952–1961, 2004.
18. Reardon LC and Macpherson DS, Hyperkalemia in outpatients using angiotensin-converting enzyme inhibitors: How much should we worry? *Arch Intern Med,* 158:26–32, 1998.
19. Palmer BF, Managing hyperkalemia caused by inhibitors of the renin-angiotensin-aldosterone system, *N Engl J Med,* 351:585–592, 2004.
20. Heart Outcomes Prevention Evaluation Study Investigators, Effects of ramipril on cardiovascular and microvascular outcomes in people with diabetes mellitus, Results of the HOPE study and MICRO-HOPE substudy, *Lancet,* 355:253–259, 2000.
21. Lindholm LH, Dahlof B, and Edelman JM et al., LIFE Study Group, Effect of losartan on sudden cardiac death in people with diabetes, Data from the LIFE study, *Lancet,* 362:619–620, 2003.
22. Haire-Joshu D, Glasgow RE, and Tibbs TL, Smoking and diabetes, *Diabetes Care,* 22:1887–1898, 1999.
23. Sawicki PT, Didjurgeit U, and Muhlhauser I et al., Smoking is associated with progression of diabetic nephropathy, *Diabetes Care,* 17:126–131, 1994.
24. Chuahirun T, Simoni J, and Hudson C et al., Cigarette smoking exacerbates and its cessation ameliorates renal injury in type-2 diabetes, *Am J Med Sci,* 327:57–67, 2004.
25. Ritz E, Ogata H, and Orth SR, Smoking: A factor promoting onset and progression of diabetic nephropathy, *Diabetes Metab,* 26(Suppl 4):54–63, 2000.
26. Cerami C, Founds H, and Nicholl I et al., Tobacco smoke is a source of toxic reactive glycation products, *Proc Natl Acad Sci USA,* 94:13915–13920, 1997.
27. The Diabetes Control and Complications Trial Research Group, The effect of intensive treatment of diabetes on the development and progression of long-term complications in insulin-dependent diabetes mellitus, *N Engl J Med,* 329:977–986, 1993.
28. UK Prospective Diabetes Study (UKPDS) Group, Intensive blood-glucose control with sulphonylureas or insulin compared with conventional treatment and risk of complications in patients with type-2 diabetes (UKPDS 33), *Lancet,* 352:837–853, 1998.
29. Shichiri M, Kishikawa H, and Ohkubo Y et al., Long-term results of the Kumamoto Study on optimal diabetes control in type-2 diabetic patients, *Diabetes Care,* 23(Suppl 2):B21–29, 2000.
30. Lorenzo V, Martn M, and Rufino M et al., Predialysis nephrologic care and a functioning arteriovenous fistula at entry are associated with better survival in incident hemodialysis patients, An observational cohort study, *Am J Kidney Dis,* 43:999–1007, 2004.
31. Collins AJ, Hao W, and Xia H et al., Mortality risks of peritoneal dialysis and hemodialysis, *Am J Kidney Dis,* 34:1065–1074, 1999.
32. Moon YS and Kashyap ML, Pharmacologic treatment of type-2 diabetic dyslipidemia, *Pharmacotherapy,* 24:1692–1713, 2004.

33. Wolfe RA, Ashby VB, and Milford EL et al., Comparison of mortality in all patients on dialysis, patients on dialysis awaiting transplantation, and recipients of a first cadaveric transplant, *N Engl J Med*, 341:1725–1730, 1999.

34. American Diabetes Association, Pancreas transplantation for patients with type-1 diabetes, *Diabetes Care*, 26:S120, 2003.

35. Fioretto P, Steffes MW, and Sutherland DE et al., Reversal of lesions of diabetic nephropathy after pancreas transplantation, *N Engl J Med*, 339:69–75, 1998.

36. Detsky AS, McLaughlin JR, and Baker JP et al., What is subjective global assessment of nutritional status? *J Parenter Enteral Nutr*, 11:8–13, 1987.

37. National Kidney Foundation, K/DOQI clinical practice guidelines for nutrition in chronic renal failure, *Am J Kidney Dis*, 35(Suppl 2):S1–136, 2000.

38. Weir MR, Impact of salt intake on blood pressure and proteinuria in diabetes: Importance of the renin-angiotensin system, *Miner Electrolyte Metab*, 24:438–445, 1998.

39. Feldstein CA, Salt intake, hypertension, and diabetes mellitus, *J Hum Hypertens*, 16(Suppl 1):S48–55, 2002.

40. American Diabetes Association Position Statement, Evidence-based nutrition principles and recommendations for the treatment and prevention of diabetes and related complications, *Diabetes Care*, 25:S50–60, 2002.

41. Fried LF, Orchard TJ, and Kasiske BL, Effect of lipid reduction on the progression of renal disease, A meta-analysis, *Kidney Int*, 59:260–269, 2001.

42. Himmelfarb J, Stenvinkel P, and Ikizler TA et al., The elephant in uremia: Oxidant stress as a unifying concept of cardiovascular disease in uremia, *Kidney Int*, 62:1524–1538, 2002.

43. National Kidney Foundation, K/DOQI clinical practice guidelines for managing dyslipidemias in chronic kidney disease, *Am J Kidney Dis*, 41(Suppl 3):S1–76, 2003.

44. Go AS, Chertow GM, and Fan D et al., Chronic kidney disease and the risks of death, cardiovascular events, and hospitalization, *N Engl J Med*, 351:1296–1305, 2004.

45. Teixeira SR, Tappenden KA, and Carson L et al., Isolated soy protein consumption reduces urinary albumin excretion and improves the serum lipid profile in men with type-2 diabetes mellitus and nephropathy, *J Nutr*, 134:1874–1880, 2004.

46. Fouque D, Why is the diet intervention so critical during chronic kidney disease? *J Ren Nutr*, 13:173, 2003.

47. Zatz R, Meyer TW, and Rennke HG et al., Predominance of hemodynamic rather than metabolic factors in the pathogenesis of diabetic glomerulopathy, *Proc Natl Acad Sci USA*, 82:5963–5967, 1985.

48. Kasiske BL, Lakatua JD, and Ma JZ et al., A meta-analysis of the effects of dietary protein restriction on the rate of decline in renal function, *Am J Kidney Dis*, 31:954–961, 1998.

49. Klahr S, Levey AS, and Beck GJ et al., Modification of Diet in Renal Disease Study Group, The effects of dietary protein restriction and blood-pressure control on the progression of chronic renal disease, *N Engl J Med*, 330:877–884, 1994.

50. Barsotti G, Cupisti A, and Barsotti M et al., Dietary treatment of diabetic nephropathy with chronic renal failure, *Nephrol Dial Transplant*, 13(Suppl 8):49–52, 1998.

51. Zeller K, Whittaker E, and Sullivan L et al., Effect of restricting dietary protein on the progression of renal failure in patients with insulin-dependent diabetes mellitus, *N Engl J Med*, 324:78–84, 1991.

52. Brouhard BH and LaGrone L, Effect of dietary protein restriction on functional renal reserve in diabetic nephropathy, *Am J Med*, 89:427–431, 1990.

53. Dullaart RP, Beusekamp BJ, and Meijer S et al., Long-term effects of protein-restricted diet on albuminuria and renal function in IDDM patients without clinical nephropathy and hypertension, *Diabetes Care*, 16:483–492, 1993.

54. Evanoff G, Thompson C, and Brown J et al., Prolonged dietary protein restriction in diabetic nephropathy, *Arch Intern Med*, 149:1129–1133, 1989.

55. Walker JD, Bending JJ, and Dodds RA et al., Restriction of dietary protein and progression of renal failure in diabetic nephropathy, *Lancet*, 2:1411–1415, 1989.

56. Ciavarella A, Di Mizio G, and Stefoni S et al., Reduced albuminuria after dietary protein restriction in insulin-dependent diabetic patients with clinical nephropathy, *Diabetes Care*, 10:407–413, 1987.

57. Pijls LT, de Vries H, and Donker AJ et al., The effect of protein restriction on albuminuria in patients with type-2 diabetes mellitus, A randomized trial, *Nephrol Dial Transplant*, 14:1445–1453, 1999.

58. Raal FJ, Kalk WJ, and Lawson M et al., Effect of moderate dietary protein restriction on the progression of overt diabetic nephropathy, A 6-month prospective study, *Am J Clin Nutr*, 60:579–585, 1994.

59. Mitch WE, Dietary protein restriction in chronic renal failure: Nutritional efficacy, compliance, and progression of renal insufficiency, *J Am Soc Nephrol*, 2:823–831, 1991.

60. Hansen HP, Tauber-Lassen E, and Jensen BR et al., Effect of dietary protein restriction on prognosis in patients with diabetic nephropathy, *Kidney Int*, 62:220–228, 2002.

61. Meloni C, Morosetti M, and Suraci C et al., Severe dietary protein restriction in overt diabetic nephropathy: Benefits or risks? *J Ren Nutr*, 12:96–101, 2002.

62. Maroni BJ, Steinman TI, and Mitch WE, A method for estimating nitrogen intake of patients with chronic renal failure, *Kidney Int*, 27:58–65, 1985.

63. Kopple JD, National Kidney Foundation K/DOQI Work Group, The National Kidney Foundation K/DOQI clinical practice guidelines for dietary protein intake for chronic dialysis patients, *Am J Kidney Dis*, 38(4 Suppl 1):S68–73, 2001.

64. Rocco MV, Paranandi L, and Burrowes JD et al., Nutritional status in the HEMO Study cohort at baseline, hemodialysis. *Am J Kidney Dis,* 39:245–256, 2002.

65. Fouque D, Nutritional requirements in maintenance hemodialysis, *Adv Ren Replace Ther,* 10:183–193, 2003.

66. Lowrie EG and Lew NL, Death risk in hemodialysis patients: The predictive value of commonly measured variables and an evaluation of death rate differences between facilities, *Am J Kidney Dis,* 15:458–482, 1990.

67. Canada-USA (CANUSA) Peritoneal Dialysis Study Group, Adequacy of dialysis and nutrition in continuous peritoneal dialysis: Association with clinical outcomes, *J Am Soc Nephrol,* 7:198–207, 1996.

68. Lindsay RM, Spanner E, and Heidenheim RP et al., Which comes first, Kt/V or PCR—chicken or egg? *Kidney Int,* 38(Suppl):S32–36, 1992.

69. Uribarri J, Levin NW, and Delmez J et al., Association of acidosis and nutritional parameters in hemodialysis patients, *Am J Kidney Dis,* 34:493–499, 1999.

70. Burrowes JD, Larive B, and Cockram DB et al., Hemodialysis (HEMO) Study Group, Effects of dietary intake, appetite, and eating habits on dialysis and non-dialysis treatment days in hemodialysis patients, Cross-sectional results from the HEMO study, *J Ren Nutr,* 13:191–198, 2003.

71. Wright MJ, Woodrow G, and O'Brien S et al., A novel technique to demonstrate disturbed appetite profiles in haemodialysis patients. *Nephrol Dial Transplant,* 16:1424–1429, 2001.

72. Blumenkrantz MJ, Gahl GM, and Kopple JD et al., Protein losses during peritoneal dialysis, *Kidney Int,* 19:593–602, 1981.

73. Davies SJ, Phillips L, and Griffiths AM et al., Analysis of the effects of increasing delivered dialysis treatment to malnourished peritoneal dialysis patients, *Kidney Int,* 57:1743–1754, 2000.

74. Rocco MV, Dwyer JT, and Larive B et al., HEMO Study Group, The effect of dialysis dose and membrane flux on nutritional parameters in hemodialysis patients, Results of the HEMO Study, *Kidney Int,* 65:2321–2334, 2004.

75. Spanner E, Suri R, and Heidenheim AP et al., The impact of quotidian hemodialysis on nutrition, *Am J Kidney Dis,* 42(Suppl 1):30–35, 2003.

76. Pecoits-Filho R, Lindholm B, and Stenvinkel P, The malnutrition, inflammation, and atherosclerosis (MIA) syndrome—the heart of the matter, *Nephrol Dial Transplant,* 17(Suppl 11):28–31, 2002.

77. Kalantar-Zadeh K, Fouque D, and Kopple JD, Outcome research, nutrition, and reverse epidemiology in maintenance dialysis patients, *J Ren Nutr,* 14:64–71, 2004.

78. Caglar K, Fedje L, and Dimmitt R et al., Therapeutic effects of oral nutritional supplementation during hemodialysis, *Kidney Int,* 62:1054–1059, 2002.

79. Coulston AM, Clinical experience with modified enteral formulas for patients with diabetes. *Clin Nutr,* 17(Suppl 2):46–56, 1998.

80. Feriani M, Dell'Aquila R, and La Greca G, The treatment of diabetic end-stage renal disease with peritoneal dialysis, *Nephrol Dial Transplant*, 13(Suppl 8):53–56, 1998.

81. Dasgupta MK, Strategies for managing diabetic patients on peritoneal dialysis, *Adv Perit Dial,* 20:200–202, 2004.

82. Grzegorzewska AE, Mariak I, and Dobrowolska-Zachwieja A et al., Effects of amino acid dialysis solution on the nutrition of continuous ambulatory peritoneal dialysis patients, *Perit Dial Int,* 19:462–470, 1999.

83. Taylor GS, Patel V, and Spencer S et al., Long-term use of 1.1% amino acid dialysis solution in hypoalbuminemic continuous ambulatory peritoneal dialysis patients, *Clin Nephrol,* 58:445–450, 2002.

84. Li FK, Chan LY, and Woo JC et al., A 3-year, prospective, randomized, controlled study on amino acid dialysate in patients on CAPD, *Am J Kidney Dis,* 42:173–183, 2003.

85. Tjiong HL, van den Berg JW, and Wattimena JL et al., Dialysate as food: combined amino acid and glucose dialysate improves protein anabolism in renal failure patients on automated peritoneal dialysis, *J Am Soc Nephrol,* 16:1486–1493, 2005.

86. Chan TM, Leung JK, and Sun Y et al., Different effects of amino acid-based and lucose-based dialysate from peritoneal dialysis patients on mesothelial cell ultrastructure and function, *Nephrol Dial Transplant,* 18:1086–1094, 2003.

87. Reimann D, Dachs D, and Meye C et al., Amino acid-based peritoneal dialysis solution stimulates mesothelial nitric oxide production, *Perit Dial Int,* 24:378-384, 2004.

88. Vychytil A, Fodinger M, and Pleiner J et al., Acute effect of amino acid peritoneal dialysis solution on vascular function, *Am J Clin Nutr,* 78:1039-1045, 2003.

89. Van Biesen W, Boer W, and De Greve B et al., A randomized clinical trial with a 0.6% amino acid/1.4% glycerol peritoneal dialysis solution, *Perit Dial Int,* 24:222-230, 2004.

90. Vande Walle J, Raes A, and Dehoorne J et al., Combined amino-acid and glucose peritoneal dialysis solution for children with acute renal failure, *Adv Perit Dial,* 20:226-230, 2004.

91. Pupim LB, Flakoll PJ, and Brouillette JR et al., Intradialytic parenteral nutrition improves protein and energy homeostasis in chronic hemodialysis patients, *J Clin Invest,* 110:483–492, 2002.

92. Capelli JP, Kushner H, and Camiscioli TC et al., Effect of intradialytic parenteral nutrition on mortality rates in end-stage renal disease care, *Am J Kidney Dis,* 23:808–816, 1994.

93. Serna-Thome MG, Padilla-Rosciano AE, and Suchil-Bernal L, Practical aspects of intradialytic nutritional support, *Curr Opin Clin Nutr Metab Care,* 5:293–296, 2002.

94. Cano N, Intradialytic parenteral nutrition: Where do we go from here? *J Ren Nutr,* 14:3–5, 2004.

95. Fouque D, Peng SC, and Shamir E et al., Recombinant human insulin-like growth factor-1 induces an anabolic response in malnourished CAPD patients, *Kidney Int,* 57:646–654, 2000.

96. Boccanfuso JA, Hutton M, and McAllister B, The effects of megestrol acetate on nutritional parameters in a dialysis population, *J Ren Nutr,* 10:36–43, 2000.

97. Matson A, Wright M, and Oliver A et al., Zinc supplementation at conventional doses does not improve the disturbance of taste perception in hemodialysis patients, *J Ren Nutr,* 13:224–228, 2003.

98. Sprenger KB, Bundschu D, and Lewis K et al., Improvement of uremic neuropathy and hypogeusia by dialysate zinc supplementation, A double-blind study, *Kidney Int,* 16(Suppl):S315–318, 1983.

99. Mahajan SK, Prasad AS, and Lambujon J et al., Improvement of uremic hypogeusia by zinc, A double-blind study, *Am J Clin Nutr,* 33:1517–1521, 1980.

100. National Kidney Foundation, K/DOQI clinical practice guidelines for bone metabolism and disease in chronic kidney disease, *Am J Kidney Dis,* 42(4 Suppl 3):S1–201, 2003.

101. Slatopolsky E, Brown A, and Dusso A, Role of phosphorus in the pathogenesis of secondary hyperparathyroidism, *Am J Kidney Dis,* 37(1 Suppl 2):S54–57, 2001.

102. Block GA, Hulbert-Shearon TE, and Levin NW et al., Association of serum phosphorus and calcium x phosphate product with mortality risk in chronic hemodialysis patients, A national study, *Am J Kidney Dis,* 31:607–617, 1998.

103. Block GA, Martin KJ, and de Francisco AL et al., Cinacalcet for secondary hyperparathyroidism in patients receiving hemodialysis, *N Engl J Med,* 350:1516–1525, 2004.

104. Makoff R, Vitamin replacement therapy in renal failure patients, *Miner Electrolyte Metab,* 25:349–351, 1999.

105. Kalantar-Zadeh K, Block G, and Humphreys MH et al., A low, rather than a high, total plasma homocysteine is an indicator of poor outcome in hemodialysis patients, *J Am Soc Nephrol,* 15:442–453, 2004.

106. National Kidney Foundation, K/DOQI clinical practice guidelines for anemia of chronic kidney disease, 2000, *Am J Kidney Dis,* 37(Suppl 1):S182–238, 2001.

107. Loureiro H, Silva RS, and Machado C et al., Kidney transplantation and posttransplantation diabetes: Nutritional evaluation, *Transplant Proc,* 35:1091–1092, 2003.

108. Clinical practice guidelines for managing dyslipidemias in kidney transplant patients, A report from the Managing Dyslipidemias in Chronic Kidney Disease Work Group of the National Kidney Foundation Kidney Disease Outcomes Quality Initiative, *Transplantation,* 4(Suppl 7):11–53, 2004.

109. Kasiske BL, Anjum S, and Shah R et al., Hypertension after kidney transplantation. *Am J Kidney Dis,* 43(6):1071–1081, 2004.

110. Miller DG, Levine SE, and D'Elia JA et al., Nutritional status of diabetic and nondiabetic patients after renal transplantation, *Am J Clin Nutr,* 44:66–69, 1986.

111. Guijarro C, Massy ZA, and Wiederkehr MR et al., Serum albumin and mortality after renal transplantation, *Am J Kidney Dis,* 27:117–123, 1996.

112. Kasiske BL, Guijarro C, and Massy ZA et al., Cardiovascular disease after renal transplantation, *J Am Soc Nephrol,* 7:158–165, 1996.

113. Adang EM, Engel GL, and van Hooff JP et al., Comparison before and after transplantation of pancreas-kidney and pancreas-kidney with loss of pancreas—a prospective controlled quality of life study, *Transplantation,* 62:754–758, 1996.

114. Becker BN, Becker YT, and Heisey DM et al., The impact of hypoalbuminemia in kidney–pancreas transplant recipients, *Transplantation,* 68:72–75, 1999.

115. Kalantar-Zadeh K, Stenvinkel P, and Pillon L et al., Inflammation and nutrition in renal insufficiency, *Adv Ren Replace Ther,* 10:155–169, 2003.

11 Nutrition Support and Hyperglycemia

Elise M. Brett

CONTENTS

CAUSES OF HYPERGLYCEMIA

Hyperglycemia in patients receiving nutrition support may be due to type-1 diabetes (T1DM), type-2 diabetes (T2DM), or stress hyperglycemia (SH). Stress hyperglycemia is defined as the presence of elevated glucose during an acute illness, in a patient without a prior diagnosis of diabetes, which normalizes after the illness. The majority of patients who receive nutrition support are hospitalized patients with acute illnesses in whom the need for nutrition support is temporary. A retrospective chart review of 1886 consecutive hospital admissions demonstrated hyperglycemia, defined as a fasting plasma glucose of > 126 mg/dL or random plasma glucose of > 200 mg/dL, in 38% of patients [1]. Of the patients that were hyperglycemic, 68% were known to have diabetes and 32% were hyperglycemic without a prior history of diabetes. In a study by Levetan et al. [2], 37.5% of medical and 33% of surgical admissions with hyperglycemia, defined as a glucose level > 200 mg/dL, did not have a prior diagnosis of diabetes. This latter group consists of patients with undiagnosed T2DM and SH. Compared with patients previously diagnosed with diabetes, patients with SH have a higher in-hospital mortality rate despite a lower average blood glucose level [1]. This suggests that new hyperglycemia in hospitalized patients may be an indicator of more severe stress.

Stress hyperglycemia results from increased gluconeogenesis, enhanced glycogenolysis, and increased insulin resistance as a result of increased counterregulatory hormones and cytokine responses [3,4]. One mechanism by which this occurs is via nuclear factor kappa-B (NF-κB)-mediated inflammatory pathways involving tumor necrosis factor-α (TNF-α) and interleukin-1 (IL-1) which interfere with insulin action [5,6]. This occurs by increased serine phosphorylation of

171

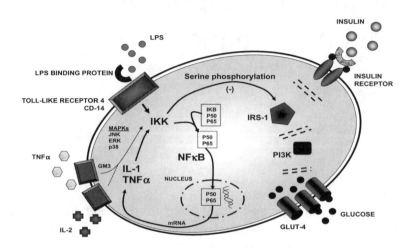

FIGURE 11.1 Inflammation-induced insulin resistance. Lipopolysaccharide (LPS) binds to LPS-binding protein and then activates the serine kinase "inhibitor κB kinase" (IKK) via toll-like receptor-4/CD14 [6]. Tumor-necrosis factor-α (TNF-α) or interleukin-1 (IL-1) can also activate IKK via various mitogen-activated protein kinase (MAPK) pathways (p30β, c-Jun N-terminal kinase [JNK], extracellular signal-regulated kinases [ERK1/2-p42/p44]) [7]. The inhibitory action of TNF-α has also been associated with ganglioside GM3 accumulation in cell membrane lipid rafts [8]. IKK controls nuclear translocation of nuclear factor κB which activates a pro-inflammatory cascade, including TNF-α and IL-1 gene expression. Serine phosphorylation of insulin receptor substrate-1 (IRS-1) by IKK decreases: (1) interaction with the insulin receptor; (2) IRS-1 tyrosine phosphorylation and binding to phosphatidylinositol-3 kinase (PI3K); and eventually (3) glucose transporter-4 (GLUT-4)-mediated glucose transport.

insulin receptor substrate (IRS) molecules that block tyrosine phosphorylation [6,7] (see Figure 11.1). Sepsis further increases insulin resistance through the production of endotoxin (lipopolysaccharide; LPS). In a prospective, controlled animal study, sustained endotoxemia led to marked down-regulation of early steps in the insulin-signaling cascade [8]. McCowen et al. [8] demonstrated reduced abundance of insulin receptors and IRS molecules during a prolonged (74 hours) endotoxin infusion. It was particularly interesting that this effect reversed with adequate nutrition, suggesting that prolonged insulin resistance may depend on concomitant malnutrition [8].

In addition to the induction of an insulin-resistant state, there are primary β-cell defects associated with hyperglycemia and stress [9]. Hyperglycemia has been shown to result in the generation of reactive oxygen species (ROS). This increases oxidative stress and causes direct cellular damage, including damage to pancreatic β-cells [10]. Another mechanism of β-cell dysfunction involves the abnormally increased glycation of insulin during periods of sustained hyperglycemia [11]. Glucose desensitization represents an adaptive, reversible refractoriness of the β-cell exocytotic apparatus to transient hyperglycemia. After prolonged hyperglycemia, the depletion of readily releasable insulin pools results in β-cell exhaustion. Glucose toxicity refers to the slowly progressive and irreversible effects of prolonged hyperglycemia on β-cell function and eventually, β-cell mass, due to apoptosis. β-cell apoptosis is mediated via death receptors and DNA damage (extrinsic pathway activated by cytokines) or mitochondrial activation (intrinsic pathway). Achieving tight glycemic control with insulin decreases inflammation and restores at least some β-cell function in SH [12]. Thus, SH requires treatment as in true diabetes, even though it typically resolves after the acute illness.

The use of nutrition support markedly increases the risk of hyperglycemia. Inzucchi et al. [13] reported an odds ratio of 14 for the development of hyperglycemia, defined as mean glucose > 150 mg/dL, in non-diabetic intensive care unit (ICU) patients receiving parenteral nutrition (PN) and an odds ratio of 3.8 for ICU patients receiving enteral nutrition (EN). In a retrospective analysis of 65 non-insulin-requiring diabetic patients requiring nutrition support, 47% of patients receiving EN eventually required insulin compared with 77% receiving PN [14]. Of the previously insulin-requiring patients, 67% receiving EN required an increased insulin dose compared with 100% receiving PN, where insulin therapy was only changed if the glucose level was > 270 mg/dL [14]. Hence, when tighter control is the goal, nearly all diabetic patients will require treatment with insulin or increases in their previous insulin requirements.

RATIONALE FOR GLYCEMIC CONTROL IN HOSPITALIZED PATIENTS

The rationale for short-term glycemic control in hospitalized patients differs from that for long-term glycemic control (i.e., the prevention of microvascular complications) and is supported by a recent spate of evidence demonstrating improved clinical outcomes. It is well known that hyperglycemia above the renal threshold of 180 mg/dL results in an osmotic diuresis, which leads to dehydration and electrolyte abnormalities complicating the management of acutely ill patients. More recently, it has been recognized that hyperglycemia increases morbidity by directly impairing immune function. *In vitro* studies with hyperglycemia show impaired superoxide production from activated neutrophils [15], impaired complement fixation [16], and impaired phagocytic killing of microorganisms [17,18]. Raising glucose levels *in vitro* also increases the expression of a complement receptor-like protein in Candida. which promotes its adhesion and blocks its phagocytosis [19]. This is particularly important in critically ill patients receiving PN who are already at higher risk for candiduria, which is associated with increased mortality [20].

Hyperglycemia also has a prothrombotic effect increasing the risk for cardiovascular complications. Plasma levels of many clotting factors are increased in diabetes [21]. Short-term hyperglycemia increases activation of platelets in patients with diabetes [22]. P-selectin expression on the endothelial cells is increased with hyperglycemia and can be blocked with insulin [23]. Acute hyperglycemia in normal subjects raises plasma levels of intracellular adhesion molecule-1 (ICAM-1), altering the adhesive properties of the endothelium. This effect appears to be due to reduced availability of nitric oxide (NO). Correction with insulin restores ICAM-1 levels to normal in diabetics [24]. Short-term treatment with insulin also decreases plasminogen activator inhibitor-1 (PAI-1) in diabetic subjects [25].

Increased ROS formation is another mechanism contributing to endothelial dysfunction and increasing the risk for ischemic events. Generation of superoxide and lipid peroxide is higher in conditions of hyperglycemia [26]. This appears to be mediated by protein kinase C [26]. Other possible sources of oxidative excess in diabetes involve inhibition of the thioredoxin ROS-scavenging function in hyperglycemia [27] and increased nicotinamide adenine dinucleotide, reduced form (NADPH) oxidase activity [28]. Hyperglycemia directly leads to activation of NF-κB in vascular smooth muscle cells, which regulates a variety of genes involved in inducing atherosclerosis [29]. Furthermore, elevation of free fatty acids and TNF-α [30], seen in insulin-resistant states or after a high-fat meal in patients with T2DM [31], impairs vasodilation via decreased production of nitric oxide (NO) [32].

Observational studies consistently show worse outcomes in hyperglycemic patients. In one of the earliest studies documenting the association between glucose control and risk of infection, Pomposelli et al. [33] showed that the incidence of post-operative infection risk in patients undergoing elective surgery was 2.7 times higher in patients with at least one glucose level greater than 220 mg/dL on the first post-operative day. The relative risk for severe infection was even higher [33].

Hyperglycemia adversely affects outcome in patients with cardiovascular disease (CVD). In patients with acute myocardial infarction, with or without a prior diagnosis of diabetes, admission hyperglycemia predicts long-term morbidity and mortality due to CVD [34]. In diabetic patients undergoing coronary artery bypass surgery, in-hospital complication rates increased by 17% for each 1 mmol/L increase in post-operative day-one glucose levels above 6.1 mmol/L[35]. In patients who undergo cardiac bypass surgery, pre-operative hyperglycemia is an independent predictor of infectious complications and total length of hospital stay [36]. Perioperative hyperglycemia has been correlated with increased length of postoperative hospital days and increased cost of hospitalization [37].

Stroke patients, another population often requiring nutrition support, also have increased morbidity with higher glucose levels, irrespective of a prior diagnosis of diabetes [38]. In patients with ischemic stroke, the likelihood of neurologic improvement decreased with higher admission glucose levels, suggesting that hyperglycemia may augment brain injury [39]. Patients who undergo reperfusion with tissue plasminogen activator (tPA) have also been shown to have poorer neurologic outcomes if a random admission blood glucose level was > 140 mg/dL [40].

The degree of hyperglycemia in critically ill patients is directly correlated with in-hospital mortality. In a retrospective review by Krinsley et al. [41], the lowest mortality (9.6%) occurred in patients with mean glucose values of 80–99 mg/dL, and was as high as 42.5% in patients with mean glucose values exceeding 300 mg/dL.

Studies demonstrating the effects of interventions to lower blood glucose are limited but show clear benefit. The primary population studied thus far has been surgical patients. The implementation of an intravenous insulin protocol to reduce blood glucose < 200 mg/dL in the immediate postoperative period, in diabetic patients undergoing cardiac surgery, significantly decreased the risk of deep sternal wound infections [42]. These authors subsequently lowered the glycemic goals to 100–150 mg/dL and have demonstrated a 60% mortality reduction in coronary artery bypass graft (CABG) patients, a decreased length of stay, and substantial cost savings [43]. In a landmark study, Van den Berghe et al. [44], from Leuven, Belgium described 1548 patients in a surgical ICU receiving mechanical ventilation plus PN, EN, or combined PN + EN. The majority of patients (63%) had undergone cardiac surgery. The patients were randomized to intensive (glucose 80–110 mg/dL) or conventional therapy (glucose 180–200 mg/dL) with intravenous insulin infusions. The average glucose in the intensive group was 103 ± 19 mg/dL vs. 153 ± 33 mg/dL in the control group. In-hospital mortality was reduced by 34% with intensive glycemic control [44]. There was a 46% reduction in sepsis, a 41% reduction in acute renal failure, a 44% reduction in critical illness polyneuropathy, as well as a reduction in the need for prolonged ventilatory support and ICU stay [44]. Grey et al. [45] showed a 3.5-fold reduction in intravascular device-related and surgical site infection in surgical ICU patients receiving nutrition support with aggressive glycemic control (mean glucose 125 ± 36 vs. 179 ± 61 mg/dL). In a prospective study using historical controls, Krinsley [46] instituted an insulin protocol in a heterogeneous population of 800 medical and surgical patients. Mean blood glucose decreased from 152 to 130.7 mg/dL and there were decreases in the development of renal failure, need for transfusion, mortality, and length of stay in the group with better glycemic control [46].

It has been argued that it may be the anti-inflammatory and profibrinolytic effects of insulin, rather than improvements in glycemic control, that are primarily responsible for these clinical benefits. Insulin is a potent anti-inflammatory agent. Insulin infusions have been shown to decrease PAI-1 and C-reactive protein (CRP) in patients with myocardial infarction [47]. Insulin lowers CRP and counteracts the effects of low mannose-binding lectin, an acute phase protein which has antimicrobial properties, in critically ill patients [48]. Insulin therapy also inhibits TNF-α-induced lipolysis and consequent pro-inflammatory changes. Moreover, insulin glargine therapy has been shown to have beneficial vasodilatory effects on endothelium [49] that are inhibited by TNF-α mediated suppression of NO production [30]. Insulin-glucose infusions have been shown to decrease long-term mortality (30% at 1 and 3.5 years), with an acceptable level of cost effectiveness [50] in diabetic patients after acute myocardial infarction [34,51–56] and in diabetic patients undergoing CABG [57].

In-depth analysis of the Leuven study shows that high glucose levels and high insulin doses were independent predictors of death, suggesting that glucose control is the key factor [58]. This is consistent with the findings of Finney et al. [59], who reported that for every level of glucose in ICU patients, those patients receiving the highest doses of insulin had the highest mortality. This group suggested mortality benefit with an upper limit for glucose of 145 mg/dL [59]. Of interest, intraoperative intensive insulinization, titrated to maintain blood glucose of 80–120 mg/dL, did not reduce the need for postoperative inotropic or antiarrhythmic support after cardiopulmonary bypass surgery [60].

Another potential benefit of insulin treatment is the optimization of nitrogen retention when used with nutrition support. Increased skeletal muscle protein synthesis and decreased proteolysis have been observed with insulin infusions in animal [61–63] and human studies [64–67]. However, even though this effect occurs with PN, it has not been demonstrated with EN [68]. This phenomenon is thought to be due to the modification and use of amino acid substrates by the liver prior to use by skeletal muscle [68].

CLINICAL PRACTICE GUIDELINES FOR GLYCEMIC CONTROL AMONG HOSPITALIZED PATIENTS

Until recently there were no guidelines for glycemic goals in hospitalized patients. It was generally accepted that glucose levels < 200 mg/dL constituted adequate control. In 2004, the American College of Endocrinology published a position statement on inpatient diabetes control [69]. The upper limit glycemic targets recommended are 110 mg/dL for ICU patients and 180 mg/dL for non-ICU patients. The American Diabetes Association (ADA) recommends that glucose levels be kept "as close to 110 mg/dL as possible and generally < 180 mg/dL" in critically ill patients [70]. For non-critically ill patients, a premeal glucose of 90–130 mg/dL and postprandial glucose < 180 mg/dL is recommended [70]. At this time, it is unknown whether the results of the Leuven study involving primarily cardiac surgery patients should be broadly applied to other patient populations such as medical ICU, general surgery, chronically critically ill, or more stable hospitalized patients. Although those authors did not report any adverse consequences to hypoglycemia, the rate of hypoglycemia was high, and the potential risks serious. For now, many institutions have adopted ICU protocols with somewhat higher target glucose levels.

NUTRITION SUPPORT

Malnutrition is associated with higher complication rates, increased cost, increased mortality, and increased length of stay in hospitalized patients [71]. All hospitalized patients should undergo nutritional screening and nutritional assessment, and nutrition support should be instituted when appropriate. Nutritional therapies are generally provided by nutrition support teams led by a physician with expertise in nutritional medicine.

Hospitalized diabetic patients who can eat should be provided with a "consistent-carbohydrate diabetes meal plan," rather than a standardized calorie-based meal plan or "ADA diet" [72]. The ADA no longer endorses any specific macronutrient composition in meals [72]. In addition, a "no concentrated sweets" diet is also considered inappropriate as the restriction of sucrose does not facilitate glycemic control [72]. Insulin and/or oral agents should be coordinated with therapy and adjusted according to fingerstick glucose measurements. Whenever possible, oral nutrition in the form of regular food or nutritional supplements should be continued in patients requiring EN or PN in patients who can tolerate it. A variety of oral supplements are marketed specifically for the diabetic patient (see Table 11.1).

TABLE 11.1
Macronutrient Content in Various Commercially Available Enteral Feeding Formulas

Product	Manu-facturer	Marketed or DM?	Cal/cc	Carb % (g/L)	Fat % (g/L)	Protein% (g/L)	mOsm/kgH20	Fiber?
INTACT PROTEIN								
DiabetaSource AC	Novartis®	Yes	1.0	36(100)	44(59)	20(60)	350	Yes
Glucerna®	Ross®	Yes	1.0	34.3(95.6)	49(54.4)	16.7(41.8)	355	Yes
Choice DM®	Novartis	Yes	1.06	40(119)	43(51)	17(45)	300	Yes
Glytrol®	Nestle®	Yes	1.0	40(100)	42(47.5)	18(45)	280	Yes
Resource Diabetic®	Novartis	Yes	1.06	36(100)	40(47)	24(63)	300	Yes
Pulmocare®	Ross	No	1.5	28.2(105.7)	55.1(93.3)	16.7(62.6)	475	No
Jevity®	Ross	No	1.0	54.3(154)	29(34.7)	16.7(44.3)	300	Yes
Jevity 1.2	Ross	No	1.2	52.5(171)	29(39)	18.5(55)	450	Yes
Osmolite®	Ross	No	1.06	57(151)	29(34.7)	14(37.1)	300	No
Promote® w/ fiber	Ross	No	1.0	50(138)	25(28.2)	25(62.5)	380	Yes
TwoCal HN	Ross	No	2.0	43.2(218.5)	40.1(90.5)	16.7(83.5)	725	Yes
Impact®	Novartis	No	1.0	53(130)	25(28)	22(56)	375	No
Isocal	Novartis	No	1.06	50(135)	37(10.5)	13(34)	270	No
Isosource®	Novartis	No	1.2	57(170)	29(39)	14(43)	490	No
SEMI-ELEMENTAL								
Peptinex	Novartis	No	1.0	65(160)	15(17)	20(50)	320	No
Peptamen®	Nestle	No	1.0	51(127)	33(39)	16(40)	270	No
Peptamen VHP	Nestle	No	1.0	42(104.5)	33(39.2)	25(62.5)	270	No
Peptamen 1.5	Nestle	No	1.5	49(188)	33(56)	18(67.6)	550	No
Perative®	Ross	No	1.3	54.5(180.3)	25(37.3)	20.5(66.7)	460	Yes
Alitraq	Ross	No	1.0	65.7(165)	13(15.5)	21.1(52.5)	575	No
Optimental	Ross	No	1.0	54.5(138.7)	25(28.4)	20.5(51.3)	540	No
Subdue®	Novartis	No	1.0	50(130)	30(34)	20(50)	330	No
ELEMENTAL								
Vivonex® RTF	Novartis	No	1.0	70(175)	10(12)	20(50)	630	No
F.A.A.	Nestle	No	1.0	70(176)	10(11.2)	20(50)	700	No
RENAL								
Nepro®	Ross	No	2.0	43(222.7)	43(95.6)	14(70)	665	No
Suplena®	Ross	No	2.0	51.6(255.2)	43(95.6)	6(30)	600	No
Novasource® Renal	Novartis	No	2.0	40(200)	45(100)	15(74)	700	No

The indications for providing nutrition support do not differ in diabetic as compared with non-diabetic patients. Malnourished or metabolically stressed patients expected to be unable to eat for > 5–7 days or normally nourished nonstressed patients expected to be unable to eat for > 7–9 days should receive nutrition support [73]. In general, EN is preferred if the gastrointestinal tract is functional; this is due to the increased risk of line sepsis and increased cost associated with PN [74]. Common indications for PN are shown in Table 11.2. Critically ill patients fed enterally often do not receive the amount of prescribed calories due to a variety of reasons, such as gastrointestinal

TABLE 11.2
Common Indications for Parenteral Nutrition Support

Critical illness with uncertain glycemic index (GI) function
Crohn's disease flare
Distal enterocutaneous fistula
Severe pancreatitis
Gastrointestinal obstruction
Perioperative for severely malnourished patients
Intractable diarrhea
Prolonged postoperative ileus
Bone marrow transplant

intolerance, problems with the feeding tube, or procedures or surgical interventions requiring temporary discontinuation of feeds. In one study of ICU patients, only 35% of patients received 80% of their measured energy expenditure enterally [75]. When nutritional needs are only partially met with EN alone, combined-modality PN and EN should be used.

PARENTERAL NUTRITION

Parenteral nutrition generally results in more hyperglycemia than enteral feeding. This is primarily due to loss of the effect of the incretin hormones, glucagon-like peptide-1 (GLP-1), and glucose-dependent insulinotropic polypeptide (GIP), which are normally released from the gut in response to orally ingested carbohydrates and are insulinotropic [76]. However, recent evidence suggests that providing glucose enterally does not, in fact, stimulate hepatic glucose uptake more efficiently than intravenous glucose in nondiabetic humans [77].

Infusions of the GLP-1 analog, exendin-4, retard gastric emptying and reduce both fasting and peak postprandial glucose in nondiabetic subjects [78]. Patients with T2DM have impaired GLP-1 secretion [79] and decreased GIP amplification of the late-phase insulin response [80]. The administration of GLP-1 to diabetic patients retards gastric emptying [81], augments the insulin response [81], improves insulin sensitivity and β-cell function [82], lowers postprandial glucose [81], decreases free fatty acids [82], decreases appetite [82], decreases energy intake [83], and reduces body weight [82,83]. One analog of GLP-1, exenatide, is now available for the treatment of T2DM via subcutaneous injection. Oral inhibitors of the dipeptidyl peptidase IV enzyme, which naturally degrades GLP-1, are currently in development [84].

When GLP-1 was given to 8 hyperglycemic subjects receiving PN there was significant insulin stimulation and a reduction in glucose levels in the majority of patients [85]. However, some patients were non-responders, and no patient had complete normalization of glucose. Further study will determine if the use of GLP-1 with PN is warranted to improve glycemic control.

MACRONUTRIENT REQUIREMENTS

Critically ill patients are markedly hypercatabolic (increased proteolysis) but not necessarily hypermetabolic (increased caloric requirements) [86]. The purpose of providing dextrose in PN is to suppress gluconeogenesis, decreasing the need for muscle breakdown as substrate, and to oxidize glucose as an energy source to decrease the need to use amino acids for energy. Consistent with this "protein-sparing effect," amino acids provided intravenously would be used exclusively for protein synthesis. However, acutely ill patients have non-suppressible gluconeogenesis and increased nitrogen excretion. Administration of glucose at a rate of 4 mg/kg/minute fails to suppress gluconeogenesis in critically ill patients [87], although increases in glucose oxidation have been shown with infusions up to 7 mg/kg/minute [88]. The administration of high glucose loads to metabolically stressed patients can result in hyperglycemia, increased CO_2 generation, and lipogenesis when the capacity for glucose oxidation is exceeded. Lipogenesis may in turn lead to hepatic steatosis and increased CO_2 generation has potential adverse effects on ventilatory function.

For critically ill patients, most nutrition societies recommend nitrogen intake between 1.2–2.0 g of amino acids/kg/day and energy intake of 25 ± 5 kcal/kg/day [89]. There is greater controversy surrounding the amount of carbohydrate that should be provided. Recommendations for glucose intake vary from 2–3 to up to 7.2 mg/kg/minute. In critically ill diabetic patients, a reasonable goal for dextrose infusion is no more than 2–3 mg/kg/minute. In nondiabetic stressed patients, the use of a hypocaloric, high-protein PN (100–200 g of dextrose and 1.5–2.0 g/kg of amino acids per day) early in acute illness avoids hyperglycemia and does not worsen nitrogen balance [90]. In a study not limited to diabetic patients, Frankenfield et al. [91] showed that hypocaloric feeding promotes endogenous lipid mobilization without adversely affecting protein metabolism. In addition, obese patients receiving only 50% of their resting energy expenditure (REE) calories in PN can achieve positive nitrogen balance [92].

Krishnan et al. [93] reported on 185 critically ill patients receiving nutrition support (69.7% EN, 19.5% EN+PN, and 10.8% PN). The average calorie intake received was only 50% of that recommended and the best outcomes (discharge alive and spontaneous ventilation) were seen in that tertile which received the middle range of calorie intake: 33–65% of calories prescribed or 9–18 kcal/kg/day. Thus, it is reasonable to conclude that hypocaloric PN has advantages over formulas providing 35–40 nonprotein kcal/day, generally considered to represent "overfeeding" but still used in many medical institutions. Estimating energy expenditure using prediction equations is often highly inaccurate [94]. When possible, indirect calorimetry should be used to avoid overfeeding. This point is illustrated by the findings of McClave and Snider [95], in which some ICU patients had inappropriately low metabolic rates, in large part due to less "work of breathing" while receiving mechanical ventilation.

Lipid emulsions in PN provide an additional source of calories and provide essential fatty acids. It has been suggested that high-fat, high-amino acid (HFHA) PN infusions can be beneficial in the immediate post-operative period in diabetic patients [96], though controlled studies with adequate power are lacking. In obese patients with large adipose stores, lipids can be withheld or severely limited. In one study of trauma patients, the provision of IV lipid in PN in the early postinjury period increased susceptibility to infection, prolonged pulmonary failure, and delayed recovery compared to a group receiving lipid-free PN [97]. It is unclear whether the benefits were due to the lack of lipid specifically or hypocaloric feeding [97]. Eventually lipids must be provided to prevent an essentially fatty acid deficiency. Approximately 500 cc of a 20% intralipid solution or 100 g/week have been shown to prevent deficiency [98]. When prescribing lipid, one must also consider whether the patient is receiving any other exogenous source of lipids such as with IV propofol. Current recommendations for macronutrient intake are shown in Table 11.3.

Diabetic patients may develop hypertriglyceridemia while receiving PN with intravenous lipids. There is some controversy as to what threshold of serum hypertriglyceridemia requires reduction in the lipid dosing. Clinical and chemical pancreatitis due to hypertriglyceridemia does not generally occur at levels less than 1000–1500 mg/dL though many clinicians have advocated lipid dose reductions at levels above 400 mg/dL. Additional strategies to control hypertriglyceridemia include addition of insulin, lowering of dextrose, and the addition of carnitine 1–3 g/day.

TABLE 11.3
Recommended Target Macronutrient Intake for Hospitalized Patients

	Amino Acid (g/day)	Dextrose (mg/kg/day)	Lipid (g/kg/day)	Total Calories (kcal/kg/day)	PN kcal/g AA
Stable	0.8–1.5	3–4	1.0	25–35	~150
Critically ill	1.2–1.8	2–3	0.5–1.0	18–25	~75

INSULINIZATION WITH PARENTERAL NUTRITION

Insulin requirements in PN are greater than insulin requirements with oral or enteral nutrition. In one study of 20 previously insulin-requiring diabetics who received their estimated basal energy expenditure in PN, no patient required less than 100% of their usual pre-hospital insulin dose [99]. The majority of patients required 200% of their usual dose to achieve glucoses < 220 mg/dL. Patients required an average of 0.22 and 0.31 units of insulin per gram of dextrose for non-infected and infected patients, respectively. In another study of 24 patients with insulin-requiring diabetes on PN, the average insulin requirement was 221 ± 109% of their pre-hospital insulin doses to achieve glucoses in the 150–250 mg/dL range [100]. In this study, type-1 diabetics received an average of 5.8 mg/kg/minute of dextrose and type-2 diabetics received an average of 4.6 mg/kg/minute of dextrose. In general, all patients with a prior diagnosis of diabetes require insulin during PN therapy.

Several protocols have been suggested for providing insulin in PN. McMahon [101] recommended starting with 0.1 units of regular insulin per gram of carbohydrate in patients previously treated with insulin or oral agents, increasing by 0.05 units of regular insulin per gram of dextrose each subsequent day until control is achieved. Gavin [102] recommended starting with approximately 25 units of regular insulin per liter of PN, assuming 25% dextrose in the PN. This is based on an estimate of 1 unit of regular insulin per hour as a basal requirement plus 3 units of regular insulin per hour for the carbohydrate infused. Michael and Sabo [103] recommended starting with no insulin in the PN if the patient was not previously insulin-requiring and then adding 2/3 of the insulin coverage amount the next day. For previously insulin-treated patients, they recommended using the following formula: 1.5 times the usual daily insulin dose multiplied by the fraction of total calorie requirements infused. Magee and Clement [104] suggested using a separate insulin infusion for the first 24 hours then adding 2/3 of the total dose administered to the next day's PN.

The principle of distinguishing basal, nutritional and correction insulin requirements either conceptually or practically is rational, particularly in patients with T1DM. Basal insulin requirements can be provided separately by subcutaneous injection while the nutritional insulin is provided in the PN. The major benefit is the continued presence of basal insulin when the insulin-containing PN infusion is interrupted. A continuous PN infusion may be interrupted unexpectedly due to loss of intravenous access, surgery, procedures, or late arrival of the PN bag. The provision of basal insulin subcutaneously avoids the risk of ketoacidosis in the insulin-deficient patient whose PN has been held.

An alternate approach is to provide both basal and nutritional insulin as a separate insulin infusion. Advantages of this approach include more rapid achievement of glucose control, more rapid achievement of caloric goals, and the ability to adjust the insulin frequently for changing requirements. Glucose desensitization, or its resolution, can dramatically alter insulin requirements over the course of a day. Also, when insulin is provided by a separate IV infusion, the need to discard a PN bag, which contains too much insulin if hypoglycemia has developed, is avoided. This approach may therefore result in cost savings [105].

Several insulin infusion protocols have now been published which allow nurses to independently manage insulin drips [43,106,107]. The primary disadvantage is the need for more frequent glucose monitoring and titration of the insulin dose. There is also a risk of hypoglycemia if the PN is discontinued and the insulin infusion is inadvertently continued. Furthermore, it increases the need for additional intravenous access and increases fluid administered. This approach is most appropriate for ICU patients, since the majority of stable patients can be managed with insulin-containing PN alone.

Successful use of continuous subcutaneous insulin infusion (CSII) has been reported in patients on cyclic nocturnal PN [108]. This method is obviously not practical for the majority of patients on PN, but represents a reasonable option for a select group of patients with T1DM who are receiving PN at home.

Due to individual and daily variations in insulin resistance and insulin secretory capacity, no standard protocol has been universally successful for the use of insulin with PN. However, some general guidelines can be offered: (1) all previously diagnosed diabetics will require insulin therapy with PN; (2) insulin requirements in PN are higher than previous subcutaneous requirements when patients are receiving full enteral calories; (3) when insulin requirements are unknown, a safe starting point which will avoid hypoglycemia and achieve a certain degree of control is 0.1 unit of insulin per gram of dextrose added to the PN; and (4) separate insulin infusions will achieve the most rapid control.

CHROMIUM CONTENT IN PARENTERAL NUTRITION

Chromium deficiency results in hyperglycemia, hypertriglyceridemia, and neuropathy. Though there is no generally accepted, reliable diagnostic test for chromium deficiency, Bahijri and Mufti [109] found that patients with T2DM responding to chromium therapy demonstrated increased urinary chromium excretion after a glucose load, compared with non-responders. Chromium therapy improves insulin binding to cells, insulin receptor number, and activates insulin receptor kinase, leading to increased insulin sensitivity [110]. In a randomized, controlled study of 180 patients with T2DM, chromium picolinate, 500 mcg po twice a day (BID), was associated with improved hemoglobin A1C (A1C) levels, lower fasting, postprandial glucose, and insulin levels, and lower total cholesterol levels [111].

The usual chromium content in standard multiple trace element (MTE) preparations is only 4–10 mcg. Therefore, the chromium content of usual PN solutions may not be adequate for severely stressed patients [112]. Chromium is available as single-entity product for addition to PN solutions, and supplemental chromium may be given empirically to facilitate glycemic control. The dosing can range from 10–200 mcg daily in addition to the routine MTE added. High-dose chromium (250 mcg daily) has been used safely in a patient with deficiency for 2 weeks [113]. There have been no proven toxic clinical effects in human studies involving supplemental chromium, despite reports of potentially toxic accumulations [114,115]. However, this is not a generally accepted claim since many experts in the field emphatically articulate concern, based on their own clinical experience and various studies in the literature, about the toxic effects of chromium [116].

ENTERAL NUTRITION

In healthy individuals, liquid diets are absorbed more rapidly and insulin and glucose responses are greater than with solid food [117]. During continuous enteral feeding in patients with T2DM, insulin and glucose oscillations are asynchronous, resulting in large peak blood glucose levels by 210 minutes followed by a steady state [118].

Modifications using nonglucose carbohydrates have been made to standard enteral formulas to try to blunt the glycemic response. Fructose is an acute regulator of liver glucose uptake and glycogen synthesis primarily by activation of hepatic glucokinase. Inclusion of fructose with an oral glucose load [119] or prior to a starchy meal [120] blunts the glucose response. In a study of 8 healthy nondiabetic subjects, insulin responses, but not postprandial glucose levels, were decreased following 25 g doses of enteral formulas containing fructose or xylitol, compared with formulas containing equivalent amounts of glucose, with or without fiber [121]. However, substitution of glucose or glucose-equivalent carbohydrates with nonglucose carbohydrates in EN formulas has not been proven to improve glycemic control or confer an outcome benefit in diabetic patients.

High-fiber (50g/day) solid diets result in lower preprandial glucose, 24-hour plasma glucose, 24-hour plasma insulin, total cholesterol, and triglycerides in diabetic patients [122]. The addition of fiber to enteral feeding formulas has not been proven to improve glucose control [123]. Gel-forming fibers cannot be used because of high viscosity and clogging of feeding tubes. The addition of hydrolyzed guar to various enteral formulas does not decrease the postprandial glucose response [124]. Although the glycemic response is not improved, the addition of fiber to enteral formulas may provide other benefits such as the provision of trophic, gut-specific fuels to the colonic mucosa [125] and decrease in diarrheal episodes [126,127].

Glucerna is a disease-specific diabetic formula containing 50% fat (enriched with monounsaturated fatty accids [MUFA]), 8% soy polysaccharide, 18% glucose oligosaccharide, and 7% fructose. This formula was compared to a standard formula Ensure HN, containing 30% fat and 53% carbohydrates, in type-1 diabetics ingesting 20 cc every 15 minutes. There was no significant rise of blood glucose with Glucerna where a steady rise was seen with Ensure HN® [128]. The investigators then needed to determine which of the potential glucose-lowering factors was responsible for the difference. They hypothesized that it may be due to (1) added fiber, (2) lower carbohydrate, (3) fructose vs. sucrose, or (4) slower gastric emptying with increased fat. They then compared five different enteral formulas in 11 subjects with T1DM and found that the postprandial glucose response directly correlated with the grams of carbohydrate present in the enteral formula [129]. Similarly, Printz et al. [130] found no difference in insulin or glucose response comparing high-fiber, high-fructose, and standard enteral formulas when the carbohydrate amount was kept constant. Sanz-Paris et al. [131] compared a single ingestion of Glucerna to another specialized diabetic formula, Precitene Diabet, which contains 54% carbohydrate, 31% fat, fructose, and fiber. The formula was ingested by ambulatory type-2 diabetic patients receiving their usual insulin or sulfonylurea dose. Mean peak plasma glucose was higher in patients who received the higher-carbohydrate Precitene Diabet formula. Of note, the insulin-treated patients were suboptimally treated with NPH alone. The same two formulas were recently compared in 104 patients with head and neck cancers or neurologic disorders receiving full enteral feeds for a median of 13 days [132]. Mean glucose was higher in the Precitene Diabet group and there was a trend toward increased triglycerides [132].

Lowering the carbohydrate content of enteral formulas necessitates an increase in fat content. The replacement of carbohydrates with MUFA in regular diets has been consistently shown to favorably affect the lipid profile, decreasing total cholesterol, very low-density lipoprotein cholesterol (VLDL-c), and triglycerides, while raising high-density lipoprotein cholesterol (HDL-c) [133]. Postprandial glucagon-like peptide-1 (GLP-1) responses were higher and triglycerides were lower in response to a meal rich in MUFA vs. saturated fat [134].

Few studies have compared outcomes in patients receiving a disease-specific vs. a standard enteral formula. Thirty stable nursing home residents with T2DM who received tube feeds with Glucerna had lower A1C and required less insulin than those patients receiving a standard formula containing fiber (Jevity) [135]. In addition, HDL-c was higher and triglycerides lower with Glucerna and there were fewer infections in the Glucerna group. Similar benefits have been seen in critically ill patients receiving a disease-specific formula with soluble fiber, MUFA, and lower carbohydrate (40%) [136].

Although use of a disease-specific formula is often helpful in achieving glycemic control, its use must be weighed against other factors for the individual patient. For example, in a patient with renal failure, the use of a formula low in volume and electrolytes (i.e., potassium, magnesium, and phosphorus), may take priority. In patients with hypoalbuminemia [137], critical illness [138], or impaired gastrointestinal absorption, use of a semi-elemental formula containing protein hydrolysates rather than an intact protein formula may be preferred. On the other hand, high-fat, low-carbohydrate enteral formulas may also improve pulmonary function in patients with chronic obstructive pulmonary disease (COPD) [139] and facilitate weaning in ventilated patients by decreasing the respiratory quotient [140].

Macronutrient Requirements

The carbohydrate content of commercially available enteral formulas ranges 28–80% and the fat content ranges 6–55%. The first step in feeding the diabetic patient is to select the most appropriate formula based on glucose levels, fluid requirements, albumin level, renal function, and status of the gastrointestinal tract. Once the most appropriate formula is selected, the goal rate of feeding is determined based on estimated caloric requirements. If additional protein is required, a modular protein powder such as ProMod or ProCel (5 g/scoop), or glutamine (0.285–0.57 g/kg/day or 15–30 g/day) [141], may be provided. As with parenteral feeding, increasing carbohydrate administration to critically ill patients fed enterally fails to suppress endogenous glucose production and stimulates *de novo* lipogenesis [142]. Overfeeding total calories can cause a significant increase in V_{CO2} and impair weaning from a ventilator [143].

Obese critically ill patients receiving enteral feeding of less than 20 kcal/kg/day of adjusted body weight had similar nitrogen balance and prealbumin levels, and shorter length of ICU stay, as compared with a group receiving 25–30 kcal/kg [144]. An adjusted body weight can be used to estimate energy requirements in obese patients by adding 25% [145] to 50% [146] of the excess body weight to the ideal body weight. Some data suggest that this approach may not be appropriate in elderly obese patients who have a limited ability to mobilize endogenous fat stores [147].

Micronutrient Supplements

Certain formulas are marketed based on claims that their micronutrient content improves the health of the diabetic patient. Despite theoretical benefits of antioxidant therapy, supplementation of vitamins C and E to patients with T2DM has not been shown to improve endothelial function or cardiovascular outcomes [148–151]. On the other hand, van Etten et al. [152] found that folic acid administration improved NO-mediated vasodilation in patients with T2DM. Indeed, the whole issue of using antioxidant micronutrition in the management of diabetes is completely unresolved [153].

Arginine is conditionally essential during stress and levels are reduced in patients with diabetes. Enteral and parenteral administration of L-arginine improves endothelial function via enhanced NO synthesis as well as NO-independent mechanisms [154]. Oral arginine supplementation has been shown to improve peripheral and hepatic insulin sensitivity in subjects with T2DM [155]. The American Diabetes Association Position Statement concluded "there is no clear evidence of benefit from vitamin or mineral supplementation in people with diabetes who do not have underlying deficiencies" [156].

Insulinization with Enteral Nutrition

As with PN, critically ill patients in the ICU receiving EN are best managed with IV insulin due to marked insulin resistance and constantly changing insulin sensitivity. Moreover, the presence of edema [157] or the use of pressor medications [158] may make absorption of subcutaneously injected insulin unreliable. The development of protocols which allow nurses to independently adjust the drips is crucial. Chase et al. [159] recently published proof of concept results utilizing a bolus-based insulin algorithm. This was based on a complex nonlinear model of time varying changes in insulin sensitivity. The equations were solved with a computationally simple linear, least-squares method. They reported successful control of blood glucose in three ICU patients receiving continuous EN. Such an algorithm is a marked improvement over fixed protocols, which often lead to dosing errors, and may set the stage for eventual closed-loop glycemic control systems in hospitalized patients.

More stable hospitalized patients receiving EN can be managed with subcutaneous insulin. Very few studies have evaluated different insulin regimens in patients receiving EN. Kerr et al. [160] reported on the use of regular insulin prior to a slow-bolus feeding of Osmolite over 4 hours, three times per day, with the addition of neutral pH–protamine–Hagedorn insulin (NPH) at bedtime.

Average insulin requirements were 45 units per 24 hours and the average glucose was 156 mg/dL [160]. There was no symptomatic hypoglycemia. Now with the availability of rapid-acting insulin analogs, control is facilitated of diabetes in patients receiving bolus feeding via syringe or gravity. Basal insulin coverage is needed in many, but not all patients with T2DM, and can be given with long- or intermediate-acting insulin.

At first glance, the use of insulin glargine or insulin detemir, which are long-acting peakless insulins, seems logical and most appropriate for continuous tube feeding. One author reported on the use of glargine in a single outpatient receiving continuous feeds [161]. There were no episodes of hypoglycemia, but it took 3 weeks to achieve adequate glycemic control [161]. In hospitalized patients, control must be achieved more rapidly. More importantly, hospitalized patients will frequently have their tube feeding held at unpredictable times for procedures or feeding intolerance (vomiting, diarrhea, abdominal pain, or distension). If the patient has been receiving full calories, there will be a substantial risk of hypoglycemia with a large dose of or detemir glargine still acting, which may be difficult to avert with IV dextrose. Furthermore, with a glargine regimen, one can only intervene once or twice a day. In patients requiring relatively low total daily doses of insulin (i.e., < 40 units per day), the use of long acting analog insulin may provide smooth control of glucose and greater convenience without a substantially increased risk of hypoglycemia. Clinical studies using insulin glargine or detemir in patients receiving EN are warranted.

For the time being, a better practice may be to use NPH, every 6–8 hours with supplemental rapid-acting insulin coverage every 3–4 hours. Nierman and Mechanick [162] used this type of regimen in chronically critically ill patients receiving continuous tube feeding. Mean glucose achieved was 115 mg/dL with an average of 40 units of insulin per day [162]. Once feeds have been tolerated at the goal rate and the patient is stable, it may be reasonable to convert the total dose into one or two daily doses of glargine or detemir for more convenient dosing and lower risk of hypoglycemia.

Glycemic control becomes more challenging when continuous feeds are cycled over part of the day. This requires more attention toward synchronizing insulin with carbohydrate provision in the EN. Such feeding regimens are commonly used when transitioning patients from enteral to oral feeding and in patients undergoing rehabilitation who need to be liberated from the feeding pump for a substantial portion of the day. An intermediate-acting insulin, with a lower dose of a rapid-acting insulin at the initiation of feeds, followed by a second smaller dose of the intermediate-acting insulin 8–12 hours later, works well with EN cycled over 12–18 hours a day.

Continuous subcutaneous insulin infusions have been used safely and effectively in the management of patients receiving continuous EN [163]. This is a reasonable, albeit more expensive, option for patients, particularly those receiving cycled, continuous feeds. We believe this treatment should be reserved for patients requiring long-term home EN, with an excellent prognosis, and who are capable of programming the pump.

Correction dose insulin is provided subcutaneously with any of the above regimens to correct an elevated glucose level. Such "sliding scales" should take into account individual variations in insulin sensitivity and may need to be modified over subsequent days. A sliding scale should not be used alone in diabetic patients who are receiving nutrition support.

The use of oral agents to control diabetes in hospitalized patients receiving EN is generally inappropriate. Insulin secretagogues (sulfonylureas and meglitinides) are often ineffective in patients with metabolic stress and glucose desensitization or glucose toxicity. Sulfonylureas are long-acting and can cause hypoglycemia if feeds are held. Nevertheless, the shorter-acting meglitinides may be used prior to bolus feeds in nonstressed patients. Metformin is contraindicated in patients with unstable renal, pulmonary, or cardiac function and in patients going for surgery or intravenous contrast procedures. Thiazolidinediones (TZD) do not act quickly enough to be effective for glucose control in the hospital. Furthermore, TZD can exacerbate fluid retention in patients with anasarca due to hypoalbuminemia.

TABLE 11.4
Special Scenarios Involving Hospitalized Patients with Hyperglycemia Receiving Enteral Nutrition

Scenario	Circumstances	Preferred Strategy
1	Continuous enteral feeds	q 6–8 Hour (NPH) or q 12–24 hour glargine or detemir
2	Cycled enteral feeds	Intermediate-acting + rapid-acting insulin analog at start; Intermediate-acting insulin 8–12 hours later
3	Continuous feeds + po nutrition	Add standing pre-meal rapid-acting insulin analog
4	Bolus feeds	Standing prebolus insulin analog; consider meglitinide if very mild hyperglycemia in stable patient with normal fasting glucose
5	Enteral + parenteral nutrition	sq Insulin for enteral carbohydrate + IV insulin in PN
6	Glucocorticoids + tube feeds	Split steroid dose; give intermediate-acting insulin with each steroid dose
7	Glucocorticoids + po nutrition	Increase standing pre-meal rapid-acting insulin analog; give intermediate-acting insulin with each steroid dose
8	Severe insulin resistance	Decrease dietary fat; cross-titrate: decrease rate of feeds while increasing insulin to decrease glucose toxicity
9	Po nutrition requiring insulin	glargine or detemir + rapid-acting insulin analog

See text for abbreviatons.

Special issues make management of diabetes exceptionally challenging in hospitalized patients receiving enteral feeding (see Table 11.4). Feeding is frequently interrupted or rates decreased due to procedures or symptoms such as vomiting, diarrhea, or abdominal distension. The development or resolution of metabolic stress, as with sepsis, alters insulin requirements. The rapid development of glucose desensitization, as mentioned previously, can result in rapid and marked deterioration of glucose control, which can take days to correct if not promptly addressed.

Frequent use of glucocorticoids for immune suppression, relative adrenal insufficiency, intracerebral edema, laryngeal edema, and other conditions will transiently and variably increase requirements in an unpredictable manner. Furthermore, when steroids are used, insulin requirements may vary throughout the day depending on the dosing regimen. For example, if steroids are given only in the morning, insulin requirements are highest in the afternoon; early morning hypoglycemia may result if insulin is dosed consistently throughout the day.

Glucose control and provision of adequate calories can be particularly problematic in the patient with gastroparesis. The presence of gastroparesis may be a result of long-standing diabetes and may predate the hospitalization. Additional factors in critically ill patients increase the risk of gastroparesis such as sepsis mediators (nitric oxide), use of narcotics and dopamine, increased intracranial pressure [164], hypovolemia, as well as the underlying disease. Hyperglycemia slows gastric emptying and may exacerbate symptoms. The prokinetic agents, metoclopramide and erythromycin, have been used successfully in patients with gastroparesis [165]. Gastric electrical stimulation is a relatively new development in the management of severe and persistent gastroparesis. Jejunal feeding can improve nutritional status and gastric function in patients with gastroparesis [166,167]. However, in those patients not responding to the above intervention, PN may be necessary.

The following are general recommendations for providing EN to a patient with abnormal glucose tolerance:

1. Consider using a disease-specific formula
2. Use insulin to control the glucose rather than oral agents

3. Be careful initiating intermediate- or long-acting insulin until the patient is clearly tolerating feeds
4. Use continuous feeds in critically ill patients
5. Use intravenous insulin in ICU patients
6. Avoid increasing feeds until adequate glycemic control is obtained
7. Avoid overfeeding
8. Monitor glucose levels frequently and provide supplemental correction insulin as needed

HYPOGLYCEMIA

Concerns about hypoglycemia limit the most aggressive insulin management. This psychological factor on the part of the treating physician has contributed to the hesitancy and reluctance to adopt contemporary guidelines for tight glycemic control. Hypoglycemia results in unpleasant symptoms for the patient (tremors, sweats, and irritability) and, at worst, can result in loss of consciousness, seizures, and even death. Furthermore, hypoglycemia can be particularly difficult to recognize in ventilated or critically ill patients who are already in high-catecholamine states. The strictest definition of hypoglycemia is a glucose level < 40 mg/dL. However, many patients will experience symptoms with glucose levels < 70 mg/dL. The goal is to bring glucose values as close to normal as possible, while avoiding dangerous or symptomatic hypoglycemia.

When hypoglycemia does occur, rapid correction of glucose is essential. If a patient is conscious and able to take oral carbohydrate, 4–8 oz of juice will generally raise plasma glucose adequately. Patients receiving nutrition support usually need to be treated differently. Patients receiving PN can be given a 50% dextrose solution intravenously. When the glucose level is in the 50–80 mg/dL range, half an ampoule of D50 (12.5 g) will generally raise glucose adequately. If the glucose is < 50 mg/dL, a full ampoule of D50 should be given. For patients receiving enteral feeds, 4 oz of juice (15 g) can be given through the feeding tube for a glucose level in the 50–80 mg/dL range and 8 oz (30 g) for lower glucose values. If the patient has altered mental status as a result of the hypoglycemia, an ampoule of D50 should be given immediately. If intravenous access is not available or the response to D50 is inadequate, intramuscular glucagon 1 mg can be given. The glucose level must be retested 15–20 minutes after the treatment. If the glucose is not increasing, the treatment should be repeated. The glucose should be rechecked until the level is greater than 80 mg/dL.

The next step is to evaluate the carbohydrate and insulin sources. If severe hypoglycemia occurs in a patient receiving PN that contains insulin, the PN will likely need to be held until the bag can be reformulated with less insulin. In patients receiving EN, one must first check that the prescribed nutrition is being delivered. If the patient is receiving the tube feeding as prescribed, and the cause of hypoglycemia was an overestimate of insulin requirements, additional dextrose should be provided intravenously (i.e., D5W or D10W) until the last insulin injection has worn off (i.e., 4–6 hours for rapid-acting, 6–10 hours for regular insulin, 12–20 hours for NPH, and 20–24 hours for glargine or detemir) [168] and then subsequent doses should be reduced. One should try to determine if the hypoglycemia was a result of too much correction insulin dosing or too much standing insulin dosing. Contrary to popular belief, abrupt discontinuation of PN, even bags containing high doses of insulin, does not typically result in hypoglycemia [169], and the common practice of routinely initiating a 10% dextrose infusion after stopping PN is unnecessary.

REFERENCES

1. Umpierrez GE, Isaacs SD, and Bazargan N et al., Hyperglycemia: An independent marker of in-hospital mortality in patients with undiagnosed diabetes, *J Clin Endocrinol Metab*, 87:978–982, 2002.

2. Levetan CS, Passaro M, and Jablonski K et al., Unrecognized diabetes among hospitalized patients, *Diabetes Care,* 21:246–249, 1998.

3. Mizock BA, Alterations in carbohydrate metabolism during stress, A review of the literature, *Am J Med,* 98:75–84, 1995.

4. McCowen KC, Malhotra A, and Bistrian BR, Stress-induced hyperglycemia, *Crit Care Clin,* 17:107–24, 2001.

5. de Alvaro, Teruel T, and Hernandez R et al., Tumor necrosis factor- produces insulin resistance in skeletal muscle by activation of inhibitor kinase in a p38 MAPK-dependent manner, *J Biol Chem,* 279:17070–17078, 2004.

6. Marik PE and Raghavan M, Stress-hyperglycemia, insulin, and immunomodulation in sepsis, *Int Care Med,* 30:748–756, 2004.

7. Le Roith D, Molecular mechanisms by which metabolic control may improve outcomes, *Endocr Pract,* 10(Suppl 2):57–62, 2004.

8. McCowen KC, Ciccarone A, and Mao Y et al., *Crit Care Med,* 29:839–846, 2001.

9. Poitout V and Robertson RP, Minireview: Secondary β-cell failure in type-2 diabetes—a convergence of glucotoxicity and lipotoxicity, *Endocrinology,* 143:339–342, 2002.

10. Evans JL, Goldfine ID, and Maddux BA et al., Are oxidative stress-activated signaling pathways mediators of insulin resistance and β-cell dysfunction? *Diabetes,* 52:1–8, 2003.

11. McKillop AM, Abdel-Wahab YH, and Mooney MH et al., Secretion of glycated insulin represents a novel aspect of β–cell dysfunction and glucose toxicity, *Diabetes Metab,* 28:3S61–3S69, 2002.

12. Weekers F, Giulietti AP, and Michalaki M et al., Metabolic, endocrine, and immune effects of SH in a rabbit model of prolonged critical illness, *Endocrinology,* 144:5329–5338, 2003.

13. Inzucchi SE, Goldberg PA, and Dziura JD et al., Risk factors for poor glycemic control in a medical intensive care unit, *Diabetes,* 52(Suppl 1):A96, 2003.

14. Park RH, Hansell DT, and Davidson LE et al., Management of diabetic patients receiving nutrition support, *Nutrition,* 8:316–320, 1992.

15. Perner A, Nielsen SE, and Rask-Madsen J, High glucose impairs superoxide production from isolated blood neutrophils, *Intensive Care Med,* 29:511-514, 2003.

16. Hennessey PJ, Black CT, and Andrassy RJ, Nonenzymatic glycosylation of immunoglobulin G impairs complement fixation, *JPEN,* 15:60–64, 1991.

17. Wilson RM and Reeves WG, Neutrophil phagocytosis and killing in insulin-dependent diabetes, *Clin Exp Immunol,* 63:478–484, 1986.

18. van Oss CJ and Border JR, Influence of intermittent hyperglycemic glucose levels on the phagocytosis of microorganisms by human granulocytes in vitro, *Immunol Commun,* 7:669–776, 1978.

19. Hostetter MK, Handicaps to host defense: Effects of hyperglycemia on C3 and Candida albicans, *Diabetes,* 39:271–275, 1990.

20. Alvarez-Lerma F, Nolla-Salas J, and Leon C et al., Candiduria in critically ill patients admitted to intensive care medical units, *Int Care Med,* 29:1069–1076, 1990.

21. Carr ME, Diabetes mellitus: A hypercoaguable state, *J Diabetes Complications,* 15:44–54, 2001.

22. Gresele P, Guglielmini G, and De Angelis M et al., Acute, short-term hyperglycemia enhances shear stress-induced platelet activation with type-II diabetes, *J Am Coll Cardiol,* 41:1013–1020, 2003.

23. Booth G, Stalker TJ, and Lefer AM et al., Elevated ambient glucose induces acute inflammatory events in the microvasculature: Effects of insulin, *Am J Physiol Endocrinol Metab,* 280:E848–856, 2001.

24. Marfella, Rafaele, and Esposito K et al., Circulating adhesion molecules in humans, *Circulation,* 101:2247, 2000.

25. Aso Y, Okumura K, and Yoshida N et al., Enhancement of fibrinolysis in poorly controlled, hospitalized type-2 diabetic patients by short-term metabolic control: Association with a decrease in plasminogen activator inhibitor 1, *Exp Clin Endocrinol Diabetes,* 112:175–180, 2004.

26. Pricci F, Leto G, and Amadio L et al., Oxidative stress in diabetes-induced endothelial dysfunction involvement of nitric oxide and protein kinase C, *Free Radic Biol Med,* 35:683–694, 2003.

27. Schulze PC, Yoshioka J, and Takahashi T et al., Hyperglycemia promotes oxidative stress through inhibition of thioredoxin function by thioredoxin-interacting protein, *J Biol Chem,* 279:30369–30374, 2004.

28. Zhang L, Zalewski A, and Liu Y et al., Diabetes-induced oxidative stress and low-grade inflammation in porcine coronary arteries, *Circulation,* 108:472–478, 2003.

29. Kumar K, Yernerni V, and Bai W et al., Hyperglycemia-induced activation of nuclear transcription factor B in vascular smooth muscle cells, *Diabetes,* 48:855–864, 1999.

30. Rask-Madsen C, Dominguez H, and Ihlemann N et al., Tumor necrosis factor-α inhibits insulin's stimulating effect on glucose uptake and endothelium-dependent vasodilation in humans, *Circulation,* 108:1815–1821, 2003.

31. Nappo F, Esposito K, and Cioffi M et al., Postprandial endothelial activation in healthy subjects and in type-2 diabetic patients: Role of fat and carbohydrate meals, *J Am Coll Cardiol,* 39:1145–1150, 2002.

32. Steinberg HO, Paradisi G, and Hook G et al., Free fatty acid elevation impairs insulin-mediated vasodilation and nitric oxide production, *Diabetes,* 49:1231–1238, 2000.

33. Pomposelli JJ, Baxter JK, and Babineau TJ et al., Early postoperative glucose control predicts nosocomial infection rate in diabetic patients, *JPEN,* 22:77–81, 1998.

34. Norhammar AM, Ryden L, and Malmberg K, Admission plasma glucose: Independent risk factor for long-term prognosis after myocardial infarction even in nondiabetic patients, *Diabetes Care,* 22:1827–1831, 1999.

35. McAlister FA, Man J, and Bistritz L et al., Diabetes and coronary artery bypass surgery: An examination of perioperative glycemic control and outcomes, *Diabetes Care,* 26:1518–1524, 2003.

36. Guvener M, Pasaoglu I, and Demircin M et al., Perioperative hyperglycemia is a strong correlate of postoperative infection in type-II diabetic patients after coronary artery bypass grafting, *Endocr J,* 49:531–537, 2002.

37. Estrada CA, Young JA, and Nifong LW et al., Outcomes and perioperative hyperglycemia in patients with or without diabetes mellitus undergoing coronary artery bypass grafting, *Ann Thorac Surg,* 75:1392–1399, 2003.

38. Capes SE, Hunt D, and Malmberg K et al., Stress hyperglycemia and prognosis of stroke in nondiabetic and diabetic patients, *Stroke,* 32:2426–2432, 2001.

39. Bruno A, Levine SR, and Frankel MR et al., Admission glucose level and clinical outcomes in the NINDS rt-PA stroke trial, *Neurology,* 59:669–674, 2002.

40. Alvarez-Sabin J, Molina CA, and Montaner J et al., Effects of admission hyperglycemia on stroke outcome in reperfused tissue plasminogen activator-treated patients, *Stroke,* 34:1235, 2003.

41. Krinsley JS, Association between hyperglycemia and increased hospital mortality in a heterogeneous population of critically ill patients, *Mayo Clin Proc,* 78:1471–1478, 2003.

42. Zerr KJ, Furnary AP, and Grunkemeier GL et al., Glucose control lowers the risk of wound infection in diabetics after open-heart operations, *Ann Thorac Surg,* 63:356–361, 1997.

43. Furnary AP, Wu Y, and Bookin SO, The Portland Diabetic Project, Effect of hyperglycemia and continuous intravenous insulin infusions on outcomes of cardiac surgical procedures, *Endocr Pract,* 10(Suppl 2):21–33, 2004.

44. van den Berghe G, Wouters P, and Weekers F et al., Intensive insulin therapy in critically ill patients, *N Engl J Med,* 345:1359–67, 2001.

45. Grey NJ and Perdrizet GA, Reduction of nosocomial infections in the surgical intensive-care unit by strict glycemic control, *Endocr Pract,* 10(Suppl 2):46–52, 2004.

46. Krinsley JS, Effect of an intensive glucose management protocol on the mortality of critically ill adult patients, *Mayo Clin Proc,* 79:992–1000, 2004.

47. Chaudhuri A, Janicke D, and Wilson MF et al., Anti-inflammatory and profibrinolytic effect of insulin in acute ST-segment elevation myocardial infarction, *Circulation,* 109:848–854, 1994.

48. Hansen TK, Thiel S, and Wouters PJ et al., Intensive insulin therapy exerts anti-inflammatory effects in critically ill patients and counteracts the adverse effect of low mannose-binding lectin levels, *J Clin Endocrinol Metab,* 88:1082–1088, 2003.

49. Vehkavaara S and Yki-Jarvinen H, 3.5 years of insulin therapy with insulin glargine improves in vivo endothelial function in type-2 diabetes, *Arterioscler Thromb Vasc Biol,* 24:325–330, 2004.

50. Almbrand B, Johannesson M, and Sjostrand B et al., Cost-effectiveness of intense insulin treatment after acute myocardial infarction in patients with diabetes mellitus, *Eur Heart J,* 21:733–739, 2000.

51. Malmberg KA, Efendic S, and Ryden LE, Feasibility of insulin-glucose infusion in diabetic patients with acute myocardial infarction, *Diabetes Care,* 17:1007–1014, 1994.

52. Malmberg K, Ryden L, and Hamsten A et al., Effects of insulin treatment on cause-specific one-year mortality and morbidity in diabetic patients with acute myocardial infarction, *Eur Heart J,* 17:1337–1344, 1996.

53. Malmberg K, Ryden L, and Efendic S et al., Randomized trial of insulin-glucose infusion followed by subcutaneous treatment in diabetic patients with acute myocardial infarction (DIGAMI Study): Effects on mortality at 1 year, *J Am Coll Cardiol,* 26:57–65, 1995.

54. Malmberg K, Norhammar A, and Weder H et al., Long-term results from the Diabetes and Insulin-Glucose Infusion in Acute Myocardial Infarction Study (DIGAMI), Glycometabolic state at admission: Important risk marker of mortality in conventionally treated patients with diabetes mellitus and acute myocardial infarction, *Circulation,* 99:2626–2632, 1999.

55. Malmberg K, DIGAMI Study Group, Prospective randomized study of intensive insulin treatment on long-term survival after acute myocardial infarction in patients with diabetes mellitus, *Br Med J,* 314:1512–1515, 1997.

56. Schnell O, Schafer O, and Kleybrink S et al., Intensification of therapeutic approaches reduces mortality in diabetic patients with acute myocardial infarction, *Diabetes Care,* 27:455–460, 2004.

57. Lazar HL, Chipkin SR, and Fitzgerald CA et al., Tight glycemic control in diabetic coronary artery bypass graft patients improves perioperative outcomes and decreases recurrent ischemic events, *Circulation,* 109:1497–1502, 2004.

58. van den Berghe G, Beyond diabetes: Saving lives with insulin in the ICU, *Int J Obesity,* 26(Suppl 3):53–58, 2002.

59. Finney SJ, Zekveld C, and Elia A et al., Glucose control and mortality in critically ill patients, *JAMA,* 290:2041–2047, 2003.

60. Groban L, Butterworth J, and Legault C et al., Intraoperative insulin therapy does not reduce the need for inotropic or antiarrhythmic therapy after cardiopulmonary bypass, *J Cardiothor Vasc Anesth,* 16:405–412, 2002.

61. Garlick PJ, Fern M, and Preedy VR, The effect of insulin infusion and food intake on muscle protein synthesis in postabsorptive rats, *Biochem J,* 210:669–676, 1983.

62. Fulks RM and Goldberg AL, Effects on insulin, glucose, and amino acids on protein turnover in rat diaphragm, *J Biol Chem,* 250:290–298, 1975.

63. Jefferson LS, Li JB, and Rannels SR, Regulation by insulin of amino acid release and protein turnover in the perfused rat hemicorpus, *J Biol Chem,* 252:1476–1483, 1977.

64. Fukagawa NK, Minaker KL, and Rowe JW et al., Insulin-mediated reduction of whole-body protein breakdown, *J Clin Invest,* 76:2306–2311, 1985.

65. Clements R, Pinson T, and Borghesi L et al., Nitrogen balance is achieved and myofibrillar protein catabolism is inhibited by insulin and total parenteral nutrition in trauma patients, *Surg Forum,* 47:147–148, 1996.

66. Flakoll PJ, Kulayalt M, and Frexes-Steed M et al., Amino acids augment insulin's suppression of whole-body proteolysis, *Am J Physiol,* 257:E839–847, 1989.

67. Valarini R, Sousa MF, and Kalil R et al., Anabolic effects of insulin and amino acids in promoting nitrogen accretion in postoperative patients, *J Parenter Enteral Nutr,* 18:214–218, 1994.

68. Clements RH, Hayes CA, and Gibbs R et al., Insulin's anabolic effect is influenced by route of administration of nutrients, *Arch Surg,* 134:274–277, 1999.

69. American College of Endocrinology Task Force on Inpatient Diabetes Control, ACE position statement on inpatient diabetes and metabolic control, *Endocr Pract,* 10:77–82, 2004.

70. American Diabetes Association, Standards of medical care in diabetes, *Diabetes Care,* 28:S4–36, 2005.

71. Correia MI and Waitzberg DL, The impact of malnutrition on morbidity, mortality, length of hospital stay, and costs evaluated through a multivariate model analysis, *Clin Nutr,* 22:235–239, 2003.

72. American Diabetes Association, Diabetes nutrition recommendations for health care institutions, *Diabetes Care,* 27:S55–57, 2004.

73. Charney P, American Society of Parenteral and Enteral Nutrition, Enteral nutrition, indications, options, and formulations, In: *The Science and Practice of Nutrition Support,* Dubuque, Iowa: Kendall-Hunt Publishing, 141–166, 2001.

74. Lipman TO, Grains or veins: Is enteral nutrition really better than parenteral nutrition? A look at the evidence, *JPEN,* 22:167, 1998

75. Engel JM, Muhling J, and Junger A et al., Enteral nutrition practice in a surgical intensive-care unit: What proportion of energy expenditure is delivered enterally? *Clin Nutr,* 22(2):187–192, 2003.

76. Vilsboll T, Krarup T, and Madsbad S et al., Both GLP-1 and GIP are insulinotropic at basal and postprandial glucose levels and contribute nearly equally to the incretin effect of a meal in healthy subjects, *Regul Pept,* 114:115–121, 2003.

77. Fery F, Tappy L, and Deviere J et al., Comparison of intraduodenal and intravenous glucose metabolism under clamp conditions, *Am J Physiol Endocrinol Metab,* 286:E176–183, 2004.

78. Edwards CMB, Stanley SA, and Davis R et al., Exendin-4 reduces fasting and postprandial glucose and decreases energy intake in healthy volunteers, *Am J Physiol Endocrinol Metab,* 281:E155–161, 2001.

79. Lugari R, Dei Cas A,and Ugolotti D et al., Evidence for early impairment of glucagons-like peptide-1-induced insulin secretion in human type-2 (non-insulin-dependent) diabetes, *Horm Metab Res,* 34:150–154, 2002.

80. Vilsboll T, Krarup T, and Madsbad S et al., Defective amplification of the late-phase insulin response to glucose by GIP in obese type-II diabetic patients, *Diabetologia,* 45:1111–1119, 2002.

81. Meier JJ, Gallwitz B, and Salmen S et al., Normalization of glucose concentrations and deceleration of gastric emptying after solid meals during intravenous glucagons-like peptide 1 in patients with type-2 diabetes, *J Clin Endocrinol Metab,* 88:2719–2725, 2003.

82. Zander M, Madsbad S, and Madsen JL et al., Effect of 6-week course of glucagon-like peptide 1 on glycaemic control, insulin sensitivity, and β-cell function in type-2 diabetes, A parallel-group study, *Lancet,* 359(9309):824–830, 2002.

83. Holst JJ and Orskov C, The incretin approach for diabetes treatment: Modulation of islet hormone release by GLP-1 agonism, *Diabetes,* 53(Suppl 3):S197–204, 2004.

84. Drucker DJ, Enhancing incretin action for the treatment of type-2 diabetes, *Diabetes Care,* 26:2929–2940, 2003.

85. Nauck MA, Walberg J, and Vethacke A et al., Blood glucose control in healthy subject and patients receiving intravenous glucose infusion or total parenteral nutrition using glucagon-like peptide 1, *Regul Pept,* 118(1–2):89–97, 2004.

86. McClave SA and Snider HL, Understanding the metabolic response to critical illness: Factors that cause patients to deviate from the expected pattern of hypermetabolism, 2(2):139–46, 1994.

87. Tappy L, Schwarz JM, and Schneiter P et al., Effects of isoenergetic glucose-based or lipid-based parenteral nutrition on glucose metabolism, de novo lipogenesis, and respiratory exchanges in critically ill patients, *J Crit Care Med,* 26:860–867, 1998.

88. Wolfe RR, O'Donnell TF, Jr, and Stone MD et al., Investigation of factors determining the optimal glucose infusion rate in total parenteral nutrition, 29:892–900, 1980.

89. Bozzeetti F and Allaria B, Nutritional support in ICU patients: Position of scientific societies, *Nutr Crit Care,* 8:279–298, 2003.

90. Patino JF, de Pimiento SE, and Vergara A et al., Hypocaloric support of the critically ill, *World J Surg,* 23:553–559, 1999.

91. Frankenfield DC, Smith JS, and Cooney RN, Accelerated nitrogen loss after traumatic injury is not attenuated by achievement of nitrogen balance, *JPEN,* 21:324–329, 1997.

92. Burge JC, Goon A, and Choban PS et al., Efficacy of hypocaloric total parenteral nutrition in hospitalized obese patients, A prospective, double-blind randomized trial, *JPEN,* 18:203–207, 1994.

93. Krishnan JA, Parce PB, and Martinez A et al., Caloric intake in medical ICU patients, *Chest,* 124:297–305, 2003.

94. Flancbaum L, Choban PS, and Sambucco S et al., Comparison of indirect calorimetry, the Fick method, and prediction equations in estimating the energy requirements of critically ill patients, *Am J Clin Nutr,* 69:461–466, 1999.

95. McClave SA and Snider HL, Understanding the metabolic response to critical illness: Factors that cause patients to deviate from the expected pattern of hypermetabolism, *New Horiz,* 2:139–146, 1994.

96. Watanabe Y, Sato M, and Abe Y et al., Fat emulsions as an ideal nonprotein energy source under surgical stress for diabetic patients, *Nutrition,* 11:734–738, 1995.

97. Battistella FD, Widergren JT, and Anderson JT et al., A prospective, randomized trial of intravenous fat emulsion administration in trauma victims requiring total parenteral nutrition, *J Trauma,* 43:52–58, 1997.

98. Jeppsen PB, Hoy CE, and Mortensen PB, Essential fatty acid deficiency in patients receiving home parenteral nutrition, *Am J Clin Nutr,* 68:126–144, 1998.

99. Hongsermeier T and Bistrian BR, Evaluation of a practical technique for determining insulin requirements in diabetic patients receiving total parenteral nutrition, *JPEN,* 17:16–19, 1993.

100. Overett TK, Bistrian BR, and Lowry SF et al., Total parenteral nutrition in patients with insulin-requiring diabetes mellitus, 5:79–89, 1986.

101. McMahon MM, Management of hyperglycemia in hospitalized patients receiving parenteral nutrition, *Nutr Clin Pract,* 12:35–38, 1997.

102. Gavin LA, Perioperative management of the diabetic patient, *Endo Metab Clin North Am,* 21:457–474, 1992.

103. Michael SR and Sabo CE, Management of the diabetic patient receiving nutritional support, *Nutr Clin Pract,* 4:179–183, 1989.

104. Magee MF and Clement S, Subcutaneous insulin therapy in the hospital setting: Issues, concerns, and implementation, *Endocr Pract,* 10(Suppl 2):81–88, 2004.

105. Sajbel TA, Dutro MP, and Radway PR, Use of separate insulin infusions with total parenteral nutrition, *JPEN,* 11:97–99, 1987.

106. Goldberg PA, Siegel MD, and Sherwin RS et al., Implementation of a safe and effective insulin infusion protocol in a medical intensive care unit, *Diabetes Care,* 27:461–467, 2004.

107. Markovitz LJ, Wiechmann RJ, and Harris N et al., Description and evaluation of a glycemic management protocol for patients with diabetes undergoing heart surgery, *Endocr Pract,* 8:10–18, 2002.

108. Beau P, Marechaud R, and Matuchansky C, Cyclic total parenteral nutrition, diabetes mellitus, and subcutaneous insulin pump, *The Lancet,* 1(8492):1272–1273, 1986.

109. Bahijri SM and Mufti AM, Beneficial effects of chromium in people with type-2 diabetes, and urinary chromium response to glucose load as a possible indicator of status, *Biol Trace Elem Res,* 85:97–109, 2002.

110. Anderson RA, Chromium in the prevention and control of diabetes, *Diabetes Metab,* 26:22–27, 2000.

111. Anderson RA, Cheng N, and Bryden NA et al., Elevated intakes of supplemental chromium improve glucose and insulin variables in individuals with type-2 diabetes, *Diabetes,* 46:1786–1791, 1997.

112. Anderson RA, Chromium, glucose intolerance, and diabetes, *J Am Coll Nutr,* 17:548–555, 1998.

113. Verhage AH, Cheong WK, and Jeejeebhoy KN, Neurologic symptoms due to possible chromium deficiency in long-term parenteral nutrition that closely mimic metronidazole-induced syndromes, 20:123–127, 1996.

114. Leung FY, Grace DM, and Alfieri MA et al., Abnormal trace elements in a patient on total parenteral nutrition with normal renal function, *Clin Biochem,* 28:297–302, 1995.

115. Prokurat S, Grenda R, and Lipowski D et al., MARS procedure as a bridge to combined liver-kidney transplantation in severe chromium-copper acute intoxications, A pediatric case report, *Liver,* 22(Suppl 2):76–77, 2002.

116. Bagchi D, Stohs SJ, and Downs BW et al., Cytotoxicity and oxidative mechanisms of different forms of chromium, *Toxicology,* 180:5–22, 2002.

117. Cashmere KA, Costill DL, and Cataland S et al., Serum endocrine and glucose response elicited from ingestion of enteral feedings, *Fed Proc,* 40:440, 1981.

118. Simon C, Brandenberger G, and Follenius M et al., Alteration in the temporal organization of insulin secretion in type-2 (non-insulin-dependent) diabetic patients under continuous enteral nutrition, *Diabetologia,* 34:435–440, 1991.

119. McGuiness OP and Cherrington AD, Effects of fructose on hepatic glucose metabolism, *Curr Opin Clin Nutr Metab Care,* 6:441–448, 2003.

120. Heacock PM, Hertzler SR, and Wolf BW, Fructose pre-feeding reduces the glycemic response to a high-glycemic index, starchy food in humans, *J Nutr,* 132:2601–2604, 2002.

121. Otto C, Sonnichsen AC, and Ritter MM et al., Influence of fiber, xylitol, and fructose in enteral formulas on glucose and lipid metabolism in normal subjects, *Clin Investig,* 71:290–293, 1993.

122. Chandalia M, Garg A, and Lutjohann D et al., Beneficial effects of high dietary fiber intake in patients with T2DM mellitus, *N Engl J Med,* 342:1392–1398, 2000.

123. Scheppach W, Burghardt W, and Bartram P et al., Addition of dietary fiber to liquid formula diets: The pros and cons, *JPEN,* 14:204–209, 1990.

124. Peters AL and Davidson MB, Addition of hydrolyzed guar to enteral feeding products in type-1 diabetic patients, *Diabetes Care,* 19:899–900, 1996.

125. Ordonez J, Garcia de Lorenzo A, and Lopez J et al., Enteral nutrition and fiber in intensive care, *Nutr Hosp,* 9:355–363, 1994.

126. Rushdi TA, Pichard C, and Khater YH, Control of diarrhea by fiber-enriched diet in ICU patients on enteral nutrition, A prospective randomized controlled trial, *Clin Nutr,* 23:1344–1352, 2004.

127. Spapen H, Diltoer M, and van Maleren C et al., Soluble fiber reduces the incidence of diarrhea in septic patients receiving total enteral nutrition, A prospective, double-blind, randomized, and controlled trial, *Clin Nutr,* 20:301–305, 2001.

128. Peters AL, Davidson MB, and Isaac RM, Lack of glucose elevation after simulated tube feeding with a low-carbohydrate, high-fat enteral formula in patients with T1DM, *Am J Med,* 87:178–182, 1989.

129. Peters AL and Davidson MB, Effects of various enteral feeding products on postprandial blood glucose response in patients with T1DM, *JPEN,* 16:69–74, 1992.

130. Printz H, Recke B, and Fehmann HC et al., No apparent benefit of liquid formula diet in NIDDM, *Exp Clin Endocrinol Diabetes,* 105:134–139, 1997.

131. Sanz-Paris A, Calvo L, and Guallard A et al., High-fat versus high-carbohydrate enteral formulae: Effect on blood glucose, C-peptide, and ketones in patients with T2DM treated with insulin or sulfonylurea, *Nutrition,* 14:840–845, 1998.

132. Leon-Sanz M, Garcia-Luna PP, and Planas M et al., Glycemic and lipid control in hospitalized type-2 diabetic patients, evaluation of two enteral nutrition formulas (low-carbohydrate-high-monounsaturated fat vs. high-carbohydrate) *JPEN,* 29:11–19, 2005.

133. Wright J, Total parenteral nutrition and enteral nutrition in diabetes, *Curr Opin Clin Nutr Metab Care,* 3:5–10, 2000.

134. Thomsen C, Storm H, and Holst JJ et al., Differential effects of saturated and monounsaturated fats on postprandial lipemia and glucagon-like peptide 1 responses in patients with T2DM, *Am J Clin Nutr,* 77:605–611, 2003.

135. Craig LD, Nicholson S, and Silverstone FA et al., Use of a reduced-carbohydrate, modified-fat enteral formula for improving metabolic control and clinical outcomes in long-term care residents with T2DM, Results of a pilot trial, *Nutrition,* 14:1998, 1998.

136. Mesejo A, Acosta JA, and Ortega C et al., Comparison of a high-protein disease-specific enteral formula with a high-protein enteral formula in hyperglycemic critically ill patients, 22:295–305, 2003.

137. Brinson RR and Kolts BE, Diarrhea associated with severe hypoalbuminemia: A comparison of a peptide-based chemically-defined diet and standard enteral alimentation, 16:130–136, 1988.

138. Heimburger DC, Geels VJ, and Bilbrey J et al., Effects of small-peptide and whole-protein enteral feedings on serum protein and diarrhea in critically ill patients, A randomized trial, *JPEN,* 21:162–167, 1997.

139. Cai B, Zhu Y, and Ma Y et al., Effect of supplementing a high-fat, low-carbohydrate enteral fomula in COPD patients, *Nutrition,* 19:229–232, 2003.

140. van den Berg, Bogaard JM, and Hop WC, High-fat, low-carbohydrate, enteral feeding in patients weaning from the ventilator, 20:470–475, 1994.

141. Ziegler TR, Benfell K, and Smith RJ et al., Safety and metabolic effects of L-glutamine administration in humans, *J Parent Enteral Nutr,* 14(4 Suppl):137S–146S, 1990.

142. Schwarz JM, Chiolero R, and Revelly JP et al., Effects of enteral carbohydrates on de novo lipogenesis in critically ill patients, *Am J Clin Nutr,* 72:940–945, 2000.

143. van den Berg B and Stam H, Metabolic and respiratory effects of enteral nutrition in patients during mechanical ventilation, *Intensive Care Med,* 14:206–211, 1988.

144. Dickerson RN, Boschert KJ, and Kudsk KA et al., Hypocaloric enteral tube feeding in critically ill obese patients, *Nutrition,* 18:241–246, 2002.

145. Cutts ME, Dowdy RP, and Ellersieck MR et al., Predicting energy needs in ventilator-dependent critically ill patients: Effect of adjusting weight for edema or adiposity, *Am J Clin Nutr,* 66:1250–1256, 1997.

146. Barak N, Wall-Alonso E, and Sitrin MD, Evaluation of stress factors and body weight adjustments currently used to estimate energy expenditure in hospitalized patients, *JPEN,* 26:231–238, 2002.

147. Liu KJ, Cho MJ, and Atten MJ et al., Hypocaloric parenteral nutrition support in elderly obese patients, *Am Surg,* 66:394–399, 2000.

148. Lonn E, Yusuf S, and Hoogwerf B et al., Effects of vitamin E on cardiovascular and microvascular outcomes in high-risk patients with diabetes, *Diabetes Care,* 25:1919–1927, 2002.

149. Beckman JA, Goldfine AB, and Gordon MB et al., Oral antioxidant therapy improves endothelial function in type-1 but not T2DM mellitus, *Am J Physiol Heart Circ Physiol,* 285:H2392–2398, 2003.

150. Darko D, Dornhorst A, and Kelly FJ et al., Lack of effect of oral vitamin C on blood pressure, oxidative stress, and endothelial function in type-II diabetes, *Clin Sci,* 103:339–344, 2002.

151. Heart Protection Study Collaborative Group, MRC/BHF Heart protection study of antioxidant vitamin supplementation in 20,536 high-risk individuals, A randomized placebo-controlled trial, *Lancet,* 360:23–33, 2002.

152. van Etten RW, de Koning EJP, and Verhaar MC et al., Impaired NO-dependent vasodilation in patients with type-II (non-insulin-dependent) diabetes mellitus is restored by acute administration of folate, *Diabetologia,* 45:1004–1010, 2002.

153. Wiernsperger NF, Oxidative stress: The special case of diabetes, *Biofactors,* 19:11–18, 2003.

154. Guoyao W and Meininger CJ, Arginine nutrition and cardiovascular function, *J Nutr,* 130:2626–2629, 2000.

155. Piatti P, Monti LD, and Valsechi G, Long-term oral L-arginine administration improves peripheral and hepatic insulin sensitivity in type-2 diabetic patients, *Diabetes Care,* 24(5):875–880, 2001.

156. American Diabetes Association, Nutrition principles and recommendations in diabetes, *Diabetes Care,* 27:S36–46, 2004.

157. Ariza-Andraca CR, Altamirano-Bustamante E, and Frati-Munari AC et al., Delayed insulin absorption due to subcutaneous edema, *Arch Invest Med (Mex),* 22:229–233, 1991.

158. Fernqvist E, Gunnarsson R, and Linde B, Influence of circulating epinephrine on absorption of subcutaneously injected insulin, *Diabetes,* 37:694–701, 1988.

159. Chase JG, Shaw GM, and Lin J et al., Adaptive bolus-based targeted glucose regulation of hyperglycaemia in critical care, *Med Eng Phys,* 27:1–11, 2005.

160. Kerr D, Hamilton P, and Cavan DA, Preventing glycaemic excursions in diabetic patients requiring percutaneous endoscopic gastrostomy (PEG) feeding after a stroke, *Diabet Med,* 19:1006–1008, 2002.

161. Putz D and Kabadi UM, Insulin glargine in continuous enteral tube feeding, *Diabetes Care,* 25:1889–1890, 2002.

162. Nierman D and Mechanick JI, Blood glucose control in the post-ICU respiratory care unit, *Chest,* 124:176S, 2003.

163. Bergman M, RaviKumar S, and Auerhahn C et al., Insulin pump therapy improves blood glucose control during hyperalimentation, *Arch Intern Med,* 144:2013–2015, 1984.

164. Moore FA and Weisbrodt NW, Gut dysfunction and intolerance to enteral nutrition in critically ill patients, *Nutr Clin Care,* 8:149–170, 2003.

165. O'Donovan D, Feinle-Bisset C, and Jones K et al., Idiopathic and diabetic gastroparesis, *Curr Treat Options Gastroenterol,* 6:299–309, 2003.

166. Devendra D, Millward BA, and Travis SPL, Diabetic gastroparesis improved by percutaneous endoscopic jejunostomy, *Diabetes Care,* 23:426, 2000.

167. Beaven K, Gastroparesis and jejunal feeding, *J Ren Nutr,* 9(4):202–205, 1999.

168. Hirsch IB, Insulin analogues, *N Engl J Med,* 352:174–183, 2005.

169. Krzywda EA, Andris D, and Whipple JK et al., Glucose response to abrupt initiation and discontinuation of total parenteral nutrition, *JPEN,* 17:64–67, 1993.

12 Nutritional Strategies for Wound Healing in Diabetic Patients

Neal G. Breit and Jeffrey I. Mechanick

CONTENTS

GENERAL DISCUSSION OF WOUND TYPES

Skin is the primary barrier to the environment and its breakdown exposes the body to infection and desiccation. Skin is composed of epithelial tissue with tightly packed sheets of cells. Membrane proteins forming "tight junctions" between cells confer integrity to this barrier function [1]. Disruption of this barrier occurs with wounds; any subsequent impairment in wound healing results in morbidity and increased mortality risk. Diabetic patients may have impaired wound healing due to a variety of different mechanisms, many of which are nutritionally responsive.

In young, healthy patients, acute superficial wounds are most common. Acute wounds are defined as a disruption of the integrity of the skin including the dermis and epidermis [2]. They generally involve subcutaneous punctures, scratches from environmental objects such as wood, plastics, stone, concrete, metal, electrical injuries, and chemical injuries [3]. Tears can also occur on extensor surfaces secondary to excessive stretching, pulling, or shear forces. These acute wounds, if kept clean, can usually heal with simple bandages and, occasionally, minor suture support.

Among lower extremity wounds, foot wounds are fairly common and the most serious. In a study by Reinherz et al. [4], 7% of all lower extremity injuries presented to an emergency department were plantar foot puncture wounds. Wounds that are poorly managed or fail to heal can lead to ulcer formation. Ulcers result when dermal breaks occur with subsequent erosion of subcutaneous tissue [5]. Shear forces are the major causes of tissue breakdown in the neuropathic foot [6]. Infections, repeated trauma mainly due to neuropathy or deformities, poor healing due to impaired vascular perfusion, and decreased nutritional states that inhibit tissue regeneration all contribute to ulcer formation [5,7]. When ulcers occur in lower extremities, especially the feet, the risk of bacterial contamination and infection increases. Wounds involving deeper tissues are at risk of deep-tissue infection and osteomyelitis. An infected diabetic foot ulcer can rapidly progress to gangrene and the need for amputation. Therefore, aggressive management of diabetic foot wounds is indicated, including early debridement, appropriate antibiotics, reduced or non-weight-bearing status, and vascular surgery [8]. Wounds that occur as the result of animal or insect bites and scratches may become infected with the respective bacterium carried by the animal or insect and typically require antibiotics.

In hospitalized patients, there are primarily two categories of wounds: (1) acute—those that are intentionally created, under sterile technique, for the purposes of achieving intravenous access or related to surgical procedures and (2) chronic—those from skin breakdown due to inadequate perfusion or prolonged pressure, yielding ischemic or pressure-induced ulcers [9]. Compared with the ambulatory patient, wounds in hospitalized or institutionalized patients are more affected by nutrition, mobility, and stress.

Burns are a form of wound that is due to thermal, chemical, radiation, or electrical injury. They generally involve a different pathophysiology in their evolution and resolution, and require different treatment modalities. Often, they are much more serious and involve a greater surface area. Treatment differences include more extensive supportive care with intravenous fluid, electrolytes, protein, and antibiotics. Additionally, thermal injury results in immunosuppression and poses a greater threat for infection—due to immunocompromise, inflammation, and fluid–electrolyte–nutrition losses—than with other types of injury [10].

Bite wounds are deep punctures, which most commonly occur from dogs and cats. They generally result in (1) crush injuries if they occur over areas such as hands, feet, or wrists where bony prominences lie shallow or (2) infections due to oral bacterial flora. Human bites can result in even more serious infections due to oral aerobic and anaerobic bacterial species [11]. Bite wound treatment and nutritional considerations should be essentially the same as with other wound types if delayed closure occurs.

Venous stasis wounds and subsequent ulcer development in the lower extremity are observed with venous obstruction and valvular incompetence, though this association is not clearly understood [12]. However, the term 'stasis' in the description of this type of ulcer may actually be a misnomer and the pathophysiology may not be due to stasis at all [13]. The clinical findings that usually precede lower extremity skin breakdown, wound formation, and ulcer development are leg heaviness, swelling, pain, dilated saphenous veins, skin stretching, and skin thinning [12].

Chronic wounds are those that do not heal at a normally expected pace. Sometimes burns and certain wounds with vascular compromise have been placed in this category, but essentially skin ulcers make up the vast majority of chronic wounds. There are numerous causes of chronic wounds (see Table 12.1) but most are rare [9]. In fact, nearly 70% of chronic wounds are comprised of the three most common types: diabetic ulcers, pressure ulcers, and venous ulcers [9].

TABLE 12.1
Classification of Chronic Wounds

Class	Associated Disease
Vascular occlusion	Venous insufficiency
	Atherosclerosis
	Antiphospholipid syndrome
	Cryofibrinogenemia/cryoglobulinemia
	Sickle cell disease
	Cholesterol emboli
Inflammation	Pyoderma gangrenosum
	Necrobiosis lipoidica diabeticorum
	Panniculitis
	Dysproteinemias
	Idiopathyic leukocytoclastic vasculitis
	Periarteritis nodosa
	Wegener's granulomatosis
	Erythema elevatum diutinum
Pressure necrosis	Decubitis ulcers
	Neuropathic ulcers
Physical agents	Radiation
	Heat
	Frostbite
	Chemicals
	Factitial
Infection	Bacterial
	Fungal
	Mycobacterial
	Tertiary syphilis
Tumors	Lymphomas
	Metastases
	Primary skin tumors

DIABETIC ULCERS

Diabetic ulcers usually occur on the feet and weight-bearing areas and can lead to lower extremity amputation [9]. They result from sensory neuropathy, large arterial vessel occlusion, and unrelieved pressure to a specific site. Many diabetic patients also have non-occlusive small-vessel disease with abnormal protein exchange and perivascular edema [9]. The failure to increase blood flow during periods of extended pressure contributes to ulcer development [14]. Thus, diabetic patients with advanced atherosclerosis and non-occlusive small-vessel disease are at particularly high risk for tissue hypoxia and the development of lower extremity ulcers.

Frequent causes of diabetic foot ulcers are trauma, neuropathy, deformity, high plantar pressures, and peripheral arterial disease [15]. Among 233 cases of diabetic foot ulcers preceded by minor trauma, 192 were associated with preceding callous formation [16]. When not discovered and managed early, diabetic foot ulcers can lead to leg amputation with associated high mortality and ulcer recurrence [17]. Approximately 15% of diabetic patients will develop foot ulceration at some time in their lives [18]. While it is known that the debridement of necrotic tissue is effective at promoting healing in diabetic foot ulcers, more effective methods have been elusive.

Pressure Ulcers

Pressure ulcers are the most common type of chronic wound [9]. They remain a problem in all healthcare settings and are a common occurrence in disabled, bed-bound, and critically ill hospitalized patients. As of 2001, the incidence of pressure ulcers ranged from 0.4–38% among hospitalized patients, from 2.2–23.9% among patients in long-term care facilities, and from 0–17% among patients dependent on long-term home care [19]. A 1996 study involving 2 hospitals and 2 nursing homes found that among 843 patients that did not have pressure ulcers when they were admitted, an overall average of 12.8% developed pressure ulcers [20]. In fact, 12.9% of activity-limited or bed-bound hospitalized patients developed a stage II or larger pressure ulcer during a median 9-day hospitalization [21]. However, in a more recent 2002 retrospective cohort study, the prevalence of pressure ulcers in patients over age 65 was 0.31–0.7% per year, with a dramatic increase in patients over age 80 [22]. Since these data reflect a healthier ambulatory population, they demonstrate the potential benefit of maintaining improved nutritional status in reducing the incidence of pressure ulcers [22]. Of note, modifiable risk factors for pressure ulcers included mobility limitations, incontinence, altered levels of consciousness, and malnutrition [23].

Pressure ulcers develop from localized areas of tissue breakdown in skin or underlying tissues caused by persistent pressure from sustained mechanical loads. This usually occurs over bony prominences but can occur elsewhere. The pressure obstructs capillary flow and can lead to tissue necrosis [24,25]. Pressure ulcers are particularly common in patients who are bedridden or restricted by wheelchair or prosthesis limitations [24]. The pathophysiology of pressure ulcer development is somewhat different from that of other ulcer types. With pressure ulcers, there is a complex interplay of external mechanical forces and internal physiology. The external forces that have been identified include pressure, immobility, friction, shearing forces, and moisture [26]. Some of the internal factors include concomitant disease, vascular impairment, immune dysfunction, poor tissue status, dehydration, and malnutrition.

Data supporting the nutritional needs of tissues affected during pressure ulcer development have been demonstrated in muscle. Muscle has higher continuous metabolic needs for oxygen and nutrients than other tissues. This is supported by several facts. Muscle is typically affected before skin with pressure ulcers [27]. Muscle also shows a higher incidence of necrosis in response to pressure opposed to the skin [24,27] and requires only half the time to develop ischemic damage when compared with skin in response to persistent pressure [24,28]. During high skin interface pressure loading, more vessels are obliterated in skin and subcutaneous tissues than muscle, but muscle sustains significantly greater damage [24,29].

Chronic disease and intercurrent infection can impair normal adaptive functions including immune function, neural function, and local microcirculatory endothelial function [30]. During illness, growth factors and metabolic substrates for tissue regeneration are diverted to support critical systems. In hospitalized patients with critical illness, concurrent diseases including diabetes, peripheral and cerebrovascular disease, and hypotension in elderly patients have been implicated in impaired wound healing [30]. Sepsis has been associated with microvascular dysfunction and decreased skin blood flow [25,30,31]. When microcirculation is disrupted by neural and endothelial dysfunction, the rate of blood, oxygen, and nutrient delivery may be impaired and result in ischemic organ damage, pressure sore development, and impaired wound healing [25,30].

The large retrospective cohort National Pressure Ulcer Long-Term Care Study (NPULS) [32,33] focused on the impact of patient and caregiver factors on pressure ulcer development in skilled nursing facilities. Risk factors for ulcer development included a body mass index (BMI) < 22 kg/M^2, weight loss of at least 5%, poor oral nutritional intake, low serum albumin (less than 2.8 g/dL in patients with existing pressure ulcers), cognitive impairment, and immobility [32]. In addition, residents with new pressure ulcers had the highest percentage of weight loss and those with existing ulcers had the lowest BMI [32]. NPULS also demonstrated an association of enteral nutrition for greater than 21 days with a decreased likelihood of pressure ulcer progression from stages I to IV

[33]. In patients who developed a stage II or greater pressure ulcer in 14 days, low albumin levels were found to be an important risk factor [33]. The association of pressure ulcers and low protein and calorie intake in nursing home patients [34] or overall nutritional status in immobilized hospitalized patients [35] has been confirmed.

VENOUS ULCERS

Venous hypertension—the failure of ambulatory venous pressure to fall to normal limits—is known to be associated with venous ulcers [9]. Venous ulcers constitute nearly 70% of all leg ulcers [9]. Perivascular fibrin accumulation with venous hypertension creates perivascular fibrin cuffs, leading to impaired oxygen delivery, nutrient delivery, and white blood cell passage [9,36]. Extravasated macromolecules in the perivascular interstitium of the dermis can bind and sequester necessary growth factors and matrix collagen proteins, thus impairing wound healing [37,38].

PRINCIPLES OF WOUND FORMATION AND HEALING

There are a variety of cellular mechanisms that contribute to injury and ulcer development. Tissue geometry and composition are inhomogeneous, so deep tissue pressures may not represent surface pressures [24]. However external loading conditions are transmitted across tissue planes and can lead to tissue breakdown via cellular deformation, cytoskeleton rearrangements, and cell volume changes [24,39–41]. Ischemia, impaired lymphatic drainage, interstitial flow [42,43], reperfusion injury [44,45], and sustained cellular deformation [46] also contribute to tissue damage and ulcer development.

In chronic wounds, persistent neutrophilic infiltration has been found as a consistent feature [47]. Proteolysis by proteases, including neutrophil-derived matrix metalloproteinase (MMP)-8 and elastase, are elevated in chronic ulcers [48]. In fact, chronic wound granulation tissue contains greater than 95% neutrophilic content [48]. Furthermore, chemotactic migration of neutrophils to the wound site increases reactive oxygen species (ROS) production, yielding extensive matrix destruction.

STAGES OF WOUND HEALING

The mammalian response to injury begins with deep tissue repair followed by re-epithelialization [49]. An early event and primary component of tissue repair is collagen synthesis and incorporation [49]. Wound healing can last up to 2 years depending on nutritional factors, metabolic states, local oxygen tension, and perfusion [50]. Even though the healing process occurs along a continuous spectrum [51] it can be classified into four stages: (1) coagulation and inflammation; (2) re-epithelialization; (3) granulation (also referred to as the "proliferative" phase); and (4) remodeling and maturation. Despite neutrophilic predominance, the late stages of chronic wounds are characterized by a shift from neutrophil to lymphoid infiltrates, which yield acute inflammatory exudates, re-epithelialization of ruptured areas, organization into granulation tissue, and fibrous repair. These events occur concomitantly in chronic wounds, rather than sequentially as in acute processes, and may be prolonged by immunocompromise, infection, malnutrition, foreign bodies, or retained necrotic tissue [52]. Digital photographs of the various stages of wound healing are given in Figure 12.1 to Figure 12.7.

Acute injury is immediately followed by coagulation, hemeostasis, and then inflammation. Mononuclear cell migration and conversion into macrophages begin on the first day and reach a peak by the fifth day [53,54]. Mast cell degranulation increases capillary permeability and chemotactic factors recruit neutrophils for bacterial lysis [54]. Wound cleansing begins within 3–12 hours after injury by monocyte-macrophage bacterial phagocytosis and neutrophilic fibrinolysis [54–56]. This process resolves within 3 days and clinically appears as warmth, swelling, erythema, and edema.

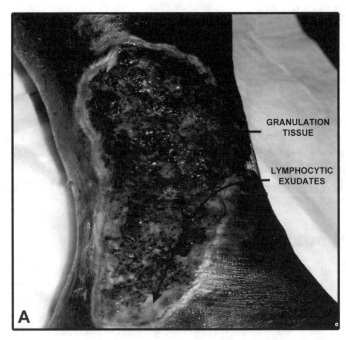

FIGURE 12.1 Panel A—Venous stasis wounds are due to venous obstruction. This results from WBC activation, venule damage, macromolecule leakage, perivascular fibrin cuffs, impairment of oxygen and nutrient delivery, and trapping of growth factors. Digital photograph provided by Dr. Harold Brem.

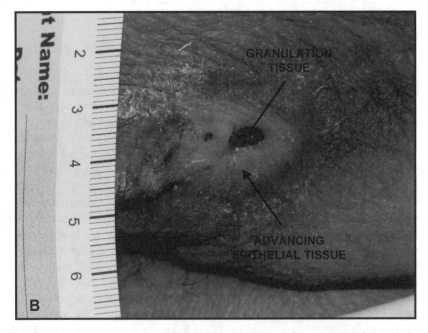

FIGURE 12.2 Panel B—Pressure ulcer healing is demonstrated by the presence of granulation tissue and advancing epithelial tissue. Digital photograph provided by Dr. Harold Brem.

February 10, 2006

Dear Customer:

Thank you for your purchase of *Nutritional Strategies for the Diabetic & Prediabetic Patient* by Jeffrey I. Mechanick and Elise M. Brett.

The color figures for Chapter 12 were left out at time of printing and an incorrect Figure 13.2 was included. The correct figures are on the following pages.

Best regards,
Taylor & Francis

ISBN 0-8247-2587-5/DK2975

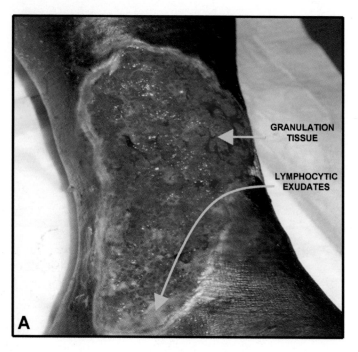

FIGURE 12.1 Panel A—Venous stasis wounds are due to venous obstruction. This results from WBC activation, venule damage, macromolecule leakage, perivascular fibrin cuffs, impairment of oxygen and nutrient delivery, and trapping of growth factors. Digital photograph provided by Dr. Harold Brem.

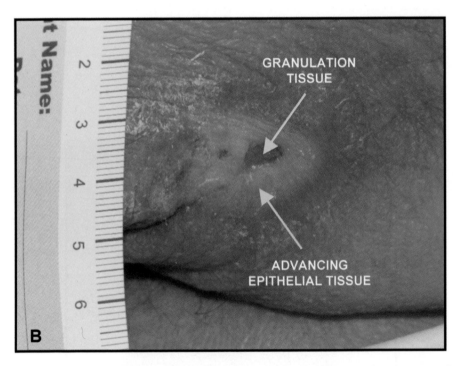

FIGURE 12.2 Panel B—Pressure ulcer healing is demonstrated by the presence of granulation tissue and advancing epithelial tissue. Digital photograph provided by Dr. Harold Brem.

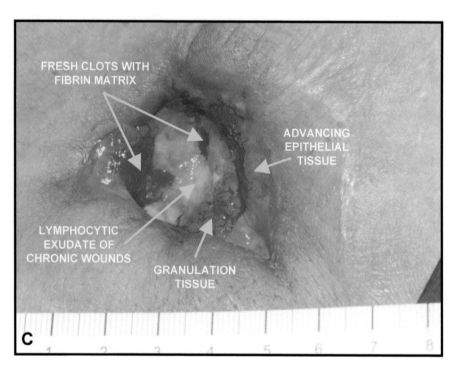

FIGURE 12.3 Panel C—Stage 1 (coagulation and inflammation) occurs at 1–5 days and is characterized by mast cell degranulation and polymorphonuclear cell attraction. Debris is removed. Monocytes arrive, become macrophages, and secrete growth factors (TGF-α, TGF-β1, FGF, VEGF, PDGF-BB), which attract fibroblasts and vascular endothelial cells for angiogenesis. TGF and IGF attract epidermal cells and stimulate fibroblasts for matrix formation. Digital photograph provided by Dr. Harold Brem.

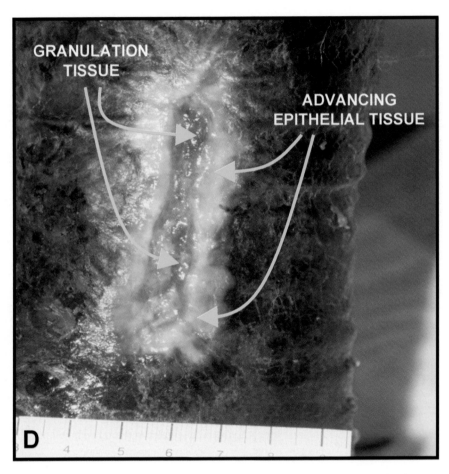

FIGURE 12.4 Panel D—Stage 2 (re-epithelialization and neovascularization) occurs at 5 days and is characterized by epidermal cell migration into the wound. Debris is removed and the epithelial cell layer is regenerated. MMP1,2,3,13, tPA and urokinase-type plasminogen activator (uPA) are secreted to allow movement between the clot and newly formed granulation tissue and to lay down basement membrane. Epithelial cell phagocytosis is followed by migration and ingrowth forming a thin barrier. Digital photograph provided by Dr. Harold Brem.

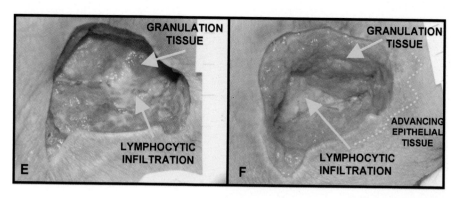

FIGURE 12.5 Panels E and F—Stage 3 (granulation and proliferation) occurs at 4–10 days and is characterized by mesenchymal cell differentiation into fibroblasts, macrophage cleansing, endothelial cell migration, angiogenesis, and then fibroblast apoptosis. A recently debrided wound is seen in panel E and the same wound 1 week later in panel F. Digital photograph provided by Dr. Harold Brem.

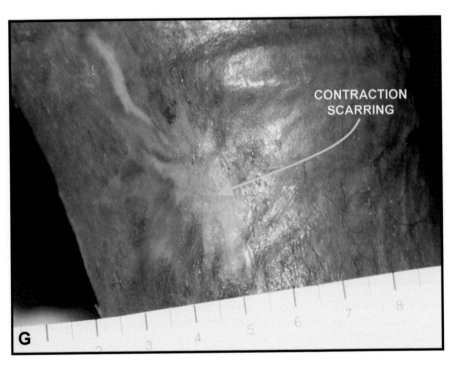

FIGURE 12.6 Panel G—Stage 4 (remodeling, maturation, and contraction) occurs at 1–2 years and is characterized by matrix reorganization, scarring, and ultimately complete healing conferring 70% of the original strength. Digital photograph provided by Dr. Harold Brem.

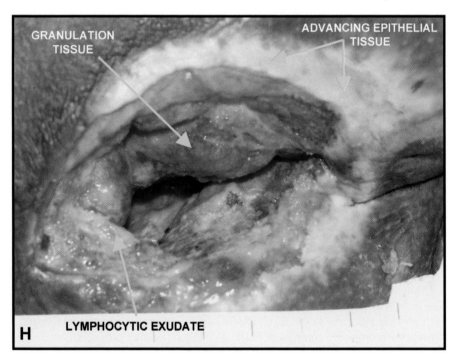

FIGURE 12.7 Panel H—Chronic wound in a diabetic patient demonstrating disordered healing: persistent neutrophilic inflammation, patchy continuous destruction, lymphcytic exudates, re-epithelialization, and granulation. Digital photograph provided by Dr. Harold Brem.

See page 226.

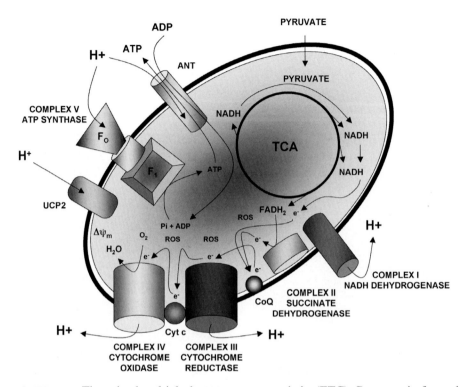

FIGURE 13.2 The mitochondrial electron transport chain (ETC). Pyruvate is formed by glycolysis and enters the tricarboxylic acid (TCA) cycle forming nicotinamide adenine dinucleotide, reduced form (NADH) and flavin adenine dinucleotide (FADH$_2$), which provide electrons to the ETC. Electrons (e$^-$) flowing along the ETC result in extrusion of protons by complexes I, III, and IV, as well as production of reactive oxygen species (ROS). This creates an electrochemical gradient across the IM ($\Delta\psi_m$). As protons diffuse back into the matrix through ATP synthase, ADP condenses with inorganic phosphate to form a high-energy bond: ATP. ATP is transported into the cytosol in exchange for ADP by the adenine nucleotide translocator (ANT). Leakage of protons through UCP2 lowers $\Delta\psi_m$ and ATP formation. Abbreviations: CoQ—coenzyme Q10; Cyt c—cytochrome-c; UCP2—uncoupling protein 2.

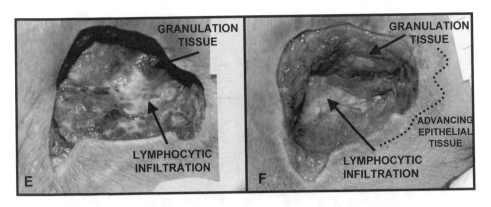

;URE 12.5 Panels E and F—Stage 3 (granulation and proliferation) occurs at 4–10 days and is characterized mesenchymal cell differentiation into fibroblasts, macrophage cleansing, endothelial cell migration, angio-esis, and then fibroblast apoptosis. A recently debrided wound is seen in panel E and the same wound 1 week r in panel F. Digital photograph provided by Dr. Harold Brem.

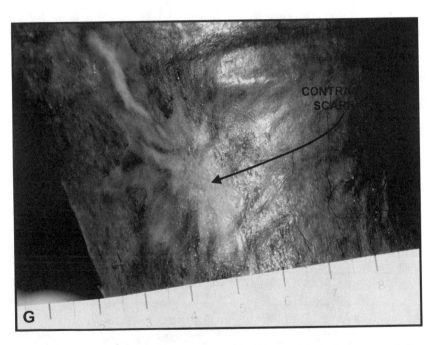

;URE 12.6 Panel G—Stage 4 (remodeling, maturation, and contraction) occurs at 1–2 years and is aracterized by matrix reorganization, scarring, and ultimately complete healing conferring 70% of the original ength. Digital photograph provided by Dr. Harold Brem.

Re-epithelialization begins within hours after the injury and consists of dissolution of desmo-mes and epithelial migration [56]. Epidermal cell integrin receptor expression coordinates extra-llular matrix fibronectin-, vitronectin-, type-1 collagen-, and fibrin-mediated eschar removal from ible regenerative tissue [56–59]. Degradation of matrix material by epidermal cell collagenase and asmin facilitates epidermal cell migration underneath the fibrin eschar and between the collagenous

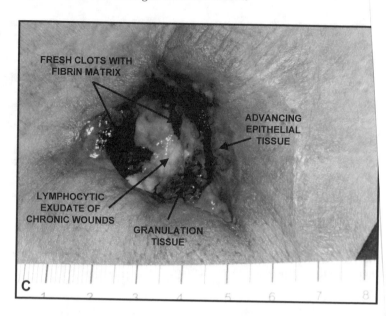

FIGURE 12.3 Panel C—Stage 1 (coagulation and inflammation) occurs at 1–5 days and is ch
mast cell degranulation and polymorphonuclear cell attraction. Debris is removed. Monocytes
macrophages, and secrete growth factors (TGF-α, TGF-β1, FGF, VEGF, PDGF-BB), which att
and vascular endothelial cells for angiogenesis. TGF and IGF attract epidermal cells and stimul
for matrix formation. Digital photograph provided by Dr. Harold Brem.

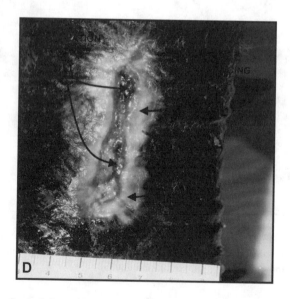

FIGURE 12.4 Panel D—Stage 2 (re-epithelialization and neovascularization) occurs at 5 days and
acterized by epidermal cell migration into the wound. Debris is removed and the epithelial cell
regenerated. MMP1,2,3,13, tPA and urokinase-type plasminogen activator (uPA) are secreted to allo
ment between the clot and newly formed granulation tissue and to lay down basement membrane. E
cell phagocytosis is followed by migration and ingrowth forming a thin barrier. Digital photograph
by Dr. Harold Brem.

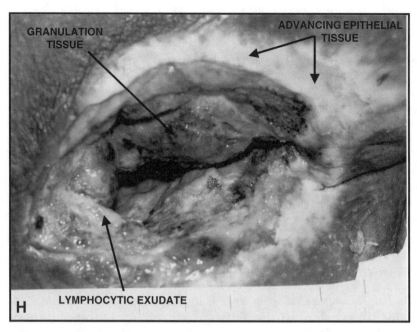

FIGURE 12.7 Panel H—Chronic wound in a diabetic patient demonstrating disordered healing: persistent neutrophilic inflammation, patchy continuous destruction, lymphcytic exudates, re-epithelialization, and granulation. Digital photograph provided by Dr. Harold Brem.

dermis [60]. Furthermore, epidermal cell-derived tissue-type plasminogen activator (tPA) generates plasmin and activates matrix metalloproteinase 1 (interstitial collagenase) (MMP-1) for collagen and matrix protein degradation [61,62]. One to two days after the initial injury, marginal epidermal cells proliferate behind the migrating epidermal cells under the influence of epidermal growth factor (EGF), transforming growth factor-α (TGF-α), and keratinocyte growth factor (KGF) [56,63–65]. A basement membrane is then reconstructed in a "zipper-like" fashion with epidermal cells attaching and reverting to their normal phenotype [56,66]. This process is repeated until the wound is completely covered by this protective barrier. However, while this layer of protection prevents desiccation, bacterial colonization, and contamination by foreign material, it remains thin, has little strength, and is easily disrupted.

The granulation stage (days 1–10 after injury) [67] is comprised of fibroplasia, angiogenesis, and neovascularization leading to the regeneration of the underlying tissues that ultimately provide structural and vascular support. Macrophages stimulate fibroplasia and angiogenesis via release of platelet-derived growth factor (PDGF), transforming growth factor β-1 (TGFβ-1), acidic fibroblast growth factor (AFGF), and basic FGF (BFGF) [56,68–73]. Proteolytic enzymes from migrated fibroblasts such as tPA, plasminogen, collagenases, gelatinase A, and stromolysin are required to clear a path for cellular migration to the cross-linked fibrin blood clot [56,62,74]. Angiogenesis and neovascularization rely on macrophage- and epidermal cell-derived vascular endothelial-cell growth factor (VEGF) [75,76]. Other recently identified important angiogenesis growth factors include angiogenin, angiotropin, angiopoietin 1, and thrombospondin, which stimulate macrophages and endothelial cells to release more VEGF and BFGF [71–73]. After migrating into the wound in response to chemotactic agents, a path is cleared by proteolysis, and fibroblasts begin synthesizing a newly formed provisional extracellular matrix [66,77]. This scaffolding perpetuates cell migration [56,78]. The provisional matrix is composed of fibrin, fibronectin, and hyaluronic acid [78,79]. The appearance of fibroblast integrin receptors that bind fibrin and fibronectin may be the rate-limiting step in the induction of granulation tissue [80,81]. Fibroblasts are responsible for synthesis, deposition, and remodeling the extracellular matrix and ultimately replacing the provisional matrix with a final collagenous matrix [56,77]. Then they stop producing collagen and undergo apoptosis, leaving an acellular scar [56,82]. Angiogenesis is completed when adequate vasculature is available to provide sufficient oxygen and nutrients to the newly formed granulation tissue [56].

During the maturation stage, the wound is strengthened via contraction, extracellular-matrix reorganization, and collagen cross-linking [56]. Collagen is made of glycine, proline, 4-hydroxyproline, and 5-hydroxylysine [83]. Procollagen is strengthened and assembled into collagen by cross-linking strands in staggered arrays. This process is catalyzed by ascorbic acid, copper, and pyridoxal phosphate [83]. Wounds gain 20% of their final strength at 3 weeks and 80% by 6 weeks [84], but never regain their original uninjured strength [85]. Wound scars are only about 70% as strong as normal skin [85] and they do not have the appearance of normal skin until about 6 months to 2 years [84].

WOUND HEALING IN DIABETIC PATIENTS

Chronic wounds represent a significant morbidity for the diabetic patient and result from disruption of the normal sequence of wound healing events described above. This is often associated with a chronic inflammatory state produced by an amplification loop between advanced glycation end products (AGE), extracellular newly identified receptor for advanced glycation end products binding protein (EN-RAGE), pro-inflammation cytokines, and proteases [53,85]. Peppa and Brem [86] found that in diabetic db/db (+/+) and db/db (+/–) mice, a low-AGE diet led to more rapid wound closure, lower skin AGE deposits, increased epithelialization, increased angiogenesis, increased inflammation, increased granulation tissue deposition, enhanced collagen organization, and improved wound contraction. Also, in diabetes, capillary permeability to macromolecules in normal tissue is reduced and can impair wound healing [87].

There are various strategies to address deranged wound healing in diabetic patients besides nutritional interventions. Standard treatment approaches include occlusive dressings that provide a clean moist environment, pressure amelioration and, where appropriate, antibiotics and surgery [88]. Sharp debridement of the wound to its bleeding margins interrupts the pathological state of chronic inflammation [89]. Recombinant human platelet-derived growth factor-BB (PDGF-BB) promotes an exaggerated, beneficial inflammatory response. This maneuver elicits a ~15% improvement in the rate of fully healed diabetic ulcers and may be due to stimulation of fibronectin and integrin receptors on wound fibroblasts [90–92]. Non-healing diabetic wounds may also respond to proteases and protease inhibitors [53,93,94], PDGF [53] or activated fibroblasts [81].

SPECIFIC NUTRITIONAL INTERVENTIONS FOR WOUND HEALING IN DIABETIC PATIENTS

Nutritional therapies to support wound healing in diabetics must target specific nutritional deficiencies critical for wound healing (see Table 12.2) and maintain adequate energy and nitrogen balance without worsening glycemic control. The following discussion includes nutrients and dietary supplements that are well-grounded in theory and experimental evidence to furnish an objective recommendation grade. Clearly, there are many other agents that have been touted as beneficial dietary substances but are not fully presented here. They may, at first glance, have indistinguishable theoretical and evidentiary attributes but, upon closer inspection of extant data, have no reasonable utility in the management of wounds in diabetic patients. Examples of these omitted substances include bromelain (an extract from the stem of the pineapple plant with proteinase and immune-modulating activity) and glucosamine (a substrate for connective tissue synthesis).

TABLE 12.2
Wound Healing Stages Targeted by Various Nutrients or Dietary Supplements

Stage	Nutrient/Dietary Supplement
1—Inflammation	Protein
	Vitamin A
	Vitamin C
2—Re-epithelialization	Protein
	Vitamin A
	Vitamin E
	Zinc
3—Proliferation	Aloe vera
	Calendula succus
	Centella asiatica
	Glucosamine
	Vitamin A
	Vitamin C
	Zinc
4—Remodeling	Protein

NITROGEN

Whole Protein

In theory, nutrition support for wound healing should contain sufficient energy and nitrogen so that there is sufficient substrate for protein synthesis to support tissue regeneration and wound healing. During the physiological adaption to stress, nitrogen requirements are also increased to support muscle catabolism, inflammation, exudative protein losses, and tissue repair [95,96]. Protein depletion delays wound healing by prolonging the inflammatory phase and inhibiting fibroplasia, collagen synthesis, proteoglycan synthesis, angiogenesis, and wound maturation [95]. In nonstressed malnourished patients with pressure ulcers, nutrition support consists of energy, 25–35 kcal/kg/day, and protein > 1.0-1.2 g/kg/day. With stress, protein needs may increase from 1.5 to over 2.1 g/kg/day [97,98].

There are no published clinical trials that specifically address intervention with dietary protein on wound healing in diabetic patients. Thus, conclusions must be extrapolated from studies involving diabetic and nondiabetic patients. A randomized, double-blind, placebo-controlled trial of 103 hip fracture patients, with or without T2DM, showed that daily supplementation with 40 g protein, 500 kcal, 6 mg L-arginine, 20 mg zinc, 500 mg vitamin C, 200 mg vitamin E, and 4 mg carotenoids did not prevent but did delay the onset and progression of pressure ulcers [99]. In a large randomized, controlled, multi-center trial of 672 critically ill patients, with or without diabetes, treatment with dietary supplements containing 30% protein for 15 days reduced the risk of pressure ulcer incidence [100]. In this study, there were significant increases in total kcal/day (1081 vs. 957) and total protein per day (45.9 vs. 38.3) in the treatment group, compared with the control group. In malnourished nursing home patients, with or without diabetes, dietary supplements containing 24% vs. 14% protein have also been associated with greater improvements in pressure ulcer healing [101]. Here, total pressure ulcer area negatively correlated with total caloric intake ($r = -0.41$; $p < 0.03$) and total protein intake ($r = -0.50$; $p < 0.05$) per kg body weight. Nevertheless, meta-analyses have not shown benefit of protein supplementation on pressure ulcer healing [102,103]. Excessive dietary protein can exacerbate diabetic nephropathy or simply increase obligate renal free water excretion and induce hypertonic dehydration (hypernatremia). Routine evaluation and monitoring of renal status in diabetic patients should limit any toxicity from deliberate protein loading to support wound healing [104]. In summary, protein supplementation data vary in quality, result from experimental power and design limitations, and are not specific for diabetic patients (evidence level 3) [105]. Nevertheless, protein supplementation for wound healing in diabetic patients is relatively safe (grade C).

Arginine

Arginine is a conditionally essential amino acid, regenerated in the urea cycle from citrulline and aspartate. Arginine is necessary for collagen deposition, wound healing, immune function, and nitric oxide (NO) generation [95,106]. L-arginine supplementation in diabetic rats improved wound healing and breaking strength via hydroxyproline synthesis [107] and NO-mediated events [108], which are disturbed in diabetic wounds. Arginine metabolism in diabetic wounds, at epithelial sites along the margins, is determined by two competing pathways: (1) arginase-1 and -2 gene expression are increased resulting in higher polyamine and collagen concentrations and (2) inducible nitric oxide synthase (iNOS) concentrations increases resulting in higher NO concentrations [109]. In streptozotocin-induced diabetic rats with burn wounds, L-arginine administration was associated with an enhanced inflammatory response, necrotic tissue shedding, epithelial cell advancement, hydroxyproline content, TGF-β concentrations, and reduced local glucose levels [110]. Moreover, angiogenesis was improved with L-arginine via increased synthesis of VEGF, NO, and TGF-β [111]. In humans, arginine enhances immune function and promotes wound healing. In a prospective randomized, double-blind, controlled study, arginine supplementation (17 g/day) for 2 weeks in 30 patients was associated with increased hydroxyproline and protein accumulation at the wound site, increased IGF-1 levels, and improved lymphocyte responses (evidence level 3) [95,112]. Arginine contains three nitrogen molecules and overdosage can therefore lead to hyperammonemia. Otherwise, it is a relatively safe dietary supplement (grade C).

Glutamine

Glutamine is a conditionally essential amino acid that is a substrate for gluconeogenesis, a gut-specific fuel and an immune system modulator. During the stress response, glutamine flux subserves various adaptive mechanisms that confer a survival advantage. Inflammatory cells within a wound use glutamine as an energy source while fibroblasts use it for protein synthesis, nucleic acid synthesis, and tissue repair [95]. In a small, randomized, controlled study of 35 elderly subjects, ingestion of a nutritional supplement containing 14 g/day glutamine, 14 g/day arginine, and 3 g/day β-hydroxy-β-methylbutyrate (a metabolite of leucine) was associated with increased collagen deposition [113]. As with arginine, excessive glutamine use is associated with hyperammonemia. There are no clinical data supporting the specific use of glutamine for wound healing in diabetic patients (evidence level 4), though there are theoretical advantages derived from preclinical data and it is relatively safe (grade C).

VITAMINS

Diabetic patients have significant oxidant stress [114–117] resulting in low plasma and erythrocyte zinc levels [114,118,119], low plasma thymulin activity [114,120], and immune dysfunction [114,120]. Impaired wound healing can result from inadequate natural antioxidant defenses. Although in theory the routine supplementation of antioxidants seems beneficial, their use in the management of wound healing in diabetic patients should be confined to those agents that are safe and efficacious.

Vitamin A

Vitamin A is known to be necessary for maintenance of the epidermis, synthesis of glycoproteins, and proteoglycans [121]. Vitamin A is required for epithelial and bone tissue growth, cellular differentiation, and immune function [95], and its deficiency delays re-epithelialization and collagen synthesis, decreases collagen stability, and increases susceptibility to wound infection [122,123]. In streptozotocin-induced diabetic rats, large quantities of vitamin A (150,000 units/kg food/day) for 7 days improved the strength and hydroxyproline content of newly healed wounds independent of glycemic status [124]. In other animal studies, increased wound tensile strength due to greater collagen cross-linkage, resulted in quicker wound healing [95]. Vitamin A levels were found to be lower in patients with chronic leg ulcers in one small observational study [121]. In addition, vitamin A, 25,000 IU/day, before and after elective surgery, reduced complications and improved wound healing [95]. There are no data demonstrating specific benefit of vitamin A therapy on wounds in diabetic patients (evidence level 4).

Vitamin A also reverses the inhibitory effects of glucocorticoids (GC) on wound healing and antagonizes many of the effects of cortisone on wound contraction and infection in clinical studies [125–128]. This beneficial effect involves replenishing TGF-β and IGF-1 levels which are depleted with GC use [129,130]. Glucocorticoids are also incorporated into a repressosome complex which inhibits keratin K6 and K16 gene expression thereby "stopping" keratinocyte proliferation/migration [131]. Vitamin A serves as a wound healing modulator through its incorporation into both repressosomes and EGF-enhanceosomes, the latter stimulating keratin K6 and K16 gene expression [131]. The important point is that experimental pretreatment with vitamin A prevents the *in vitro* inhibitory effects of the GC repressosome on wound healing [131].

Vitamin A toxicity is infrequent but can occur with doses of 50,000–100,000 IU over periods of weeks to years [95]. Excessive vitamin A is associated with hepatic dysfunction, bone hyperresorption, and hypercalcemia [132]. In patients with renal insufficiency and increased levels of retinol-binding protein, toxicity may be more likely. In contrast, low levels of retinol-binding protein occur with severe malnutrition, resulting in low levels of serum vitamin A. This could be misinterpreted as representing a vitamin A deficiency state. Overall, vitamin A therapy poses a potential risk with overdosing and its routine use in the management of diabetic wounds is unproven and not recommended (grade D). On the contrary, vitamin A therapy in steroid-induced nonhealing wounds has proven benefit (grade C).

Vitamin C

Vitamin C is water-soluble and acts as a cofactor in hydroxylation reactions, which are critical for collagen, proteoglycan, and intracellular matrix synthesis in connective tissues [95,133]. Vitamin C deficiency leads to decreased adhesion of endothelial cells, alterations in the extracellular matrix resulting in decreased fibrous tissue strength, and fragile granulation tissue [95,134]. In collagen, vitamin C is essential for efficient hydroxylation of collagen proline and lysine residues that allow stable triple-helix structures [95]. Humans lack the ability to store vitamin C; hence, subclinical deficiencies are suspected in patients who are malnourished or stressed [95].

Among the many effects of vitamin C are its antioxidant properties [95]. Studies have identified lower levels of vitamin C, with elevation in markers of free radical damage, in the tissues of healing wounds as compared with normal tissue [95]. In an observational study of 21 elderly hospitalized patients admitted with femoral neck fracture, the only measured nutritional marker that distinguished those who developed pressure ulcers from those that did not was the leukocyte vitamin C concentration [135].

Vitamin C improves markers of immune function in humans and therefore can potentially reduce chronic infectious complications in wounds [95]. In humans, vitamin C, 2–3 g/day for several weeks, increased neutrophilic chemotactic sensitivity and improved lymphocyte transformation [95,136]. Other studies observed similarly increased immune function with only 1 g/day [95]. In fact, in patients with hip fracture and pressure ulcers, treatment with as little as 600 mg/day of vitamin C, along with arginine, zinc, vitamin E, and protein supplementation, was associated with improved wound healing [99]. There were no significant adverse events observed at these doses [95]. These clinical data are weak (evidence level 3) and do not specifically address the role of vitamin C on wound healing in diabetic patients. Vitamin C toxicities, including gastrointestinal distress and hyperoxaluria, are rare and associated with high doses (> 3–4 g/day) [95]. Patients with diabetes and impaired renal function (serum creatinine > 2 mg/dL) are cautioned against using vitamin C in doses > 200 mg/day, which correspond to amounts that are associated with maximal plasma and lymphocyte levels [137]. Overall, vitamin C use is rational and safe but as yet unproven as a specific measure to manage wounds in diabetic patients (grade C).

Vitamin E

Vitamin E is a lipid-soluble vitamin comprised of eight compounds known as tocopherols and tocotrienols. The tocopherols are the physiologically active forms and are designated as α, β, γ, or δ based on the location of a methyl group [133]. α-tocopherol is the most common form and is found in high abundance in dietary sources [133]. Each of these compounds has antioxidant properties but they differ in structure, dietary source, and potency [138].

The primary role of vitamin E is free radical scavenging but it also enhances cell mediated immunity, especially in elderly patients [133,139]. Vitamin E deficiency is rare and is generally observed with diseases associated with fat malabsorption, such as cystic fibrosis, cholestatic liver disease, short bowel syndrome, and abetalipoproteinemia [133]. Vitamin E deficiency states yield the clinical symptoms of muscle weakness, ataxia, and hemolysis [133]. Doses in the range of 200–800 mg daily are typically without adverse effects [133].

Vitamin E levels are diminished in the wounds in aged rats that had delayed closure [140]. In a murine model of diabetes, raxofelast (a vitamin E analogue) reduced malondialdehyde and myeloperoxidase activity, improved wound angiogenesis, epithelialization, synthesis, and maturation of extracellular matrix, and increased wound breaking strength and collagen content [141,142]. In addition, α-tocopherol also reduced malondialdehyde levels while increasing glutathione peroxidase activity and accelerating wound closure in diabetic rats [138]. When given to prevent scar formation, vitamin E is thought to act by preventing lipid peroxidation resulting in more stable membranes [95]. Vitamin E has been shown to enhance wound healing in irradiated rat skin [121]. However, similar to glucocorticoids, vitamin E can stabilize lysosomal membranes, inhibit inflammatory responses, impair collagen synthesis, and decrease tendon repair [95,96]. In various animal models, vitamin E impairs wound healing [95,143,144].

In humans, parenteral vitamin E treatment is associated with decreased lipid peroxidation and improved membrane stability, leading to quicker healing of purulent soft tissue wounds (evidence level 3) [145]. One potential mechanism for this effect in diabetic patients might be the reduction of neutral endopeptidase (NEP; a membrane-bound metallopeptidase) by vitamin E [146,147]. *In vitro* studies demonstrate that NEP activation by hyperglycemia and hyperlipidemia blunts the early, beneficial, inflammatory response to injury [146,147]. Potential adverse effects of vitamin E are vitamin K deficiency and, with large doses (> 200 IU/day), necrotizing enterocolitis [148]. In light of the potential for impaired wound healing and the absence of conclusive beneficial effects, the routine use of vitamin E for wound healing in diabetic patients is not recommended (grade D).

MINERALS AND TRACE ELEMENTS

Boron

Boron is an essential ultratrace mineral in humans with effects on bone metabolism and joint disorders [149,150]. Using cell-free systems of transcription and translation, boron was found to induce expression of VEGF and TGF-β genes and translation of their functional mRNAs [151]. Boron was also found to increase TNF-α-mediated phosphorylation activity [152], keratinocyte migration [153], and gene expression of the gelatinases MMP-2 and -9 involved in granulation tissue remodeling *in vitro* [152]. In animals, boron affects proteoglycan, collagen, and protein synthesis *in vitro*, mimics the effects of TNF-α and induces proteoglycan release, and augments protein phosphorylation and endoprotease activity [154]. These effects are more pronounced with hyperglycemia, leading to the theory that boron therapy should improve wound healing in diabetic patients [154]. Boron toxicity (associated with ingestion > 500 mg/day) is manifested by nausea, diarrhea, skin rashes, and fatigue. Overall, there are theoretical beneficial effects of boron on wound healing but no clinical data on wound healing in diabetics (evidence level 4) along with a potential for adverse effects (grade D).

Calcium

Wound healing is initiated by a local influx of calcium into cells [155,156] and calcium treatment improves fibroblast migration [156], keratinocyte proliferation, and keratinocyte differentiation [157]. In the early stage of wound repair, calcium participates in the coagulation cascade and, in later stages, is a required element in regeneration [157]. Nevertheless, there are no clinical data to suggest a potential therapeutic advantage of routine calcium dosing in diabetic patients to promote wound healing (evidence level 4, grade D).

Copper

Copper nutriture is related to ultimate scar strength and resistance. In animals, copper is released early in the tissue healing process with a measurable rise in serum levels [158]. Copper neutralizes tolmetin (a nonselective cyclooxygenase-2 inhibitor)-induced impairments on the tensile strength of newly healed wounds [259]. In keratinocyte monolayer cultures, copper gluconate upregulates integrin-α_2, -α_6, and -β_1 gene expression in differentiated keratinocytes during the final re-epithelialization phase of wound healing [160]. Copper also has a role in VEGF-mediated angiogenesis, extracellular matrix remodeling, and dermal wound contracture and closure [161]. Potential adverse effects of copper supplementation include hemolytic anemia, jaundice, nausea, vomiting, abdominal pain, headache, weakness, diarrhea, hepatopathy, and hemochromatosis. There are no clinical data on the routine use of copper supplementation for wound healing in diabetic patients (evidence level 4, grade D).

Magnesium

Based on animal studies, magnesium plays an important role in the activation of integrin- and E-cadherin mediated cell migration, oxidative stress, and collagen synthesis during wound healing [162,163]. In humans, magnesium increases endothelial cell proliferation and migration in a dose-dependent fashion [164]. Magnesium deficiency, which has been associated with diabetes in nursing home residents, has the opposite effect of inhibiting cell migration and proliferation [164]. Adverse effects of magnesium supplementation include drowsiness, weakness, and lethargy. Overall, there is insufficient evidence to recommend magnesium supplementation in diabetic patients with wounds (grade D). However, hypomagnesemia should be adequately treated in diabetic patients with or at risk for wounds (grade C).

Zinc

Zinc deficiency is associated with decreased gene expression of inhibitory-κBα (IκBα), decreased NF-κB translocation to the nucleus, decreased gene expression of IL-1β and TNF-α, and thus decreased wound healing [165]. During the initial inflammatory stage, zinc tissue concentrations can also transiently fall in response to IL-6, TNF-α, and calprotectin, a zinc-binding protein [166,167]. This facilitates and prolongs inflammation during the early stage [166]. However, in the late phase zinc levels rise, possibly due to EGF [168], and exert anti-inflammatory effects on phagocytic cells [165], promoting late-phase healing and wound closure [166,167]. Moreover, zinc participates in the synthesis or activation of at least 70 metalloenzymes, many of which are involved in the later stages of wound healing, such as granulation, maturation and tissue generation [166]. Wound fluids were found to contain positively charged zinc complexes that may be important for zinc transport into cells [169].

Breslow et al. [170] found no association of plasma zinc levels with pressure ulcers in a study of 26 nursing home tube-fed patients. This study was confirmed by data from Henderson et al. [171]. Various interventional studies have also failed to demonstrate any benefit of zinc therapy with pressure ulcer healing [98,172–175]. Other studies that demonstrated benefit also contained methodological flaws [165,176–178]. Nevertheless, Williams et al. [179] and Gengenbacher et al. [180] demonstrated an association of zinc deficiencies with pressure ulcer occurrence. Also, chronic leg ulcers in the elderly have been associated with diminished serum zinc levels [121]. Utilizing the Cochrane Database, Wilkinson and Hawke [181] found no evidence for the use of oral zinc therapy in the treatment of chronic leg ulcers, though there was a trend toward benefit in patients with zinc deficiency (evidence level 2, no benefit). Langer et al. [182] also performed a Cochrane Database Systematic Review of enteral and parenteral nutrition, including zinc therapy, and wound healing and found that methodological inconsistencies precluded meta-analysis of the data.

Decreased absorption of zinc and hyperzincuria has been described in patients with T2DM and borderline zinc levels [183]. Furthermore, zinc deficiency has been linked with decreased immune function in patients with T2DM [184]. Zinc status is extremely difficult to assess. In the nonstressed patient, serum and plasma zinc levels are helpful. However, the levels may be reduced by 50% with inflammation. More specific functional markers are not readily available, though a low alkaline phosphatase level would suggest a functional zinc deficiency [185]. Hence, the greater risk for zinc deficiency in patients with T2DM confers potential benefit of zinc therapy for wound healing [186]. Yet, this is still an unproven claim (evidence level 4).

Oral zinc is 20% bioavailable, therefore oral dosages of 200–220 mg daily should be adequate to provide the RDI of 11 mg/day for men and 8 mg/day for women. Parenteral zinc is 100% bioavailable and doses should be reduced and administered accordingly. Zinc administration is not without risk and includes copper deficiency, anemia, neutropenia, adverse low-density lipoprotein cholesterol (LDL-c)/high-density lipoprotein cholesterol (HDL-c) ratios, gastrointestinal distress, suppressed immunity, and infection [187,188]. In summary, the clinical evidence does not support any benefit of zinc therapy for patients with T2DM and wounds. However, zinc therapy is safe, possibly effective in wound healing, and rational in diabetic patients shown to have a zinc deficiency (grade C) (see Table 12.3).

INSULIN

Insulin is an anabolic growth factor that stimulates uptake of both glucose and branched-chain amino acids (valine, leucine, and isoleucine) [196]. Insulin also inhibits intracellular degradation of proteins [196]. In wound healing, insulin participates in glucose homeostasis and acts as a trophic factor to stimulate tissue growth and regeneration [197]. Insulin also enhances peripheral nerve regeneration possibly via effects on nerve growth factor [198]. In diabetic patients, tight glycemic control with insulinization is associated with preservation of lean body mass [199], increased neutrophil phagocytosis [200], reduced infection rates [200], and stage-III pressure sore healing [201]. *In vitro* and animal studies demonstrate decreased protein breakdown [202–205] and increased protein synthesis [202,206] by insulin. Moreover, insulin therapy improves wound healing in rats [207] and diabetic mice [208].

In humans, perioperative glucose-insulin-potassium infusions that achieved tight glycemic control (blood glucose 125–200 mg/dL), compared with usual practice (blood glucose < 250 mg/dL), were associated with decreased infectious complications of wounds in post-operative diabetic coronary artery bypass graft patients [209]. Nevertheless, glycemic control does not appear to influence collagen deposition in acute wounds in patients T1DM or T2DM [210]. In critically ill burn patients, a 7-day continuous insulin infusion, at a maximal dose of 25–49 units/hour, improved

TABLE 12.3
Clinical Evidence Supporting Oral Zinc Therapy for Wound Healing in the General Population[a]

Reference	Experimental Design	Result	Level
181	Systematic review of 6 randomized trials 210–215	No effect Limited evidence of benefit with low zinc levels	2
189	Zinc sulfate 220 mg/day × 16 weeks N = 18 completed study nonhealing venous stasis ulcers measure re-epithelialization	5/18 Healed completely	3
190	Zinc sulfate 220 mg qD – BID × 4 weeks N = 8 randomized, double-blind trial	No benefit of treatment	3
191	Zinc sulfate 220 mg qD – BID × 10 months N = 42 randomized, double-blind trial	No benefit	3
192	Zinc sufate 200 mg TID × 18 weeks N = 27 (selection bias) randomized, double-blind trial arterial and venous ulcers	No deficiency: 14% healed with zinc Zinc deficient: 71% healed with zinc	3
193	Zinc sulfate 200 mg TID × 14 months N = 30 (selection bias) randomized trial ischemic leg ulcers	Zinc treatment beneficial More rapid healing with zinc deficiency	3
194	Zinc sulfate 200 mg TID × 12 weeks N = 36 randomized, double-blind trial venous stasis ulcers Typical therapy also used (possible confounder)	Zinc treatment: 73% healed Placebo: 52% healed Statistically significant	3
195	Zinc sulfate 200 mg TID × > 16 weeks N = 38 randomized, double-blind trial	No benefit with zinc deficiency	3
99	Zinc-containing supplement (also contained protein and arginine) N = 103 hip fracture patients randomized, double-blind trial	Delayed onset and progression of leg ulcers	3

[a] These data do not support any claim that zinc therapy has a specific benefit in diabetic patients with wounds.

nitrogen balance and stimulated a 350% increase in protein synthesis in healthy muscle and a 50% increase in protein synthesis in wound tissue [211]. However, the protein synthesis was also accompanied by increased muscle breakdown, which was thought to be due to an inadequate supply of administered amino acids [210]. Lower insulin infusion rates have been found to elicit less protein breakdown with similar improvements in nitrogen balance and protein synthesis [212,213]. This dose-dependent effect on anabolism was observed with parenteral nutrition containing insulin, and not insulin in conjunction with enteral nutrition [202,214]. Insulin has also been found to increase type-IV collagen synthesis [215].

These level 2 and 3 data support beneficial direct effects of insulin on wound healing in diabetic and nondiabetic patients. Thus, consideration should be given to the use of insulin in all diabetic patients with wounds even if previously well-controlled with oral agents (grade B). This recommendation is buttressed by the premise that, compared with endogenous hyperinsulinemia in

TABLE 12.4
Summary of Nutrient and Dietary Supplement Interventions for Wound Healing in Diabetic Patients

Nutrient/Dietary Supplement	Safe Doses	Recommendation Grade
Nitrogen		
Whole protein supplement[a]	30–60 g/day	C
Arginine	6–17 g/day	C
Glutamine	0.285–0.570 g/kg/day IV[b]	C
	15–45 mg/day po	
Vitamins		
Vitamin A	10,000–25,000 units/day perioperative	D (no steroid exposure)
	(4000 units/day with pregnancy or	C (steroid exposure)
	childbearing age)	
Vitamin C	500–2000 mg/day	C
Vitamin E	50–800 mg/day	D
Minerals		
Boron	3 mg/day	D
Calcium	1000–1500 mg/day	D
Copper	2 mg/day	D
Zinc	200–220 mg qD–TID	C (especially with zinc deficiency)

[a] Beyond sufficient dietary protein to meet needs of the patient (0.8–1.5 g/kg/day).

[b] *Source*: From Reference [216].

patients with T2DM primarily found in the portal circulation, exogenous insulinization creates a state of systemic hyperinsulinemia which positively affects wound healing.

AN INTEGRATED NUTRITIONAL APPROACH TO WOUND HEALING IN DIABETIC PATIENTS

Diabetic patients with nonhealing wounds should be managed aggressively. The mainstay of a comprehensive approach is tight glycemic control, though the specific target glucose level is not evidence-based. This is a theory-driven concept based on clinical data demonstrating that impaired wound healing is associated with hyperglycemia. Thus, since insulin has direct beneficial effects on wound healing, an optimal approach would be to achieve as close to normal glycemic status as possible using insulin and not oral agents or diet alone.

Diabetic patients with wounds must also be nourished aggressively. If patients are unable to meet their energy, protein, and/or micronutrient needs with oral intake, then nutrition support must be initiated. In general, patients should receive roughly 30 total kcal/kg/day and 0.8–2.1 g protein/kg/day with the following caveats. Obese patients should be maintained in negative energy balance (15–20 kcal/kg/day) to promote lipolysis and weight loss while providing adequate protein, which is based on the adjusted body weight {(([actual weight − ideal weight] × 0.25) + actual weight}. Stressed patients may require more total kcal per day but care must be taken not to overfeed or induce hyperglycemia. The use of specific nutrients and dietary supplements should be based on the clinical evidence and is summarized in Table 12.4. Recommendation grades for these substances are ultimately based on the presence of safety, since proven clinical benefit is generally lacking or weak. A prudent treatment strategy would include (1) one multivitamin; (2) protein supplementation to achieve optimal nitrogen retention; (3) arginine and/or glutamine provided ammonia and blood urea nitrogen levels are acceptable; (4) vitamin A if there is steroid exposure; (5) vitamin C; (6) and zinc, especially if there is clinical or biochemical evidence of zinc deficiency.

Biochemical testing should be performed to detect and avoid nutrient deficiencies and monitor the response to nutrition support. This is particularly important for maintaining optimal nitrogen retention and consideration of zinc therapy, which seems to work best in the setting of zinc deficiency. Unquestionably, conventional wound care strategies must be incorporated, including infection control, regular debridement, adequate pressure relief, and appropriate use of growth factors and other pharmacologic agents. Creating and utilizing a multidisciplinary wound care team, including a nutrition specialist, are recommended.

REFERENCES

1. Campbell NA, *Biology*, 2nd ed., California: Benjamin/Cummings, 1990.
2. Moy LS, Management of acute wounds, *Dermatol Clin,* 11(Suppl 4):759–766, 1993.
3. Newcomer VD and Young EM Jr., Unique wounds and wound emergencies, *Dermatol Clin,* 11(Suppl 4):715–727, 1993.
4. Reinherz RP, Hong DT, and Tisa LM et al., Management of puncture wounds of the foot, *J Foot Surg,* 24:288, 1985.
5. Sumpio BE, Foot ulcers, *New Eng J Med,* 343(Suppl 11):787–793, 2000.
6. Habershaw G and Chzran J, Biomechanical considerations of the diabetic foot, In: Kozak GP, Campbell DR, and Frykberg RG et al., Eds., *Management of Diabetic Foot Problems*, 2nd ed., Philadelphia: WB Saunders, 1995:53–65.
7. American Diabetes Association, Preventive foot care in people with diabetes, *Diabetes Care*, 22(Suppl 1):S54–55, 1999.
8. Levin ME, Prevention and treatment of diabetic foot wounds, *J Wound Ostomy Continence Nurs*, 25(Suppl 3):129–146, 1998.
9. Eaglstein WH and Falanga V, Wound healing, chronic wounds, *Surg Clin North Am*, 77(Suppl 3):689–700, 1997.
10. Arturson G, Pathophysiology of the burn wound and pharmacological treatment, The Rudi Hermans Lecture, 1995, *Burns*, 22(Suppl 4):255–274, 1996.
11. Bower MG, Evaluating and managing bite wounds, *Adv Skin Wound Care*, 15(Suppl 2):88–90, 2002.
12. Black SB, Venous stasis ulcers, A review, *Ostomy Wound Manage*, 41(Suppl 8):20–22, 24–26, 28–30, passim, 1995.
13. Scwhartzberg JB and Kirsner RS, Stasis in venous ulcers: A misnomer that should be abandoned, *Dermatol Surg*, 26(Suppl 7):683–684, 2000.
14. Sanada H, Nagakawa T, and Yamamoto M et al., The role of skin blood flow in pressure ulcer development during surgery, *Adv Wound Care*, 10(Suppl 6):29–34, 1997.
15. Frykberg RG, Diabetic foot ulcers: Pathogenesis and management, *Am Fam Physician*, 66(Suppl 9):1655–1662, 2002.
16. Sage RA, Webster JK, and Fisher SG, Outpatient care and morbidity reduction in diabetic foot ulcers associated with chronic pressure callous, *J Am Podiatr Med Assoc*, 91(Suppl 6):275–279, 2001.
17. Jeffcoate WJ and Harding KG, Diabetic foot ulcers, *Lancet*, 361(Suppl 9368):1545–1551, 2003.
18. Smith J, Debridement of diabetic foot ulcers, *Cochrane Database Syst Rev*, 4:CD003556, 2002.
19. Cuddigan J, Ayello EA, and Sussman C et al., Eds., *Pressure Ulcers in America: Prevalence, Incidence, and Implications for the Future,* Reston, VA: National Pressure Ulcer Advisory Panel, 2001.
20. Bergstrom N, Braden B, and Kemp M et al., Multi-site study of incidence of pressure ulcers and the relationship between risk level, demographic characteristics, diagnoses, and prescription of preventive interventions, *J Am Geriatr Soc*, 44(Suppl 1):22–30, 1996.
21. Allman RM, Goode PS, and Patrick MM et al., Pressure ulcer risk factors among hospitalized patients with activity limitation, *JAMA*, 274(Suppl 13):1014–1015, 1995.
22. Margolis DJ, Bilker W, and Knauss J et al., The incidence and prevalence of pressure ulcers among elderly pataients in general medical practice, *Ann Epidemiol*, 21(Suppl 5):321–325, 2002.

23. Allman RM, Pressure ulcer prevalence, incidence, risk factors, and impact, *Clin Geriatr Med*, 13(Suppl 3):421–436, 1997.
24. Bouton CV, Oomens CW, and Baaijens FP et al., The etiology of pressure ulcers: Skin-deep or muscle-bound? *Arch Phys Med Rehabil*, 84(Suppl 4):616–619, 2003.
25. Lyder CH, Pressure ulcer prevention and management, *JAMA*, 289(Suppl 2):223–226, 2003.
26. Reuler JB and Cooney TG, The pressure sore: Pathophysiology and principles of management, *Lancet*, 94(Suppl 5):661–666, 1981.
27. Nola GT and Vistnes LM, Differential response of skin and muscle in the experimental production of pressure sores, *Plast Reconstr Surg*, 66(Suppl 5):728–733, 1980.
28. Daniel RK, Priest DL, and Wheatley DC, Etiologic factors in pressure sores: An experimental model, *Arch Phys Med Rehabil,* 81(Suppl 10):492–498, 1962.
29. Hussain T, Experimental study of some pressure effects on tissue, with reference to the bed-sore problem, *J Pathol Bacteriol*, 66(Suppl 2):347–363, 1953.
30. Bliss MR, Hyperaemia, *J Tissue Viability*, 8(Suppl 4):4–13, 1998.
31. Schubert V, Hypotension as a risk factor for the development of pressure sores in elderly subjects, *Age Ageing*, 20(Suppl 4):255–261, 1991.
32. Horn SD, Bender SA, and Ferguson ML et al., The National Pressure Ulcer Long-Term Care Study, Pressure ulcer development in long-term care residents, *J Am Geriatr Soc*, 52(Suppl 3):359–367, 2004.
33. Horn SD, Bender SA, and Bergstrom N et al., Description of the national pressure ulcer long-term care study, *J Am Geriatr Soc*, 50(Suppl 11):1816–1825, 2002.
34. Bergstrom N and Braden B, A prospective study of pressure sore risk among institutionalized elderly, *J Am Geriatr Soc*, 40:747–758, 1992.
35. Reed RI, Hepburn K, and Adelson R et al., Low serum albumin levels, confusion, and fecal incontinence: Are these risk factors for pressure ulcers in mobility-impaired hospitalized adults? *Gerontology*, 49(Suppl 4):255–259, 2003.
36. Browse NL and Burnand KG, The cause of venous ulceration, *Lancet*, 2(Suppl 8292):243–245, 1982.
37. Higley H, Ksander GA, and Gerhardt CO et al., Extravasation of macromolecules and possible trapping of transforming growth factor-beta in venous ulceration, *Br J Dermatol*, 132(Suppl 1):79–85, 1995.
38. Falanga V and Eaglstein WH, The "trap" hypothesis of venous ulceration, *Lancet*, 341(Suppl 8851):1006–1008, 1993.
39. Vandeberg JS and Rudolph R, Pressure (decubitus) ulcer: Variation in histopathology—a light and electron microscope study, *Hum Pathol*, 26:195–200, 1995.
40. Landsman AS, Meaney DF, and Cargill RS et al., High strain rate tissue deformation, A theory on the mechanical etiology of diabetic foot ulcerations, *Am Podiatr Med Assoc*, 85:519–527, 1995.
41. Bouten CV, Knight MM, and Lee DA et al., Compressive deformation and damage of muscle cell subpopulations in a model system, *Ann Biomed Eng*, 29:153–163, 2001.
42. Miller GE and Seale J, Lymphatic clearance during compressive loading, *Lymphology*, 14:161–166, 1981.
43. Reddy NP, Patel H, and Krouskop TA, Interstitial fluid flow as a factor in decubitus ulcer formation, *J Biomech*, 14:879–881, 1981.
44. Herrman EC, Knapp CF, and Donofrio JC et al., Skin perfusion responses to surface pressure-induced ischemia: Implication for the developing pressure ulcer, *J Rehabil Res Dev*, 36:109–120, 1999.
45. Peirce SM, Skalak TC, and Rodheaver GT, Ischemia-reperfusion injury in chronic pressure ulcer formation: A skin model in the rat, *Wound Repair Regen*, 8:68–76, 2000.
46. Ryan TJ, Cellular responses to tissue distortion, In: Bader DL, Ed., *Pressure Sores: Clinical Practice and Scientific Approach*, London: MacMillan Press, 1990:141–152.
47. Yager DR and Nwomeh BC, The proteolytic environment of chronic wounds, *Wound Repair Regen*, 7(Suppl 6):433–441, 1999.
48. Diegelmann RF, Excessive neutrophils characterize chronic pressure ulcers, *Wound Repair Regen*, 11(Suppl 6):490–495, 2003.
49. Heughan C and Hunt TK, Some aspects of wound healing research, A review, *Can J Surg*, 18(Suppl 2):118–126, 1975.
50. Hunt TK, The physiology of wound healing, *Ann Emerg Med*, 17(Suppl 12):1265–1273, 1988.
51. Hunt TK, Hopf H, and Hussain Z, Physiology of wound healing, *Adv Skin Wound Care*, 13(Suppl 2):6–11, 2000.

52. Wheater PR, Burkitt HG, and Stevens A et al., *Basic Histopathology—A Colour Atlas and Text*, 2nd ed., United Kingdom: Churchill Livingstone Longman Group UK Limited, 1992.
53. Leibovich SJ and Ross R, The role of macrophages in wound repair, A study with hydrocortisone and antimacrophage serum, *Am J Pathol*, 78(Suppl 1):71–100, 1975.
54. Ross R and Odland G, Human wound repair, II, Inflammatory cells, epithelial-mesenchymal interrelations, and fibrogenesis, *J Cell Biol*, 39(Suppl 1):152–168, 1968.
55. Odland G and Ross R, Human wound repair, I, Epidermal regeneration, *J Cell Biol*, 39(Suppl 1):135–151, 1968.
56. Singer AJ and Clark RAF, Cutaneous wound healing, *NEJM*, 341(Suppl 10):738–746, 1999.
57. Pierce GF, Inflammation in nonhealing diabetic wounds, the space-time continuum does matter, *Am J Pathol*, 159(Suppl 2):399–403, 2001.
58. Clark RA, Fibronectin matrix deposition and fibronectin receptor expression in healing and normal skin, *J Invest Dermatol*, 94(Suppl 6):128S–134S, 1990.
59. Larjava H, Salo T, and Haapasalmi K et al., Expression of integrins and basement membrane components by wound keratinocytes, *J Clin Invest*, 92:1425–1435, 1993.
60. Pilcher BK, Dumin JA, and Sudbeck BD et al., The activity of collaagenase-1 is required for keratinocyte migration in a type-1 collagen matrix, *J Cell Biol*, 137:1445–1457, 1997.
61. Bugge TH, Kombrinck KW, and Flick MJ et al., Loss of fibrinogen rescues mice from the pleiotropic effects of plasminogen deficiency, *Cell*, 87:709–719, 1996.
62. Mignatti P, Rifkin DB, and Welgus HG et al., Proteinases and tissue remodeling, In: Clark RAF, Ed., *The Molecular and Cellular Biology of Wound Repair*, 2nd ed., New York: Plenum Press, 427–474, 1996.
63. Nanney LB and King LE, Jr, Epidermal growth factor and transforming growth factor alpha, In: Clark RAF, Ed., *The Molecular and Cellular Biology of Wound Repair*, 2nd ed., New York: Plenum Press, 171–194, 1996.
64. Werner S, Smola H, and Liao X, The function of KGF in morphogenesis of epithelium and reepithelialization of wounds, *Science,* 266:819–822, 1994.
65. Abraham JA and Klagsbrun M, Modulation of wound repair by members of the fibroblast growth factor family, In: Clark RAF, Ed., *The Molecular and Cellular Biology of Wound Repair*, 2nd ed., New York: Plenum Press, 195–248, 1996.
66. Clark RAF, Lanigan JM, and DellaPelle P et al., Fibronectin and fibrin provide a provisional matrix for epidermal cell migration during wound reepithelialization, *J Invest Dermatol,* 79:264–269, 1982.
67. Ross R, Everett NB, and Tyler R, Wound healing and collagen formation, VI, The origin of the wound fibroblast studies in parabiosis, *J Cell Biol*, 44:645, 1970.
68. Hunt TK, Ed., Wound healing and wound infection: Theory and surgical practice, New York: Appleton-Century-Crofts, 1980.
69. Heldin C-H and Westermark B, Role of platelet-derived growth factor in vivo, In: Clark RAF, Ed., *The Molecular and Cellular Biology of Wound Repair*, 2nd ed., New York: Plenum Press, 249–273, 1996.
70. Roberts AB and Sporn MB, Transforming growth factor-beta, In: Clark RAF, Ed., *The Molecular and Cellular Biology of Wound Repair*, 2nd ed., New York: Plenum Press, 275–308, 1996.
71. Folkman J and D'Amore PA, Blood vessel formation: What is its molecular basis? *Cell*, 87:1153–1155, 1996.
72. Iruela-Arispe ML and Dvorak HF, Angiogenesis: A dynamic balance of stimulators and inhibitors, *Thromb Haemost*, 78:672–677, 1997.
73. Risau W, Mechanisms of angiogenesis, *Nature*, 386:671–674, 1997.
74. Vaalamo M, Mattila L, and Johansson N, Distinct populations of stromal cells express collagenase-3 (MMP-13) and collagenase-1 (MMP-1) in chronic ulcers but not in normally healing wounds, *J Invest Dermatol*, 109:96–101, 1997.
75. Nissen NN, Polverini PJ, and Koch AE et al., Vascular endothelial growth factor mediates angiogenic activity during the proliferative phase of wound healing, *Am J Pathol*, 152:1445–1452, 1998.
76. Brown LF, Yeo K-T, and Berse B, Expression of vascular permeability factor (vascular endothelial growth factor) by epidermal keratinocytes during wound healing, *J Exp Med*, 176:1375–1379, 1992.

77. Welch MP, Odland GF, and Clark RAF, Temporal relationships of F-actin bundle formation, collagen and fibronectin matrix assembly, and fibronectin receptor expression to wound contraction, *J Cell Biol*, 110:133–145, 1990.

78. Greiling D and Clark RAF, Fibronectin provides a conduit for fibroblast transmigration from collagenous stroma into fibrin clot provisional matrix, *J Cell Sci*, 110:861–870, 1997.

79. Toole BP, Proteoglycans and hyaluronan in morphogenesis and differentiation, In: Hay ED, Ed., *Cell Biology of Extracellular Matrix*, 2nd ed., New York, Plenum Press, 305–341, 1991.

80. Xu J and Clark RAF, Extracellular matrix alters PDGF regulation of fibroblast integrins, *J Cell Biol*, 132:239–249, 1996.

81. McClain SA, Simon M, and Jones E et al., Mesenchymal cell activation is the rate-limiting step of granulation tissue induction, *Am J Pathol*, 149:1257–1270, 1996.

82. Desmouliere A, Redard M, and Darby I et al., Apoptosis mediates the decrease in cellularity during the transition between granulation tissue and scar, *Am J Pathol*, 146:56–66, 1995.

83. Stryer L, Connective-tissue proteins, In: Stryer L, Ed., *Biochemistry*, 3rd ed., New York: W.H. Freeman, 261–281, 1988.

84. Howes EL and Harvey SC, The strength of the healing wound in relation to the holding strength of the catgut suture, *NEJM*, 200:1285, 1929.

85. Levenson SM, Geever EF, and Crowley LV et al., The healing of rat skin wounds, *Ann Surg*, 161:293–308, 1965.

86. Peppa M, Brem H, and Ehrlich P et al., Adverse effects of dietary glycotoxins in wound healing in genetically diabetic mice, *Diabetes*, 52:2805–2813, 2003.

87. Taussig SJ and Batkin S, Bromelain, the enzyme complex of pineapple (ananas comosus) and its clinical application, An update, *J Ethnopharmacol*, 22(Suppl 2):191–203, 1988.

88. Murad H and Tabibian MP, The effect of an oral supplement containing glucosamine, amino acids, minerals, and antioxidants on cutaneous aging, A preliminary study, *J Dermatolog Treat*, 12(Suppl 1):47–51, 2001.

89. Steed DL, Donohoe D, and Webster MW et al., Diabetic Ulcer Study Group, Effect of extensive debridement and treatment on the healing of diabetic foot ulcers, J *Am Coll Surg*, 183:61–64, 1996.

90. Pierce GF, Tarpley J, and Yanagihara D et al., PDGF-BB, TGF Beta-1, and basic FGF in dermal wound healing: Neovessel and matrix formation and cessation of repair, *Am J Pathol*, 140:1375–1388, 1992.

91. Smiell JM, Wierman TJ, and Steed DL et al., Efficacy and safety of becaplermin (recombinant human platelet-derived growth factor-BB) in patients with nonhealing, lower extremity diabetic ulcers, A combined analysis of four randomized studies, *Wound Repair Regen*, 7:335–346, 1999.

92. Gailit J, Xu J, and Bueller H et al., Platelet-derived growth factor and inflammatory cytokines have differential effects on the expression of integrins alpha 1 beta 1 and alpha 5 beta 1 by human dermal fibroblasts in vitro, *J Cell Physiol*, 169:281–289, 1996.

93. Pilcher BK, Wang M, Qin XJ, Parks WC, Senior RM, and Welgus HG, Role of matrix metalloproteinases and their inhibition in cutaneous wound healing and allergic contact hypersensitivity, *Ann NY Acad Sci*, 878:12–24, 1999.

94. Madlener M, Parks WC, and Werner S, Matrix metalloproteinases (MMPs) and their physiological inhibitors (TIMPs) are differentially expressed during excisional skin wound repair, *Exp Cell Res*, 242:201–210, 1998.

95. MacKay D and Miller A, Nutrition support for wound healing, *Alternative Medicine Review*, 8:359–377, 2003.

96. Dickerson RN, Estimating energy and protein requirements of thermally injured patients: Art or science? *Nutrition*, 18:439–442, 2002.

97. Mechanick JI, Practical aspects of nutritional support for wound-healing patients, *Am J Surg*, 188(Suppl 1A):52–56, 2004.

98. Mathus-Vliegen EMH, Old age, malnutrition, and pressure sores: An ill-fated alliance, *J Gerontol A Biol Sci Med Sci*, 59(Suppl 4):355–360, 2004.

99. Houwing RH, Rozendaal M, and Wouters-Wesseling W et al., A randomized, double-blind assessment of the effect of nutritional supplementation on the prevention of pressure ulcers in hip-fracture patients, *Clinical Nutr*, 22(Suppl 4):401–405, 2003.

100. Bourdel-Marchasson I, Barateau M, and Rondeau V et al., GAGE Group, Groupe Aquitain Geriatrique d'Evaluation, A multi-center trial of the effects of oral nutritional supplementation in critically ill older inpatients, *Nutrition*, 16:1–5, 2000.
101. Breslow RA, Hallfrisch J, and Guy DG et al., The importance of dietary protein in healing pressure ulcers, *J Am Geriatr Soc*, 41:357–362, 1993.
102. Thomas DR, Improving outcome of pressure ulcers with nutritional interventions, A review of the evidence, *Nutrition*, 17:121–125, 2001.
103. Mitchell SL, Kiely DK, and Lipsitz LA, The risk factors and impact on survival of feeding tube placement in nursing home residents with severe cognitive impairment, *Arch of Int Med*, 157(Suppl 3):327–332, 1997.
104. Ikizler TA, Greene JH, and Wingard RL et al., Spontaneous dietary protein intake during progression to chronic renal failure, *J Am Soc Nephrol*, 6(Suppl 5):1386–1391, 1995.
105. Avenell A and Handoll HH, A systematic review of protein and energy supplementation for hip fracture aftercare in older people, *Eur J Clin Nutr*, 57(Suppl 8):895–903, 2003.
106. Singer P, Nutritional care to prevent and heal pressure ulcers, *Isr Med Assoc J*, 4(Suppl 9):713–716, 2002.
107. Shi HP, Most D, and Efron D et al., Supplemental L-arginine enhances wound healing in diabetic rats, *Wound Repair and Regen*, 11(Suppl 3):198–203, 2003.
108. Witte M, Thornton FJ, and Tantry U et al., L-Arginine supplementation enhances diabetic wound healing: Involvement of the nitric oxide synthase and arginase pathways, *Metabolism*, 51:1269–1273, 2002.
109. Kamfer H, Pfeilschifter J, and Frank S, Expression and activity of arginase isoenzymes during normal and diabetes impaired skin repair, *The J of Invest Derm*, 121(Suppl 6):1544–1551, 2003.
110. Ge K, Lu SL, and Qing C et al., A study promoting the effect of L-arginine on the burn wound healing of rats with diabetes, *Zhonghua Shao Shang Za Zhi*, 19(Suppl):11–14, 2003.
111. Ge K, Lu SL, and Qing C et al., The influence of L-arginine on the angiogenesis in burn wounds in diabetic rats, *Zhonghua Shao Shang Za Shi*, 20(Suppl 4):210–213, 2004.
112. Kirk SJ, Hurson M, and Regan MC et al., Arginine stimulates wound healing and immune function in elderly human beings, *Surgery*, 114(Suppl 2):155–159, 1993.
113. Williams JZ, Abumrad N, and Barbul A, Effect of a specialized amino acid mixture on human collagen deposition, *Ann Surg*, 236(Suppl 3):369–374, 2002.
114. DiSilvestro RA, Zinc in relation to diabetes and oxidative stress, *J Nutr*, 130:1509S–1511S, 2000.
115. Lyons TJ, Oxidized low-density lipoproteins: A role in the pathogenesis of atherosclerosis in diabetes? *Diab Med*, 8:411–419, 1991.
116. Oberley LW, Free radicals and diabetes, *Free Radic Biol Med*, 5:113–124, 1988.
117. Sinclair AJ, Lunec J, Girling J, and Barnett AH, Modulators of free radical activity in diabetes mellitus: Role of ascorbic acid, *Free Radic Aging*, 2:342–352, 1992.
118. Mooradian AD and Morely JE, Micronutrient status in diabetes mellitus, *Am J Clin Nutr*, 45:877–895, 1986.
119. Pai L and Prasad AS, Cellular zinc in patients with diabetes mellitus, *Nutr Res*, 8:889–897, 1988.
120. Moutschen MP, Scheen AJ, and Lefebvre PJ, Impaired immune responses in diabetes mellitus: Analysis of the factors and mechanisms involved: Relevance to the increased susceptibility of diabetic patients to specific infections, *Diab Metab*, 18:187–201, 1992.
121. Rojas AI and Phillips TJ, Patients with chronic leg ulcers show diminished levels of vitamins A and E, carotenes, and zinc, *Dermatol Surg*, 25:601–604, 1999.
122. Frieman M, Seifter E, Connerton C, and Levenson SM, Vitamin A deficiency and surgical stress, *Surg Forum*, 21:81–82, 1970.
123. Hunt TK, Vitamin A and wound healing, *J Am Acad Dermatol*, 15:817–821, 1986.
124. Seifter E, Rettura G, and Padawer J et al., Impaired wound healing in streptozotocin diabetes, Prevention by supplemental vitamin A, *Ann Surg*, 194(Suppl 1):42–50, 1981.
125. Ehrlich HP and Hunt TK, Effects of cortisone and vitamin A on wound healing, *Ann Surg*, 167:324–328, 1968.
126. Hunt TK, Ehrlich HP, and Garcia JA et al., Effect of vitamin A on reversing the inhibitory effect of cortisone on healing of open wounds in animals and man, *Ann Surg*, 170:633–641, 1969.

127. Ehrlich HP, Tarver H, and Hunt TK, Effects of vitamin A and glucocorticoids upon inflammation and collagen synthesis, *Ann Surg*, 177:222–227, 1973.

128. Anstead GM, Steroids, retinoids, and wound healing, *Adv Wound Care*, 11(Suppl 6):277–285, 1998.

129. Roberts SB and Sporn MB, The transforming growth factor betas, In: *The Handbook of Experimental Pharmacology*, Vol. 95/I: Peptide growth factors and their receptors, Berlin: Springer-Verlag, 1990:419–472.

130. Wicke C, Halliday B, and Allen D et al., Effects of steroids and retinoids on wound healing, *Arch Surg*, 135:1265–1270, 2000.

131. Lee B, Vouthounis C, and Stojadinovic O et al., From an enhanceosome to a repressosome: Molecular antagonism between glucocorticoids and EGF leads to inhibition of wound healing, *J Mol Biol*, 345:1083–1097, 2005.

132. Barker ME and Blumsohn A, Is vitamin A consumption a risk factor for osteoporotic fracture? *Proc Nutr Soc*, 62(Suppl 4):845–850, 2003.

133. Fairfield KM and Fletcher RH, Vitamins for chronic disease prevention in adults, *JAMA*, 287(Suppl 23):3116–3126, 2002.

134. Russell L, The importance of patients' nutritional status in wound healing, *Br J Nurs*, 10(Suppl 6):S42, 44–49, 2001.

135. Goode HF, Burns E, and Walker BE, Vitamin C depletion and pressure sores in elderly patients with femoral neck fracture, *BMJ*, 305(Suppl 6859):925–927, 1992.

136. Anderson R, Oosthuizen R, and Maritz R, The effects of increasing weekly doses of ascorbate on certain cellular and humoral immune function in normal volunteers, *Am J Clin Nutr*, 33:71–76, 1980.

137. Hendler SS and Rorvik D, Eds., *PDR for Nutritional Supplements, Medical Economics,* Thomson Healthcare, Montvale NJ, 2001:486–498.

138. Musalmah M, Fairuz AH, and Gapor MT et al., Effect of vitamin E on plasma malondialdehyde, antioxidant enzyme levels and the rates of wound closures during wound healing in normal and diabetic rats, *Asia Pac J Clin Nutr*, 11 Suppl 7:S448–451, 2002.

139. Meydani SN, Meydani M, and Blumberg JB, Vitamin E supplementation and in vivo immune response in healthy elderly subjects, A randomized controlled trial, *JAMA*, 277:1380–1386, 1997.

140. Rasik AM and Shukla A, Antioxidant status in delayed healing type of wounds, *Int J Exp Pathol*, 81(Suppl 4):257–263, 2000.

141. Galeano M, Torre V, and Deodato B et al., Raxofelast, a hydrophilic vitamin E-like antioxidant, stimulates wound healing in genetically diabetic mice, *Surgery*, 129(Suppl 4):467–477, 2001.

142. Altavilla D, Saitta A, and Cucinotta D et al., Inhibition of lipid peroxidation restores impaired vascular endothelial growth factor expression and stimulates wound healing and angiogenesis in the genetically diabetic mouse, *Diabetes*, 50(Suppl 3):667–674, 2001.

143. Ehrlich HP, Tarver H, and Hunt TK, Inhibitory effects of vitamin E on collagen synthesis and wound repair, *Ann Surg*, 175:235–240, 1972.

144. Greenwald DP, Sharzer LA, and Padawer J, Zone II flexor tendon repair: Effects of vitamins A, E, beta-carotene, *J Surg Res*, 49:98–102, 1990.

145. Efiendev VM, Kuliev RA, and Babaev RF et al., The possibilities for correcting lipid peroxidation in suppurative wounds in diabetic patients, *Vestn Khir Im IIGrek*, 151(Suppl 7–12):84–86, 1993.

146. Muangman P, Spenny ML, and Tamura RN et al., Fatty acids and glucose increase neutral endopeptidase activity in human microvascular endothelial cells, *Shock*, 19(Suppl 6):508–512, 2003.

147. Muangman P, Tamura RN, and Gibran NS, Antioxidants inhibit fatty acid and glucose-mediated induction of neutral endopeptidase gene expression in human microvascular endothelial cells, *J Am Coll Surg*, 200:208–215, 2005.

148. Johnson L, Bowen FW, and Abbasi S, Relationship of prolonged pharmacological serum levels of vitamin E to incidence of sepsis and necrotizing enterocolitis in infants with birth weight 1500 grams or less, *Pediatrics*, 75:619, 1985.

149. Nielsen FH, Hunt CD, and Mullen LM et al., Effect of dietary boron on mineral, estrogen, and testosterone metabolism in postmenopausal women, *FASEB*, 1(Suppl 5):394–397, 1987.

150. Newnham RE, Essentiality of boron for healthy bones and joints, *Environ Health Perspect*, 102 Suppl 7:83–85, 1994.

151. Dzondo-Gadet M, Mayap-Nzietchueng R, and Hess K et al., Action of boron at the molecular level: Effects on transcription an translation in an acellular system, *Biol Trace Elem Res*, 85(Suppl 1):23–33, 2002.

152. Nzietcheung RM, Dousset B, and Franck P et al., Mechanisms implicated in the effects of boron on wound healing, *J Trace Elem Med Biol*, 16(Suppl 4):239–244, 2002.

153. Chebassier N, Ouijja el H, and Viegas I et al., Stimulatory effect of boron and manganese salts on keratinocyte migration, *Acta Derm Venereol*, 84(Suppl 3):191–194, 2004.

154. Benderdour M, Hess K, and Gadet MD et al., Effect of boric acid solution on cartilage metabolism, *Biochem Biophys Res Commun*, 234(Suppl 1):263–268, 1997.

155. Stanisstreet M, Smedley MJ, and Veltkamp CJ, Effects of calcium antagonists and calcium-buffered salines on wound healing in xenopus early embryos, *Cytobios*, 46(Suppl 184):25–35, 1986.

156. Weimann BI and Hermann D, Studies on wound healing: Effects of calcium D-pantothenate on the migration, proliferation, and protein synthesis of human dermal fibroblasts in culture, *Int J Vitam Nutr Res*, 69(Suppl 2):113–119, 1999.

157. Lansdown AB, Calcium: A potential central regulator in wound healing in the skin, *Wound Repair Regen*, 10(Suppl 5):271–285, 2002.

158. Vaxman F, Olender S, and Maldonado H et al., Variations of magnesium, iron, copper, and zinc during the colonic wound-healing process: Experimental study on rabbits, *Eur Surg Res*, 12(Suppl 5):283–290, 1992.

159. Somayaji SN, Jacob AP, and Bairy KL, Effect of tolmeting and its copper complex on wound healing, *Indian J Exp Biol*, 33(Suppl 3):201–204, 1995.

160. Tenaud I, Sainte-Marie I, and Jumbou O et al., *In vitro* modulation of keratinocyte wound healing integrins by zinc, copper, and manganese, *Br J Dermatol*, 140(Suppl 1):26–34, 1999.

161. Sen CK, Khanna S, and Venojarvi M et al., Copper-induced vascular endothelial growth factor expression and wound healing, *Am J Physiol Heart Circ Physiol*, 282(Suppl 5):H1821–1827, 2002.

162. Grzesiak JJ and Pierschbacher MD, Shifts in the concentrations of magnesium and calcium in early porcine and rat wound fluids activate the cell migratory response, *J Clin Invest*, 95(Suppl 1):227–233, 1995.

163. Shivakumar K and Kumar BP, Magnesium deficiency enhances oxidative stress and collagen synthesis in the aorta of rats, *Int J Biochem Cell Biol*, 29(Suppl 11):1273–1278, 1997.

164. Banai S, Haggroth L, and Epstein SE et al., Influence of extracellular magnesium on capillary endothelial cell proliferation and migration, *Circ Res*, 67(Suppl 3):645–650, 1990.

165. Lim Y, Levy M, and Bray TM, Dietary zinc alters early inflammatory responses during cutaneous wound healing in weanling CD-1 mice, *J Nutr*, 134:811–816, 2004.

166. Gray M, Does oral zinc supplementation promote healing of chronic wounds, *J WOCN*, 30:295–299, 2003.

167. Henzel JH, DeWeese MS, and Lichti EL, Zinc concentrations within healing wounds, Significance of post-operative zincuria on availability and requirements during tissue repair, *Arch Surg*, 100(Suppl 4):349–357, 1970.

168. Gonul B, Soylemezoglu T, and Yanicoglu L et al., Effects of epidermal growth factor on serum zinc and plasma prostaglandin E2 levels of mice with pressure sores, *Prostaglandins*, 45(Suppl 2):153–157, 1993.

169. Jones PW, Taylor DM, and Williams DR, Analysis and chemical speciation of copper and zinc in wound fluid, *J Inorg Biochem*, 81(Suppl 1–2):1–10, 2000.

170. Breslow RA, Hallfrisch J, and Goldberg AP, Malnutrition in tubefed nursing home patients with pressure sores, *J Parenter Enteral Nutr*, 15(Suppl 6):663–668, 1991.

171. Henderson CT, Trumbore LS, and Mobarhan S et al., Prolonged tube feeding in long-term care: Nutritional status and clinical outcomes, *J Am Coll Nutr*, 11(Suppl 3):309–325, 1992.

172. Brewer RD Jr, Leal JF, and Mihaldzic N, Preliminary observations on the effect of oral zinc sulfate on the healing of decubitus ulcers, *Proc Annu Clin Spinal Cord Inj Conf*, 15:93–96, 1966.

173. Brewer RD Jr, Mihaldzic N, and Dietz A, The effect of oral zinc sulfate on the healing of decubitus ulcers in spinal cord injured patients, *Annu Clin Spinal Cord Inj Conf*, 16:70–72, 1967.

174. Lansdown AB, Zinc in the healing wound, *Lancet*, 347:706–707, 1996.

175. Lewis B, Zinc and Vitamin C in the aetiology of pressure sores, A review, *J Wound Care*, 5:483–494, 1996.

176. Kohn S, Kohn D, and Schiller D, Effect of zinc supplementation on epidermal Langerhans' cells of elderly patients with decubitus ulcers, *J Dermatol*, 27(Suppl 4):258–263, 2000.

177. Cohen C, Zinc sulphate and bedsores, *Br Med J*, 2(Suppl 604):561, 1968.

178. Abbott DF, Exton-Smith AN, and Millard PH et al., Zinc sulphate and bedsores, *Br Med J*, 2(Suppl 607):763, 1968.

179. Williams CM, Lines CM, and McKay EC, Iron and zinc status in multiple sclerosis patients with pressure sores, *Eur J Clin Nutr*, 42(Suppl 4):321–328, 1988.

180. Gengenbacher M, Stahelin HB, and Scholer A et al., Low biochemical nutritional parameters in acutely ill hospitalized elderly patients with and without stage III to IV pressure ulcers, *Aging Clin Exp Res*, 14(Suppl 5):420–423, 2002.

181. Wilkinson AJ and Hawke CI, Does oral zinc aid in the healing of leg ulcers? *Arch Dermatol*, 134:1556–1560, 1998.

182. Langer G, Schloemer G, and Knerr A et al., Nutritional interventions for preventing and treating pressure ulcers, *Cochrane Database Syst Rev*, (Suppl 4):CD003216, 2003.

183. Kinlaw WB, Levine AS, and Morley JE et al., Abnormal zinc metabolism in type-2 diabetes mellitus, *Am J Med*, 75:273–277, 1983.

184. Niewoehner CB, Allen JI, and Boosalis M et al., Role of zinc supplementation in type-2 diabetes mellitus, *Am J Med*, 81:63–68, 1986.

185. Prasad AS, Zinc deficiency in human subjects, *Prog Clin Biol Res*, 129:1–33, 1983.

186. Morley JE and Silver AJ, Nutritional issues in nursing home care, *Annals of Int Med*, 123(Suppl 11):850–859, 1995.

187. Houston S, Haggard J, and Williford J, Jr, et al., Adverse effects of large-dose zinc supplementation in an institutionalized older population with pressure ulcers, *JAGS*, 49(Suppl 8):1130–1132, 2001.

188. Fosmire G, Zinc toxicity, *Am J Clin Nutr*, 51(Suppl 2):225–227, 1990.

189. Greaves MW and Skillen AW, Effects of long-continued ingestion of zinc sulfate in patients with venous leg ulceration, *Lancet*, 2(Suppl 7679):889–891, 1970.

190. Clayton RJ, Double-blind trial of oral zinc sulphate in patients with leg ulcers, *Br J Clin Prac*, 26(Suppl 8):368–370, 1972.

191. Phillips A, Davidson M, and Greaves MW, Venous leg ulceration: Evaluation of zinc treatment, serum zinc, and rate of healing, *Clin Exp Dermat*, 2(Suppl 24):395–399, 1977.

192. Hallbook T and Lanner E, Serum-zinc and healing of venous ulcers, *Lancet*, 2(Suppl 7781):780–782, 1972.

193. Haeger K and Lanner E, Oral zinc sulphate and ischemic leg ulcers, *VASA*, 3(Suppl 1):77–81, 1974.

194. Haeger K, Lanner E, and Magnusson PO, Oral zinc sulphate in the treatment of venous leg ulcers, *VASA*, 1(Suppl 1):62–69, 1972.

195. Greaves MW and Ive FA, Double-blind trial of zinc sulphate in the treatment of chronic venous leg ulceration, *Br J Dermatol*, 87(Suppl 6):632–634, 1972.

196. Stryer L, Integration of metabolism: Hormonal regulators of fuel metabolism, In: Stryer L, Ed., *Biochemistry*, 3rd ed., New York: W.H, Freeman, 26:636–637, 1988.

197. Vogt PM, Lehnhardt M, and Wagner D et al., Growth factors and insulin-like growth factor binding proteins in acute wound fluid, *Growth Horm IGF Res*, 8(Suppl B):107–109, 1998.

198. Ozkul Y, Sabuncu T, and Yazgan P et al., Local insulin injection improves median nerve regeneration in NIDDM patients with carpal tunnel syndrome, *Eur J Neurol*, 8(Suppl 4):329–334, 2001.

199. Thomas SJ, Morimoto K, and Herndon DN et al., The effect of prolonged euglycemic hyperinsulinemia on lean body mass after severe burn, *Surgery*, 132(Suppl 2):341–347, 2002.

200. Rassias AJ, Marrin CA, and Aarruda J et al., Insulin infusion improves neutrophil function in diabetic cardiac surgery patients, *Anesth Analg*, 88(Suppl 5):1011–1016, 1999.

201. Zhou DP, Lu LQ, and Mao XL, Insulin and hyperosmotic glucose solution external used for treating pressure sore, *Hunan Yi Ke Da Xue Bao*, 26(Suppl 5):475–476, 2001.

202. Clements RH, Hayes CA, and Gibbs ER et al., Insulin's anabolic effect is influenced by route of administration of nutrients, *Arch Surg*, 134:274–277, 1999.

203. Lundholm K and Schers T, Determination *in vitro* of the rate of protein synthesis and degradation in human-skeletal-muscle tissue, *Eur J Biochem*, 60:1–6, 1975.

204. Fulks RM and Goldberg AL, Effects on insulin, glucose, and amino acids on protein turnover in rat diaphragm, *J Biol Chem*, 250:290–298, 1975.

205. Jefferson LS, Li JB, and Rannals SR, Regulation by insulin of amino acid release and protein turnover in the perfused rat hemicorpus, *J Biol Chem*, 252:1476–1483, 1977.
206. Garlick PJ, Fern M, and Preedy VR, The effect of insulin infusion and food intake on muscle protein synthesis in postabsorbtive rats, *Biochem J*, 210:669–676, 1983.
207. Madibally SV, Solomon V, and Mitchell RN et al., Influence of insulin therapy on burn wound healing in rats, *J Surg Res*, 109(Suppl 2):92–100, 2003.
208. Weringer EJ, Kelso JM, and Tamai IY et al., Effects of insulin on wound healing in diabetic mice, *Acta Endocrinol*, 99(Suppl 1)101–108, 1982.
209. Lazar HL, Chipkin SR, and Fitzgerald CA et al., Tight glycemic control in diabetic coronary artery bypass graft patients improves perioperative outcomes and decreases recurrent ischemic events, *Circulation*, 109(Suppl 12):1497–1502, 2004.
210. Black E, Vibe-Petersen J, and Jorgensen LN et al., Decrease of collagen deposition in wound repair in type-1 diabetes independent of glycemic control, *Arch Surg*, 138:34–40, 2003.
211. Sakurai Y, Aarsland A, and Herndon DN et al., Stimulation of muscle protein synthesis by long-term insulin infusion in severely burned patients, *Ann Surg*, 222(Suppl 3):283–297, 1995.
212. Ferrando AA, Chinkes DL, and Wolf SE et al., A submaximal dose of insulin promotes net skeletal muscle protein synthesis in patients with severe burns, *Ann Surg*, 229(Suppl 1):11–18, 1999.
213. Fukagawa NK, Minaker KL, and Rowe JW, Insulin-mediated reduction of whole body protein breakdown, *J Clin Invest*, 76:2306–2311, 1985.
214. Clements R, Pinson T, and Borghesi L et al., Nitrogen balance is achieved and myofibrillar protein catabolism is inhibited by insulin and total parenteral nutrition in trauma patients, *Surg Forum*, 47:147–148, 1996.
215. Pierre EJ, Barrow RE, and Hawkins HK et al., Effects of insulin on wound healing, *J Trauma*, 44(Suppl 2):342–345, 1998.
216. Ziegler TR, Benfell K, and Smith RJ et al., Safety and metabolic effects of L-glutamine administration in humans, *J Parenter Enteral Nutr*, 14(Suppl 4):137S–146S, 1990.

13 Mitochondrial Function in Diabetes: Pathophysiology and Nutritional Therapeutics

Jeffrey I. Mechanick

CONTENTS

INTRODUCTION

Diabetes mellitus is a disease resulting from a variety of genetic abnormalities and environmental factors that generate a common phenotype of hyperglycemia. Type-1 diabetes (T1DM) and type-2 diabetes (T2DM) result from nuclear genomic mutations, and transmission depends on maternal and paternal genotypes according to Mendelian genetics. "Mitochondrial diabetes" (MTDM) results from mutations in both the nuclear genome (Mendelian genetics) and the mitochrondrial genome which are inherited primarily as a maternal trait [1]. Almost no paternal mitochondrial DNA (mtDNA) is inherited, since sperm mitochondria are localized in the tail and disappear during fertilization. Identical twins do not manifest concordance in mtDNA mutations because there is unequal distribution of mitochondria during meiosis. Depending on ethnicity, up to 10% of patients with T2DM have MTDM, and the phenotype depends on how many mutated mitochondria are present [2,3].

Mitochondrial dysfunction is associated with many diseases (see Table 13.1) and with the diabetic state in a variety of ways (see Table 13.2). Generally speaking, diabetes can result from true MTDM, or from a multitude of cytosolic or nuclear derangements that directly or indirectly affect mitochondrial physiology. Food choices and nutritional therapies can be tailored to target specific mitochondrial abnormalities. This can be accomplished by providing different substrates for energy and micronutrients that affect intermediary metabolism and mitochondrial physiology, antioxidants that affect the apoptosis cascade, and nutritional pharmacologic agents that modulate mitochondrial genetics.

MITOCHONDRIAL PHYSIOLOGY

Mitochondria are structurally composed of an outer membrane (OM), intermembrane space, inner membrane (IM), and matrix. They perform functions that ultimately produce energy—including pyruvate oxidation—reducing power generation in the Krebs cycle, fatty acid metabolism, and amino acid metabolism. Mitochondria are also responsible for the coupling of energy liberated by the electron transport chain (ETC) with formation of high-energy phosphate bonds and ATP production (OXPHOS) (see Figure 13.1).

The primary function of mitochondria is formation and provision of energy to drive metabolic processes and sustain a continuous supply of substrate for life. Teleologically, not only is the survival of the individual dependent on competent mitochondrial function, but human evolution is the byproduct of the capacity to generate high-energy compounds, such as ATP. OXPHOS is the process that captures the energy liberated by the formation of water in the ETC and redirects it to synthesize the high-energy chemical bond in ATP. Availability of ADP and, to a lesser extent, reducing equivalents and inorganic phosphate, controls OXPHOS activity. The adenine-nucleotide translocator (ANT) on the inner mitochondrial membrane (IM) exchanges ADP for ATP. Inorganic phosphate is provided by the H^+/Pi symporter, Pi/OH^- antiporter and creatine phosphate shuttle. Reducing equivalents reflect the metabolic state of the individual and are derived from the oxidation of fatty acid in the mitochondria, amino acid in the cytosol, and glucose in the cytosol. These cytosolic-reducing equivalents are transported to the mitochondria via the α-glycophosphate, malate-aspartate, and malate-citrate shuttles. Therefore, OXPHOS is intimately related to the nutritional status of the cell and is regarded as "nutritionally responsive" [5]. During catabolism and increased fatty acid synthesis, less ATP is synthesized and less ATP is consumed for anabolism [6]. With a protein-deficient, fat-deficient, but carbohydrate-sufficient diet, glycolysis, lipogenesis, and fatty acid oxidation are stimulated with little protein synthesis [6]. This produces an early rise in ATP followed by a decline with protein depletion [6].

Regulated, programmed cell death (apoptosis) results from mitochondrial dysfunction and is associated with the chronic hyperglycemic state observed in DM (see Figure 13.2) [7]. According to the "endosymbiont hypothesis," mitochondria provide high-energy chemical bonds in the form of ATP in exchange for physical protection and substrate. There is also a functional relationship between nDNA and mtDNA. However, when physical protection fails and mitochondria are exposed to noxious substances, mitochondrial apoptotic pathways are activated, which are curiously similar to the molecular events accompanying bacterial sporulation [8].

TABLE 13.1
Mitochondrial Diseases

Type of Defect	Effect
Krebs cycle	α-Ketoglutarate deficiency
	Aconitase deficiency
	Di-OH-lipoyldehydrogenase deficiency
	Fumarase deficiency
	Succinate dehydrogenase deficiency
Fatty acid oxidation	Carnitine cycle deficiencies
	Carnitine transport deficiencies
	Carnitine palmityltransferase I deficiency
	Carnitine palmityltransferase II deficiency
	Translocase deficiency
Respiratory chain	Glutaric acidemia II deficiency
Oxidative phosphorylation nuclear DNA	Friedrich's ataxia
	AR hereditary spastic paraplegia
	Wilson's disease
	Leigh's disease
	Optic atrophy and ataxia
	Autosomal dominant progressive external ophthalmoplegia (ADPEO)
	Mitochondrial neurogastrointestinal encephalopathy (MNGIE)
	Chronic progressive external ophthalmoplegia (CPEO)
	Kearns Sayre syndrome (KSS)
	Maternally inherited diabetes and deafness syndrome (MIDD)
	Pearson's bone marrow-pancreas syndrome
	Migraine
	Stroke
Point mutation protein	Leber's hereditary optic neuropathy (LHON)
	LHON/dystonia
	Neurogenic weakness, ataxia, and retinitis pigmentosa (NARP)
	Leigh's disease
tRNA	Mitochondrial encephalopathy, lactic acidosism, and stroke-like episodes (MELAS)
	Myoclonic epilepsy and ragged red fiber disease (MERRF)
	Maternally inherited myopathy with cardiac involvement (MIMyCa)
	MIDD
	Encephalomyopathy
	Leigh's disease
rRNA	Nonsyndromic sensorineural deafness
	Aminoglycoside induced nonsyndromic deafness
Undefined	Luft's disease
	Alpers' disease

Source: Adapted from Reference [4].

In T1DM, autoimmune mechanisms acting through various cytokines such as interleukin-1β (IL-1β), tumor necrosis factor-α (TNF-α), and interferon-γ (IFN-γ) induce nitric oxide (NO) production, disruption of mitochondrial function and release of proapoptotic factors [9]. In MTDM, β-cell apoptosis, leading to decreased glucose-stimulated insulin secretion (GSIS), results from cellular stress or withdrawal of growth factors (e.g., insulin-like growth factor-1 [IGF-1]), via an intrinsic pathway, and not from "death receptors" involving Fas (CD95; APO-1) and tumor necrosis factor (TNF-α) receptor I and II, via an extrinsic pathway [10,11]. It is noteworthy that inhibitors of apoptosis protein (IAP) family members, which bind and inhibit caspases and have been investigated as potential therapies for malignancies and neurodegenerative disorders, could also be potential targets for MTDM therapeutics [12,13].

TABLE 13.2
Summary of Effects of Mitochondrial Dysfunction in Diabetes and Prediabetes

Decreased glucose-stimulated insulin secretion (GSIS)
nDNA mutations
Mitochondrial proteins
Cytosolic proteins affecting mitochondrial function
mtDNA mutations
Primary mtDNA inheritance
Secondary to nDNA mutations (dual-genome defect)
Age-related accumulation due to environmental and dietary factors
Single-nucleotide polymorphisms and decreased enzyme activity
AMPK-PGC1α cascade
Decreased β-cell mass (apoptosis)
Glucose toxicity
Lipotoxicity
Decreased insulin action
Diabetic complications
ROS – NO – peroxynitrite formation
PARP – GADPH pathway
Polyol pathway
AGE formation
PK-C activation
Hexosamine pathway

Abbreviations: AMPK—5-adenosine monophosphate activated protein kinase; PGC1-α—peroxisome proliferators activated receptor-γ coactivators 1α; ROS—reactive oxygen species; NO—nitric oxide; PARP—poly(ADP-ribose)polymerase; GADPH—glyceraldehydes-3-phosphate dehydrogenase; AGE—advanced glycation endproducts; PK-C—protein kinase-C.

The mitochondrial genome, often referred to as a "thrifty genome," differs in structure and function from the nuclear genome in many ways (see Table 13.3) Many mitochondrial diseases have been pinpointed to loci on the mitochondrial genome (see Figure 13.3) and principally affect organs dependent on ATP generation: endocrine, central nervous system (CNS), sensory organs, skeletal muscle, and the heart. The principles for phenotypic expression of mitochondrial disease are complex and will be briefly summarized. One mtDNA mutation can be associated with multiple diseases and one disease can be caused by mtDNA mutations in different mitochondrial genes. Moreover, mitochondrial diseases affect multiple tissue types and organ systems due to the ubiquitous distribution of mitochondria in cells throughout the body. Syndromic differences are recognized by a specific distribution of organs being affected. The proportion of mutated/nonmutated mtDNA copies in the mitochondria is termed "degree of heteroplasmy" and the disproportionate distribution of mutated mtDNA in a certain tissue type is termed "skewed heteroplasmy." Since mtDNA is not replicated in synchrony with cellular division, there is also a random and unequal distribution of mtDNA mutations among cells within the same tissue and among various tissues within the same individual; this is termed "mitotic segregation." Since the appearance of mitochondrial dysfunction in a particular tissue depends on that tissue's metabolic rate, there is a "threshold effect" correlating to the ratio of mutated:nonmutated mtDNA. A good example of this involves the mtDNA mutation of base pair 8993 in the ATPase gene: a mutation rate < 60% produces MTDM, 60–90% produces NARP, and > 90% produces Leigh's disease [48].

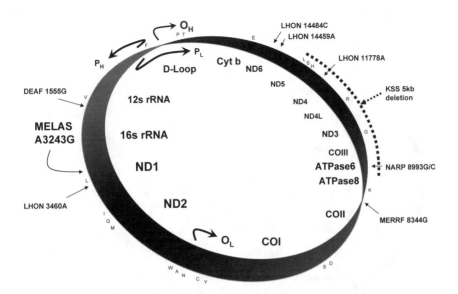

FIGURE 13.1 Human mitochondrial genome and loci for mutations. mtDNA is composed of heavy (main coding) and light strands and contains 16,568 base pairs of which only 6% are noncoding (97% of which are in the two controller regions (OL—origin of replication for the light strand; D-Loop—displacement loop which containts the origin of transcription for the heavy strand [OH])). Six genes share coding nucleotides. Complex I genes code for NADH dehydrogenases (ND1, ND2, ND3, ND4, ND4L, ND5, and ND6). Complex III genes code for ubiquinol:cytochrome-c oxidoreductase (Cyt b). Complex IV genes code for cytochrome-c oxidase (COI, COII, and COIII). Complex V genes code for ATP synthase (ATPase 6 and ATPase 8). The 22 tRNA sequences are designated by the small capital letters outside the loop. There are two genes encoding ribosomal RNA (12s rRNA and 16s rRNA). Straight arrows indicate approximate positions of mtDNA mutations corresponding to the indicated diseases. Abbreviations: LHON—Leber's hereditary optic neuropathy; KSS—Kearns Sayre Syndrome; NARP—Neurogenic weakness, ataxia and retinitis pigmentosa; MERRF—Myoclonic epilepsy and ragged red fibers disease; MELAS—Mitochondrial encephalopathy, lactic acidosis and stroke-like episodes.

MITOCHONDRIAL DIABETES

PATHOPHYSIOLOGY OF MITOCHONDRIAL DIABETES

Mitochondrial diabetes can resemble T2DM, in which there is impaired insulin secretion and insulin resistance, or T1DM, in which there is more severe impairment of insulin secretion. In the consensus model of GSIS, abnormalities among several key mitochondrial enzymes could produce MTDM [21]. The various mtDNA mutations that have been associated with MTDM are given in Table 13.4. In addition to diabetes resulting directly from inherited mitochondrial genomic mutations, defects in mitochondrial functions governing glucose homeostasis can arise from age-related accumulations of mtDNA mutations. These low-level mutations can decrease respiratory chain capacity, increase free radical production and oxidative damage, and then further compromise respiratory chain capacity in a vicious cycle [49].

Mitochondrial diabetes, due to mutations in mtDNA, primarily affects GSIS in the β-cell rather than peripheral glucose utilization. As a result, GSIS is lost in association with decreased glucose oxidation, increased lactate production, and NADH accumulation, but is only marginally associated with decreased glucose utilization and not associated with glibenclamide-induced changes [50].

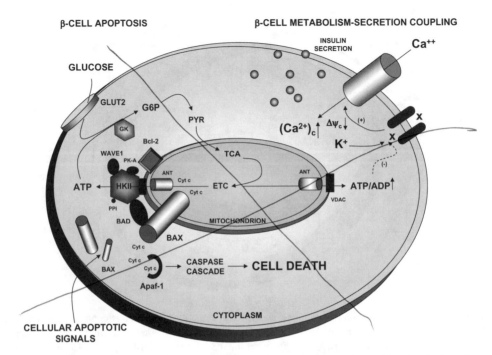

FIGURE 13.2 The mitochondrial electron transport chain (ETC). Pyruvate is formed by glycolysis and enters the tricarboxylic acid (TCA) cycle forming nicotinamide adenine dinucleotide, reduced form (NADH) and flavin adenine dinucleotide ($FADH_2$), which provide electrons to the ETC. Electrons (e^-) flowing along the ETC result in extrusion of protons by complexes I, III, and IV, as well as production of reactive oxygen species (ROS). This creates an electrochemical gradient across the IM ($\Delta\psi_m$). As protons diffuse back into the matrix through ATP synthase, ADP condenses with inorganic phosphate to form a high-energy bond: ATP. ATP is transported into the cytosol in exchange for ADP by the adenine nucleotide translocator (ANT). Leakage of protons through UCP2 lowers $\Delta\psi_m$ and ATP formation. Abbreviations: CoQ—coenzyme Q10; Cyt c—cytochrome-c; UCP2—uncoupling protein 2.

These findings are consistent with β-cell OXPHOS defects causing abnormal GSIS, or "metabolism-secretion coupling" (see Figure 13.2).

The term "glucose toxicity" describes the phenomenon of adverse effects of hyperglycemia on insulin target tissue and pancreatic β-cells. Mitochondrial and extramitochondrial mechanisms of glucose toxicity on the pancreatic β-cells are nonphysiologic, potentially irreversible, and result from chronic exposure of hyperglycemia (see Table 13.5). On the other hand, "glucose desensitization" is generally reversible and results from repeated exposure to hyperglycemia. Because chronic oxidative stress represents a common thread in these mechanisms, nutritional antioxidant therapies can potentially abrogate the feed-forward loop of glucose toxicity that accelerates the evolution from impaired glucose tolerance (IGT) to frank diabetes [64]. Impairment of OXPHOS is the central defect in MTDM and couples glucose metabolism, insulin synthesis, and insulin release [65–67]. Patients with MTDM initially have a T2DM phenotype but can progress and require insulin replacement. Defects in critical cytosolic enzyme systems, encoded by nDNA and that control OXPHOS, can contribute to MTDM. One important example is the "glucose sensor" FAD-linked human mitochondrial glycerol-3-phosphate dehydrogenase (hmGPD). This enzyme catalyzes the rate-limiting step in the glycerol-phosphate shuttle, reoxidizes cytosolic NADH generated by glycolysis, and is impaired in patients with T2DM [68] and in some women with gestational diabetes (GDM) [69]. In addition, patients with GDM may possess one of several

Correct image for figure 13.2, page 226.

Disregard figure printed in book.

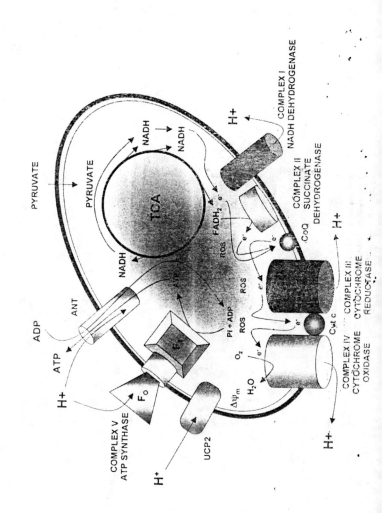

TABLE 13.3
Unique Features of Mitochondrial DNA Compared with Nuclear DNA

No introns or exons
Circular
Tiny
Long primary transcripts of several genes
Small amount of "control DNA"
Little space between genes
Each transcript encodes the pertinent tRNA, rRNA, and mRNA for gene expression
Many mitochondrial codons differ from nuclear codons
Maternally inherited mutations
Deleted mutations rarely transmitted
High rate of mtDNA mutation fixation due to absence of histones and an effective repair system
Vicious cycle: mutated mtDNA causes increases free radicals, which cause more mtDNA mutations
Heteroplasmy: an individual can carry several allelic forms of mtDNA (mixture of mutated:nonmutated mtDNA)
Skewed heteroplasmy: unequal distribution of mutant:nonmutant mtDNA among tissue types
Postmitotic tissue with high-energy demands (e.g., endocrine tissue) are highly sensitive to mtDNA mutations
Rapidly dividing tissue (e.g., bone marrow) are rarely affected by mtDNA mutations
Mitotic segregation
Threshold effect
New mtDNA alleles arise only from spontaneous mutations

Source: Adapted from Reference [4].

mtDNA mutations: C3254A, A3399T, G3316A, T3394C, T3398C, and A3243G [70]. It is also unclear to what extent the development of diabetes in the elderly may reflect the age-related decline in OXPHOS efficiency resulting from accumulated mtDNA mutations [6]. The phenotypic expression of T2DM later in life may also be due to an integration and accumulation of mitochondrial defects arising from nDNA mutations.

Uncoupling proteins (UCP) are members of the ANT family of anion mitochondrial carriers. They are found on the IM and generically serve as a proton shunt to decrease mitochondrial ROS [71]. Uncoupling proteins can also mediate the effects of free radicals on mitochondrial function. UCP1 parcels protons across the IM and diverts energy from OXPHOS. Single-nucleotide polymorphisms in UCP1 have been associated with T2DM [72]. UCP2 is widely expressed and found in pancreatic β-cells. UCP2 is directly activated by the ROS superoxide and indirectly by fatty acids [73,74]. UCP2 activation increases mitochondrial proton leak and decreases mitochondrial membrane potential [74,75]. This leads to decreased ATP levels and GSIS [74,75]. A negative feedback loop is generated when ROS production declines with the decreased mitochondrial membrane potential leading to a steady state [76]. Superoxide-induced activation of UCP2 is therefore important in the pathogenesis of MTDM. In addition to regulating ROS, UCP2 may also be responsible for peroxisome proliferators-activated receptor α (PPAR-α)-independent exportation of free fatty acids from the mitochondria [77–79]. UCP3 is expressed selectively in skeletal muscle and regulates fatty acid metabolism via mitochondrial thioesterase (MTE-1) gene expression and by stimulating glucose transport [80]. Both UCP3 and MTE1 remove fatty acids from the mitochondrial matrix, which liberates coenzyme A (CoA), allowing higher rates of fatty acid oxidation [81]. Dietary fat, via PPAR-α, and insulin stimulate UCP3 gene expression [77].

In contrast to other mitochondrial diseases that require a relatively high ratio of mutated:nonmutated mtDNA, MTDM becomes symptomatic with relatively small amounts of mutated mtDNA [82]. This has been explained by interactions among energy production (respiratory chain efficiency), the glucose sensor [83], NADH shuttle [84,85], and uncoupling proteins [72,86]. On the other hand, when diabetes and deafness occur as part of the diabetes insipidus, diabetes mellitus, optic atrophy, deafness (DIDMOAD) and MIDD syndromes, biochemical defects that directly

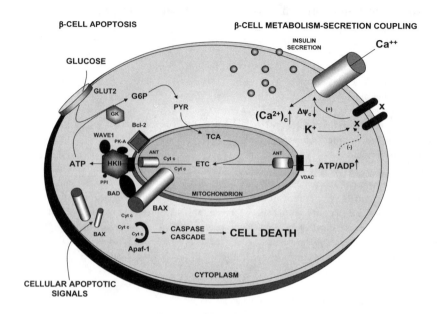

FIGURE 13.3 Apoptosis and metabolism-secretion coupling in a β-cell mitochondrion. Left: Cellular apoptotic signals (hormonal, cytokine, noxious agents) induce BAX translocation from the cytosol to the mitochondrial membrane where it is activated by BAD and inactivated by Bcl-2. Cytochrome-c can be released from the mitochondria into the cytosol via [1] nonspecific leakage as a result of matrix swelling, [2] leakage through BAX oligomerization channels, [3] BAX regulation of voltage-dependent anion channel (VDAC)-adenine nucleotide translocator (ANT) permeability transition pore (mPTP) size, or [4] BAX-induced membrane instability (Reference 14). Cytosolic cytochrome-c interacts with apoptosis protease-activating factor-1 (Apaf-1) and initiates the caspase cascade and eventual apoptosis. Recruitment of hexokinase II (HKII) by insulin and other factors to the mitochondrial membrane forms a functional holoenzyme complex with protein linase-A (PK-A), protein phosphatase 1 (PPI), Wiskott–Aldrich family member, kinase-anchoring protein (WAVE1), and BAD. During normal cellular respiration, terminal oxidation steps in OXPHOS generate ATP, which is shuttled through the PT pore to initiate glucose-6 phosphorylation and formation of glucose-6-phosphate (G6P), the rate-limiting step of glycolysis. The active HKII prevents the mPTP from leaking cytochrome-c. Right: Normal cellular respiration produces an increased ATP/ADP ratio which closes ATP-dependent potassium channels, depolarizes the cell membrane, opens the voltage-activated calcium channel, increases intracellular calcium, and then facilitates insulin secretion.

result from the associated mutant mtDNA are insufficient to cause significant mitochondrial dysfunction [87,88]. Table 13.6 summarizes several mitochondrial diabetes syndromes.

Non-T1DM is classified as polygenic or monogenic. Monogenic DM results from a nDNA mutation, a mtDNA mutation, one of the maturity-onset diabetes of the young (MODY) mutations, or atypical diabetes mellitus of African-Americans (ADM). When maternal transmission of T2DM and features suggestive of a mitochondrial disease are evident, screening for one of the mtDNA mutations associated with MTDM should be performed [89]. This strategy is reinforced by the recent observation by Petersen et al. [90], that insulin-resistant offspring of patients with T2DM harbored demonstrable OXPHOS defects. Thus, an increased awareness of mitochondria-targeted nutritional therapy in DM is justified.

TABLE 13.4
Forty-Three mtDNA Mutations Associated with Diabetes Mellitus

Mutation Type	Gene	Mutation (ref)	Clinical Features	A3243G Mutation Present
rRNA				
	12S rRNA	C946A(15)	HC	+
		A1041G(15)	HC	+
		C1310T(16)	DF	n/a
		G1438A(16)	DF	n/a
	16S rRNA	G1888A(17)	MERRF, DF, LHON	−
		C3093G(18)	MELAS, CM, HT	+
tRNA				
	tRNA^Leu (UUR)	A3243G(19,20)	MELAS, DF, CPP	+
		A3252G(15,21)	MM	−
		C3254A(15,21)		n/a
		C3256T(22)	MM, LHON	−
		A3260G(15,21)	MM, CM	−
		T3264C(23,24)	MT, MERRF, CPEO, DF	−
		T3271C(15,21)	MELAS	−
tRNA^ile		G4284A(25)	PSP	−
tRNA^Lys		A8296G(26-28)	MERRF, MELAS, DF	−
		A8344G(29)	MERRF	−
		T8356C(30)	MERRF	−
		G8363A(26)	MERRF	−
		A8381G(17)	DF	n/a
tRNA^Ser		C12258A(31)	USHIII	−
tRNA^Glu		7472insC(32,33)	EPC, DF	−
		T14709C(17,34)	MM, DF	−
		A14693G(35)	MELAS	+
Complex I (NADH dehydrogenase)				
	ND1	G3316A(36)	—	−
		T3394C(37,38)	HC, LHON	+
		A3397G(39)	LHON	+
		T3398C(40)		n/a
		A3399T(15,21)		n/a
		T4216G(17)	MERRF, DF, LHON	−
	ND2	G4491A(15,21)	HC	+
		A4833G(41)	FHH	−
		A4917G(18)	MERRF, DF, LHON	−
		Mt5178C(42)	—	−
		A5466G(43)	DF, CM, CSA	−
	ND4	G11963A(15)	HC	+
		A12026G(16)	DF	n/a
	ND4L	T10601C(43)	DF, CM, CSA	−
	ND6	T14577C(44)	—	−
Complex III (cytochrome b)				
	Cyt b	A15662G(40)		
		G15812A(40)		
Complex IV (cytochrome-c oxidase)				
	COXII	G7912A(43)	DF, CM, CSA	−
Complex V ATP synthase				
	ATPase 8	A8381G(15,21)	DF	−
D-loop		T16189C(45–47)	—	−

Abbreviations: HC—hypertrophic cardiomyopathy; CM—cardiomyopathy; HT—hypothyroidism; MT—multiple tumors; PSP—"pure" spastic paraparesis; DF—sensineural hearing loss; CPP—chronic progressive ptosis; EPC—epilepsia partialis continua; MM—mitochondrial myopathy; FHH—familial hypocalciuric hypercalcemia; CSA—central sleep apnea; see Table 13.1, appendix II, and text for other abbreviations.

Source: Reference adapted from Rosenbloom et al. [15] and Maechler and Wollheim [21].

TABLE 13.5
Mitochondrial and Extramitochondrial Mechanisms of Glucose Toxicity and Desensitization in Pancreatic β-cells

Glucose toxicity

Mitochondrial	*Extramitochondrial*
NAD(P)H depletion	GK overactivity (glucose overload)
ATP depletion	Increased CREM-17X expression (suppresses insulin gene promoter)
ROS buildup	Increased C/EBP-β expression (suppresses E47 dimerization and insulin gene activity)
Oxidative inury	Decreased STF-1 binding (decreases insulin gene transcription)
Increased UCP2	Decreased RIPE-3b1 binding (decreases insulin gene transcription)
Apoptosis	Post-translational defect in IPF-1/PDX-1 mRNA maturation (decreases insulin gene transcription)
	Protein glycation (decreased insulin gene transcription)
	Increased glycated insulin (less biologic activity)
	Activation of NF-κB
	AMPK activation – malonyl CoA fuel sensor – CPT-I

Glucose desensitization

Mitochondrial	*Extramitochondrial*
Decreased "metabolism-secretion coupling" via Ca^{++} uniporter	Decreased insulin translational rates
	Decreased GK gene expression
	Impaired insulin exocytosis

Abbreviations: NAD(P)H—nicotinamide adenine dinucleotide phosphate, reduced form; GK—glucokinase; CREM—cAMP response element modulator; C/EBP—CCAAT/enhancer-binding protein; ROS—reactive oxygen species; UCP2—uncoupling protein-2; STF—somatostatin transcription factor; RIPE—rat insulin promoter element; IPF—insulin promoter factor; PDX—pancreatic duodenal homeobox; NF-κB—nuclear transcription factor; AMPK—5-adenosine monophosphate-activated protein kinase; CPT—carnitine palmitoyltransferase.

Source: References 51–63.

GENERAL TREATMENT STRATEGIES FOR PRIMARY MITOCHONDRIAL DISEASES

Treatment options for mitochondrial disease are profoundly inadequate. Patients are generally treated with conventional medical therapy for the individual phenotypic features of the disease and offered genetic counseling. However, treatment of the proximate cause of the disease—mitochondrial dysfunction—is elusive. Others strategies consist of dietary supplements and nutraceuticals designed to target specific mitochondrial pathways thought to be contributing to the disease process. Specifically, many nutritional therapies are offered to patients based on sound theory and data from preclinical studies, but are derived from clinical studies with varying levels of scientific substantiation [91]. Unfortunately, many patients who are not deriving any benefit from conventional therapy are offered therapies that are not based on any rational theory, have no proven benefit, have varying levels of risk, result from profiteering, and represent frank quackery [91]. Ryan et al. [92] found that 31% of diabetic patients take alternative-care medications, a figure comparable to the 37% of nondiabetics who take alternative-care medications. In general, therapeutic strategies for mitochondrial disorders, amenable to nutritional intervention, include the use of artificial electron acceptors, cofactors, and metabolites to (1) remove noxious compounds; (2) reduce ROS formation; and (3) enhance OXPHOS efficiency.

Gene therapy efforts are encouraging but challenged by the need to target specific organelles in affected cells. Current gene therapy strategies target selective destruction of mutant mtDNA

Table 13.6
Genetic, Biochemical, and Clinical Features of Some Mitochondrial Diabetes Syndromes

Syndrome	Genetics	Biochemical Features	Clinical Features
MODY	Autosomal dominant nDNA mutations in insulin gene transcription factors (HNF-1α, -1β, -4α; IPF1/PDX1; NEUROD1/BETA2) and GK (HKIV)	Impaired insulin gene expression, GSIS, and anti-apoptosis	1–5% all DM; presents < age 25 years; primary insulinopenia; absence of obesity; nonketotic; slowly progressive
ADM	Autosomal dominant mtDNA point mutation in T3308C mtDNA; A8296G mutation; nDNA mutation in GK nDNA; missense mutation Gly574Ser in HNF-1α	Severe β-cell defect	5–10% DM in children; initially insulin-dependent; eventually non-insulin-dependent; obesity prevalent
MIDD, or Ballinger–Wallace syndrome	mtDNA A3243G point mutation encoding tRNA^{LEU} heteroplasmic T14709C mtDNA mutation	Impaired GSIS inactive aldehyde dehydrogenase 2; atypical alcohol dehydrogenase 2; no peripheral insulin resistance; increased degradation of mitochondrial proteins	1–2% DM in Europe and Japan; T1DM or T2DM phenotypes; T2DM patients become insulin requiring; present < age 35 years; low BMI; hearing loss, cardiomypathy, neurologic symptoms, renal insufficiency
DIDMOAD, or Wolfram syndrome	nDNA mutation in WFS1 gene encoding wolframin mtDNA polymorphisms LHON-associated mtDNA Point mutation	nDNA mutation predisposes mtDNA to deletions and mutations via a susceptibility factor (dual-genome defect); wolframin is an ER Ca channel in β-cells and neurons	Juvenile-onset DM, presents in first decade
MELAS	mtDNA A3243G mutation mtDNA T3271C mutation	Impaired GSIS	Mitochondrial encephalomyopathy, lactic acidosis, stroke-like episodes
MERFF	mtDNA A83446, G8363A, and T8356C mutations; encoding tRNA^{LYS} (terminates translation)	Formation of truncated mitochondrial peptides impaired GSIS	Myoclonic epilepsy with red ragged fibers
KSS	Large-scale mtDNA deletions and duplications	Impaired GSIS	Ocular myopathy and pigmentary retinopathy; heart block; ataxia; endocrinopathy (GH deficiency, hypogonadism, DM, hypoparathyroidism, adrenal insufficiency)

(continued)

Table 13.6 (continued)
Genetic, Biochemical, and Clinical Features of Some Mitochondrial Diabetes Syndromes

Syndrome	Genetics	Biochemical Features	Clinical Features
Pearson bone marrow– pancreas syndrome	Large-scale mtDNA deletion	Impaired GSIS	T1DM picture; small birth weight; anemia, tubulopathy (renal Fanconi syndrome); lactic acidosis and complex organic aciduria
Usher syndrome Type-III-like	mtDNA C12258A mutation encoding the MTTS2 gene (second mitochondrial tRNA^{SER})	Impaired GSIS	Cerebellar ataxia; cataracts; DM

via (1) introduction of the gene for a restriction endonuclease (e.g., Sma I) that can be imported by mitochondria to selectively destroy the mutant mtDNA [93]; (2) replacement of the mutant mtDNA-encoded protein with a genetically engineered nDNA-encoded equivalent protein (allotropic expression) [94–96]; (3) replacement of a defective respiratory chain complex (resulting from a mutant mtDNA or nDNA) with an nDNA-encoded equivalent complex from another organism [97]; and (4) mitochondrial importation of normal cytoplasmic tRNA with an altered aminoacylation identity to compensate for mutant mtDNA-encoded mitochondrial tRNA [98]. "Gene shifting" can reduce heteroplasmy (mutated:nonmutated mtDNA) and has been accomplished in patients with KSS and myopathy through the use of concentric exercise training [99].

GENERAL OVERVIEW OF NUTRITIONAL THERAPIES TARGETING MITOCHONDRIAL FUNCTION OR USED FOR MITOCHONDRIAL DIABETES

Patients with MTDM typically have the phenotypic appearance of T2DM. Therefore, they are treated with conventional approaches for all T2DM: an appropriate diet, oral agents, and insulin depending on the severity of the glucose intolerance and idiosyncratic factors. Treatment of MODY1, MODY3, and MODY4 is with oral hypoglycemic agents, MODY5 and MODY6 with insulin, and MODY2 with diet and exercise [100]. Proven specific nutritional therapies for MTDM are lacking. For the most part, the medical literature discusses nutritional agents based on theoretical actions on mitochondrial physiology and limited scientific evidence.

Nutritional therapies that are recommended to patients with MTDM are generally extrapolated from experience, both anecdotal and scientifically investigated, involving mitochondrial cytopathies [101]. Broad therapeutic strokes target bioenergetic augmentation and free radical reduction. The overarching presumption is that mitochondria harboring mutated DNA and impaired OXPHOS must have relative, or "functional," deficiencies in certain micronutrients acting as cofactors. According to this paradigm, simple dietary replacement of these cofactors would have a salutary effect. This assertion, however, is supported by relatively weak clinical evidence.

In general, pancreatic β-cells have relatively low levels of antioxidant, cytoprotective enzymes such as catalase, glutathione peroxidase, and superoxide dismutase [102,103]. In the Third National Health and Nutrition Examination Survey of 8808 U.S. adults, the metabolic syndrome was associated with suboptimal concentrations of antioxidants [104]. In addition, the antioxidant status in T1DM and T2DM correlates with lipid status and dietary intake of saturated fat and cholesterol, but not the dietary intake of the respective antioxidant [105]. In diabetic C57BL/KsJ-db/db mice, in which chronic hyperglycemic induces apoptosis and reduced β-cell mass, the antioxidants N-acetyl-L-cysteine, vitamin C, and vitamin E suppress apoptosis and improve GSIS [106]. Antioxidant therapy plays a central role in the various nutritional strategies for patients with

MTDM. Polyphenolics (chrysin, quercetin, catechin, and caffeic acid) derived from certain teas, fruits, and vegetables can function as pro- or anti-oxidants [107]. "Symptomatic" therapies, involving various antioxidants, are differentiated from "causal" antioxidant therapies that target the pathological formation of ROS during OXPHOS. Examples of causal therapies are protein kinase β isoform inhibition (LY 333531), poly(ADP-ribose)polymerase (PARP) inhibition (PJ34), and peroxynitrate inhibition (FP15) [108]. Overall, the use of antioxidant preconditioning and therapy in DM is based on theory and clinical data demonstrating associations rather than causal effects [109,110].

On the other hand, a sequence of discoveries over the last decade linking fatty acid metabolism and mitochondrial bioenergetics with obesity and diabetes has directed therapies toward optimal intake of fat and carbohydrate. These discoveries are: (1) muscle insulin resistance predicting the development of T2DM; (2) β-cell dysfunction preceding frank hyperglycemia; (3) muscle and liver lipid accumulation also preceding clinical onset of T2DM; (4) thiazolidinedione-induced delay in β-cell dysfunction and prevention of T2DM onset, via interaction with PPAR-γ; (5) association of a polymorphism of PPAR-γ coactivator-1 (PGC-1) with T2DM and obesity; and (6) the demonstration of mitochondrial gene mutations linking defects in muscle and β-cells in T2DM [111].

TECHNICAL REVIEW OF SPECIFIC NUTRITIONAL THERAPIES TARGETING MITOCHONDRIAL FUNCTION IN DIABETIC AND PREDIABETIC PATIENTS

Due to the paucity of large, well-designed clinical trials, nutritional therapy of MTDM has relied on extrapolation from evidence of related conditions. Additionally, the medical literature is populated with reviews espousing alternative medicine approaches. The technical reviews that follow serve to prioritize scientific evidence in clinical decision making and rational implementation of available therapeutic agents. Levels of scientific substantiation and recommendation grades are given in Appendix 2.

PROTEIN AND AMINO ACIDS

Certain amino acids (arginine, citrulline, glycine, taurine, and histidine), small peptides (glutathione and carnosine), and nitrogenous metabolites (creatine and uric acid) directly scavenge ROS [112]. Although leucine can stimulate insulin release and is directly used by mitochondria to form acetyl CoA [113], there are no clinical data demonstrating benefits of leucine-enriched diets in patients with MTDM. Low-protein diets are associated with zinc deficiency and iron overload, which contribute further to oxidative injury [114,115]. On the other hand, high-protein diets increase ROS generation and inducible nitric oxide synthase (iNOS) [116–118]. Though there are data indicating that a diet with 30% protein, 40% carbohydrate, and 30% fat is associated with improved glycemic control—compared with a diet with 15% protein, 55% carbohydrate, and 30% fat—there are no data to support the notion that protein can directly improve mitochondrial function [119].

Taurine, a naturally occurring sulfur-containing amino acid, is abundant in mammalian plasma and tissues but not a component of protein. Taurine has pleiotropic effects, including modulation of calcium fluxes, maintenance of photoreceptor cells, modulation of neuronal excitability, osmoregulation, inhibition of iNOS, and cell proliferation [118,120]. In addition, taurine is normally incorporated into tRNA at the first uridine anticodon position to confer precise codon recognition during translation [121]. Suzuki et al. [121] discovered that in patients with the mitochondrial diseases, MELAS and MERRF, there is an absence of normal post-transcriptional modification of the tRNA[LEU(UUR)] (with the A3243G or U3271C mtDNA mutations) and tRNA[LYS] (with the A8344G mtDNA mutation). Thus, deficient decoding arising from this modification defect, along with the point mutation, contributes to mitochondrial dysfunction [121]. There are no clinical data demonstrating any role of dietary taurine adjustments on mitochondrial disorders or diabetes.

Overall, there is no proven role for high-protein diets or any other manipulation of the dietary protein content that targets mitochondrial function in the management of DM or, more specifically, MTDM (conflicting level 3 evidence; recommendation grade D).

FATTY ACIDS

Polyunsaturated fatty acids (PUFA) are susceptible to oxidation by ROS [122]. In pancreatic β-cells, inducible iNOS gene expression is increased with dietary saturated fatty acids as extracellular fatty acid and low-density lipoprotein (LDL) concentrations rise [118,123]. In rats, a high-fat diet reduces gene expression governing free radical scavenging; despite this, mitochondrial function in skeletal muscle remains unaltered [124]. PUFA with ω-3 structure (docosahexaenoic acid, eicosapentaenoic acid, and α-linolenic acid) inhibit free radical formation, inhibit iNOS expression, and increase expression of antioxidant (glutathione-S-transferases, UCP-2, and manganese superoxide dismutase [Mn-SOD]) and lipid catabolism genes via PPAR-α activation [125–127]. PPAR-δ activation has also been associated with beneficial effects on insulin resistance and the metabolic syndrome [128].

Another hypothesis, which has been asserted but not elucidated, is that a β-cell defect in insulin secretion, leading to hyperinsulinemia and the insulin resistance syndrome, involves dietary fat and the malonyl-CoA-acetyl-CoA carboxylase (ACC) fuel sensor [129,130]. Historically, the Randle hypothesis asserts that fatty acids induce insulin resistance via inhibition of pyruvate dehydrogenase (PDH) [131]. A novel alternative hypothesis asserts that fatty acids sequentially induce (1) malonyl CoA generation by the ACC isoform 2 (ACC2); (2) inhibition of the mitochondrial carnitine shuttle; (3) accumulation of intracellular fatty acid metabolites; (4) activation of the serine kinase cascade; (5) reduction of insulin receptor substrate-1 (IRS-1; an intracellular docking protein involved in insulin and insulin-like growth factor [IGF] signaling), tyrosine phosphorylation, and phosphatidylinositol-3-kinase (PI3K) activity; and (6) reduction of GLUT4 activity [132,133].

Dietary influences and mitochondrial gene mutations induce an increase in *de novo* fatty acid synthesis, gluconeogenesis, glycogen storage, and cholesterol synthesis, followed by impaired glucose tolerance and then eventually renal disease [134–137]. In the diabetes-prone BHE/Cdb rat, there is an amino acid substitution in the complex V (F_1F_0ATPase) anchoring subunit 6, which confers susceptibility of the F_0 portion to mitochondrial membrane fluidity changes [138]. This strain of rats has impaired β-cell insulin release, age-related impaired glucose tolerance, diabetic nephropathy and aberrant metabolic control [66,139–141]. When fed a diet high in hydrogenated coconut oil (high in trans-fatty acids [TFA]), membrane viscosity increases and ATP production becomes impaired [5,21]. On the other hand, when fed a diet high in sardine oil (high in omega-3 fatty acids [n-3 FA]), ATP production was increased [5,21]. Other animal studies have confirmed that dietary TFA lowers mitochondrial OXPHOS [142].

Earlier studies conducted by Stein et al. [143] demonstrate that GSIS is influenced, not only by ambient glucose levels, but by free fatty acid (FFA) chain length and degree of saturation (see Table 13.7). Specifically, a high ratio of saturated to unsaturated fatty acid in the plasma pool acutely (< 6 hours) promotes insulin hypersecretion [143,144]. With chronic elevation of plasma fatty acids (24–48 hours), lipotoxicity occurs in patients with T2DM [145–147]. It should be noted that the pro-apoptotic and deleterious GSIS effects of hyperlipidemia are only observed in the setting of preexisting hyperglycemia [148]. In addition, conflicting *in vitro* and clinical data demonstrate a stimulatory effect of FFA on GSIS after 48–72 hours [149,150]. One could postulate that this augmentation of insulin secretion prevents the onset of T2DM in the > 80% of obese patients with FFA-induced insulin resistance [151]. The saturated fat palmitic acid activates the apoptotic mitochondrial pathway in β-cells via ceramide formation and suppression of Bcl-2 gene expression [152]. On the other hand, monounsaturated fatty acids (MUFA) prevent this effect and can promote β-cell proliferation [152].

TABLE 13.7

Quantitative Potency of Various Dietary Fatty Acids on First- and Second-Phase GSIS from Perfused Pancreas of Fasted Rats

Fatty Acid	Fold Increase in Total Insulin Secretion[a]
Octanoate ($C_{8:0}$)	3.4
Linoleate ($C_{18:2\ cis/cis}$)	5.3
Oleate ($C_{18:1\ cis}$)	9.4
Palmitate ($C_{16:0}$)	16.2
Stearate ($C_{18:0}$)	21.0

[a] Control insulin secretion is 6.7 ng during 12.5 mM glucose infusion; fatty acid was added to medium at a concentration of 0.5 mM.

Source: From Reference [143] with permission.

Energy-controlled high-MUFA diets have beneficial effects on LDL particle size, endothelial activation, inflammation, blood pressure, coagulation, thermogenic capacity, and obesity in diabetic patients [153]. Oleic acid (cis C18:1 n-9) accounts for over 90% of MUFA in MUFA-containing foods (see Table 13.8). The plasma fatty acid pool and GSIS are also influenced by adipocyte differentiation induced by conjugated linoleic acid-mediated PPAR-γ activation [154,155]. This observation can be extrapolated to humans and account for the epidemiologic association of dietary saturated fat overconsumption with heart disease, obesity, β-cell defects, insulin resistance, metabolic syndrome, and aging [156–162].

Certain fatty acids have also been demonstrated to rescue HNF-4α mutant activity and therefore show promise in patients with MODY1, though no clinical data are available yet [163]. A patient with MELAS and the A3243G mtDNA mutation was reported who demonstrated improvement in auditory disturbance, cerebellar ataxia, and glycemic control following treatment with eicosapentaenoic acid ethyl ester (EPA-E), 2700 mg daily [164]. Overall, mitochondrial physiology (theory), abundant pre-clinical evidence, and limited clinical evidence support the use of dietary ω-3 FA and MUFA, reduction of saturated fats, and elimination of TFA in the nutritional management of MTDM (conflicting level 3 evidence; recommendation grade C).

COENZYME Q10

Coenzyme Q10 (CoQ10; ubiquinone) acts as an electron shuttle from complex I (NADH dehydrogenase) and complex II (succinate dehydrogenase) to complex III. It is also an essential cofactor in the proton-pumping action of uncoupling proteins [165] and an inhibitor of the mitochondrial permeability transition pore (mPTP), which plays a role in the early phases of apoptosis [166]. CoQ10 also localizes in other endomembranes, including Golgi apparatus and endoplasmic reticulum [167], where it serves as an antioxidant by reducing the α-tocopherolfree radical and, as a result, the pro-oxidant activity of vitamin E [168]. CoQ10 redox activity is also found in lysosomal [169] and plasma membrane [170] electron transport systems. Overall, CoQ10 can be envisioned as a proton translocator and free radical source that regulates the cytoplasmic redox potential with a specific efficiency that varies based on the biomembrane upon which it acts [171]. In rabbits fed a diet enriched with TFA, CoQ10 improves fasting and postprandial insulin levels [172]. In some diabetics, CoQ10 stores become deficient [173] and correlate with poor glycemic control and the development of diabetic complications [174]. Purported antiatherogenic properties of CoQ10 have also been described [175]. Chew and Watts [176] postulate a beneficial effect of CoQ10 during oxidative stress whereby endothelial NOS is "recoupled" with OXPHOS. This attenuates endothelial injury and can theoretically potentiate the beneficial effects of TZD, statins, and fibrates.

TABLE 13.8
Dietary Sources with High MUFA Content

Dietary Source	Energy (MJ)	Fat (g)	SFA (g)	MUFA (g)	PUFA (g)
Vegetable oils					
Sunflower oil (100 g)	3.7	100	9.7	83.6	3.8
Safflower oil (100 g)	3.7	100	6.2	74.6	14.4
Olive oil (100 g)	3.7	100	13.5	73.7	8.4
Canola oil (100 g)	3.7	100	7.1	58.9	29.6
Nuts					
Macadamia nuts (100 g)	3.0	75.8	12.1	58.9	1.5
Hazelnuts (100 g)	2.6	60.7	4.5	45.7	7.9
Pecans (100 g)	2.9	72.0	6.2	40.8	21.6
Almonds (100 g)	2.4	50.6	3.9	32.2	12.2
Cashews (100 g)	2.4	46.4	9.2	27.3	7.8
Peanuts (100 g)	2.4	49.2	6.8	24.4	15.6
Pistachios (100 g)	2.3	44.4	5.4	23.3	13.4
Fruit					
Avocado (100 g)	0.7	15.3	2.4	9.6	2.0
Olives (100 g)	0.5	10.7	1.4	7.9	0.9
Animal products					
Ground beef (100 g)	1.3	26.6	10.8	11.6	1.1
Fried eggs (2)	0.8	15.0	4.2	6.0	2.8
Butter (25 g)	0.8	20.2	12.6	5.9	0.8
Fried bacon (3 slices)	0.5	9.4	3.3	4.5	1.1

Abbreviations: SFA—saturated fatty acid; MFA—monounsaturated fatty acid; PUFA—polyunsaturated fatty acid.

Source: From Reference [153] with permission.

In animal studies, CoQ10 dosing can improve antioxidant status and decrease the susceptibility of mPTP opening with calcium and oxidative stress, but CoQ10 can also worsen the hepatic effect of diabetes [177–179]. Based on several uncontrolled clinical trials, McCarty [180] proposed that correction of suboptimal CoQ10 status could improve β-cell function. However, in a randomized, double-blind, placebo-controlled study of patients with T2DM, there was no demonstrable benefit of CoQ10 [181]. Eriksson et al. [182] also failed to demonstrate an effect of CoQ10 on metabolic control in a randomized, placebo-controlled trial of 23 patients with T2DM. In a randomized, double-blind, placebo-controlled 2×2 factorial intervention study of fenofibrate and CoQ10 in 74 patients with T2DM, CoQ10 supplementation was associated with improved blood pressure and long-term glycemic control [183]. The beneficial effects of CoQ10 on endothelial function were demonstrated by Watts et al. [184] in a randomized, double-blind, placebo-controlled trial of 40 patients with T2DM. In a subsequent randomized, placebo-controlled study of 80 dyslipidemic patients with T2DM, beneficial effects of fenofibrate and CoQ10 on circulation were demonstrated [185].

Data examining the role of CoQ10 in patients with MTDM are very limited. Some case reports have described variable benefit in patients with MTDM with treatment regimens that incorporate CoQ10 [186–190]. In a study of 50 patients with the A3243G mutation (28 with MIDD, 7 with impaired glucose tolerance, and 15 with normal glucose tolerance), CoQ10 treatment improved glucagon-induced C-peptide secretion and 24-hour urinary C-peptide excretion in the MIDD patients compared with controls [191]. This study was not placebo-controlled or adequately randomized.

Finally, CoQ10 is a natural lipid antioxidant and not water soluble. This fact essentially precludes its efficacy as a therapeutic agent and seriously challenges any of the above medicinal claims. CoQ10 analogs have been developed to circumvent this problem. For example, the short-chain CoQ10 analog, idebenone, increases ROS formation [192] while the CoQ10 analog, decylubiquinone, decreases ROS production, mPTP opening, and apoptosis [193]. Therefore, based on (1) the above clinical data with a single, unconfirmed level 2 study involving MTDM; (2) extrapolation from the use of CoQ10 in mitochondrial myopathies; (3) extrapolation from the use of CoQ10 in T2DM; (4) the dubious nature of any significant benefit of CoQ10 due to poor water solubility; and (5) no significant adverse effects, CoQ10 may have limited benefit in the management of MTDM with a preference for the CoQ10 analogs that are well-absorbed (recommendation grade C).

α-LIPOIC ACID

α-Lipoic acid (LA; thioctic acid) is an eight-carbon disulfide compound with a single chiral carbon and is easily reduced to a dithiol form, dihydrolipoic acid. The most abundant plant sources of LA are spinach, broccoli, and tomatoes [194]. LA is responsible for (1) protein repair, primarily of oxidized methionine, cysteine and tyrosine residues; (2) free radical scavenging; (3) elevation of glutathione and regeneration of vitamins C and E; and (4) chelation of metals [195]. In humans, LA is synthesized in the liver, where it also functions as a cofactor in multienzyme dehydrogenase complexes, such as PDH, localized in the mitochondria [196]. In a study by Korotchkina et al. [197], various thiol compounds (low-molecular-weight glutathione and cysteine > LA) protect against lipid peroxidation products that mediate mitochondrial free radical damage. In rats, LA partially reverses age-related oxidative stress, mitochondrial dysfunction, and apoptosis [198–200] via (1) increasing reduced glutathione and vitamins C and E; (2) increasing the activity of mitochondrial dehydrogenases and cytochrome-c oxidase; and (3) stimulating mitochondrial Ca^{++} release and mitochondiral permeability transition pore (mPTP) opening [194,200].

LA has been used to safely treat diabetic peripheral neuropathy and cardiovascular autonomic neuropathy in doses up to 1800 mg/day [201–203]. In the α-lipoic acid in diabetic neuropathy (ALADIN) [204] and ALADIN II [205] trials, short-term (3 weeks) and long-term (2 years) use of 600–1200 mg daily of LA were associated with beneficial effects on nerve conduction. However, in the ALADIN III [206] trial, a 3-week intravenous course followed by a 6-month oral course of LA, 600 mg daily, failed to significantly improve neuropathic symptoms, though favorable effects on neuropathic deficits were demonstrated. In the SYDNEY trial [207] a randomized, parallel, placebo-controlled, double-blind study of 120 T1DM or T2DM patients with A1C < 12%, LA, 600 mg daily for 5 days/week for 14 treatments, rapidly and significantly improved neuropathic sensory symptoms. This effect was due to improved neurophysiology and not increased nerve fiber regeneration [207]. In a series of 39 patients with T2DM, LA corrected the oxidative stress-related impairment of NO-mediated vasodilation [208]. When administered with acetyl-L-carnitine (ALCAR), LA decreases age-associated mitochondrial decay in the rat heart [209].

Other studies have demonstrated effects of LA on insulin sensitivity [210–213] via stimulation of GLUT1 and GLUT4, increased tyrosine phosphorylation, oxidation of thiol groups in the β-subunit of the insulin receptor and in IRS-1, and increased PI3K and protein kinase B (PKB) activities [194,210–214]. Specifically, LA induces GLUT4 translocation and p38 mitogen-activating protein kinase (MAPK)-mediated regulation of GLUT4 intrinsic activity [215]. LA increases oxidative and nonoxidative glucose metabolism which reduces insulin resistance in rats [216]. In a study by Midaoui et al. [217], LA prevents the increase in heart mitochondrial ROS formation, AGE formation, hypertension, and hyperglycemia in chronically glucose-fed insulin-resistant rats. In contrast to insulin effects in muscle, LA can act as a mild pro-oxidant, uncouple OXPHOS and ROS generation, and increase glucose oxidation, but also inhibit glycogen synthesis [218]. In a small, single-arm, observational study of 21 patients with T2DM, controlled-release LA—900 mg daily for 6 weeks, and then 1200 mg daily for 6 weeks—was well-tolerated and associated with a significant reduction in fructosamine levels in 15 patients [219]. Overall, there is evidence to support the use of LA in diabetes, especially in the treatment of peripheral neuropathy, due to its effects on mitochondrial function (evidence level 3). Adverse effects are not significant (recommendation grade C).

CARNITINE

Carnitine is a dipeptide derived from dietary sources, such as meat and dairy products, or from endogenous synthesis by combining the essential amino acids methionine and lysine. Carnitine participates in a variety of biochemical processes, such as:

1. β-oxidation of long-chain fatty acids in mitochondria
2. β-oxidation of very long-chain fatty acids in peroxisomes
3. Transfer of acetyl and other short-chain acyl groups from peroxisomes to mitochondria
4. Re-esterification of triacylglycerol in endoplasmic reticulum before secretion as very-low-density lipoproteins (VLDL)
5. Stimulation of pyruvate and branched-chain amino acid oxidative metabolism
6. Removal and scavenging of toxic acyl groups
7. Deacylation and reacylation for erythrocyte membrane phospholipid remodeling
8. Metabolism of neuronal phospholipid and triglyceride fatty acids
9. Synthesis and elongation of polyunsaturated fatty acids
10. Stabilization of proteins and membranes
11. Protection of membranes from denaturing solute effects and osmotic stress [220,221]

Insulin regulation of carnitine palmitoyltransferase I (CPT I) is a critical step in mitochondrial fatty acid-glucose crosstalk [222]. This step is modulated by fasting, high-carbohydrate diets, high-fat diets, and diabetes [220]. CPT I is an outer mitochondrial membrane enzyme that catalyzes the formation of long-chain acylcarnitines. Carnitine-acyl-carnitine translocase (CACT) transports long-chain acylcarnitines across membranes. Carnitine palmitoyltransferase II (CPT II) is an IM enzyme that reconverts long-chain acylcarnitines into their long-chain acyl CoA thioesters. These long-chain acyl CoAs are β-oxidized into acetyl CoA, which activates gluconeogenesis via pyruvate decarboxylase. Malonyl CoA mediates glucose toxicity and regulates β-cell GSIS via allosteric inhibition of CPT I [63,129,130]. Malonyl CoA fuel sensing is influenced by insulin, glucose, exercise, and AMPK activation [63,130].

In rats, carnitine administration also improves glycemic status [223], vascular function [224], and mitochondrial antioxidant activity [225]. In humans, insulin sensitivity is associated with long-chain acyl CoA content and intracellular lipid accumulation [226]. Obesity-related insulin resistance is associated with CPT I and CACT activities [227,228]. Children [229] and adults [230] with DM have decreased plasma-free carnitine levels. Pharmacologic administration of carnitine, producing an acute hypercarnitinemia, induces nonoxidative glucose disposal [231,232] and oxidative glucose consumption with hypoglycemia [233,234]. In a study of 18 patients with T2DM, acylcarnitine administration increased glucose oxidation during hyperinsulinemic euglycemic clamp conditions [235]. In a 6-month, randomized, double-blind controlled trial of 94 patients with newly diagnosed T2DM, carnitine, 1 g po twice a day (BID), lowered lipoprotein (a) levels without effects on serum cholesterol levels, serum triglyceride levels, or glycemic control [236]. In addition, reversible CPT I inhibitors (carnitine derivatives) are being developed that lower acetyl CoA levels, reduce gluconeogenesis, and thus serve as hypoglycemic agents in patients with T2DM [237].

Mutations in the CPT II gene are reported in association with several mitochondrial disorders: MELAS, MERRF, NARP, MIMyCa, LHON, Pearson bone marrow-pancreas syndrome, and MTDM [238]. Oral carnitine administration has been associated with improvements in lipid metabolism and neuromuscular symptoms in various mitochondrial disorders [221,239–242]. Silvestre-Aillaud et al. [186] found no improvement in glycemic status in a patient with MTDM due to the A3243G mutation treated with CoQ10, 150 mg/day, and carnitine, 2 g/day, for 6 months. In another patient with MTDM on hemodialysis with the same mutation, Matsumura et al. [243] found improvements in lactate accumulation and cardiac function with carnitine, 500 mg/day for 5 months, but did not comment on glycemic status. Overall, there is no evidence to support the use of carnitine therapy in the treatment of MTDM (evidence level 4). Adverse effects are not significant and therapy may still be rational for improvement of mitochondrial function and glycemic status (recommendation grade C).

CREATINE

Creatine is used as a therapeutic intervention targeting mitochondrial function in the management of diabetes. In order to compensate for an abnormal redox state resulting from mitochondrial dysfunction, high-energy phosphate is transferred from ATP to creatine to form phosphocreatine via mitochondrial creatine kinase (MtCK). Phosphocreatine is transported to the cytosol to provide phosphate for the formation of cytosolic ATP and subsequent activation of glycogenolysis and glycolysis. The expression of MtCK is ubiquitous with highest expression in the brain, gut, and kidney [244]. Substrate channeling occurs among MtCK, ANT, and OXPHOS in a tightly coupled functional microcompartment in the mitochondrial intermembrane space that, via creatine, ultimately protects mitochondria from mPTP opening and a pro-apoptotic cascade [245]. This microcompartment concept has been challenged, however, by data from Lipskaya and Savchenko [246]. A creatine transport system (CRT) localizing to the IM, and inhibited by arginine and lysine, accounts for subcellular compartmentalization of the creatine/phosphocreatine pool [247].

In a case report of a patient with MELAS, creatine, 20 g/day × 4 weeks, was associated with improvements in neurologic function [248]. In an uncontrolled study of 5 patients with mitochondrial encephalopathies, creatine (0.08–0.35 g/kg/day × 9 months to 4 years) was associated with improved aerobic oxidative function [249]. In a double-blind, placebo-controlled trial of 22 healthy volunteers, creatine monohydrate (5–20 g/day for 12 weeks) prevented an immobilization-related decline in GLUT4 and increased rehabilitation-related improvements in GLUT4 by 40% [250]. Potential adverse effects on renal function should be considered in those patients with preexisting nephropathy. The use of creatine as a modulator of mitochondrial function in patients with DM is supported only by level 3 evidence with risks applicable to patients with nephropathy (recommendation grade C [no nephropathy] and D [nephropathy present]).

THIAMIN

Thiamin (vitamin B_1) is critical for glucose utilization and insulin secretion. Approximately 40% of thiamin requirements are provided by the ingestion of fiber-containing foods such as whole grain products, unprocessed rice, and legumes [251]. A significant contribution to thiamin requirements can also be provided by meats, especially pork (27.1%), dairy products (8.1%), fruits (4.4%), and eggs (2.0%) [252]. The three main enzymes in glucose metabolism that are thiamin-dependent are PDH, α-ketoglutarate dehydrogenase, and transketolase. Decreased glucose oxidation in isolated pancreatic islets from thiamin-deficient rats is associated with decreased insulin secretion [253].

In "thiamin-responsive megaloblastic anemia" (TRMA), the saturable component of the thiamin transporter (THTR1) is absent [254]. This component is similar to the reduced-folate transporter and is encoded by a member of the solute carrier gene superfamily, the SLC19A2 gene, in chromosome 1q23.3 [255,256]. Several different mutations in the SLC19A2 gene have been associated with TRMA [257]. TRMA is similar to "Rogers syndrome," which is associated with DM and sensorineural deafness, and responds to pharmacologic doses of thiamin [258–260].

In a murine model, targeted disruption of the SLC19A2 gene produced TRMA with DM and reduced insulin secretion that resolved with thiamin repletion [261]. In a family with TRMA described by Gritli et al. [262], a 287delG mutation in the SLC19A2 gene was associated with insulin-requiring DM, dilated cardiomyopathy, anemia, and deafness. The DM was thought to result from β-cell apoptosis [262]. Bappal et al. [263] discussed two patients with TRMA and T1DM, presenting with diabetic ketoacidosis, in which insulin cessation resulted from oral thiamin treatment (200 mg/day). Valerio et al. [264] conducted a small randomized, double-blind, placebo-controlled study in which 5 children with T1DM were treated with thiamin, 50 mg/day for 3 months, and later found to have a significant improvement in A1C levels and insulin requirements. However, in a review of the literature, benefit from thiamin treatment with respect to T1DM was inconsistent [265].

In sum, the clinical features of TRMA closely resemble features of mitochondrial disorders and thiamin treatment; perhaps simply enriching the diet with fiber-containing foods [266] appears to be a rational approach to the patient with MTDM. Although there are no data to support the use of thiamin supplements in the treatment of MTDM (evidence level 4), the use of thiamin is rational, based on potential benefits on mitochondrial function, and there are no significant risks (recommendation grade C).

RIBOFLAVIN

The chief source of intramitochondrial flavin cofactors flavin adenine dinucleotide (FAD) and riboflavin-5-phosphate, flavin mononucleotide (FMN) is provided by riboflavin (Rf) uptake from the cytosol. Riboflavin itself has little intrinsic activity. Mitochondrial Rf pools are regulated by the Rf/FAD cycle which involves Rf kinase, FAD synthase, FAD pyrophosphatase, FMN phosphohydrolase, Rf transporter, FAD transporter, and flavinylation-stimulating factor [267]. FAD and FMN serve as redox cofactors for various mitochondrial dehydrogenases and oxidases involved in bioenergetics. Recently, it was determined that the principal ROS generation site in the ETS is the FMN group of complex I and not the ubiquinone group of complex III as previously thought [268]. Furthermore, increased fatty acid accumulation resulting from a Rf-responsive, multiple acylcoenzyme A dehydrogenase (RR-MAD) deficiency is associated with upregulation of UCP3 [269].

Increased mitochondrial respiration in pancreatic β-cells responds to glucose uptake via the glucose sensor FAD-linked hmGPD [270]. Defects in the FAD-binding domain of hmGPD have been associated with T2DM [68,271,272], emphasizing the potential role of flavin cofactors in mediating mitochondrial events that lead to the diabetic state. Following the addition of glucose to clonal pancreatic β-cells and the subsequent glucose phosphorylation, flavin nucleotide reduction ensues. This is followed by increased O_2 consumption rate, ATP/ADP ratio, cellular pH, and cytosolic free Ca^{2+} [273]. Nevertheless, studies in Goto-Kakizaki rats fail to demonstrate decreased hmGPD activity having a primary role in impaired GSIS [273].

Thus, theoretical benefits of Rf therapy on mitochondrial function can be inferred from the above studies. These benefits include decreased ROS production, decreased pancreatic β-cell apoptosis and increased GSIS. Riboflavin therapy can increase complex I activity alone [275], with carnitine [276,277] or with nicotinamide [278]. Riboflavin therapy has also resulted in improvement of clinical symptoms in patients with mitochondrial myopathy without consistent effects on complex I activity [279]. In a patient with MELAS, but without DM, Rf and idebenone (a short-chain CoQ10 analog) restored metabolic impairments [280]. There are no clinical studies specifically evaluating the effects of Rf in patients with MTDM (evidence level 4), though Rf therapy has a rational theoretic basis without significant risks (recommendation grade C).

NIACIN

Niacin refers to nicotinic acid (NA; pyridine-3-carboxylic acid) and its derivatives, which produce biologic effects qualitatively similar to nicotinamide (nicotinic acid amide). Niacin is synthesized from the essential amino acid tryptophan via the kynurenine pathway and quinolinate phosphoribosyltransferase. This biosynthetic pathway is inhibited by deficiencies in vitamin B_6, Rf, or iron, and enhanced with restricted protein intake [281]. Nicotinamide is the essential moiety in the coenzymes nicotinamide adenine dinucleotide (NAD) and NAD phosphate (NADP), which serve as electron acceptors or hydrogen donors in many biologic redox reactions.

Niacin is a safe and efficacious treatment for dyslipidemia in patients with T2DM but has been associated with deterioration of glycemic control in some patient cohorts [282–284]. In the diabetes-prone NOD mouse, NA feeding is associated with inhibition of insulitis [285]. In rats, NA lowers FFA, lowers UCP2 and UCP3 gene expression in oxidative muscles [286], and completely ablates GSIS [143]. This same effect of NA on GSIS is observed in humans, but it is an indirect effect via lowering of FFA and not a direct effect of NA on β-cells [287,288]. In healthy, nonobese subjects, NA-induced decline in FFA are associated with decreased gluconeogenesis and increased glycogenolysis [289]. In T1DM, NA administration is associated with elevated insulin, non-esterified fatty acid, ketone body, and glycerol levels [290]. Nicotinic acid also activates glycogen synthase which could normalize the impaired glycogen synthesis typically found in T2DM [291]. Apoptosis results from gradual depletion of intracellular NAD via (1) decreased nicotinamide phosphoribosyltransferase (NAPRT) regulation of NAD synthesis, (2) catabolic reactions, and (3) increased poly(ADP-ribose) polymerase (PARP) activity [292]. Both NA and nicotinamide block this apoptotic effect [292].

In MELAS, the A3243G mtDNA mutation eradicates a transcription termination sequence in the tRNA$^{LEU(UUR)}$ gene yielding an abnormally large 16 S rRNA derivative and defective translation [293]. As a result of the 7 (out of 41) defective complex I (NADH:Q oxidoreductase) subunits, NADH affinity is decreased, leading to lactic acidosis and the clinical phenotype [293]. Oral NA therapy, 1 g QID × 5 months, increased erythrocyte NAD content and induces a 50% decrease in blood lactate and pyruvate concentrations [293]. There are no reported cases of benefit in MTDM with NA therapy in the literature (evidence level 4). Niacin use has been associated with myopathy, hepatopathy, hyperuricemia, gout, and deterioration of glycemic control. Therefore, until clinical evidence demonstrates benefits that outweigh the above risks, niacin therapy is not recommended to improve glycemic control in MTDM (recommendation grade D).

Biotin

Biotin is an essential cofactor for four carboxylases that catalyze the incorporation of bicarbonate into a substrate as a carboxyl group. All four carboxylases are found in mitochondria. Acyl-CoA carboxylase (ACC) incorporates bicarbonate into acetyl CoA to form malonyl CoA. Pyruvate carboxylase (PC) incorporates bicarbonate into pyruvate to form oxaloacetate. Methylcrotonyl CoA carboxylase (MCC) catalyzes an essential step in the degradation of leucine. Propionyl CoA carboxylase (PCC) catalyzes the incorporation of bicarbonate into propionyl CoA to form methylmalonyl CoA. Biotinylation of the ε-amino group of a specific lysyl residue of mitochondrial apocarboxylase is catalyzed by mitochondrial holocarboxylase synthetase (HCS). In rodents, biotin increases PCC, PC, and HCS gene expression [294] and glucokinase synthesis [295], as well as improving glucose tolerance [296,297].

In T2DM patients, ACC, PC, and PCC activities are similar to those of nondiabetic patients; biotin therapy, which increases carboxylase activity, is not associated with changes in glucose, insulin, triacylglycerol, cholesterol, or lactate levels [298]. On the other hand, small clinical studies of biotin therapy (9–16 mg daily) have been associated with salutary effects on glycemic control (evidence level 3). It has even been suggested, but not proven, that biotin and chromium therapy be used together in patients with T2DM to improve glycemic control [174]. There are no clinical studies evaluating the use of biotin in MTDM but there are also no clinically significant risks associated with biotin therapy (recommendation grade C).

SELENIUM

Selenium (as sodium selenite) is an essential trace element in the human diet. Monomethylated forms of selenium compounds are selenomethionine and selenocysteine; the latter is a component of the antioxidants glutathione peroxidase and thioredoxin reductase. Selenium supplementation is associated with immunomodulatory [299] and antineoplastic [300] activities. In physiologic concentrations, selenium can act as insulin by stimulating glucose transport, ribosomal S_6 protein phosphorylation, and regulation of caspase-3 via a redox mechanism [301–303].

Selenium also participates in a complex network that regulates apoptosis. Selenium compounds and analogs upregulate the anti-apoptotic protein Bcl-2 via activation of the anti-apoptotic PI3K/Akt-dependent pathway and inhibition of the pro-apoptotic ASK1/JNK pathway [304–306]. Protein kinase B (Akt) is activated by IRS-2, IGF-1, and membrane docking catalyzed by PI3K [307,308]. ROS activates apoptosis signal-regulating kinase 1 (ASK1) which then activates the c-Jun N-terminal kinase (JNK) pathway [309]. Recent studies have also implicated JNK activation in nucleo-cytoplasmic PDX-1 translocation [310] and other mitochondrial apoptotic pathways [311] that induce diabetes. Therefore, selenium compounds can maintain the mitochondrial membrane potential, activate glycolysis, increase glucose uptake, increase β-cell mass, and ultimately protect β-cells from oxidative stress and preserve GSIS.

However, in higher concentrations, selenium promotes apoptosis, DNA damage, and ROS generation [312–315]. In rats and human hepatoma cells, toxic levels of selenium induce apoptosis by thiol oxidation, ROS generation, and mPTP opening [316,317] In an *in vitro* study of NIH 3T3 cells, Zhou et al. [318] demonstrated that selenite-induced apoptosis involved the formation of DNA topoisomerase II (Top II) cleavage complexes and "ataxia-telangiectasia mutated protein" (ATM)/p53 activation. These pharmacologic effects of selenium contribute to the prevention of age-related tissue damage and cancer chemoprevention.

There is a paucity of experimental data involving selenium use and diabetes. In streptozotocin-induced diabetic rats, selenium normalizes blood glucose levels via glucose-6-phosphate dehydrogenase (G6PDH) and fatty acid synthase (FAS) gene expression in a manner similar to insulin administration [319]. In an uncontrolled study of 43 patients with T2DM, a selenium-enriched diet was associated with reductions in blood glucose [320]. There are no reports of selenium use in the treatment of MTDM (evidence level 4). Adverse effects are limited to rare toxic hepatopathies (selenosis). The relative safety and theoretical benefit of selenium on mitochondrial function, as well as a single level 3 study in patients with T2DM, support a recommendation grade C.

ZINC

The theoretical foundation for the use of zinc in targeting mitochondrial function in patients with diabetes is predicated on the significant role of copper zinc-superoxide dismutase and ROS scavenging [321]. However, zinc has also been demonstrated to act as a paracrine death effector in β-cells following streptozotocin [322]. Supplementation with zinc alone [323] or in combination with chromium [324] was associated with increased antioxidant activity but no effects on glucose homeostasis or A1C levels. Injudicious supplementation with zinc can induce a copper deficiency. Thus, there is an increased risk-benefit ratio for the use of zinc targeting mitochondrial function in DM (recommendation grade D).

COPPER

Copper therapy in patients with mitochondrial disorders has also been based on (1) the role of copper zinc-superoxide dismutase activity and ROS scavenging [321]; (2) incorporation of copper as a prosthetic group in complex IV; and (3) along with pantothenic acid (vitamin B_5) and pyridoxine (vitamin B_6), the role of copper mediating the insertion of heme-α into complex IV [325]. In addition, copper supplementation is an adjunctive therapy in patients with mutations in the nuclear gene SCO2 (cytochrome-c oxidase [COX] assembly gene). Human SCO2 maps to chromosome 22 and mutations are associated with a fatal infantile COX deficiency disorder with muscular hypotonia, hypertrophic cardiomyopathy, and encephalopathy [326]. The SCO2 gene encodes a protein (Sco2) with a mitochondrial targeting sequence that participates in the assembly of COX [327]. SCO2 contains a putative copper-binding motif, acts as a copper chaperone, and transports copper to the Cu_A site on the Cox II subunit [327,328]. Interestingly, in myoblasts from patients with mutated SCO2, treatment with copper-histidine [329] or $CuCl_2$ [330] rescued COX activity. However, animal studies suggest that the presence of diabetes confers increased risk of oxidative injury with copper intake [331]. As a result of the lack of any data demonstrating benefit on MTDM (evidence level 4) and the potential for harm, copper therapy is not recommended in patients with MTDM (grade D).

Vitamin A

Vitamin A interacts with the retinoic acid receptor (RAR) and retinoid X receptor (RXR) in cellular differentiation. The cellular retinoic acid-binding protein-II (CRABP-II) converts vitamin A into retinoic acid, and polymorphisms in the CRABP-II promoter have been implicated in the pathogenesis of T2DM [332]. These receptors form complexes with other factors, such as Jun and Fos, and can both stimulate and inhibit nuclear gene expression. In the mitochondria, gene expression can be governed by 9-cis-retinoic acid activation of a heterodimerical complex of mitochondrial retinoid x receptor (mt-RXR) and a mitochondrial truncated triiodothyronine receptor c-Erb Aa1 (p43) [333]. mt-RXR is produced after intramitochondrial enzymatic cleavage of the nuclear receptor RXR-α [333]. All-trans-retinoic acid (atRA) is an uncompetitive inhibitor of ANT and induces Ca^{2+}-dependent mPTP opening and apoptosis [334]. Pro-apoptotic effects of retinoids also involve decreased Bcl-2 levels [335]. Moreover, retinoids are potent activators of UCP1, UCP2, and UCP3 [336,337]. The mitochondrial pro-oxidant properties of retinoids localize to a quinine-binding site in complex I and center O of complex III [338].

In patients with T2DM, retinoid levels are lower compared with healthy subjects [339]. In the same study, retinoid levels were positively correlated with A1C levels possibly reflecting β-cell toxicity of elevated retinoids [339]. However, in a study of patients with T1DM, retinoid levels negatively correlated with A1C levels [340].

In the BHE/Cdb rat model of MTDM, in which there is a maternally inherited mutation in the ATPase 6 mitochondrial gene, increasing dietary vitamin A can improve OXPHOS activity [341–343] This occurs via interaction with retinoic acid receptor (RAR), increased mtTFA, and increased ATPase 6 gene expression yielding gluconeogenesis downregulation and glucose tolerance improvement [341–343]. Overall, the rational basis for using vitamin A in mitochondrial disorders remains to be clarified and there is no clinical evidence supporting its use in MTDM (evidence level 4). Vitamin A overdosing can lead to hepatopathy, hypercalcemia, and metabolic bone disease (grade D).

Vitamin C

Vitamin C (ascorbate) is an antioxidant and is also necessary for the biosynthesis of carnitine. Many of the benefits of a diet high in fruits and vegetables have been attributed to the therapeutic effects of vitamin C but this association is still controversial [344,345]. After donating electrons to scavenge intramitochondrial free radicals, recycle α-tocopherol, or reduce ferricytochrome-c at complex IV, ascorbate is fully oxidized to dehydroascorbic acid (DHA) [346–348]. Mitochondria must recycle DHA back to vitamin C, via cytochrome-b_5, LA and NADH-dependent dehydrogenases, to replenishing stores of ascorbate [349]. This DHA-sparing function occurs at a complex III locus exposed to the outer surface of the IM [348]. DHA has also been found to be a selective regulator of H_2O_2- and Fas-dependent apoptosis [350,351]. *In vitro* loading with vitamin C protects monocyte cell lines from mitochondrial damage due to the soluble Fas ligand [352].

Ascorbic acid is transported into cells by sodium-dependent membrane-bound proteins [353]. However, DHA is transported into cells by facilitative glucose transporters and this process is competitively inhibited by hyperglycemia [353]. Therefore, a state of functional vitamin C deficiency occurs during periods of hyperglycemia [354]. In T2DM patients with oxidative stress and endothelial dysfunction, serum vitamin C levels are dimished [355]. In ob/ob mice, vitamin C administration decreases insulin glycation that could improve insulin action and glycemic control [356]. In streptozotocin-induced diabetic rats, vitamins C and E completely corrected markers of oxidative stress [357]. In a randomized, blinded study of 35 patients with T2DM, vitamin C, 1.5 g/day for 3 weeks, did not improve markers of oxidative stress [358]. However, in another placebo-controlled study of 20 patients with T2DM, vitamin C, 1 g/day for 6 weeks, improved endothelial function and reduced oxidative stress [359]. There is no clinical evidence supporting the role of vitamin C in MTDM (evidence level 4). Preclinical evidence supports the role of vitamin C in improving mitochondrial function and vitamin C therapy is safe (grade C).

Vitamin E

The eight vitamin E compounds refer to the four forms (α, β, δ, and γ) of the tocopherols and the tocotrienols. The principal role of vitamin E is to scavenge free radicals and protect cell membrane PUFAs, cytoskeleton and membrane thio-rich proteins, and nucleic acids from oxidative damage. Specifically, α-tocopherol prevents ROS oxidative damage and mitochondrial dysfunction by maintaining normal thiol status [360]. The vitamin E analog, α-tocopheryl succinate (TOS), has pro-apoptotic activity via mitochondrial membrane destabilization [361]. Another vitamin E analog, γ-tocopheryl quinine (γ-TQ), induces apoptosis via mitochondrial membrane destabilization as well as a feedback amplication loop between caspase-9 and the caspase-8/BID pathway [362]. Once reacting with a ROS, tocopherol is converted into a tocopheroxyl radical, which is then reduced back to tocopherol by vitamin C, glutathione, or ubiquinone. Increased mitochondrial α-tocopherol concentrations in rats are associated with decreased liver mitochondrial susceptibility to oxidative injury [363]. Furthermore, vitamin E has been shown to prevent alloxan-induced ROS-mediated mitochondrial damage, GSIS inhibition and apoptosis [364]. In mice, CoQ10 administration not only augments total and mitochondrial CoQ concentrations but also augments mitochondrial α-tocopherol concentrations [365].

In children with poorly controlled T1DM, plasma—but not erythrocyte—vitamin E levels positively correlate with A1C levels [366]. In adults with T1DM, vitamin E levels are higher than healthy controls due to increased glucose autoxidation and a lower exercise-induced oxidation rate of α-tocopherol [367]. There may also be a protective effect of α-tocopherol on the incidence of T2DM [368,369]. This effect is demonstrable within the range of vitamin E intake available from food, but not within the range of intake from high-dose vitamin E supplements [368,370]. Ylonen et al. [370] found an inverse association of α-tocopherol intake with first-phase insulin secretion in men and fasting plasma glucose concentrations in women. While other studies [371–375] have also demonstrated an association of vitamin E with glycemic control, several studies [376–377] have failed to demonstrate this association. In addition, though vitamin E has a presumed beneficial symptomatic effect on oxidative stress in diabetic patients, there are no data to support a role in "causal" antioxidant therapy [108,378]. It has been asserted that antioxidant enzymes have a more relevant role than vitamin E in free radical scavenging and protection against oxidative stress in diabetes [379]. The risks associated with vitamin E therapy are uncommon and include nonspecific GI symptoms, decreased vitamins A and K absorption, decreased vitamin K metabolism and, in infants, sepsis and necrotizing enterocolitis. Overall, vitamin E therapy could have a potential role as part of an overall antioxidant strategy in patients with MTDM but this approach remains unproven (evidence level 4) and is associated with potential hazards (grade D).

Vitamin K

K is responsible for post-translational γ-carboxylation of glutamic acid (Gla) residues. Vitamin K-dependent Gla-containing proteins are involved in clotting and coagulation (factors VII, IX, and X; proteins C and S), bone formation (osteocalcin), calcification inhibition (matrix Gla protein), and nephrolithiasis inhibition (nephrocalcin). Vitamin K_1 (phylloquinone) is isolated from green plants, vitamin K_2 (menaquinone) is synthesized by intestinal bacteria, and vitamin K_3 is a synthetic compound used pharmacologically as a chemotherapeutic agent for malignancy.

Phylloquinone mediates cell signaling, replication, and transformation via specific interaction as ligands with receptor tyrosine kinases (RTK) [380]. Menadione is metabolized by flavoprotein reductase to semiquinone, oxidized back to quinine by molecular oxygen, and ultimately generates ROS [381]. Menadione elicits apoptosis via cytosolic Ca^{2+} elevation [381], mPTP opening [381,382], cytochrome-c release with caspase activation [170], Jun kinase and FasL expression [383], and Fas-independent mitochondrial events associated with ATP depletion [382,383]. Bcl-2 acts as a survival antiapoptotic protein and can delay menadione-induced cytotoxicity [384]. Deprenyl, an inhibitor of mitochondrial monoamine oxidase B, inhibits menadione-induced mPTP opening [385]. In pancreatic β-cells, catalase, mitochondrial Mn-superoxide dismutase (Mn-SOD), cytosolic Cu/Zn-SOD and glutathione peroxidase overexpression protect against menadione-induced cytotoxicity [386,387].

There is one report of a patient with a complex III defect who responded clinically (improved myopathy) and biochemically (improved OXPHOS) to menadione and vitamin C therapy [388,389]. However there is no evidence to support the use of vitamin K in the treatment of MTDM (evidence level 4). Furthermore, there does not even appear to be a rational, theoretical justification for the empiric use of vitamin K, particularly menadione, in the treatment of MTDM (grade D).

CONCLUSIONS

It is apparent that an increasing number of patients with DM actually have primary MTDM resulting from a mtDNA mutation that significantly impairs mitochondrial function and GSIS. These patients have a family history consistent with a maternal inheritance pattern and should have genetic testing for mtDNA mutations. It is important to specifically diagnose MTDM in order to provide specific pharmacologic and nutritional therapy, as well as provide appropriate genetic counseling. Physicians should also be aware of the syndromic, phenotypic features that accompany many mtDNA mutations in patients with MTDM. Conventional pharmacologic therapy should be delivered according to established protocols along with nutritional therapies designed to target involved mitochondrial defects. It is also apparent that a great number of molecular mechanisms mediating the diabetic state localize to mitochondrial physiology. These include β-cell function, insulin action, intermediary metabolism and fuel utilization, and diabetic complications. Nutritional therapies that target these biochemical processes serve to buttress a comprehensive dietary prescription for all types of DM. Specific nutritional interventions targeting mitochondrial function are summarized in Table 13.9. Unfortunately, the majority of these dietary maneuvers are not supported by strong clinical evidence, so clinical judgement must prevail and potential risks should always be weighed against realistic benefit.

TABLE 13.9
Synopsis of Evidence-Based Nutritional Strategies for Patients with MTDM

Nutritional Intervention	Dosing	Comments	Rec./Grade
High-protein diet	≥ 30% total daily calories	Scavenges ROS	D
Taurine	6–12 g/day po; 30/mg/kg/day po (children)	Improves mitochondrial protein synthesis	D
n-3 fatty acids	3–5 g/day po	Improves OXPHOS	C
Monounsaturated fatty acid	Up to 40% energy from fat	Antiapoptotic	C
Reduced saturated fatty acid	< 10% total daily calories	Decreases lipotoxicity and apoptosis	C
Reduced trans-fatty acid	As little as possible	Improves OXPHOS	C
Coenzyme Q10	60–600 mg/day po; 4.3–15 mg/kg/day po	Scavenges ROS; improves OXPHOS	C
α-lipoic acid	600–1200 mg/day po	Improves peripheral neuropathy	C
Carnitine	500 – 3000 mg/day po; 100 mg/kg/day po	Improves insulin action and mitochondrial function	C
Creatine	5–20 g/day po; 0.08–0.35 g/kg/day po	Antiapoptotic	C
Thiamin	50–200 mg/day po	Improves OXPHOS	C
Riboflavin	50–600 mg/day po	Scavenges ROS, antiapoptosis, and GSIS	C
Niacin	20–4000 mg/day po	Lowers FFA and indirectly stimulates GSIS	D
Biotin	9–16 mg/day po	Improves mitochondrial function	C
Selenium	50–200 mg/day po	Scavenges ROS; antiapoptotic; increases GSIS	C
Zinc	15 mg/day po (elemental)	Scavenges ROS	D
Vitamin A	5,000–10,000 IU/day po	Improves OXPHOS	D
Vitamin C	500–1500 g/day po	Scavenges ROS	C
Vitamin E	100–400 mg/day po (d-α); 200–800 mg/day po (dl-α)	Scavenges ROS; antiapoptotic; increases GSIS	D
Vitamin K	up to 10 mg/d po	Affects mitochondrial function	D

REFERENCES

1. Giles RE, Blanc H, and Cann HM et al., Maternal inheritance of human mtDNA. *Proc Natl Acad Sci USA*, 77:6715–6719, 1980.
2. Isshiki G, Impaired glucose tolerance in the young, Nippon Rinsho 1997; 54:2766–2772.
3. Mathews CE and Berdanier CD, Non-insulin-dependent diabetes mellitus as a mitochondrial genomic disease, *Proc Soc Exp Biol Med*, 219:97–108, 1998.
4. Singhal NN, Gupta BS, and Saigal RR et al., Mitochondrial diseases: An overview of genetics, pathogenesis, clinical features, and an approach to diagnosis and treatment, *J Postgrad Med*, 46:224–230, 2000.
5. Kim MJC and Berdanier CD, Nutrient-gene interactions determine mitochondrial function: Effect of dietary fat. *FASEB J*, 12:243–248, 1998.
6. Berdanier CD. Diabetes and nutrition: The mitochondrial part, *J Nutr*, 131:344S–353S, 2001.
7. Vincent AM, Brownlee M, and Russell JW, Oxidative stress and programmed cell death in diabetic neuropathy, *Ann N Y Acad Sci*, 959:368–383, 2002.
8. Frank S, Robert EG, and Youle RJ. Scission, spores, and apoptosis: A proposal for the evolutionary origin of mitochondria in cell death induction, *Biochem Biophys Res Communic*, 304:481–486, 2003.
9. Rabinovitch A, An update on cytokines in the pathogenesis of insulin-dependent diabetes mellitus. *Diabetes Metab Rev*, 14:129–151, 1998.

10. Gallaher BW, Hille R, and Raile K et al., Apoptosis: Live or die—hard work either way! *Horm Metab Res*, 33:511–519, 2001.

11. Grodzicky T and Elkon KB, A case where too much or too little can lead to autoimmunity, *Mt Sinai J Med*, 69:208–219, 2002.

12. Fukagawa NK, Li Muyao, and Timblin CR et al., Modulation of cell injury and survival by high-glucose and advancing age, *Free Rad Biol Med*, 31:1560–1569, 2001.

13. Liston P, Fong WG, and Korneluk RG, The inhibitors of apoptosis: There is more to life than Bcl2, *Oncogene*, 22:8568–8580, 2003.

14. Lim MLR, Lum MG, and Hansen TM et al., On the release of cytochrome-c from mitochondria during cell death signaling, *J Biomed Sci*, 9:488–506, 2002.

15. Rosenbloom AL, Joe J, and Young RS et al., Emerging epidemic of type-2 diabetes in youth, *Diabetes Care*, 22:345–353, 1999.

16. Tawata M, Ohtaka M, and Iwase E et al., New mitochondrial DNA homoplasmic mutations associated with Japanese patients with type-2 diabetes, *Diabetes*, 47:276–277, 1998.

17. Perucca-Lostanlen D, Narbonne H, and Hernandez JB et al., Mitochondrial DNA variations in patients with maternally inherited diabetes and deafness syndrome, *Biochem Biophys Res Commun*, 277:771–775, 2000.

18. Hsieh RH, Li JY, and Pang CY et al., A novel mutation in the mitochondrial 16S rRNA gene in a patient with MELAS syndrome, diabetes mellitus, hyperthyroidism and cardiomyopathy, *J Biomed Sci*, 8:328–335, 2001.

19. van den Ouwenland JMW, Lemkes HHPJ, and Ruitenbeck W et al., Mutation in mitochondrial tRNA$^{Leu(UUR)}$ gene in a large pedigree with maternally transmitted type-II diabetes mellitus and deafness, *Nat Genet*, 1:368–371, 1992.

20. Thajeb P, Lee HC, and Pang CY et al., Phenotypic heterogeneity in a Chinese family with mitochondrial disease and A3243G mutation of mitochondrial DNA, *Zhonghua Yi Xue Za Zhi (Taipei)*, 63:71–76, 2000.

21. Maechler P and Wollheim CB, Mitochondrial signals in glucose-stimulated insulin secretion in the β-cell, *J Physiol*, 529:49–56, 2000.

22. Hirai M, Suzuki S, and Onoda M et al., Mitochondrial deoxyribonucleic acid 3256C-T mutation in a Japanese family with non-insulin-dependent diabetes mellitus, *J Clin Endocrinol Metab*, 83:992–994, 1998.

23. Suzuki Y, Suzuki S, and Hinokio Y et al., Diabetes associated with a novel 3264 mitochondrial tRNA (leu) (UUR) mutation, *Diabetes Care*, 20:1138–1140, 1997.

24. Suzuki Y, Suzuki S, and Taniyama M et al., Multiple tumors in mitochondrial diabetes associated with tRNALeu (UUR) mutation at position 3264, *Diabetes Care*, 26:1942–1943, 2003.

25. Corona P, Lamantea E, and Greco M et al., Novel heteroplasmic mtDNA mutation in a family with heterogeneous clinical presentations, *Ann Neurol*, 51:118–122, 2002.

26. Sakuta R, Honzawa S, and Murakami N et al., Atypical MELAS associated with mitochondrial tRNA (Lys) gene A8296G mutation, *Pediatr Neurol*, 27:397–400, 2002.

27. Arenas J, Campos Y, and Bornstein B et al., A double mutation (A8296G andG8363A) in the mitochondrial DNA tRNA (Lys) gene associated with myoclonus epilepsy with ragged-red fibers, *Neurology*, 52:377–382, 1999.

28. Kameoka K, Isotani H, and Tanaka K et al., Novel mitochondrial DNA mutation in tRNA(Lys) (8296AG) associated with diabetes, *Biochem Biophys Res Commun*, 245:523–527, 1998.

29. Tryoen-Toth P, Richert S, and Sohm B et al., Proteomic consequences of a human mitochondrial tRNA mutation beyond the frame of mitochondrial translation, *J Biol Chem*, 278:24314–24323, 2003.

30. Masucci JP, Schon EA, and King MP, Point mutations in the mitochondrial tRNA (Lys) gene: Implications for pathogenesis and mechanism, *Mol Cell Biochem*, 174:215–219, 1997.

31. Lynn S, Wardell T, and Johnson MA et al., Mitochondrial diabetes: Investigation and identification of a novel mutation, *Diabetes*, 47:1800–1802, 1998.

32. Schuelke M, Bakker M, and Stoltenburg G et al., Epilepsia partialis continua associated with a homoplasmic mitochondrial tRNA$^{Ser(UCN)}$ mutation, *Ann Neurol*, 44:700-704, 1998.

33. Toompuu M, Yasukawa T, and Suzuki T et al., The 7472insC mitochondrial DNA mutation impairs the synthesis and extent of aminoacylation of rRNA$^{Ser(UCN)}$ but not its structure or rate of turnover, *J Biol Chem*, 277:22240–22250, 2002.

34. Vialettes BH, Paquis-Flucklinger V, and Pelissier JF et al., Phenotypic expression of diabetes secondary to a T14709C mutation of mitochondrial DNA: Comparison with MIDD syndrome (A3243G mutation), A case report, *Diabetes Care,* 20:1731–1737, 1997.

35. Tzen CY, Thajeb P, and Wu TY et al., Melas with point mutations involving tRNALeu (A3243G) and tRNAGlu (A14693G), *Muscle Nerve,* 28:575–581, 2003.

36. Nakagawa Y, Ikegami H, and Yamato E et al., A new mitochondrial DNA mutation associated with non-insulin-dependent diabetes mellitus, *Biochem Biophys Res Commun,* 209:664–668, 1995.

37. Chen Y, Liao WX, and Roy AC et al., Mitochondrial gene mutations in gestational diabetes mellitus, *Diabetes Res Clin Pract,* 48:29–35, 2000.

38. Ohkubo K, Yamamo A, and Nagashima M et al., Mitochondrial gene mutations in the tRNA (Leu(UUR)) region and diabetes: Prevalence and clinical phenotypes in Japan, *Clin Chem,* 47:1641–1648, 2001.

39. Cavelier L, Erikson I, and Tammi M et al., MtDNA mutations in maternally inherited diabetes: Presence of the 3397 ND1 mutation previously associated with Alzheimer's and Parkinson's disease, *Hereditas,* 135:65–70, 2001.

40. Finsterer J, Bittner R, and Bodingbauer M et al., Complex mitochondriopathy associated with four mtDNA transitions, *Eur Neurol,* 44:37–41, 2000.

41. Ohkubo K, Aida K, and Chen J et al., A patient with type-2 diabetes mellitus associated with mutations in calcium sensing receptor gene and mitochondrial DNA, *Biochem Biophys Res Commun,* 278:808–813, 2000.

42. Uchigata Y, Okada T, and Gong JS et al., A mitochondrial genotype associated with the development of autoimmune-related type-1 diabetes, *Diabetes Care,* 25:2106, 2002.

43. Sakaue S, Ohmuro J, and Mishina T et al., A case of diabetes, deafness, cardiomyopathy, and central sleep apnea: Novel mitochondrial DNA polymorphisms, *Tohoku J Exp Med,* 196:203–211, 2002.

44. Tawata M, Hayashi JI, and Isobe K et al., A new mitochondrial DNA mutation at 14577 T/C is probably a major pathogenic mutation for maternally inherited type-2 diabetes, *Diabetes,* 49:1269–1272, 2000.

45. Takada Y and Mukaida M, Polymorphism of hypervariable region in D-loop of mitochondrial DNA, *Nippon Hoigaku Zasshi,* 53:199–206, 1999.

46. Khogali SS, Mayosi BM, and Beattie JM et al., A common mitochondrial DNA variant associated with susceptibility to dilated cardiomyopathy in two different populations, *Lancet,* 357:1265–1267, 2001.

47. Ji L, Gao L, and Han X, Association of 16189 variant (T C transition) of mitochondrial DNA with genetic predisposition to type-2 diabetes in Chinese populations, *Zhonghua Yi Xue Za Zhi,* 81:711–714, 2001.

48. Berdanier CD, Mitochondrial gene expression in diabetes mellitus: Effect of nutrition, *Nutr Rev,* 59:61–70, 2001.

49. Mecocci P, MacGarvey U, and Kaufman AE et al., Oxidative damage to mitochondrial DNA shows marked age-dependent increases in human brain, *Ann Neurol,* 34:609–616, 1993.

50. Noda M, Yamashita S, and Takahashi N et al., Switch to anaerobic glucose metabolism with NADH accumulation in the β-cell model of mitochondrial diabetes: Characteristics of betaHC9 cells deficient in mitochondrial DNA transcription, *J Biol Chem,* 277:41817–41826, 2002.

51. Robertson RP, Harmon J, and Tran PO et al., Glucose toxicity in β-cells: Type-2 diabetes, good radicals gone bad, and the glutathione connection, *Diabetes,* 52:581–587, 2003.

52. Robertson RP, Olson LK, and Zhang HJ, Differentiating glucose toxicity from glucose desensitization: A new message from the insulin gene, *Diabetes,* 43:1085–1089, 1994.

53. Gleason CE, Gonzalez M, and Harmon JS et al., Determinants of glucose toxicity and its reversibility in the pancreatic islet β-cell line: HIT-T15, *Am J Physiol Endocrinol Metab,* 279:E997–1002, 2000.

54. Maechler P, Kennedy ED, and Wang H et al., Desensitization of mitochondrial Ca^{2+} and insulin secretion responses in the β-cell, *J Biol Chem,* 273:20770–20778, 1998.

55. Wu L, Nicholson W, and Knobel SM et al., Oxidative stress is a mediator of glucose toxicity in insulin-secreting pancreatic islet cell lines, *J Biol Chem,* 279:12126–12134, 2004.

56. Zhou YP, Marlen L, and Palma JF et al., Overexpression of repressive cAMP response element modulators in high glucose and fatty acid-treated rat islets: A common mechanism for glucose toxicity and lipotoxicity? *J Biol Chem,* 278:51316–51323, 2003.

57. Lu M, Seufert J, and Habener JF, Pancreatic β-cell-specific repression of insulin gene transcription by CCAAT/enhancer-binding protein β, *J Biol Chem,* 272:28349–28359, 1997.

58. Moran A, Zhang HJ, and Olson LK et al., Differentiation of glucose toxicity from β–cell exhaustion during the evolution of defective insulin gene expression in the pancreatic islet cell line: HIT-T15, *J Clin Invest,* 99:534–539, 1997.

59. Matsuoka T, Kajimoto Y, and Watada H et al., Glycation-dependent, reactive oxygen species-mediated suppression of the insulin gene promoter activity in HIT cells, *J Clin Invest,* 99:144–150, 1997.

60. McKillop AM, Abdel-Wahab YH, and Mooney MH et al., Secretion of glycated insulin from pancreatic β-cells in diabetes represents a novel aspect of β-cell dysfunction and glucose toxicity, *Diabetes Metab,* 28:3S61–3S69, 2002.

61. Nishikawa T, Edelstein D, and Du XL et al., Normalizing mitochondrial superoxide production blocks three pathways of hyperglycemia damage, *Nature,* 404:787–790, 2000.

62. Krauss S, Zhang CY, and Scorrano L et al., Superoxide-mediated activation of uncoupling protein 2 causes pancreatic β–cell dysfunction, *J Clin Invest,* 112:1831–1842, 2003.

63. Saha AK and Ruderman NB, Malonyl-CoA and AMP-activated protein kinase: An expanding partnership, *Mol Cell Biochem,* 253:65–70, 2003.

64. Brownlee M, A radical explanation for glucose-induced β cell dysfunction, *J Clin Invest,* 112:1788–1790, 2003.

65. Malaisse WJ, Glucose sensing by the pancreatic 36 cell: The mitochondrial part, *Int J Biochem,* 24:693–701, 1992.

66. Liang Y, Bonner-Weir S, and Wu YJ et al., In situ glucose uptake and glucokinase activity of pancreatic islets in diabetic and obese rodents, *J Clin Investig,* 93:2473–2481, 1994.

67. Matschinsky FM, A lesson in metabolic regulation inspired by the glucokinase glucose sensor paradigm, *Diabetes,* 45:223–241, 1996.

68. Gudayol M, Fabregat ME, and Rasschaert J et al., Site-directed mutations in the FAD-binding domain of glycerophosphate dehydrogenase: Catalytic defects with preserved mitochondrial anchoring of the enzyme in transfected COS-7 cells, *Mol Genet Metab,* 75:168–173, 2002.

69. Vidal J, Corominola H, and Cardona F et al., Low mitochondrial glycerophosphate dehydrogenase activity in lymphocytes of women with gestational diabetes, *Horm Metab Res,* 29:60–62, 1997.

70. Chen Y, Liao WX, and Roy AC et al., Mitochondrial gene mutations in gestational diabetes mellitus, *Diabetes Res Clin Pract,* 48:29–35, 2000.

71. Rousset S, Alves-Guerra M-C, and Mozo J et al., The biology of mitochondrial uncoupling proteins, *Diabetes,* 53(Suppl 1):S130–135, 2004.

72. Mori H, Okazawa H, and Iwamoto K et al., A polymorphism in the 5 untranslated region and a Met229 Leu variant in exon 5 of the human UCP1 gene are associated with susceptibility to type-II diabetes mellitus, *Diabetologia,* 44:373–376, 2001.

73. Lameloise N, Muzzin P, and Prentki M et al., Uncoupling protein 2: A possible link between fatty acid excess and impaired glucose-induced insulin secretion? *Diabetes,* 50:803–809, 2001.

74. Krauss S, Zhang CY, and Scorrano L et al., Superoxide-mediated activation of uncoupling protein 2 causes pancreatic β cell dysfunction, *J Clin Invest,* 112:1831–1842, 2003.

75. Chan CB, De Leo D, and Joseph JW et al., Increased uncoupling protein-2 levels in β-cells are associated with impaired glucose-stimulated insulin secretion, *Diabetes,* 50:1302–1310, 2001.

76. Echtay KS, Roussel D, and St-Pierre J et al., Superoxide-activated mitochondrial uncoupling proteins, *Nature,* 415:96–99, 2002.

77. Young ME, Patil S, and Ying J et al., Uncoupling protein 3 transcription is regulated by peroxisome proliferator-activated receptor α in the adult rodent heart, *FASEB J,* 15:833–845, 2001.

78. Li X, Cobb CE, and May JM, Mitochondrial recycling of ascorbic acid from dehydroascorbic acid: Dependence on the electron transport chain, *Arch Biochem Biophys,* 403:103–110, 2002.

79. Joseph JW, Koshkin V, and Zhang CY et al., Uncoupling protein 2 knockout mice have enhanced insulin secretory capacity after a high-fat diet, *Diabetes,* 51:3211–3219, 2002.

80. Clapham JC, Coulthard VH, and Moore GB, Concordant mRNA expression of UCP-3, but not UCP-2, with mitochondrial thioesterase-1 in brown adipose tissue and skeletal muscle in db/db diabetic mice, *Biochem Biophys Res Commun,* 287:1058–1062, 2001.

81. Harper ME, Dent RM, and Bezaire V et al., UCP3 and its putative function: Consistencies and controversies, *Biochem Soc Trans,* 29:768-773, 2001.

82. DiMauro S, Bomilla E, and Davidson M et al., Mitochondria in neuromuscular disorders, *Biochim Biophys Acta,* 1366:199–210, 1998.

83. Matschinsky FM, Glaser B, and Magnuson MA, Pancreatic β-cell glucokinase: Closing the gap between theoretical concepts and experimental realities, *Diabetes,* 47:307–315, 1998.

84. Eto K, Tsubamoto Y, and Terauchi Y et al., Role of NADH shuttle system in glucose-induced activation of mitochondrial metabolism and insulin secretion, *Science,* 283:981–985, 1999.

85. Eto K, Suga S, and Wakui M et al., NADH shuttle system regulates K_{ATP} channel-dependent pathway and steps distal to cytosolic Ca^{2+} concentration elevation in glucose-induced insulin secretion, *J Biol Chem,* 274:25386–25392, 1999.

86. Langin D, Diabetes, insulin secretion, and the pancreatic β-cell mitochondrion, *N Engl J Med,* 345:1772–1774, 2001. [Erratum, *N Engl J Med,* 346:634, 2002.]

87. Jackson MJ, Bindoff LA, and Weber K et al., Biochemical and molecular studies of mitochondrial function in diabetes insipidus, diabetes mellitus, optic atrophy, and deafness, *Diabetes Care,* 17:728–733, 1994.

88. Perucca-Lostanlen D, Narbonne H, and Hernandez JB et al., Mitochondrial DNA variations in patients with maternally inherited diabetes and deafness syndrome, *Biochem Biophys Res Commun,* 277:771–775, 2000.

89. Choo-Kang ATW, Lynn S, and Taylor GA et al., Defining the importance of mitochondrial gene defects in maternally inherited diabetes by sequencing the entire mitochondrial genome, *Diabetes,* 51:2317–2320, 2002.

90. Petersen KF, Befroy D, and Dufour S et al., Mitochondrial dysfunction in the elderly: Possible role in insulin resistance, *Science,* 300:1140–1142, 2003.

91. Mechanick JI, Brett EM, and Chausmer AB et al., American association of clinical endocrinologists' medical guidelines for the clinical use of dietary supplements and nutraceuticals, *Endocr Pract,* 9:417–470, 2003.

92. Ryan EA, Pick ME, and Marceau C, Use of alternative medicines in diabetes mellitus, *Diab Med,* 18:242–245, 2001.

93. Tanaka M, Borgeld HJ, and Zhang J et al., Gene therapy for mitochondrial disease by delivering restriction endonuclease SmaI into mitochondria, *J Biomed Sci,* 9:534–541, 2002.

94. Guy J, Qi X, and Pallotti F et al., Rescue of a mitochondrial deficiency causing Leber Hereditary Optic Neuropathy, *Ann Neurol,* 52:534–542, 2002.

95. Manfredi G, Fu J, and Ojaimi J et al., Rescue of a deficiency in ATP synthesis by transfer of MTATP6, a mitochondrial DNA-encoded gene, to the nucleus, *Nat Genet,* 30:394–399, 2002.

96. Ojaimi J, Pan J, and Santra S et al., An algal nucleus-encoded subunit of mitochondrial ATP synthase rescues a defect in the analogous human mitochondrial-encoded subunit, *Mol Biol,* 13:3836–3844, 2002.

97. Bai Y, Hajek P, and Chomyn A et al., Lack of complex I activity in human cells carrying a mutation in MtDNA-encoded ND4 subunit is corrected by the Saccharomyces cerevisiae NADH-quinone oxidoreductase (NDI1) gene, *J Biol Chem,* 276:38808–38813, 2001.

98. Kolesnikova OA, Entelis NS, and Mireau H et al., Suppression of mutations in mitochondrial DNA by tRNAs imported from the cytoplasm, *Science,* 289:1931–1933, 2000.

99. Taivassalo T, Fu K, and Johns T et al., Gene shifting: A novel therapy for mitochondrial myopathy, *Hum Mol Genet,* 8:1047–1052, 1999.

100. Fajans SS, Bell GI, and Polonsky KS, Molecular mechanisms and clinical pathophysiology of maturity-onset diabetes of the young, *N Engl J Med,* 345:971–980, 2001.

101. Gold DR and Cohen BH, Treatment of mitochondrial cytopathies, *Sem Neurol,* 21:309–325, 2001.

102. Lenzen S, Drinkgern J, and Tiedge M, Low antioxidant enzyme gene expression in pancreatic islets compared with various other mouse tissues, *Free Rad Biol Med,* 20:463–466, 1996.

103. Tiedge M, Lortz S, and Drinkgern J et al., Relation between antioxidant enzyme gene expression and antioxidative defense status of insulin-producing cells, *Diabetes,* 46:1733-1742, 1997.

104. Ford ES, Mokdad AH, and Giles WH et al., The metabolic syndrome and antioxidant concentrations, *Diabetes,* 52:2346–2352, 2003.

105. Dierckx N, Horvath G, and van Gils C et al., Oxidative stress status in patients with diabetes mellitus: Relationship to diet, *Eur J Clin Nutr,* 57:999–1008, 2003.

106. Kaneto H, Kajimoto Y, and Miyagawa J et al., Beneficial effects of antioxidants in diabetes, Possible protection of pancreatic β–cells against glucose toxicity, *Diabetes,* 48:2398–2406, 1999.
107. Lapidot T, Walker MD, and Kanner J, Antioxidant and prooxidant effects of phenolics on pancreatic β–cells *in vitro, J Agric Food Chem,* 50:7220–7225, 2002.
108. Ceriello A, New insights on oxidative stress and diabetic complications may lead to a "causal" antioxidant therapy, *Diabetes Care,* 26:1589–1596, 2003.
109. Liou CW, Huang CC, and Lee CF et al., Low antioxidant content and mutation load in mitochondrial DNA A3243G mutation-related diabetes mellitus, *J Formos Med Assoc,* 102:527–533, 2003.
110. Orzechowski A, Justification for antioxidant preconditioning (or how to protect insulin-mediated actions under oxidative stress), *J Biosci,* 28:39–49, 2003.
111. Taylor R, Causation of type-2 diabetes—the Gordian knot unravels, *New Engl J Med,* 350:639–641, 2004.
112. Fang YZ, Yang S, and Wu G, Free radicals, antioxidants, and nutrition, *Nutrition,* 18:872–879, 2002.
113. Prentki M, New insights into pancreatic β-cell metabolic signaling in insulin secretion, *Eur J Endocrinol,* 134:272–286, 1996.
114. Machlin LJ and Bendich A, Free radical tissue damage: Protective role of antioxidant nutrients, *FASEB J,* 1:441–5, 1987.
115. Dempster WS, Sive AA, and Rosseau S et al., Misplaced iron in kwashiorkor, *Eur J Clin Nutr,* 49:208–210, 1995.
116. Wu G, Flynn NE, and Flynn SP et al., Dietary protein or arginine deficiency impairs constitutive and inducible nitric oxide synthesis by young rats, *J Nutr,* 129:1347–1354, 1999.
117. Mohanty P, Ghanim H, and Hamouda W et al., Both lipid and protein intakes stimulate increased generation of reactive oxygen species by polymorphonuclear leukocytes and mononuclear cells, *Am J Clin Nucl,* 75:767–772, 2002.
118. Wu G and Meininger CJ, Regulation of nitric oxide synthesis by dietary factors, *Annu Rev Nutr,* 22:61–86, 2002.
119. Gannon MC, Nuttall FQ, and Saeed A et al., An increase in dietary protein improves the blood glucose response in persons with type-2 diabetes, *Am J Clin Nutr,* 78:734–741, 2003.
120. Huxtable RJ, Physiologic actions of taurine, *Physiol Rev,* 72:101–163, 1992.
121. Suzuki T, Suzuki T, and Wada T et al., Taurine as a constituent of mitochondrial tRNAs: New insights into the functions of taurine and human mitochondrial diseases, *EMBO J,* 21:6581–6589, 2002.
122. Hennig B, Toborek M, and McClain CJ, High-energy diets, fatty acids, and endothelial cell function: Implications for atherosclerosis, *J Am Coll Nutr,* 20:97–105, 2001.
123. Wan G, Ohnomi S, and Kato N, Increased hepatic activity of inducible nitric oxide synthase in rats fed on a high-fat diet, *Biosci Biotechnol Biochem,* 64:555–561, 2000.
124. Sreekumar R, Unnikrishnan J, and Fu A et al., Impact of high-fat diet and antioxidant supplement on mitochondrial functions and gene transcripts in rat muscle, *Am J Physiol Endocrinol Metab,* 282:E1055–1061, 2002.
125. Khair-El-Din T, Sicher SC, and Vazquez MA et al., Transcription of the murine iNOS gene is inhibited by docosahexaenoic acid, a constituent of fetal and neonatal sera as well as fish oils, *J Exp Med,* 183:1241–1246, 1996.
126. Ohata T, Fukuda K, and Takahashi M et al., Suppression of nitric oxide production in lipopolysaccharide-stimulated macrophage cells by omega-3 polyunsaturated fatty acids, *Jpn J Cancer Res,* 88:234–237, 1997.
127. Takahashi M, Tsuboyama-Kasaoka N, and Nakatani T et al., Fish oil feeding alters liver gene expressions to defend against PPAR-α activation and ROS production, *Am J Physiol Gastrointest Liver Physiol,* 282:G338–348, 2002.
128. Tanaka T, Yamamoto J, adn Iwasaki S et al., Activation of peroxisome proliferators-activated receptor δ induces fatty acid β-oxidation in skeletal muscle and attenuates metabolic syndrome, *Proc Natl Acad Sci,* 100:15924–15929, 2003.
129. Ruderman NB, Saha AK, and Vavvas D et al., Malonyl-CoA, fuel sensing, and insulin resistance, *Am J Physiol,* 276:E1–18, 1999.
130. Ruderman NB, Saha AK, and Kraegen EW, Minireview: Malonyl CoA, AMP-activated protein kinase, and adiposity, *Endocrinology,* 144:5166–5171, 2003.

131. Randle PJ, Garland PB, and Hales CN et al., The glucose fatty acid cycle: Its role in insulin sensitivity and the metabolic disturbances of diabetes mellitus, *Lancet,* 1:785–789, 1963.

132. Petersen KF and Shulman GI, Pathogenesis of skeletal muscle insulin resistance in type-2 diabetes mellitus, *Am J Cardiol,* 90:11G–18G, 2002.

133. Abu-Elheiga L, Oh W, and Kordari P et al., Acetyl-CoA carboxylase 2 mutant mice are protected against obesity and diabetes induced by high-fat/high-carbohydrate diets, *Proc Natl Acad Sci,* 100:10207–10212, 2003.

134. Berdanier CD, Tobin RB, and DeVore V, Studies on the control of lipogenesis: Strain differences in hepatic metabolism, *J Nutr,* 104:247–260, 1979.

135. Berdanier CD and McNamara S, Aging and mitochondrial activity in BHE and Wistar rats, *Exp Gerontol,* 15:519–525, 1980.

136. Berdanier CD, Rat strain differences in gluconeogenesis by isolated hepatocytes, *Proc Soc Exp Biol Med,* 169:74–79, 1982.

137. Lakshmanan MK, Berdanier CD, and Veech RL, Comparative studies on lipogenesis and cholesterogenesis in lipemic BHE rats and normal Wistar rats, *Arch Biochem Biophys,* 183:355–360, 1977.

138. Cross RL and Duncan TM, Subunit rotation in F0F1-ATP syntheses as a means of coupling proton transport through F0 to the binding changes in F1, *Bioenerg Biomembr,* 28:403–408, 1996.

139. Berdanier CD, NIDDM in the nonobese BHE/Cdb rat, In: Shafrir E, Ed., *Lessons from Animal Diabetes,* Smith-Gordon, London: Smith-Gordon, 231–246, 1994.

140. Berdanier CD, Kras K, and Wickwire K et al., Progressive glucose intolerance and renal disease in aging rats, *Int J Diab,* 5:27–38, 1997.

141. Wickwire K, Kras K, and Gunnett C et al., Menhaden oil feeding increases potential for renal free radical production in the BHE/Cdb rat, *Proc Soc Exp Biol Med,* 209:397–402, 1995.

142. Lamson DW and Plaza SM, Mitochondrial factors in the pathogenesis of diabetes: A hypothesis for treatment, *Alt Med Rev,* 7:94–111, 2002.

143. Stein DT, Stevenson BE, and Chester MW et al., The insulinotropic potency of fatty acids is influenced profoundly by their chain length and degree of saturation, *J Clin Invest,* 100:398–403, 1997.

144. Sako Y and Grill VE, A 48-hour lipid infusion in the rat time-dependently inhibits glucose-induced insulin secretion and β-cell oxidation through a process likely coupled to fatty acid oxidation, *Endocrinology,* 127:1580–1589, 1990.

145. Zhou YP and Grill VE, Long-term exposure of rat pancreatic islets to fatty acid inhibits glucose-induced insulin secretion and biosynthesis through a glucose fatty acid cycle, *J Clin Invest,* 93:870–876, 1994.

146. Hawkins M, Tonelli J, and Kishore P et al., Contribution of elevated free fatty acid levels to the lack of glucose effectiveness in type-2 diabetes, *Diabetes,* 52:2748–2758, 2003.

147. Kashyap S, Belfort R, and Gastaldelli A et al., A sustained increase in plasma free fatty acids impairs insulin secretion in nondiabetic subjects genetically predisposed to develop type-2 diabetes, *Diabetes,* 52:2461–2474, 2003.

148. Robertson RP, Harmon J, and Tran POT et al., β-cell glucose toxicity, lipotoxicity, and chronic oxidative stress in type-2 diabetes, *Diabetes,* 53(Suppl 1):S119–124, 2004.

149. Bollheimer LC, Skelley RH, and Chester MW et al., Chronic exposure to free fatty acids reduced pancreatic β cell insulin content by increasing basal insulin secretion that is not compensated for by a corresponding increase in proinsulin biosynthesis translation, *J Clin Invest,* 101:1094–1101, 1998.

150. Boden G, Chen X, and Rosner J, and Barton M, Effects of a 48-h fat infusion on insulin secretion and glucose utilization, *Diabetes,* 44:1239–1242, 1995.

151. Boden G and Carnell LH, Nutritional effects of fat on carbohydrate metabolism, *Best Pract Res Clin Endocrinol Metab,* 17:399–410, 2003.

152. Maedler K, Oberholzer J, and Bucher P et al., Monounsaturated fatty acids prevent the deleterious effects of palmitate and high glucose on human pancreatic β-cell turnover and function, *Diabetes,* 52:726–733, 2003.

153. Ros E, Dietary cis-monounsaturated fatty acids and metabolic control in type-2 diabetes, *Am J Clin Nutr,* 78(3 Suppl):617S–625S, 2003.

154. Roche HM, Noone E, and Sewter C, et al., Isomer-dependent metabolic effects of conjugated linoleic acid, *Diabetes,* 51:2037–2044, 2002.

155. Brown JM and McIntosh MK, Conjugate linoleic acid in humans: Regulation of adiposity and insulin sensitivity, *J Nutr,* 133:3041–3046, 2003.

156. Grundy SM and Denke MA, Dietary influences on serum lipids and lipoproteins, *J Lipid Res,* 31:1149–1172, 1990.

157. Maron DJ, Fair JM, and Haskell WL, Saturated fat intake and insulin resistance in men with coronary artery disease. The Stanford coronary risk intervention project investigators and staff, *Circulation,* 84:2020–2027, 1991.

158. Mayer EJ, Newman B, and Quesenberry CP, Jr, et al., Usual dietary fat intake and insulin concentrations in healthy women twins, *Diabetes Care,* 16:1459–1469, 1993.

159. Parker DR, Weiss ST, and Troisi R et al., Relationship of dietary fatty acids and body habitus to serum insulin concentrations: The normative aging study, *Am J Clin Nutr,* 58:129–136, 1993.

160. Hannah JS and Howard BV, Dietary fats, insulin resistance, and diabetes, *J Cardiovasc Risk,* 1:31–37, 1994.

161. McGarry JD, Disordered metabolism in diabetes: Have we underemphasized the fat component? *J Cell Biochem,* 55(Suppl):29–38, 1994.

162. Rasmussen O, Lauszus FF, and Christiansen C et al., Differential effects of saturated and monounsaturated fat on blood glucose and insulin responses in subjects with non-insulin-dependent diabetes mellitus, *Am J Clin Nutr,* 63:249–253, 1996.

163. Hertz R, Ben-Haim N, and Petrescu AD et al., Rescue of MODY-1 by agonist ligands of hepatocyte nuclear factor-4α, *J Biol Chem,* 278:22578–22585, 2003.

164. Hattori Y, Matsuda M, and Eizawa T et al., A case of mitochondrial myopathy, encephalopathy, lactic acidosis and stroke-like episodes (MELAS), showing temporary improvement during the treatment with eicosapentaenoic acid ethyl ester, *Rinsho Shinkeigaku,* 41:668–672, 2001.

165. Echtay KS, Winkler E, and Klingenberg M, Coenzyme Q is an obligatory cofactor for uncoupling protein function, *Nature,* 408:609–613, 2000.

166. Walter L, Nogueira V, and Leverve X et al., Three classes of ubiquinone analogs regulate the mitochondrial permeability transition pore through a common site, *J Biol Chem,* 275:29521–29527, 2000.

167. Kalen A, Norling B, and Appelkvist EL et al., Ubiquinone biosynthesis by the microsomal fraction from rat liver, *Biochim Biophys Acta,* 926:70–78, 1987.

168. Thomas SR, Neuzil J, and Stocker R, Co-supplementation with coenzyme Q prevents the prooxidant effect of α-tocopherol and increase in the resistance of LDL to transition metal-dependent oxidation initiation, *Arterioscler Thromb Vasc Biol,* 16:687–696, 1996.

169. Gille L and Nohl H, The existence of a lysosomal redox chain and the role of ubiquinone, *Arch Biochem Biophys,* 375:347–354, 2000.

170. Sun YL, Zhao Y, and Hong X et al., Cytochrome-c release and caspase activation during menadione-induced apoptosis in plants, *FEBS Lett,* 462:317–321, 1999.

171. Nohl H, Staniek K, and Kozlov AV et al., The biomolecule ubiquinone exerts a variety of biological functions, *Biofactors,* 18:23–31, 2003.

172. Niaz MA, Singh RB, and Rastogi SS, Effect of hydrosoluble coenzyme Q10 on the lipoprotein (a) and insulin sensitivity in rabbits receiving transfatty acid-rich diet, *J Trace Elem Exp Med,* 11:275–288, 1998.

173. Jameson S, Coenzyme Q_{10} alpha-tocopherol, and free cholesterol levels in sera from diabetic patients. In: Folkers K, Littarru G, and Yamagami T, Eds., *Biochemical and Clinical Aspects of Coenzyme Q,* Amsterdam: Elsevier Science, 151–158, 1991.

174. McCarty MF, High-dose biotin, an inducer of glucokinase expression, may synergize with chromium picolinate to enable a definitive nutritional therapy for type-II diabetes, *Med Hypothesis,* 52:401–406, 1999.

175. Thomas SR, Witting PK, and Stocker R, A role for reduced coenzyme Q in atherosclerosis? *Biofactors,* 9:207–224, 1999.

176. Chew GT and Watts GF, Coenzyme Q10 and diabetic endotheliopathy: Oxidative stress and the "recoupling hypothesis." *Q J Med,* 97:537–548, 2004.

177. Rauscher FM, Sanders RA, and Watkins JB, Effects of coenzyme Q10 treatment on antioxidant pathways in normal and streptozotocin-induced diabetic rats, *J Biochem Mol Toxicol,* 15:41–46, 2001.

178. Coldiron AD, Jr, Sanders RA, and Watkins JB, III, Effects of combined quercetin and coenzyme Q(10) treatment on oxidative stress in normal and diabetic rats, *J Biochem Mol Toxicol,* 16:197–202, 2002.

179. Ferreira FM, Seica R, and Oliveira PJ et al., Diabetes induces metabolic adaptations in rat liver mitochondria: Role of coenzyme Q and cardiolipin contents, *Biochim Biophys Acta,* 1639:113–120, 2003.

180. McCarty MF, Can correction of sub-optimal coenzyme Q status improve β-cell function in type-II diabetics? *Med Hypoth,* 52:397–400, 1999.

181. Henriksen JE, Andersen CB, and Hother-Nielsen O et al., Impact of ubiquinone (coenzyme Q_{10}) treatment on glycaemic control, insulin requirement, and well-being in patients with type-1 diabetes mellitus, *Diab Med,* 16:312–318, 1999.

182. Eriksson JG, Forsen TJ, and Mortensent SA et al., The effect of coenzyme Q10 administration on metabolic control in patients with type-2 diabetes, *Biofactors,* 9:315–318, 1999.

183. Hodgson JM, Watts GF, and Playford DA et al., Coenzyme Q_{10} improves blood pressure and glycaemic control, A controlled trial in subjects with type-2 diabetes, *Eur J Clin Nutr,* 56:1137–1142, 2002.

184. Watts GF, Playford DA, and Croft KD et al., Coenzyme Q_{10} improves endothelial function of the brachial artery in type-II diabetes mellitus, *Diabetologia,* 45:420–426, 2002.

185. Playford DA, Watts GF, and Croft KD et al., Combined effect of coenzyme Q_{10} and fenofibrate on forearm microcirculatory function in type-2 diabetes, *Atherosclerosis,* 168:169–179, 2003.

186. Silvestre-Aillaud P, BenDahan D, and Paquis-Fluckinger V et al., Could coenzyme Q10 and L-carnitine be a treatment for diabetes mellitus secondary to 3243 mutation of mtDNA, *Diabetologia,* 38:1485–1486, 1995.

187. Usui T, Sawa S, and Inoue A et al., A case of 3243 point mutation of mitochondrial gene with diabetes mellitus treated with coenzyme Q, *Nippon Naika Gakkai Zasshi,* 84:1904–1906, 1995.

188. Suzuki Y, Kadowaki H, and Atsumi Y et al., A case of diabetic amyotrophy associated with 3243 mitochondrial tRNA (Leu; UUR) mutation and successful therapy with coenzyme Q10, *Endocr J,* 42:141–145, 1995.

189. Suzuki Y, Kadowaki H, and Taniyama M et al., Insulin edema in diabetes mellitus associated with 3243 mitochondrial tRNA(Leu; UUR) mutation, Case reports, *Diabetes Res Clin Pract,* 29:137–142, 1995.

190. Liou CW, Huang CC, and Lin TK et al., Corrrection of pancreatic β-cell dysfunction with coenzyme Q(10) in a patient with mitochondrial encephalomyopathy, lactic acidosis, and stroke-like episodes syndrome and diabetes mellitus, *Eur Neurol,* 43:54–55, 2000.

191. Suzuki S, Hinokio Y, and Ohtomo M et al., The effects of coenzyme Q_{10} treatment on maternally inherited diabetes mellitus and deafness, and mitochondrial DNA 3243 (A to G) mutation, *Diabetologia,* 41:584–588, 1998.

192. Genova ML, Pich MM, and Biondi A et al., Mitochondrial production of oxygen radical species and the role of coenzyme Q as an antioxidant, *Exp Biol Med,* 228:506–513, 2003.

193. Armstrong JS, Whiteman M, and Rose P et al., The coenzyme Q_{10} analog decylubiquinone inhibits the redox-activated mitochondrial permeability transition, *J Biol Chem,* 278:49079–49084, 2003.

194. Moini H, Packer L, and Saris NEL, Antioxidant and prooxidant activities of α-lipoic acid and dihydrolipoic acid, *Toxicol Appl Pharmacol,* 182:84–90, 2002.

195. Evans JL and Goldfine ID, α-lipoic acid: A multifunctional antioxidant that improves insulin sensitivity in patients with type-2 diabetes, *Diab Tech Ther,* 2:401–413, 2000.

196. Morikawa T, Yasuno R, and Wada H, Do mammalian cells synthesize lipoic acid? Identification of a mouse cDNA encoding a lipoic acid synthase located in mitochondrial, *FEBS Letters,* 498:16–21, 2001.

197. Korotchkina LG, Yang H-S, Tirosh O, Packer L, and Patel MS, Protection by thiols of the mitochondrial complexes from 4–hydroxy-2-nonenal, *Free Rad Biol Med,* 30:992–999, 2001.

198. Lykkesfeldt J, Hagen TM, and Vinarsky V et al., Age-associated decline in ascorbic acid concentration, recycling, and biosynthesis in rat hepatocytes—reversal with (R)-alpha-lipoic acid supplementation, *FASEB J,* 12:1183–1189, 1998.

199. Hagen TM, Ingersoll RT, and Lykkesfeldt J et al., (R)-alpha-lipoic acid-supplemented old rats have improved mitochondrial function, decreased oxidative damage, and increased metabolic rate, *FASEB J,* 13:411–418, 1999.

200. Arivazhagan P, Ramanathan K, and Panneerselvam C, Effect of DL-α-lipoic acid on mitochondrial enzymes in aged rats, *Chem Biol Interact,* 138:189–198, 2001.
201. Bienwenga G, Haenen GR, and Bast A, The role of lipoic acid in the treatment of diabetic polyneuropathy, *Drug Metab Rev,* 29:1025–1054, 1997.
202. Ziegler D and Gries FA, Alpha-lipoic acid in the treatment of diabetic peripheral and cardiac autonomic neuropathy. *Diabetes,* 46(Suppl 2):S62–66, 1997.
203. Ziegler D, Reljanovic M, and Mehnert H et al., Alpha-lipoic acid in the treatment of diabetic polyneuropathy in Germany: Current evidence from clinical trials, *Exp Clin Endocrinol Diabetes,* 107:421–430, 1999.
204. Ziegler D, Hanefeld M, and Ruhnau KJ et al., Treatment of symptomatic diabetic peripheral neuropathy with the anti-oxidant alpha-lipoic acid. A 3-week multicentre randomized controlled trial (ALADIN Study), *Diabetologia,* 38:1425–1433, 1995.
205. Reljanovic M, Reichel G, and Rett K et al., Alpha Lipoic in diabetic neuropathy: Treatment of diabetic polyneuropathy with the antioxidant thioctic acid (alpha-lipoic acid), A two-year multicenter randomized double-blind placebo-controlled trial (ALADIN II), *Free Radic Res,* 31:171–179, 1999.
206. Ziegler D, Hanefeld M, and Ruhnau KJ et al., ALADIN III Study Group, Treatment of symptomatic diabetic polyneuropathy with the antioxidant α–lipoic acid, *Diabetes Care,* 22:1296–1301, 1999.
207. SYDNEY Trial Study Group, The sensory symptoms of diabetic polyneuropathy are improved with α-lipoic acid, *Diabetes Care,* 26:770–776, 2003.
208. Heitzer T, Finckh B, and Albers S et al., Beneficial effects of α-lipoic acid and ascorbic acid on endothelium-dependent, nitric oxide-mediated vasodilation in diabetic patients: Relation to parameters of oxidative stress, *Free Rad Biol Med,* 31:53–61, 2001.
209. Hagen TM, Moreau R, and Suh JH et al., Mitochondrial decay in the aging rat heart, *Ann NY Acad Sci,* 959:491–507, 2002.
210. Jacob S, Henriksen EJ, and Schiemann AL et al., Enhancement of glucose disposal in patients with type-2 diabetes by alpha-lipoic acid, *Arzneimittel-Forschung,* 45:872–874, 1995.
211. Jacob S, Henriksen EJ, and Tritschler HJ et al., Improvement of insulin-stimulated glucose disposal in type-2 diabetes after repeated parenteral administration of thioctic acid, *Exp Clin Endocrinol Diabetes,* 104:284–288, 1996.
212. Jacob S, Ruus P, and Hermann R et al., Oral administration of RAC-alpha-lipoic acid modulates insulin sensitivity in patients with type-2 diabetes mellitus, A placebo-controlled pilot trial, *Free Rad Biol Med,* 27:309–314, 1999.
213. Konrad T, Vicini P, and Kusterer K et al., Alpha-lipoic acid treatment decreases serum lactate and pyruvate concentrations and improves glucose effectiveness in lean and obese patients with type-2 diabetes, *Diabetes Care,* 22:280–287, 1999.
214. Yaworsky K, Somwar R, and Ramlal T et al., Engagement of the insulin-sensitive pathway in the stimulation of glucose transport by alpha-lipoic acid in 3T3-L1 adipocytes, *Diabetologia,* 43:294–303, 2000.
215. Konrad D, Somwar R, and Sweeney G et al., The antihyperglycemic drug α-lipoic acid stimulates glucose uptake via both GLUT4 translocation and GLUT4 activation, *Diabetes,* 50:1464–1471, 2001.
216. Jacob S, Streeper RS, and Fogt DL et al., The antioxidant alpha-lipoic acid enhances insulin-stimulated glucose metabolism in insulin-resistant rat skeletal muscle, *Diabetes,* 45:1024–1029, 1996.
217. Midaoui AEL, Elimadi A, and Wu L et al., Lipoic acid prevents hypertension, hyperglycemia, and the increase in heart mitochondrial superoxide production, *Am J Hypertension,* 16:173–179, 2003.
218. Dicter N, Madar Z, and Tirosh O, α-lipoic acid inhibits glycogen synthesis in rat soleus muscle via its oxidative activity and the uncoupling of mitochondria, *J Nutr,* 132:3001–3006, 2002.
219. Evans JL, Heymann CJ, and Goldfine ID et al., Pharmacokinetics, tolerability, and fructosamine-lowering effects of a novel, controlled-release formulation of alpha-lipoic acid, *Endocr Pract,* 8:29–35, 2002.
220. Reda E, D'Iddio S, and Nicolai R et al., The carnitine system and body composition, *Acta Diabetol,* 40:S106–113, 2003.
221. Evangeliou A and Vlassapoulos D, Carnitine metabolism and deficit—when supplementation is necessary? *Curr Pharm Biotechnol,* 4:211–219, 2003.
222. Eaton S, Control of mitochondrial beta-oxidation flux, *Prog Lipid Res,* 41:197–239, 2002.

223. Yoshikawa Y, Ueda E, and Sakurai H et al., Anti-diabetes effect of Zn(II)/carnitine complex by oral administration, *Chem Pharm Bull,* 51:230–231, 2003.
224. Kumaran S, Deepak B, and Naveen B et al., Effects of levocarnitine on mitochondrial antioxidant systems and oxidative stress in aged rats, *Drugs R D,* 4:141–147, 2003.
225. Irat AM, Aktan F, and Ozansoy G, Effects of L-carnitine treatment on oxidant/antioxidant state and vascular reactivity of streptozotocin-diabetic rat aorta, *J Pharm Pharmacol,* 55:1389–1395, 2003.
226. Ellis BA, Poynten A, and Lowy AJ et al., Long-chain acyl CoA esters as indicators of lipid metabolism and insulin sensitivity in rat and human muscle, *Am J Physiol Endocrinol Metab,* 279:E554–560, 2000.
227. Simoneau JA, Veerkamp JH, and Turcotte LP et al., Markers of capacity to utilize fatty acidsin human skeletal muscle: Relation to insulin resistance and obesity and effects of weight loss, *FASEB J,* 13:2051–2060, 1999.
228. Peluso G, Petillo O, and Margarucci S et al., Decreased skeletal muscle carnitine translocase impairs utilization of fatty acids in insulin-resistant human muscle, *Front Biosci,* 7:A109–116, 2002.
229. Coker M, Coker C, and Darcan S et al., Carnitine metabolism in diabetes mellitus, *J Ped Endocrinol Metab,* 15:841–849, 2002.
230. Tamamogullari N, Silig Y, and Icagasioglu S et al., Carnitine deficiency in diabetes mellitus complications, *J Diab Compl,* 13:251–253, 1999.
231. De Gaetano A, Mingrone G, and Castagneto M et al., Carnitine increases glucose disposal in humans, *J Am Coll Nutr,* 18:289–295, 1999.
232. Mingrone G, Greco AV, and Capristo E et al., L-carnitine improves glucose disposal in type-2 diabetes patients, *J Am Coll Nutr,* 18:77-82, 1999.
233. Uziel G, Garavaglia B, and Di Donato S, Carnitine stimulation of pyruvate dehydrogenase complex (PDIIC) in isolated human skeletal muscle mitochondria, *Muscle Nerve,* 11:720–724, 1988.
234. Angelini A, Imparato L, and Landi C et al., Variation in levels of glycaemia and insulin after infusion of glucose solutions with or without added l-carnitine, *Drugs Exp Clin Res,* 19:219–222, 1993.
235. Giancaterini A, De Gaetano A, and Mingrone G et al., Acetyl-L-carnitine infusion increases glucose disposal in type-2 diabetic patients, *Metabolism,* 49:704–708, 2000.
236. Derosa G, Cicero AFG, and Gaddi A et al., The effects of L-carnitine on plasma lipoprotein(a) levels in hypercholesterolemic patients with type-2 diabetes mellitus, *Clin Therap,* 25:1429–1439, 2003.
237. Giannessi F, Pessotto P, and Tassoni E et al., Discovery of a long-chain carbamoyl aminocarnitine derivative, a reversible carnitine palmitoyltransferase inhibitor with antiketotic and antidiabetic activity, *J Med Chem,* 46:303–309, 2003.
238. Zeviani M, Mariotti C, and Antozzi C et al., OXPHOS defects and mitochondrial DNA mutations in cardiomyopathy, *Muscle Nerve,* 3:S170–174, 1995.
239. Campos Y, Huertas R, and Lorenzo G et al., Plasma carnitine insufficiency and effectiveness of L-carnitine therapy in patients with mitochondrial myopathy, *Muscle Nerve,* 16:150–153, 1993.
240. Hsu CC, Chuang YH, and Tsai JL et al., CPEO and carnitine deficiency overlapping in MELAS syndrome, *Acta Neurol Scand,* 92:252–255, 1995.
241. Munoz-Malaga A and Bautista J, Tratamiento de las enfermedades mitocondriales, *Rev Neurol (Barc),* 26(Suppl 1):87–91, 1998.
242. Munoz-Malaga A, Bautista J, and Salazar JA et al., Lipomatosis, proximal myopathy, and the mitochondrial 8344 mutation: A lipid storage myopathy? *Muscle Nerve,* 23:538–542, 2000.
243. Matsumura M, Nakashima A, and Araki T et al., L-carnitine supplementation in a hemodialysis patient with a mutation in the mitochondrial tRNA(Leu(UUR)) gene, *Nephron,* 85:275–276, 2000.
244. Payne RM and Strauss AW, Expression of the mitochondrial creatine kinase genes, *Mol Cell Biochem,* 133–134:235, 1994–243.
245. Dolder M, Walzel B, and Speer O et al., Inhibition of the mitochondrial permeability transition by creatine kinase substrates, *J Biol Chem,* 278:17760–17766, 2003.
246. Lipskaya TY and Savchenko MS, Once again about the functional coupling between mitochondria creatine kinase and adenine nucleotide translocase, *Biochemistry,* 68:68–79, 2003.
247. Walzel B, Speer O, and Zanolla E et al., Novel mitochondrial creatine transport activity, *J Biol Chem,* 277:37503–37511, 2002.
248. Barisic N, Bernert G, and Ipsiroglu O et al., Effects of oral creatine supplementation in a patient with MELAS phenotype and associated nephropathy, *Neuropediatrics,* 33:157–161, 2002.

249. Komura K, Hobbiebrunken E, and Wilichowski EKG et al., Effectiveness of creatine monohydrate in mitochondrial encephalopathies, *Pediatr Neurol*, 28:53–58, 2003.
250. Op 't Eijnde B, Urse B, and Richter EA et al., Effect of oral creatine supplementation on human muscle GLUT4 protein content after immobilization, *Diabetes*, 50:18–23, 2001.
251. Baum RA and Iber FL, Thiamin—the interaction of aging, alcoholism, and malabsorption in various populations, *World Rev Nutr Diet*, 44:85–116, 1984.
252. Rindi G, In: Ziegler EE and Filer LJ, Eds., *Present Knowledge in Nutrition*, ILSI Press, Washington, DC, 160–166, 1996.
253. Rathanaswami P, Pourany A, and Sundaresan R, Effects of thiamine deficiency on the secretion of insulin and the metabolism of glucose in isolated rat pancreatic islets, *Biochem Int*, 25:577–583, 1991.
254. Rindi G and Laforenza U, Thiamine intestinal transport and related issues: Recent aspects, *Proc Soc Exp Biol Med*, 224:246–255, 2000.
255. Neufeld EJ, Mandel H, and Raz T et al., Localization of the gene for thiamine-responsive megalobastic anemia syndrome, on the long arm of chromosome 1, by homozygosity mapping, *Am J Hum Genet*, 61:1335–1341, 1997.
256. Fleming JC, Tartaglini E, and Steinkamp MP et al., The gene mutated in thiamine-responsive anaemia with diabetes and deafness (TRMA) encodes a functional thiamine transporter, *Nat Genet*, 22:305–308, 1999.
257. Raz T, Labay V, and Baron D et al., The spectrum of mutations, including four novel ones, in the thiamine-responsive megaloblastic anemia gene SLC19A2 of eight families, *Hum Mutation*, 16:37–42, 2000.
258. Rogers L, Porter R, and Sidbury JJ, Thiamine-responsive megaloblastic anemia, *J Pediat*, 74:494–504, 1967.
259. Neufeld EJ, Fleming JC, and Tartaglini E et al., Thiamine-responsive megaloblastic anemia syndrome: A disorder of high-affinity thiamine transport, *Blood Cell Mol Dis*, 27:135–138, 2001.
260. Baron D, Assaraf YG, and Drori S et al., Disruption of transport activity in a D93H mutant thiamine transporter 1, from a Rogers syndrome family, *Eur J Biochem*, 270:4469–4477, 2003.
261. Oishi K, Hofmann S, and Diaz GA et al., Targeted disruption of SLC19A2, the gene encoding the high-affinity thiamin transporter Thtr-1, causes diabetes mellitus, sensorineural deafness, and mega-loblastosis in mice, *Hum Mol Genet*, 11:2951–2960, 2002.
262. Gritli S, Omar S, and Tartaglini E et al., A novel mutation in the SLC19A2 gene in a Tunisian family with thiamine-responsive megaloblastic anaemia, diabetes, and deafness syndrome, *Br J Haematol*, 113:508–513, 2001.
263. Bappal B, Nair R, and Shaikh H et al., Five years followup of diabetes mellitus in two siblings with thiamine-responsive megaloblastic anemia, *Indian Pediat*, 38:1295–1298, 2001.
264. Valerio G, Franzese A, and Poggi V et al., Lipophilic thiamine treatment in long-standing insulin-dependent diabetes mellitus, *Acta Diabetol*, 36:73–76, 1999.
265. Stagg AR, Fleming JC, and Baker MA et al., Defective high-affinity thiamine transporter leads to cell death in thiamine-responsive megaloblastic anemia syndrome fibroblasts, *J Clin Invest*, 103:723–729, 1999.
266. Bakker SJ, Gans RO, and ter Maaten JC et al., The potential role of adenosine in the pathophysiology of the insulin resistance syndrome, *Atherosclerosis*, 155:283–290, 2001.
267. Barile M, Brizio C, Valenti D, De Virgilio C, and Passarella S, The riboflavin/FAD cycle in rat liver mitochondria, *Eur J Biochem*, 267:4888–4900, 2000.
268. Liu Y, Fiskum G, and Schubert D, Generation of reactive oxygen species by the mitochondrial electron transport chain, *J Neurochem*, 80:780–787, 2002.
269. Russell AP, Schrauwen P, and Somm E et al., Decreased fatty acid beta-oxidation in riboflavin-responsive, multiple acylcoenzyme A dehydrogenase-deficient patients is associated with an increase in uncoupling protein-3, *J Clin Endocrinol Metab*, 88:5912–5926, 2003.
270. Civelek VN, Deeney JT, and Shalosky NJ et al., Regulation of pancreatic β-cell mitochondrial metabolism: Influence of Ca^{2+}, substrate, and ADP, *Biochem J*, 318:615–621, 1996.
271. Gudayol M, Vidal-Taboada JM, and Usac EF et al., Detection of a new variant of the mitochondrial glycerol-3-phosphate dehydrogenase gene in Spanish type-2 DM patients, *Biochem Biophys Res Comm*, 263:439–445, 1999.

272. Gudayol M, Vidal J, and Usac EF et al., Identification and functional analysis of mutations in FAD-binding domain of mitochondrial glycerophosphate dehydrogenase in caucasian patients with type-2 diabetes mellitus, *Endocrine*, 16:39–42, 2001.

273. Civelek VN, Deeney JT, and Kubik K et al., Temporal sequence of metabolic and ionic events in glucose-stimulated clonal pancreatic β-cells (HIT), *Biochem J*, 315:1015–1019, 1996.

274. Ueda K, Tanizawa Y, and Ishihara H et al., Overexpression of mitochondrial FAD-linked glycerol-3-phosphate dehydrogenase does not correct glucose-stimulated insulin secretion from diabetic GK rat pancreatic islets, *Diabetologia*, 41:649–653, 1998.

275. Scholte HR, Busch HF, and Bakker HD et al., Riboflavin-responsive complex I deficiency, *Biochim Biophys Acta*, 24:75–83, 1995.

276. Bakker HD, Scholte HR, and Jeneson JA et al., Vitamin-responsive complex I deficiency in a myopathic patient with increased activity of the terminal respiratory chain and lactic acidosis, *J Inherit Metab Dis*, 17:196–204, 1994.

277. Bernsen PL, Gabreels FJ, and Ruitenbeek W et al., Successful treatment of pure myopathy, associated with complex I deficiency, with riboflavin and carnitine, *Arch Neurol*, 48:334–338, 1991.

278. Penn AM, Lee JW, and Thuillier P et al., MELAS mutation with mitochondrial tRNA (Leu)(UUR) mutation: Correlation of clinical state, nerve conduction, and muscle 31P magnetic resonance spectroscopy during treatment with nicotinamide and riboflavin, *Neurology*, 42:2147–2152, 1992.

279. Bernsen PL, Gabreels FJ, and Ruitenbeek W et al., Treatment of complex I deficiency with riboflavin, *J Neurol Sci*, 118:181–187, 1993.

280. Napolitano A, Salvetti S, and Vista M et al., Long-term treatment with idebenone and riboflavin in a patient with MELAS, *Neurol Sci*, 21(Suppl 5):S981–982, 2000.

281. van Eys J, Niacin, In: Machlin LH, Ed., *Handbook of Vitamins*, 2nd ed., New York: Marcel Dekker, 311–340, 1991.

282. Garg A and Grundy SM, Nicotinic acid as therapy for dyslipidemia in non-insulin-dependent diabetes mellitus, *JAMA*, 264:723–726, 1990.

283. Grundy SM, Vega GL, and McGovern ME et al., Diabetes Multicenter Research Group, Efficacy, safety, and tolerability of once-daily niacin for the treatment of dyslipidemia associated with type-2 diabetes, *Arch Int Med*, 162:1568–1576, 2002.

284. Elam MB, Hunninghake DB, and Davis KB et al., ADMIT Investigators, Effect of niacin on lipid and lipoprotein levels and glycemic control in patients with diabetes and peripheral arterial disease, *JAMA*, 284:1263–1270, 2000.

285. Reddy S, Bibby NJ, and Wu D et al., A combined casein-free-nicotinamide diet prevents diabetes in the NOD mouse with minimum insulitis, *Diab Res Clin Pract*, 29:83–92, 1995.

286. Samec S, Seydoux J, and Dulloo AG, Interorgan signaling between adipose tissue metabolism and skeletal muscle uncoupling protein homologs, *Diabetes*, 47:1693–1698, 1998.

287. Dobbins RL, Chester MW, and Daniels MB et al., Circulating fatty acids are essential for efficient glucose-stimulated insulin secretion after prolonged fasting in humans, *Diabetes*, 47:1613–1618, 1998.

288. Boden G, Chen X, and Iqbal N, Acute lowering of plasma fatty acids lowers basal insulin secretion in diabetic and nondiabetic subjects, *Diabetes*, 47:1609–1612, 1998.

289. Chen X, Iqbal N, and Boden G, The effects of free fatty acids on gluconeogenesis and glycogenolysis in normal subjects, *J Clin Invest*, 103:365–372, 1999.

290. Hale PJ and Nattrass M, The short-term effect of nicotinic acid on intermediary metabolism in insulin-dependent diabetes mellitus, *Ann Clin Biochem*, 28:39–43, 1991.

291. Groop LC and Ferrannini E, Insulin action and substrate competition, *Baillieres Clin Endocrinol Metab*, 7:1007–1032, 1993.

292. Hasmann M and Schemainda I, FK866, a highly specific noncompetitive inhibitor of nicotinamide phosphoribosyltransferase, represents a novel mechanism for induction of tumor cell apoptosis, *Cancer Res*, 63:7436–7442, 2003.

293. Majamaa K, Rusanen H, and Remes A et al., Metabolic interventions against complex I deficiency in MELAS syndrome, *Mol Cell Biochem*, 174:291–296, 1997.

294. Rodriguez-Melendez R, Cano S, and Mendez ST et al., Biotin regulates the genetic expression of holocarboxylase synthetase and mitochondrial carboxylases in rats, *J Nutr*, 131:1909–1913, 2001.

295. Hsich YTL and Mistry SP, Effect of biotin on the regulation of glucokinase in the intact rat, *Nutr Res*, 12:787–799, 1992.

296. Reddi A, DeAngelis B, and Frank O, Biotin supplementation improves glucose and insulin tolerances in genetically diabetic KK mice, *Life Sci,* 42:1323–1330, 1988.

297. Zhang H, Osada K, and Maebashi M et al., A high-biotin diet improves the impaired glucose tolerance of long-term spontaneously hyperglycemic rats with non-insulin-dependent diabetes mellitus, *J Nutr Sci Vitaminol (Tokoyo),* 42:517–526, 1996.

298. Baez-Saldana A, Zendejas-Ruiz I, and Revilla-Monsalve C et al., Effects of biotin on pyruvate carboxylase, acetyl-CoA carboxylase, propionyl-CoA carboxylase, and markers for glucose and lipid homeostasis in type-2 diabetic patients and nondiabetic subjects, *Am J Clin Nutr,* 79:238–243, 2004.

299. Shilo S, Aronis A, and Komarnitsky R et al., Selenite sensitizes mitochondrial permeability transition pore opening *in vitro* and *in vivo*: A possible mechanism for chemo-protection, *Biochem J,* 370:283–290, 2003.

300. Shen HM, Ding WX, and Ong CN, Intracellular glutathione is a cofactor in methylseleninic acid-induced apoptotic cell death of human hepatoma $HEPG_2$ cells, *Free Rad Biol Med,* 33:552–561, 2002.

301. Ezaki O, The insulin-like effects of selenate in rat adipocytes, *J Biol Chem,* 265:1124–1128, 1990.

302. Stapleton SR, Garlock GL, and Foellmi-Adams L et al., Selenium: Potent stimulator of tyrosyl phosphorylation and activator of MAP kinase, *Biochim Biophys Acta,* 1355:259–269, 1997.

303. Park HS, Huh HS, and Kim Y et al., Selenite negatively regulates caspase-3 through a redox mechanism, *J Biol Chem,* 275:8487–8491, 2000.

304. Yoon SO, Kim MM, and Park SJ et al., Selenite suppresses hydrogen peroxide-induced cell apoptosis through inhibition of ASKi/JNK and activation of PI3-K/Akt pathways, *FASEB J,* 16:111–113, 2002.

305. Sarker KP, Biswas KK, and Rosales JL et al., Ebselen inhibits NO-induced apoptosis of differentiated PC12 cells via inhibition of ASK1-p38, MAPK-p53, and JNK signaling and activation of p44/42 MAPK and Bcl-2, *J Neurochem,* 87:1345–1353, 2003.

306. Yoshizumi M, Fujita Y, and Izawa Y et al., Ebselen inhibits tumor necrosis factor-alpha-induced c-Jun N-terminal kinase activation and adhesion molecule expression in endothelial cells, *Exp Cell Res,* 292(Suppl 1):1–10, 2004.

307. Whiteman EL, Cho H, and Birnbaum MJ, Role of Akt/protein kinase B in metabolism, *Trends Endocrinol Metab,* 13:444–451, 2002.

308. Wang Z, Jiang C, and Ganther H et al., Antimitogenic and proapoptotic activities of methylseleninic acid in vascular endothelial cells and associated effects on PI3K-AKT, ERK, JNK, and p38 MAPK signaling, *Cancer Res,* 61:7171–7178, 2001.

309. Goldman EH, Chen L, and Fu H, Activation of apoptosis signal-regulating kinase 1 by reactive oxygen species through dephosphorylation at Ser967 and 14-3-3 dissociation, *J Biol Chem,* 279:10442–10449, 2004.

310. Kawamori D, Kajimoto Y, and Kaneto H et al., Oxidative stress induces nucleo-cytoplasmic translocation of pancreatic transcription factor PDX-1 through activation of c-Jun NH_2-terminal kinase, *Diabetes,* 52:2896–2904, 2003.

311. Bennett BL, Satoh Y, and Lewis AJ, JNK: A new therapeutic target for diabetes, *Curr Op Pharmacol,* 3:420–425, 2003.

312. Yan L, Yee JA, and Boylan LM et al., Effect of selenium compounds and thiols on human mammary tumor cells, *Biol Trace Elem Res,* 30:145–162, 1991.

313. Thompson HJ, Wilson AC, and Lu J et al., Comparison of the effects of an organic and an inorganic form of selenium on a mammary carcinoma cell line, *Carcinogenesis,* 15:183–186, 1994.

314. Davis RL and Spallholz JE, Inhibition of selenite-catalyzed superoxide generation and formation of elemental selenium (Se(o)) by copper, zinc, and aurintricarboxylic acid (ATA), *Biochem Pharmacol,* 51:1015–1020, 1996.

315. Stewart MS, Davis RL, and Walsh LP et al., Induction of differentiation and apoptosis by sodium selenite in human colonic carcinoma cells (HT29), *Cancer Lett,* 117:35–40, 1997.

316. Kim TS, Yun BY, and Kim IY, Induction of the mitochondrial permeability transition by selenium compounds mediated by oxidation of the protein thiol groups and generation of the superoxide, *Biochem Pharmacol,* 66:2301–2311, 2003.

317. Shilo S and Tirosh O, Selenite activates caspase-independent necrotic cell death in Jurkat T cells and J774.2 macrophages by affecting mitochondrial oxidant generation, *Antioxid Redox Signal,* 5:273–279, 2003.

318. Zhou N, Xiao H, and Li T-K et al., DNA damage-mediated apoptosis induced by selenium compounds, *J Biol Chem,* 278:29532–29537, 2003.

319. Berg EA, Wu JY, and Campbell L et al., Insulin-like effects of vanadate and selenate on the expression of glucose-6-phosphate dehydrogenase and fatty acid synthase in diabetic rats, *Biochimie,* 77:919–924, 1995.

320. Skripchenko ND, Sharafetdinov KhKh, and Plotnikova OA et al., Effect of selenium enriched diet on lipid peroxidation in patients with diabetes mellitus type-2, *Vopr Pitan,* 72:14–17, 2003.

321. Aydin A, Orhan H, and Sayal A et al., Oxidative stress and nitric oxide related parameters in type-II diabetes mellitus: Effects of glycemic control, *Clin Biochem,* 34:65–70, 2001.

322. Chang I, Cho N, and Koh JY et al., Pyruvate inhibits zinc-mediated pancreatic islet cell death and diabetes, *Diabetologia,* 46:1220–1227, 2003.

323. Roussel AM, Kerkeni A, and Zouari N et al., Antioxidant effects of zinc supplementation in Tunisians with type-2 diabetes mellitus, *J Am Coll Nutr,* 22:316–321, 2003.

324. Anderson RA, Roussel AM, and Zouari N et al., Potential antioxidant effects of zinc and chromium supplementation in people with type-2 diabetes mellitus, *J Am Coll Nutr,* 20:212–218, 2001.

325. Ames BN, Delaying the mitochondrial decay of aging, *Ann NY Acad Sci,* 1019:406–411, 2004.

326. Papadopoulou LC, Sue CM, and Davidson M et al., Fatal infantile cardioencephalomyopathy with COX deficiency and mutations in SCO2, a COX assembly gene, *Nat Genet,* 23:333–337, 1999.

327. Paret C, Ostermann K, and Krause-Buchholz U et al., Human members of the SCO1 gene family: Complementation analysis in yeast and intracellular localization, *FEBS Lett,* 447:65–70, 1999.

328. Dickinson EK, Adams DL, and Schon EA et al., A Human SCO2 mutation helps define the role of Sco1p in the cytochrome oxidase assembly pathway, *J Biol Chem,* 275:26780–26785, 2000.

329. Jaksch M, Paret C, and Stucka R et al., Cytochrome-c oxidase deficiency due to mutations in SCO2, encoding a mitochondrial copper-binding protein, is rescued by copper in human myoblasts, *Hum Mol Genet,* 10:3025–3035, 2001.

330. Salviati L, Hernandez-Rosa E, and Walker WF et al., Copper supplementation restores cytochrome-c oxidase activity in cultured cells from patients with SCO2 mutations, *Biochem J,* 363:321–327, 2002.

331. Galhardi CM, Diniz YS, and Faine LA et al., Toxicity of copper intake: Lipid profile, oxidative stress and susceptibility to renal dysfunction, *Food Chem Toxicol,* 42:2053–2060, 2004.

332. Salazar J, Ferre R, and Vallve JC et al., Two novel single-nucleotide polymorphisms in the promoter of the cellular retinoic acid-binding protein II gene (CRABP-II), *Mol Cell Probes,* 17:21–23, 2003.

333. Casa F, Daury L, and Grandemange S et al., Endocrine regulation of mitochondrial activity: Involvement of truncated RXR-α and c-Erb Aα1 proteins, *FASEB J,* 17:426–436, 2003.

334. Notario B, Zamora M, and Vinas O et al., All-trans-retinoic acid binds to and inhibits adenine nucleotide translocase and induces mitochondrial permeability transition, *Mol Pharmacol,* 63:224–231, 2003.

335. Pratt MAC and Niu MY, Bcl-2 controls caspase activation following a p53-dependent cyclin D1-induced death signal. *J Biol Chem,* 278:14219–14229, 2003.

336. Rial E, Gonzalez-Barroso M, and Fleury C et al., Retinoids activate proton transport by the uncoupling proteins UCP1 and UCP2, *EMBO J,* 18:5827–5833, 1999.

337. Echtay KS, Esteves TC, and Pakay JL et al., A signaling role for 4-hydroxy-2-nonenal in regulation of mitochondrial uncoupling, *EMBO J,* 22:4103–4110, 2003.

338. Hail N and Lotan R, Mitochondrial respiration is uniquely associated with the prooxidant and apoptotic effects of N-(4-hydroxyphenyl)retinamide, *J Biol Chem,* 276:45614–45621, 2001.

339. Yamakoshi Y, Fukasawa H, and Yamauchi T et al., Determination of endogenous levels of retinoic acid isomers in type II-diabetes mellitus patients, Possible correlation with HgbA1C values, *Biol Pharm Bull,* 25:1268–1271, 2002.

340. Granado F, Olmedilla B, and Botella F et al., Retinol and α-tocopherol in serum of type-1 diabetic patients with intensive insulin therapy, A long-term follow-up study, *Nutrition,* 19:128–132, 2003.

341. Berdanier CD, Kras K, and Wickwire K et al., Whole-egg diet delays the age-related impaired glucose tolerance of BHE/Cdb rats, *Proc Soc Exp Biol Med,* 219:28–36, 1998.

342. Berdanier CD, Everts HB, and Hermoyian C et al., Role of vitamin A in mitochondrial gene expression, *Diab Res Clin Pract,* 54(Suppl 2):S11–27, 2001.

343. Everts HB and Berdanier CD, Nutrient-gene interactions in mitochondrial function: Vitamin A needs are increased in BHE/Cdb rats, *IUBMB Life,* 53:289–294, 2002.

344. Heart Protection Study Collaborative Group, MRC/BHF heart protection study of antioxidant vitamin supplementation in 20536 high-risk individuals, A randomized placebo-controlled trial, *Lancet,* 360:23–33, 2002.

345. Padayatty SJ, Katz A, and Wang Y et al., Vitamin C as an antioxidant: Evaluation of its role in disease prevention, *J Am Coll Nutr,* 22:18–35, 2003.

346. Packer JE, Slater TF, and Wilson RL, Direct observation of a free radical interaction between vitamin E and vitamin C, *Nature,* 278:7373–738, 1979.

347. Myer YP, Thallam KK, and Pande A, Kinetics of the reduction of horse heart ferricytochrome-c: Ascorbate reduction in the presence and absence of urea, *J Biol Chem,* 255:9666–9673, 1980.

348. Li LX, Skorpen F, and Egeberg K et al., Induction of uncoupling protein 2 mRNA in β-cells is stimulated by oxidation of fatty acids but not by nutrient oversupply, *Endocrinology,* 143:1371–1377, 2002.

349. Li X, Cobb CE, and Hill KE et al., Mitochondrial uptake and recycling of ascorbic acid, *Arch Biochem Biophys,* 387:143–153, 2001.

350. Gruss-Fisher T and Fabian I, Protection by ascorbic acid from denaturation and release of cytochrome-c, alteration of mitochondrial membrane potential, and activation of multiple caspases induced by H_2O_2, in human leukemia cells, *Biochem Pharmacol,* 63:1325–1335, 2002.

351. Puskas F, Gergely P, and Niland B et al., Differential regulation of hydrogen peroxide and Fas-dependent apoptosis pathways by dehydroascorbate, the oxidized form of vitamin C, *Antioxid Redox Signal,* 4:357–369, 2002.

352. Perez-Cruz I, Carcamo JM, and Golde DW, Vitamin C inhibits FAS-induced apoptosis in monocytes and U937 cells, *Blood,* 102:336–343, 2003.

353. Rumsey SC and Levine M, Absorption, transport, and disposition of ascorbic acid in humans, *J Nutr Biochem,* 9:116–130, 1998.

354. Price KD, Price CSC, and Reynolds RD, Hyperglycemia-induced ascorbic acid deficiency promotes endothelial dysfunction and the development of atherosclerosis, *Atherosclerosis,* 158:1–12, 2001.

355. Skrha J, Prazny M, and Hilgertova J et al., Serum α-tocopherol and ascorbic acid concentrations in type-1 and type-2 diabetic patients with and without angiopathy, *Clin Chim Acta,* 329:103–108, 2003.

356. Abdel-Wahab YHA, O'Harte FPM, and Mooney MH et al., Vitamin C supplementation decreases insulin glycation and improves glucose homeostasis in obese hyperglycemic (ob/ob) mice, *Metabolism,* 51:514–517, 2002.

357. Koo JR and Vaziri ND, Effects of diabetes, insulin, and antioxidants on NO synthase abundance and NO interaction with reactive oxygen species, *Kidney Int,* 63:195–201, 2003.

358. Darko D, Dornhorst A, and Kelly FJ et al., Lack of effect of oral vitamin C on blood pressure, oxidative stress, and endothelial function in type-II diabetes, *Clin Sci,* 103:339–344, 2002.

359. Evans M, Anderson RA, and Smith JC et al., Effects of insulin lispro and chronic vitamin C therapy on postprandial lipaemia, oxidative stress, and endothelial function in patients with type-2 diabetes mellitus, *Eur J Clin Invest,* 33:231–238, 2003.

360. Ramanathan K, Shila S, and Kumaran S et al., Ascorbic acid and α-tocopherol as potent modulators on arsenic induced toxicity in mitochondria, *J Nutr Biochem,* 14:416–420, 2003.

361. Weber T, Dalen H, and Andera L et al., Mitochondria play a central role in poptosis induced by α-tocopheryl succinate, an agent with antineoplastic activity: Comparison with receptor-mediated pro-apoptotic signaling, *Biochemistry,* 42:4277–4291, 2003.

362. Calviello G, Di Nicuolo F, and Piccioni E et al., γ-tocopheryl quinine induces apoptosis in cancer cells via caspase-9 activation and cytochrome-c release, *Carcinogenesis,* 24:427–433, 2003.

363. Sukalski KA, Pinto KA, and Berntson JL, Decreased susceptibility of liver mitochondria from diabetic rats to oxidative damage and associated increase in alpha-tocopherol, *Free Radic Biol Med,* 14:57–65, 1993.

364. Sakurai K, Katoh M, and Someno K et al., Apoptosis and mitochondrial damage in INS-1 cells treated with Alloxan, *Biol Pharm Bull,* 24:876–882, 2001.

365. Zalov S, Sumien N, and Forster MJ et al., Coenzyme Q intake elevates the mitochondrial and tissue levels of coenzyme Q and α–tocopherol in young mice, *J Nutr,* 133:3175–3180, 2003.

366. Campoy C, Baena RM, and Blanca E et al., Effects of metabolic control on vitamin E nutritional status in children with type-1 diabetes mellitus, *Clin Nutr,* 22:81–86, 2003.

367. Davison GW, George L, and Jackson SK et al., Exercise, free radicals, and lipid peroxidation in type-1 diabetes mellitus, *Free Rad Biol Med*, 33:1543–1551, 2002.
368. Mayer-Davis EJ, Costacou T, and King I et al., Plasma and dietary vitamin E in relation to incidence of type-2 diabetes, *Diabetes Care*, 25:2172–2177, 2002.
369. Montonen J, Knekt P, and Jarvinen R et al., Dietary antioxidant intake and risk of type-2 diabetes, *Diabetes Care*, 27:362–366, 2004.
370. Ylonen K, Alfthan G, and Groop L et al., Botnia Research Group, Dietary intakes and plasma concentrations of carotenoids and tocopherols in relation to glucose metabolism in subjects at high risk of type-2 diabetes: The Botnia Dietary Study *Am J Clin Nutr*, 77:1434–1441, 2003.
371. Boeing H, Weisgerber UM, and Jeckel A et al., Association between glycated hemoglobin and diet and other lifestyle factors in a nondiabetic population: Cross-sectional evaluation of data from the Potsdam cohort of the European Prospective Investigation into Cancer and Nutrition Study, *Am J Clin Nutr*, 71:1115–1122, 2000.
372. Paolisso G, Gambardella A, and Giugliano D et al., Chronic intake of pharmacological doses of vitamin E might be useful in the therapy of elderly patients with coronary heart disease, *Am J Clin Nutr*, 61:848–852, 1995.
373. Bhathena SJ, Berlin E, and Judd JT et al., Effects of ω3 fatty acids and vitamin E hormones involved in carbohydrate and lipid metabolism in men, *Am J Clin Nutr*, 54:684–688, 1991.
374. Paolisso G, Di Maro G, and Galzerano D et al., Pharmacologic doses of vitamin E and insulin action in elderly subjects, *Am J Clin Nutr*, 59:1291–1296, 1994.
375. Paolisso G, D'Amore A, and Galzerano D et al., Daily vitamin E supplements improve metabolic control but not insulin secretion in elderly type-II diabetic patients, *Diabetes Care*, 16:1433–1437, 1993.
376. Shoff SM, Mares-Perlman JA, and Cruickshank KJ et al., Glycosylated hemoglobin concentrations and vitamin E, vitamin C, and β-carotene intake in diabetic and nondiabetic older adults, *Am J Clin Nutr*, 58:412–416, 1993.
377. Sanchez-Lugo L, Mayer-Davis EJ, and Howard G et al., Insulin sensitivity and intake of vitamins E and C in African-American, Hispanic, and non-Hispanic white men and women: The Insulin Resistance and Atherosclerosis Study (IRAS), *Am J Clin Nutr*, 66:1224–1231, 1997.
378. Cuzzocrea S, Riley DP, and Caputi AP et al., Antioxidant therapy: A new pharmacological approach in shock, inflammation, and ischemia/reperfusion injury, *Pharmacol Rev*, 53:135–159, 2001.
379. Faure P, Protective effects of antioxidant micronutrients (vitamin E, zinc, and selenium) in type-2 diabetes mellitus, *Clin Chem Lab Med*, 41:995–998, 2003.
380. Saxena SP, Israels ED, and Israels LG, Novel vitamin-K-dependent pathways regulating cell survival, *Apoptosis*, 6:57–68, 2001.
381. Monks TJ, Hanzlik RP, and Cohen GM et al., Quinone chemistry and toxicity, *Toxicol Appl Pharmacol*, 112:2–16, 1992.
382. Gerasimenko JV, Gerasimenko OV, and Palejwala A et al., Menadione-induced apoptosis: Roles of cytosolic Ca^{2+} elevations and the mitochondrial permeability transition pore, *J Cell Sci*, 115:485–497, 2002.
383. Laux I and Nel A, Evidence that oxidative stress-induced apoptosis by menadione involves Fas-dependent and Fas-independent pathways, *Clin Immunol*, 101:335–344, 2001.
384. Paul C and Arrigo AP, Comparison of the protective activities generated by two survival proteins: Bcl-2 and Hsp27 in L929 murine fibroblasts exposed to menadione or staurosporine, *Exp Gerontol*, 35:757–766, 2000.
385. De Marchi U, Pietrangeli P, and Marcocci L et al., L-Deprenyl as an inhibitor of menadione-induced permeability transition in liver mitochondria, *Biochem Pharmacol*, 66:1749–1754, 2003.
386. Tiedge M, Lortz S, and Munday R et al., Complementary action of antioxidant enzymes in the protection of bioengineered insulin-producing RINm5F cells against the toxicity of reactive oxygen species, *Diabetes*, 47:1578–1585, 1998.
387. Lortz S and Tiedge M, Sequential inactivation of reactive species by combined overexpression of SOD isoforms and catalase in insulin-producing cells, *Free Rad Biol Med*, 34:683–688, 2003.
388. Eleff S, Kennaway NG, and Buist NR et al., 31P NMR study of improvement in oxidative phosphorylation by vitamins K and C in a patient with a defect in electron transport at complex III in skeletal muscle, *Proc Natl Acad Sci USA*, 81:3529–3533, 1984.

389. Argov Z, Bank WJ, and Maris J et al., Treatment of mitochondrial myopathy due to complex III deficiency with vitamins K3 and C, A 31P-NMR followup study, *Ann Neurol,* 19:598–602, 1986.

14 The Rational Use of Dietary Supplements, Nutraceuticals, and Functional Foods for the Diabetic and Prediabetic Patient

Jeffrey I. Mechanick

CONTENTS

Standard approaches to the management of diabetic and prediabetic patients incorporate diet, exercise and, as needed, pharmaceuticals. Nevertheless, the use of dietary supplements, nutraceuticals, and functional foods (DS/N-FF) in clinical medicine has grown enormously in recent years. This phenomenon owes its popularity to a variety of factors: (1) desire by the public to "self-treat" and avoid doctors' visits and pharmaceuticals; (2) enthusiastic, bordering on fanatical, media coverage and marketing; (3) profiteering by unscrupulous practitioners; and (4) governmental policies that permit and even encourage these practices. Many aspects of diabetology are targeted by DS/N-FF therapy and will be reviewed in this chapter. However, the important point to bear in mind is that DS/N-FF should only be recommended to patients when there is an acceptable level of scientific evidence favoring benefit greater than risk (recommendation grades A, B, or C), and

265

when commercial products can be obtained that deliver accurate amounts of the intended ingredient without interfering or deleterious substances. Patients will undoubtedly inquire about DS/N-FF, and therefore physicians must be prepared with knowledge and a willingness to discuss the issues openly and plainly.

COMPLEMENTARY AND ALTERNATIVE MEDICINE (CAM)

Various terms have been employed to describe the practice of recommending therapies not approved by the Food and Drug Administration (FDA) for treatment of disease. These include "unconventional" and "alternative" and, when combined with FDA-approved or "traditional" therapies, the terms "complementary" or "integrative" are used (see Table 14.1). More preferable terms, which are less biased and based on the scientific evidence at hand, are "proven" vs. "unproven." There is clearly a gray area blurring the distinction between alternative and traditional therapies that incorporates therapeutic agents substantiated by various gradations of clinical evidence. Thus, in order to objectively recommend DS/N-FF, an *a priori* evidence-rating scale and recommendation-grading system based on the scientific evidence, and used for "evidence-based medicine" by traditional physicians, is applied (see Appendix 2). This approach is not without criticism [1–5], though the critical point is that even when subjective factors weigh in, there must be some level of scientific substantiation behind all of the medical decision-making. Simply put, the use of DS/N-FF must be guided by clinical evidence.

Perhaps the greatest impetus driving the popularization of DS/N-FF was the 1994 Dietary Supplement Health and Education Act (DSHEA). This act was intended to increase "self-healing" among Americans and save healthcare dollars through the use of DS/N-FF based on their presumed safety and efficacy. Dietary supplements are commercially processed products, derived from natural foods, and containing one or more specifically marketed ingredients. DSHEA defines dietary supplements and governs the way they are marketed and used (see Table 14.2). Nutraceuticals, on the other hand, are regarded as concentrated presumed bioactive substances, originally derived from a food, but now in a nonfood matrix and used to promote health in dosages far greater than those found in normal foods [6]. Functional foods are whole foods in their natural state that confer therapeutic or beneficial properties beyond basic nutritional needs. Examples of functional foods are given in Table 14.3. For example, fish is a functional food, fish oil is a dietary supplement, and concentrated n-3 fatty acid in capsule form is a nutraceutical.

From 1990 to 1997, expenditures for alternative medicine professional services increased 45% to $21 billion with $12 billion out-of-pocket [8]. In addition, 72% of patients receiving alternative care failed to disclose this to their physicians [9]. Among diabetics, 78% take prescribed diabetes medication, 44% take over-the-counter (OTC) medications and DS/N-FF and 31% take alternative medicines (herbs and unconventional minerals) [10]. These proportions are comparable to a non-diabetic control group that was interviewed. The most common OTC medications used by patients with diabetes were multivitamins, vitamin E, vitamin C, calcium, and aspirin [10]. In fact, in a study by Ford [11], vitamin use was found to protect subjects from the development of diabetes. Among patients with diabetes, multivitamin and mineral supplement use was associated with a reduction in the incidence of infection and absenteeism [12]. Adverse events associated with routine multivitamin use are rare (recommendation grade C for routine multivitamin use in diabetes).

Common alternative medicines used by diabetic patients are garlic (11.6%), echinacea (8.9%), herbal mixtures (8.5%), and glucosamine (5.8%) [10]. Patients with diabetes spent nearly as much on OTC and alternative medicines as they did on prescribed medications [10]. The case for an ethnomedical approach to diabetes was made by Oubré et al. [13] in which pharmaceutical research is based on the use of medicinal plants in traditional cultures that target specific genetically determined factors. This contrasts with the Western biomedical model in which random high-throughput screening of phytochemicals are performed by the pharmaceutical industry.

TABLE 14.1
Features of Alternative Medicine

Use of non-FDA-approved therapies
Use of unproven therapies
Generally not taught in U.S. medical schools
Generally target complaints and not diagnoses

TABLE 14.2
Regulation of Dietary Supplements by DSHEA

Labeling

Nutrient content ("high in calcium")

Structure–function ("calcium builds strong bones")

Disease claims ("calcium used to treat osteoporosis")—must be approved by the FDA based on evidence

Disclaimer for nutrient content and structure-function claims

"This statement has not been evaluated by the FDA. This product has not been intended to diagnose, treat, cure, mitigate, or prevent any disease."

FDA can issue warnings about adverse events

"No regulatory process for quality control in manufacturing."

TABLE 14.3
Functional Foods Useful in Patients with Diabetes

Source	Food	Function
Plant	Oats	Decrease LDL-c and CHD risk
	Soy	Decrease CHD risk
	Flaxseed	Decrease LDL-c and platelet aggregation
	Tomatoes	Contains lycopene, reduces risk for MI
	Garlic	Antihypertensive, cholesterol-lowering, antidiabetic
	Tea	Contains catechins, decreased CHD risk
	Wine	Contains phenolics, decreased CHD and diabetes risks
Animal	Fish	Contains n-3 FA, decreased risk total CVD mortality
	Dairy	Fermented milk has cholesterol-lowering effects
	Beef	Conjugated linoleic acid has anti-obesity effects

See text for abbreviations.

Source: From Reference [7] with permission.

ANTI-DIABETIC BOTANICALS

The potential uses for botanicals include improvement in glycemic control, weight management, lipid-lowering, risk reduction for diabetic complications and treatment of diabetic complications [14] (see Table 14.4). Other botanicals with demonstrable hypoglycemic activity in animals, but with little or no clinical evidence (grade D) are given in Table 14.5. Diabetic patients seeking out "naturopathy," a form of alternative medicine specializing in the use of "natural" substances to promote health, may be taking one or more of these botanical agents.

The concept of using botanicals in diabetes management is not unlike other branches of medicine where traditional pharmaceuticals are derived from plant extracts. In fact, the biguanide metformin was derived from the guanidine-rich medicinal plant *Galega officinalis* (goat's rue or

TABLE 14.4
Antidiabetic Botanicals with Recommendation Grade C[a]

Common Name	Botanical Name
Aloe vera	*Aloe vera*
American ginseng	*Panax quinquefolius*
Asian ginseng	*Panax ginseng*
Basil	*Ocimum sanctum*
Bilberry	*Vaccinium myrtillus*
Cinnamon	*Cinnamomum cassia*
Cranberry juice	*Vaccinium macrocarpon*
Curry	*Murraya koeingii*
Fenugreek	*Trigonella foenum graecum*
Fig leaf	*Ficus carica*
Flaxseed	*Linum usitatissimum*
Garlic	*Allium sativum*
Green tea	*Camellia sinensis*
Oolong tea	*Camellia sinensis*
Gudmar	*Gymnema sylvestre*
Indian malabar	*Pterocarpus marsupium*
Ivy guard	*Coccinia indica*
Jangli amla	*Phyllanthus niruri*
Milk thistle	*Silybum marianum*
Onion	*Allium cepa*
Prickly pear cactus	*Opuntia streptacantha*

[a] All have some conclusive level-III benefit with little risk based on clinical evidence.

French lilac). Many of the anti-diabetic botanicals have been researched extensively in India, but these represent only a small proportion of the over 400 reported in literature [18], and even a smaller proportion of the over 250,000 estimated higher plants with potential medicinal activity [17]. Adusumilli et al. [19] conducted a survey of 2,186 respondents undergoing elective surgery and found that 57% admitted to using herbal remedies (most common: echinacea [48%], aloe vera [30%], ginseng [28%], garlic [27%], and ginkgo biloba [22%]) but herbal use was relatively low among diabetic patients (odds ratio 0.46).

HERBS

Both American and Asian ginseng have hypoglycemic actions attributed to the steroidal saponin ginsenoside Rb-2 as well as panaxans I, J, K, and L [20–24]. Clinical studies have demonstrated (1) a reduction in hemoglobin A1C (A1C) from 6.5% to 6.0% in patients with type-2 diabetes mellitus (T2DM) on 200 mg daily, compared with no change with placebo (but A1C improvements may be due to the weight loss in the treatment group) [25]; (2) decreased postprandial glucose 40 minutes after a 3-g dose of American ginseng [26]; and (3) beneficial effects on mood, physical activity, and body weight [25]. Potential mechanisms of action include decreased carbohydrate absorption [27], decreased nitric oxide (NO) mediated glucose transport [28], and increased NO-mediated glucose-stimulated insulin secretion [29]. Adverse effects include agitation, estrogen-like actions, interference with warfarin, and interactions with monoamine oxidase inhibitors [14]. Recommended doses are 1–3 g of the crude root or 200–600 mg of extract for 3 months [30]. Overall, the recommendation grade for ginseng is C based on level 3 evidence demonstrating benefit with no significant risks.

Antidiabetic actions have been identified in alcohol-extracted charantin and peptides from the fruit *Momordica charantia*, also known as bitter melon, balsam pear, or karela. Improved glucose

TABLE 14.5
Botanicals with Hypoglycemic Activity in Animals but with Little or No Clinical Evidence (Grade D)[a]

Common Name	Botanical Name
Alfalfa	*Medicago sativum*
Alpine ragwort	*Senecio nemorensis*
Allspice	*Pimenta officinalis*
Amarta	*Tinospora cordifolia*
Anjani	*Memecylon umbellatum*
Athalaki	*Momordica cymbalaria*
Banana	*Musa sapientum*
Bay leaf	*Laurus nobilis*
Bean pod	*Phaseolus vulgaris*
Behen	*Moringa oleifera*
Betelnut	*Areca catechu*
Bitter apple	*Citrullus colocynthis*
Bitter melon	*Momordica charantia*
Black berry	*Syzigium cumini*
Black catnip	*Phyllanthus amarus*
Black tea	*Camellia sinensis*
Buckwheat	*Fagopyrum esculentum*
Burma cutch	*Acacia catechu*
Caper plant	*Capparis deciduas*
Caturang	*Lantana camara*
Centaury	*Centaurium erythraea*
Chirata	*Swertia chirayita*
Clove	*Syzigium aromaticum*
Cocoa	*Theobroma cacao*
Cowitch	*Mucuna pruriens*
Cumin	*Cuminum cyminum*
Dandelion	*Taraxacum officinale*
Davana	*Artemisia pallens*
Divi-divi	*Caesalpinia bonducella*
Eucalyptus	*Eucalyptus globulus*
European goldenrod	*Solidago virgaurea*
Fever nut	*Caesalpinia bonducella*
Garden beet	*Beta vulgaris*
German sarsaparilla	*Carex arenaria*
Ginger	*Zingiber officinale*
Greek sage	*Salvia triloba*
Guar gum	*Cyamopsis tetragonoloba*
Holy fruit tree	*Aegle marmelose*
Indian banyan tree	*Ficus bengalenesis*
Indian gum arabic tree	*Acacia arabica*
Jambolan	*Syzygium cumini*
Kutki	*Picrorrhiza kurroa*
Laksmana	*Biophytum sensitivium*
Lotus	*Nelumbo nucifera*
Madagascar periwinkle	*Catharanthus roseus*
Mango	*Mangifera indica*
Mountain ash berry	*Sorbus aucuparia*
Mushroom, shitake	*Lentinus edodes*
Mushroom, white	*Agaricus bisporus*

(continued)

TABLE 14.5 (continued)
Botanicals with Hypoglycemic Activity in Animals but with Little or No Clinical Evidence (Grade D)[a]

Common Name	Botanical Name
Mustard	*Brassica juncea*
Neem	*Azadirachia indica*
Noni	*Morinda citrifolia*
Nutmeg	*Myristica fragrans*
Oats	*Avena sativa*
Oregano	*Origanum vulgare*
Papaya	*Carica papaya*
Pitica	*Salacia reticulata*
Plantain	*Musa paradisiacal*
Poley	*Teucriumj polium*
Pomegranate	*Punica granatum*
Ponkoranti	*Salacia oblonga*
Red silk cotton tree	*Bombax ceiba*
Red gram	*Cajanus cajan*
Reed herb	*Phragmites communis*
Sage	*Salvia officinalis*
Sakkargand	*Ipomoea batatas*
Salt bush	*Atriplex halimus*
Shoe flower	*Hibiscus rosa-sinesis*
Stevia	*Stevia rebaudiana*
Stinging nettle	*Urtica dioica*
Surinam cherry	*Eugenia uniflora*
Triticum	*Agropyron repens*
Turmeric	*Curcuma domestica*
White mulberry	*Morus alba*
Wild service tree	*Sorbus torminalis*
Witch hazel	*Hammamelis virginiana*

[a] Demonstrable clinical safety insufficient for a recommendation grade C.

Source: Adapted from References [15–17].

tolerance [31] and A1C levels (8.37% to 6.95%) [32] have been demonstrated in patients with T2DM. Both of these studies were small and poorly designed and controlled, and therefore inconclusive (evidence level 4). *Momordica charantia* is thought to have insulin-like actions [33] and inhibit gluconeogenesis [34]. Usual doses range from 100–200 mg po three times a day (TID) of a standardized extract. Adverse effects involving liver and testicular lesions have been reported in animal studies (grade D) [14].

Extracts from the bark of *Pterocarpus marsupium* contain the flavanoid (-)-epicatechin which stimulates hepatic lipid metabolism (anti-obesity effect) [35], prevents β-cell damage (via antioxidant effects) [36], reduces interleukin-1β (IL-1β)/interferon-γ (IFN-γ)-induced nitric oxide production [37], and promotes β-cell regeneration in animals [38,39]. Anti-diabetic flavanols are also found in *Camellia sinensis* (green tea polyphenols) and *Acacia catechu* (Burma cutch). In a 12-week multi-center open trial involving 97 T2DM patients, *Pterocarpus marsupium*, 2 g/day, was associated with improved fasting glucose levels (151 mg/dL to 119 mg/dL), postprandial glucose levels (216 mg/dL to 171 mg/dL), and A1C levels (9.8% to 9.4%), but not lipid levels (evidence level 3) [40]. Diabetic symptoms improved with treatment and adverse effects were not reported (grade C).

Vaccinium myrtillus (Bilberry or European blueberry) has been associated with improvements in glycemic control, hyperlipidemia, retinopathy, and other microvascular complications of diabetes in animal models with little human data available [41–44]. The active ingredients are thought to be anthrocyanosides and the dosage for bilberry, which is not exact, is 80–160 mg TID of a 25% anthrocyanoside extract [14]. A related botanical, *Vaccinium macrocarpon*, or cranberry, is also a rich source of anthrocyanins and flavonoids. These compounds are also found in red wine and *Aronia melanocarpa* (chokeberry) and have been associated with decreased lipid oxidation and protein glycosylation [45]. In a randomized placebo-controlled study of 27 patients with T2DM, 240 cc of cranberry juice cocktail for 12 weeks was not associated with any improvement in diabetic or lipid parameters (evidence level 3—no benefit) [46]. There were no adverse effects in this clinical study (grade C).

The Israeli plant *Atriplex halimus* (salt bush) has been associated with improvements in glycemic control [14]. It has been used and investigated because when sand rats are deprived of this plant, they develop diabetes [47]. Salt bush also contains vitamins A, C, and D, as well as chromium. Nevertheless, salt bush cannot be recommended (grade D) for diabetes due to the lack of clinical safety and efficacy data. Other Israeli plants used for diabetes remedies, but without sufficient clinical data on safety or efficacy (grade D) are: *Achillea fragrantissima, Ammi visnaga, Capparis spinosa, Ceratonia siliqua, Cleome droserifolia, Eryngium creticum, Inula viscose, Matricaria aurea, Origanum syriaca, Paronychia argentea, Prosopis farcta, Sarcopoterium spinosum,* and *Teucrium polium* [48].

On the Arabian peninsula, *Aloe vera* (aloe) dried sap is used to treat diabetes. The protective effects on the liver and kidney and the antidiabetic effects of aloe are described in animal models [49–52]. Notably, the beneficial effects of aloe on diabetic wound healing may be mediated via altering basic fibroblast growth factor-2 (FGF-2) signaling [53]. Various reports in the literature demonstrate glucose- and lipid-lowering effects of aloe in T2DM patients [54–56]. The results of a limited number of controlled trials in diabetics, demonstrating promise but with insufficient data, may be found in a systematic review on the clinical effectiveness of aloe by Vogler et al. [57] (evidence level 3—inconclusive benefit). The dose of aloe is 1 tablespoon of juice twice a day (BID) with no adverse effects reported (grade C) [14].

Flaxseed (*Linum usitatissimum*) contains mucilages (soluble fiber), various fatty oils such as linolenic, linoleic, and oleic acids, proteins, cyanogenic glycosides, phenylpropane derivatives, and lignans, which have antioxidant properties similar to soy isoflavones. Flaxseed use was associated with decreased area under the glucose tolerance curve by 28% in healthy women (evidence level 3) [58]. Soy isoflavones, such as daidzein and genistein, decrease intestinal glucose uptake leading to decreased postprandial glucose levels but clinical studies are lacking (evidence level 4) [59]. Genistein decreases Glucose-stimulated insulin secretion (GSIS), islet cell proliferation, and tyrosine kinase activity [60]. Flaxseed and soy isoflavones are safe (grade C).

Ficus carica (fig leaf) normalizes antioxidant status in diabetic rats [61]. *Ficus carica* also lowered postprandial glucose excursions (145 mg/dL to 157 mg/dL in treatment group vs. 197 mg/dL to 294 mg/dL in control group) and insulin requirements (12% less with treatment) in a small (N=10) crossover study of patients with type-1 diabetes mellitus (T1DM) in which there were no adverse effects (evidence level 3; grade C) [62]. *Ficus relegiosa* increases β-cell insulin release in rabbits [63]. *Ficus bengalensis* contains the flavonoids leucopelargonin and leucocyanin, which have antioxidant properties [64], and leucodelphinidin, which has insulin secretagogue properties [65].

Consumption of broiled stems from the prickly pear cactus (*Opuntia streptacantha* [nopal]), a popular treatment for diabetes among the Mexican population, was associated with decreased fasting blood glucose (about 50 mg/dL) and insulin levels (about 50%) based on 6 short-term metabolic trials of patients with T2DM (evidence level 3) [66–71]. This botanical has a high soluble fiber and pectin content that can decrease intestinal glucose absorption, and no significant adverse effects have been reported (grade C).

Silymarin, or milk thistle (*Silibum marianum*), is best known for its beneficial effects in patients with viral or alcoholic hepatitis. Silymarin contains polyphenolic flavonoids and antioxidants that act to decrease glutathione oxidation, stabilize membranes, and normalize malondialdehyde concentrations [72]. Velussi et al. [73] conducted a 12-month open controlled study of 60 patients with insulin-requiring T2DM and alcoholic cirrhosis, receiving silymarin, 600 mg/day. They demonstrated improved glycemic control (decreased mean glucose from 202 mg/dL to 172 mg/dL and A1C from 8% to 7.2%) and decreased insulin requirements (55 to 42 units/day) with the treatment (evidence level 3) [73]. In another multi-center prospective randomized controlled trial (PRCT), a new oral formuation of silybin-β-cyclodextrin given to 60 patients with T2DM and alcoholic hepatitis was associated with improved fasting glucose (174 mg/dL to 148 mg/dL) (evidence level 3) [74]. Silymarin may also hold promise for patients with T1DM. Silymarin induces β-cell cytoprotection and improves GSIS by inhibiting cytokine-induced NO production and suppressing c-Jun N-terminal kinase (JNK) and Janus kinase (JAK)/signal transducers and activators of transcription (STAT) pathways [75]. The relative safety of silymarin has been demonstrated in clinical studies (grade C).

AYURVEDA

The Indian remedy fenugreek is derived from the defatted seed of *Trigonella foenum graecum* and contains fiber (galactomannin), nicotine, coumarin, and the alkaloid trigonelline. Other active compounds in fenugreek with antidiabetic action include 4-hydroxyisoleucine (stimulates GSIS), furostanol saponins and steroidal sapogenins (increase peripheral glucose utilization) [76]. Fenugreek has also been found to decrease gastric emptying and delay glucose absorption, reverse gluconeogenic, glycolytic, and lipogenic activity in the kidney and liver, and reduce lipid peroxidation and oxidative injury [76]. In a small double-blind, placebo-controlled trial of patients with T2DM, fenugreek decreased insulin levels by 7%, increased insulin sensitivity by 56%, and decreased serum triglyceride levels by 53 mg/dL (evidence level 3) [77]. In another small randomized, controlled study of 10 patients with T1DM, fenugreek reduced the mean fasting glucose by 76 mg/dL as well as significantly decreasing total cholesterol, triglyceriders, and low-density lipoprotein cholesterol (LDL-c) (evidence level 3) [78]. Patients are cautioned to avoid taking this botanical, which slows drug absorption, at the same time as oral medication [14]. Otherwise, fenugreek is safe (grade C).

Gymnema sylvestre, or gurmar, is another Indian remedy that has been referred to as a "sugar blocker" in the U.S. market. In an uncontrolled study of 22 T2DM patients, administration of 400 mg of Gymnema sylvestre extract (GS4) for 18–20 months improved glycemic control (decreased fasting glucose, from 174 mg/dL to 124 mg/dL, and A1C, from 11.9% to 8.48%), lipid status (decreased total cholesterol from 260 mg/dL to 231 mg/dL) and was associated with reductions in oral hypoglycemic medication dosing [79]. Five of 22 patients in this study needed to discontinue oral hypoglycemics to avoid hypoglycemia (evidence level 3) [79]. In another uncontrolled study of 27 patients with T1DM by the same research group in Madras, India, the same GS4 extract amount was associated with decreased insulin requirements (25% after 6–8 months and 50% after 26–30 months), short-term improvements in fasting glucose (232 mg/dL to 177 mg/dL), A1C (12.8% to 9.5%), and increased endogenous insulin production via increased β-cell function (evidence level 3) [80]. These beneficial effects of GS4 are thought to be mediated via improved β-cell permeability and insulin-dependent glucose utilization pathways [76]. There were no significant adverse effects of *Gymnema sylvestre* extract in the above clinical studies (grade C).

Ivy guard (*Coccinia indica*) is a botanical found in India and used in traditional Ayurveda and Unani systems of medicine for the treatment of diabetes, rashes, glossitis, and earaches. This botanical has been studied in a variety of animal models and found to exert a hypoglycemic action via reduction of the hepatic gluconeogenic enzymes glucose-6-phosphatase and fructose-1,6-phosphatase [81]. In a small double-blind, controlled 6-week trial of 16 patients with T2DM, ivy guard treatment was associated with significant decreases in fasting glucose levels (179 mg/dL to 122 mg/dL) and 2-hour postprandial glucose levels (245 mg/dL to 187 mg/dL) (evidence level 3) [82]. Similar biochemical effects and improvements in glycemic control, but without significant adverse effects, have also been demonstrated in other small controlled and uncontrolled clinical studies (grade C) [83–86].

Jangli Amla (*Phyllanthus niruri*) is another Ayurveda herb and its use has been associated with mild hypoglycemic effects in diabetic and nondiabetic subjects without adverse effects (evidence level 3; grade C) [87]. In a well-designed, single-center, double-blind, placebo-controlled study of 36 subjects with T2DM, a "pancreas tonic" was associated with a reduction of mean A1C from 10.1 to 8.8 (p = 0.04) [88]. The tonic was composed of the following ingredients:

- *Aegle marmelose* (leaves)
- *Pterocarpus marsupium* (heartwood)
- *Syzigium cumini* (fruit)
- *Momordica charantia* (seeds)
- *Gymnema sylvestre* (leaves)
- *Trigonella foenum graecum* (seeds)
- *Azadirachta indica* (seeds)
- *Ficus racemosa*
- *Tinospora cordifolia* (stem)
- *Cinnamomum tamala* (leaves)

TRADITIONAL CHINESE MEDICAL SYSTEM

The paradigm of herbal treatment in the Chinese medical system is to typically combine herbs so that the action of the main herb is enhanced and the potential toxicities reduced. Seven of the antidiabetic herbal products approved for clinical use in China are presented in Table 14.6. The clinical data demonstrating benefit are based on studies with evidence levels 2–3 and are reviewed by Jia et al. [89].

A more extensive review of individual and combined Chinese herbal antidiabetic remedies are given in Li et al. [90]. Liu et al. [91] conducted a metareview of 66 randomized trials involving 8302 patients and found the methodological quality to be generally low. Herbs demonstrating benefit were holy basil leaves, Xianzhen Pian, Qidan Tongmai, Huoxue Jiangtang Pingzhi, Inolter, Bushen Jiangtang Tang, Composite Trichosanthis, Jiangtang Kang, Ketang Ling, Shenqi Jiangtang Yin, Xiaoke Tang, and Yishen Huoxue Tiaogan. The reported adverse effects of these herbal combinations are minimal (grade C).

CULINARY BOTANICALS

Onions (*Allium cepa*) and garlic (*Allium sativum*) are functional foods that have glucose-lowering effects in animals and humans owing to the presence of certain volatile oils (evidence level 3) [92,93]. Dietary garlic use has also been associated with lower blood pressures in studies based on questionnaires [94], but stronger evidence supporting this link is lacking. The active ingredients are allyl propryl disulfide (in onions) and diallyl disulfide ("allicin" in garlic). It is postulated that these compounds compete with insulin, also a disulfide, for hepatic insulin-inactivating sites causing release of free insulin [95]. Other mechanisms of action include antioxidant [96] and vascular [97] effects. *Allium cepa* is generally dosed as one 400-mg capsule daily and *Allium sativum* as 4 g of fresh garlic or 8 mg of essential oil daily [14]. Significant adverse effects have not been reported; however, garlic use can interfere with anticoagulants and anti-platelet drugs and therefore increase the risk of bleeding (grade C).

TABLE 14.6
Chinese Medical System Antidiabetic Phytotherapies

Product	Ingredients
Yi-jin	*Panax ginseng* (Ginseng)
	Atractylodes macrocephala (Largehead Atractylodes Rhizome)
	Poria cocos (Indian Bread)
	Opuntia dillenii (Cactus)
Ke-le-nin	*Radix astragalus* (Milkvetch Root)
	Rehmannia glutinosa (Chinese Foxglove Root)
Yu-san-xiao	*Radix astragalus* (Milkvetch Root)
	Scrophularia ningpoensis (Figwort Root)
	Anemarrhena asphodeloides (Common Anemarrhena Rhizome)
	Rehmannia glutinosa (Chinese Foxglove Root)
Qi-zhi	*Radix astragalus* (Milkvetch Root)
	Rehmannia glutinosa (Chinese Foxglove Root)
	Hirudo nipponia (Leech)
Shen-qi	*Panax ginseng* (Ginseng)
	Radix astragalus (Milkvetch Root)
	Rehmannia glutinosa (Chinese Foxglove Root)
	Hirudo nipponia (Leech)
	Dioscora opposite (Common Yam Rhizome)
	Coptis chinensis (Coptis Root)
	Cornus officinalis (Asiatic Cornelian Cherry Fruit)
Jinqi	*Lonicera japonica* (Honeysuckle Flower)
	Radix astragalus (Milkvetch Root)
	Coptis chinensis (Coptis Root)
Xiao-ke-an	*Radix astragalus* (Milkvetch Root)
	Hirudo nipponia (Leech)
	Pueraria lobata (Lobed Kudzuvine Root)
	Ophiopogon japonicus (Dwarf Lilyturf Tuber)

Source: From Reference [89] with permission.

There are several other culinary botanicals that have proven hypoglycemic activity. *Marraya koeingii* (curry leaf tree) increases hepatic glycogen stores, through inhibition of glycogenolysis, and increases lecithin cholesterol acyl transferase (LCAT) activity in animals [98]. In patients with T2DM, curry reduces fasting and postprandial sugars after 15 days of treatment, but without changes in A1C levels or lipid status (evidence level 3) [99]. Basil leaves have also been found to have hypoglycemic effects. In a randomized, placebo-controlled, crossover, single-blind trial of holy basil (*Ocimum sanctum* and *Ocimum album*), patients with T2DM experienced 17.6%, 7.3%, and 6.5% decreases in fasting blood glucose, postprandial blood glucose, and total cholesterol, respectively (evidence level 3) [100]. No significant adverse effects were reported in these studies (grade C).

Pimentol, from allspice, and biflorin, from clove, have antioxidant properties which could decrease advanced glycation endproducts (AGE) formation in patients with diabetes [101]. No clinical trials have supported these claims. Ginger (*Zingiber officinale*) has antidiabetic effects, possibly via 5-hydroxytryptamine (5-HT) receptors, in rats [102] but does not have an effect on blood glucose in healthy nondiabetic human subjects [103]. Along with garlic, ginkgo, and ginseng, ginger may increase the bleeding time and should not be used in patients taking warfarin. Witch hazel, nutmeg, oregano, sage, and bay leaf have insulin-like biologic activity [104].

Bioactive compounds isolated from cinnamon potentiate insulin activity via (1) stimulation of autophosphorylation of a truncated form of the insulin receptor; (2) activation of phosphatidylinositol-3-kinase (PI3K); (3) inhibition of protein-tyrosine phosphatase-1 (PTP-1) that inactivates the insulin receptor; and (4) inhibition of glycogen synthase kinase-3β, which increases glycogen synthesis [105,106]. In a randomized, placebo-controlled trial of 60 patients with T2DM, cinnamon intake of 1, 3, or 6 g/day for 40 days, reduced fasting blood glucose by 18–29%, triglycerides by 23–30%, LDL-c by 7–27%, and total cholesterol by 12–26 (evidence level 3) [106]. No significant adverse effects were reported (grade C). The active antidiabetic and antioxidant compounds found in cinnamon have been characterized as water-soluble polyphenol polymers [107]. Their very high insulin-enhancing biologic activity is due to type-A procyanidin oligomers of catechins and epicatechins.

Dark chocolate consumption (100 g/day) has been associated with improvements in insulin sensitivity, blood pressure, blood flow, and LDL-c levels [108,109]. Cocoa powder flavorings have also been associated with increased postprandial insulinemia [110]. Experimentally, these clinical findings are thought to be mediated by NO-synthase regulation, immunomodulation, and IκB/NF-κβ activation [111]. These effects have been attributed to the flavanol class of polyphenols (catechins, epicatechins, and procyanidins) in cocoa products (derived from *Theobroma cacao*) though over 600 phytochemicals have been identified in dark chocolate. High concentrations of flavanols are also found in tea, grapes, and grapefruit. The total polyphenol content of dark chocolate is approximately 500 mg/100 g and flavanol content is 88 mg/100 g. Moreover, chocolate is a magnesium-rich food ($\approx$ 100 mg/100 g) which could also account for beneficial effects on glycemic control and the cardiovascular system. The sugar content of dark chocolate may be replaced by sorbitol or isomalt to reduce the glycemic effect of diabetic confectioneries, though increased gastrointestinal symptoms, such as flatulence, may be observed [112,113]. Pre-clinical data from rats has also demonstrated that antioxidative activity in cocoa might also decrease cataract formation [114]. Potential adverse effects of dark chocolate include dental caries, obesity, calciuria, and oxaluria [115]. Thus, even with emerging data supporting a potential clinical benefit of dark chocolate on glycemic control and cardiovascular health (evidence level 3), the high fat and high caloric content, as well as unknown optimal dosing, precludes an evidence-based prescription for diabetic patients to eat dark chocolate (grade C: no objection to limited consumption provided body weight, glycemic control, and lipid status are controlled).

TEA AND COFFEE

Green and black teas were also found to have antidiabetic activity *in vitro* [116]. Oolong is a third type of tea that is partially fermented, compared with green (not fermented) and black (fully fermented) teas. In a randomized, crossover-designed study of 20 patients with T2DM treated with oral agents, oolong tea use, 1500 cc/day × 30 days, was associated with lower fasting blood glucose levels (229 mg/dL–162 mg/dL) and fructosamine levels (410 μmol/L–323 μmol/L) compared with placebo (1500 cc/day water) (evidence level 3) [117]. There were no reports of significant adverse effects in this study (grade C). The amount of polymerized polyphenols, with antidiabetic activity found in teas are related to the extent of fermentation. The green tea flavonoid, epigallocatechin gallate (EGCG), induces glucose lowering by (1) increasing tyrosine phosphorylation of the insulin receptor and insulin receptor substrate-1 (IRS-1); (2) reducing PI3K-induced phosphoenolpyruvate carboxykinase (PEPCK) gene expression; and (3) modulating the redox state of the cell [118]. EGCG also has insulin-like activity by increasing PI3K, mitogen-activating protein kinase (MAPK), and 70kDa ribosomal s6 kinase (p70^{s6k}) activities [118]. Caffeine is another compound found in teas, and it increases hypoglycemic awareness in patients with T1DM without affecting glycemic control or the frequency of hypoglycemia [119,120]. Caffeine has also been associated with decreased risk for developing T2DM [120].

WINE AND OTHER ALCOHOLIC BEVERAGES

Diabetes is associated with increased oxidative stress, so the incorporation of dietary antioxidants has potential benefit. Because wine has antioxidant properties, some clinicians have encouraged wine consumption for diabetic patients. In fact, the majority of Americans consume alcohol. Alcohol is a food and in persons consuming one drink per day (12 oz beer ≈ 5 oz wine ≈ 1.5 oz liquor ≈ 0.5 oz alcohol ≈ 15 g; × 7.1 kcal/g alcohol; ≈ about 100 kcal/drink), alcohol represents approximately 5% of a typical 2000 kcal/day American diet.

Alcohol is not stored in the body and its oxidation by alcohol dehydrogenase (ADH), microsomal ethanol oxidizing system (MEOS), and to a lesser extent, catalase, is prioritized over carbohydate and fat oxidation [121]. Alcohol dehydrogenase oxidizes ethanol to acetaldehyde and nicotinamide adenine dinucleotide, reduced form (NADH). Excess NADH participates in the following three pathways: (1) diverts pyruvate into lactic acid formation and away from gluconeogenesis, thus predisposing the person to hypoglycemia; (2) synthesizes glycerol and fatty acids (lipogenesis), thus increasing adiposity; and (3) utilization in mitochondrial electron transport chain for the formation of 5-adenosine tiphosphate (ATP)—but this inhibits fatty acid oxidation, thus increasing ketosis, hepatic fat accumulation, and hyperlipidemia. Acetaldehyde also impairs hepatic mitochondrial function, leading to hepatitis and cirrhosis, and affects central neurotransmitter physiology, leading to addiction. Certain polymorphisms that inactivate aldehyde dehydrogenase-2 (ALDH2), which metabolizes acetaldehyde into acetate, exacerbate these deleterious effects of acetaldehyde. This polymorphism can be detected with genetic testing, and affected persons should avoid alcohol. Excess acetate production further impairs fatty acid oxidation and fat mobilization from adipose tissue, and thus promotes obesity.

A full hour is required to metabolize a serving of alcohol and during this time, there is little satiation and compensatory inhibition of food intake [121]. In fact, food intake increases shortly after alcohol consumption [122]. Potential physiologic mechanisms of this orectic effect of alcohol include (1) altered hepatic redox state and reduction of fatty acid oxidation [122]; (2) inhibition of afferent signal pathways (leptin—neuropeptide Y [NPY] axis) [123,124], glucagon-like peptide-1 (GLP-1) [123], and serotonin (5HT) [125]; and (3) activation of γ-aminobutyric acid (GABA) [126] and opioid [127] neurotransmitter signals (THT).

Before proceeding with a more detailed discussion on the benefits of alcohol in general, and wine in particular, it is extremely important to review the dangers associated with irresponsible and/or excessive alcohol use. Medical issues associated with excessive alcohol use include liver disease, pancreatitis, peripheral neuropathy, certain types of cancers (liver, head, neck, and esophageal), heart disease, stroke, and alcoholism [128]. Moreover, heavy drinking may eventually cause loss of appetite, vitamin deficiencies, gastrointestinal symptoms, skin problems, sexual dysfunction, obesity, neurological damage including memory loss, and psychological disorders [128]. When the oral intake calories are not reduced in the setting of alcohol consumption, the risk for obesity is increased [121]. Most significantly, heavy drinking increases the risk for mortality from motor vehicle accidents, work injuries, recreational injuries, violence, homicide, and suicide. In addition, alcohol abuse is associated with absenteeism from work with negative economic impact. Hence, patients advised to completely abstain from alcohol use include pregnant women, those with a medical condition likely to become worse with alcohol consumption, those with a personal or family history of alcoholism, those taking medications that may interact with alcohol, those planning to engage in activities requiring alertness including routine driving, and those under the legal drinking age [128]. Because alcohol use is associated with a high rate of traumatic injury and death, especially in young adults, and that there are proven preventive strategies for a healthy lifestyle, including diet, physical activity, and smoking cessation, it is not recommended that anyone start to drink, or increase the amount of drinking, on the basis of health considerations [129].

Notwithstanding the above warnings, alcohol use has been associated with certain health benefits specifically applicable to patients with diabetes. Alcoholic beverages in general inhibit gluconeogenesis and may increase insulin sensitivity. In postmenopausal, nondiabetic women, alcohol decreases fasting insulin and triglyceride levels [130] and improves postprandial insulin sensitivity (after a low-carbohydrate meal) and energy expenditure (after a low- or high-carbohydrate meal) [131]. Consistent with this are the findings by Rimm et al. [132] and Conigrave et al.

[133] that alcohol consumption (including heavy drinkers) lowers the risk of developing T2DM. In a study by Kao et al. [134], heavy (> 21 drinks per week), but not light (≤ 1 drink/week), consumption of alcohol was associated with increased risk of developing T2DM. This effect was observed in men, but not women, and was primarily due to the consumption of spirits, rather than beer or wine [134]. Moreover, among men consuming > 14 drinks of spirits per week, the relative odds for incident T2DM was 1.82, signifying increased risk [134]. These results were similar to a population-based cross-sectional study of Swedish men in which heavy alcohol consumption (> 12 drinks per week) was associated with an odds ratio of 2.1 (increased risk) for T2DM compared with moderate alcohol consumption (7–12 drinks per week) which was associated with an odds ratio of 0.7 (decreased risk) [135]. Wannamethee et al. [136] demonstrated a protective effect of light-to-moderate alcohol consumption (5–30 g/day) on the development of T2DM. The protective effect of light-to-moderate alcohol use in decreasing the risk of T2DM has also been demonstrated in obese persons (body mass index [BMI] 45.3 ± 7 kg/M^2, range 34–77 kg/M^2) [137]. When insulin resistance parameters were measured in association with alcohol use in a longitudinal study of 1856 men and 1529 women, alcohol intake was only associated with improvements in high-density lipoprotein cholesterol (HDL-c) and worsened fasting blood glucose, body mass index, waist circumference, and systolic blood pressure [138]. In T1DM, evening alcohol consumption (dry white wine 0.75 g/kg alcohol) is associated with decreased nocturnal growth hormone (GH) levels and next-morning fasting and postprandial hypoglycemia [139]. The European Prospective Investigation of Cancer (EPIC)-Norfolk Study [140], a population-based cohort study, demonstrated an inverse relationship between alcohol intake and A1C levels among diabetic patients. Interestingly, this association was demonstrable with only wine among men, whereas the association was demonstrable with wine, beer, and spirits among women. Moderate (two glasses) prandial red wine does not adversely affect glycemic control owing to its tannin and phytate content [141] despite changes in lactate production, ketogenesis, and the redox state [142]. In sum, light-to-moderate consumption (5–15 g/day) of alcohol is not associated with any adverse effect on glycemic status. Therefore, in patients with diabetes, or at risk for diabetes, who choose to consume alcoholic beverages, the American Diabetes Association recommends no more than one drink per day for women and two drinks per day for men (grade B) [143]. Alcohol should be consumed with food to minimize the likelihood of experiencing a hypoglycemic episode, due to increased insulin sensitivity [143].

The ethanol component of alcoholic beverages decreases platelet aggregation [144] and increases HDL-c via ApoAI and ApoAII gene expression [145,146]. Ethanol also stimulates hepatic lipogenesis [147], triglyceride formation [146], and small dense atherogenic LDL-c formation [148]. A consensus viewpoint, derived from the critical examination of over 50 epidemiologic studies, recognizes that moderate ethanol intake significantly reduces mortality when compared with abstinence [149]. However, intake beyond moderate use was associated with increased mortality. It should be recognized, however, that the bulk of these data are observational and do not definitively disclose a causal relationship between alcohol use and health benefits. Furthermore, the cardioprotective effects of light-to-moderate consumption of alcoholic beverages are small and appear to be independent of the type of alcoholic beverage [140,150,151].

The health benefits of wine consumption, primarily the reduction of atherosclerotic heart disease ("The French Paradox"), have prompted great interest in the effects of alcohol and other phytochemicals found in wine on patients with diabetes [152]. Wine is the yeast fermentation product of fruit juice, predominantly grape, which changes the organic acids and phenolic compounds. Examples of these compounds include the nonflavonoid hydroxybenzoic and hydroxycinnamic acids, flavonols (quercetin, myricetin, kamempfero,l and rutin), flavanols (catechin, epicatechin, and procyanidins), and anthocyanins (see review by German and Walzem [153] for complete list and quantities of these compounds found in red and white wine). Wine typically contains ethanol 8–15% by weight and:

- Water
- Phenolic acids

- Polyphenols
- Carbohydrates
    - Glucose
    - Fructose
    - Arabinose, rhamnose, and xylose
    - Pectin
    - Inositol
    - Fucose
- Methyl alcohol, 2-, 3-butylene glycol, and acetoin
- Glycerol
- Aldehyde
- Other organic acids
- Amino acids, ammonia, amides, and protein humin
- Minerals [153]

The phenolic antioxidant content of 1 glass of red wine is equivalent to 12 glasses of white wine, 1 pint of beer, 2 cups of tea, 7 glasses of orange juice, 20 glasses of apple juice, or 5 apples [154].

Among healthy volunteers, meals that include red wine confer more plasma antioxidant activity than meals without red wine [155]. The beneficial effects of red wine on hemostatic cardiovascular risk factors complement those of the Mediterranean diet [156]. Experimental studies have identified several components of wine or whiskey contributing to antioxidant activity: phenolics, ethanol, and trace metals such as copper [157].

In patients with T2DM, wine also decreases the total radical-trapping antioxidant parameter (TRAP), with a greater benefit observed *in vitro* with red wine compared to white wine [158], while also reducing prothrombin fragments 1 and 2, activating factor VII, and reducing overall thrombosis [159]. In a study by Tessari et al. [160] of 6 patients with T1DM, red wine consumption (Red Tocai, 12% alcohol by volume, ≈300 mL over 4 hours) was associated with increased fibrinogen synthesis, glucagon levels, and first-pass splanchnic uptake of leucine and phenylalanine, without effects on endogenous proteolysis or albumin synthesis.

Anthocyanins from Cabernet-type red wine lower blood glucose levels and reactive oxygen species (ROS) generation following streptozotocin in an experimental model of diabetes in rats [161]. In another study using streptozotocin-induced diabetes in rats, a Chardonnay white wine enriched with polyphenols (catechin, epicatechin, procyanidins dimmers B1-B4, gallic acid, cafeic acid, and caftaric acid) normalized plasma antioxidant capacity [162]. The polyphenols quercetin and glabridin stabilize platelet-derived aryl esterase activity, which circulates in association with LDL-c and prevents endothelial LDL-c oxidation [163]. In a prospective study, conducted from 1986 through 1998 involving 34,492 postmenopausal women, dietary (+)-catechin and (+)-epicatechin intake, from sources such as wine and apples but not teas (catechins in the form of gallates), was associated with coronary heart disease risk reduction [164]. Catechins may partially account for the cardio-protective effects of the Mediterranean diet, which is high in fruits, vegetables, and red wine. Of note, EGCG consumption from green tea has been associated with increased tyrosine phospho-rylation of the insulin receptor and IRS-1, reduction of PEPCK gene expression via PI3K, MAPK, and p70(s6k) activation [118], and improved renal physiology due to altered prostaglandin metab-olism [165]. (-)Epicatechin possesses antioxidant properties; it increases erythrocyte glutathione levels, which are typically reduced in patients with T2DM [166]. (-)Epicatechin also mimics insulin by increasing erythrocyte membrane acetylcholinesterase activity, which is also typically low in patients with T2DM [167]. Furthermore, the antiproliferative actions of (-)epicatechin may result from its inhibitory effects on membrane Na/H antiport activity[168]. Other beneficial effects of wine polyphenols include slowed lipid oxidation, reduction of atherosclerotic plaques, and improved endothelial function and hemodynamics [153]. Polyphenols in red wine, but not white wine or rosé, decrease endothelin-1 (ET-1) gene expression [169]. In addition, red wine, but not ethanol, activates the endothelium-dependent vasodilatory nitric oxide (NO)-cGMP pathway [170] via endothelial nitric-oxide synthase (eNOS) activation [171]. Red wine polyphenols reduce intracellular adhesion molecule-1 (ICAM-1), NF-κB, monocyte chemotactic protein-1 (MCP-1), and platelet-derived growth factor β receptor (PDGFR) levels [172]. The salutary effects of polyphenols in wine are far less in populations consuming a diet rich in fruits and vegetables that also contains phenolic acids and polyphenols, such as the Mediterranean diet [173].

MINERALS

CHROMIUM

Chromium is an essential micronutrient in humans. There are several loci of action impacting intermediary metabolism, glucose homeostasis, insulin action and lipid metabolism by chromium which were first attributed to "glucose-tolerance factor" (GTF) (see Table 14.7). GTF is found in brewer's yeast and though it has never been isolated, is thought to contain trivalent chromium bound to nicotinic acid, glycine, cysteine, and glutamic acid [174]. The oligopeptide chromodulin binds chromium and the activated insulin receptor, stimulating its kinase activity [175]. Chromium is poorly absorbed from the glycemic index (GI) tract and is bound to transferrin and albumin in the blood. Chromium is stored in four compartments in bone, spleen, liver, and kidney with a half-life ranging from 1 day to 1 year. Even though patients with T2DM fail to retain chromium normally [176], the routine use of chromium in diabetes remains unsubstantiated.

A popular DS/N-FF is chromium picolinate which contains trivalent chromium (Cr^{3+}). Several evidence level 2 studies on chromium in T2DM patients have been conducted with varying degrees of demonstrable benefit (see Table 14.8). A large meta-analysis of trivalent chromium supplementation and diabetes, involving 20 PRCTs and 618 subjects with T2DM, was unable to demonstrate a conclusive benefit (evidence level 1—no benefit) [181]. There are no conclusive adverse effects of oral chromium in the dosages recommended and used in these studies. Sporadic adverse event reports describe rhabdomyolysis, rash, nephritis, anemia, liver dysfunction, and weight loss with chromium use [174]. There may be interactions of chromium with beta-blockers (increased HDL cholesterol), increased chromium absorption with ascorbate, and decreased chromium absorption with foods rich in phytic acid [174]. Normal dietary intakes of chromium are 25 g daily with typical supplement doses ranging from 50–200 g daily [174]. Therefore, chromium should not be recommended to patients with T2DM, but those who wish to take it may continue to do so with little risk (grade C).

TABLE 14.7
Physiological Effects of Chromium in Glucose and Lipid Homeostasis

Increase	Decrease
Insulin binding	Fasting glucose levels
Insulin receptor number	Tyrosine phosphatase
Insulin receptor phosphorylation	Hepatic extraction of insulin
Protein kinase activity with insulin	Insulin levels
Glucose uptake	Total cholesterol
Glucose tolerance	Triglycerides
HDL cholesterol	

TABLE 14.8
Summary of Controlled Trials on Chromium Use in T2DM Patients

Design	Evidence Findings	Reference	Effect	Level
PRCT, crossover N=43, 4 months Brewer's yeast/GTF Placebo-controlled	No effect on glucose	Rabinowitz et al. [177]	+	2
PRCT, crossover N=28, 2 months Chromium picolinate (200 g Cr/day) Placebo-controlled	No effect on glucose, 17.4% TG reduction, no adverse effects	Lee and Reasner [178]	+	2
PRCT N=180, 4 months Cr picolinate (500 g BID) Placebo-controlled	Decreased fasting BG, postprandial BG, total cholesterol, and improved A1C	Anderson et al. [179]	+	2
PRCT, crossover N=78, 8 weeks Brewer's yeast (23.3 g Cr/day) CrCl$_3$ (200 g Cr/day) Placebo-controlled	Decreased fasting BG, postprandial BG, fructosamine, TG no adverse effects	Bahijri et al. [180]	+	2

Abbreviations: BG—blood glucose; GTF—glucose tolerance factor; TG—triglyceride.

In a controlled study of 26 elderly (aged 65–74 years) subjects with impaired glucose tolerance, 160 g Cr/day failed to improve glucose tolerance or lipid levels [182]. These results are at odds with an earlier study of 24 elderly subjects (mean age 78 years with 8 "mildly non-insulin-dependent diabetics") who had improved glucose tolerance and total cholesterol levels with chromium-rich brewer's yeast compared with chromium-poor torula yeast [183]. Nevertheless, there is insufficient evidence to recommend chromium to prevent diabetes.

Vanadium

Vanadium has insulin-like properties resulting from inhibition of protein-tyrosine phosphatases (PTP), which are inactivators of IRS-1, PI3K, and insulin receptor function [184]. This transition metal has intrigued nutrition specialists because of its essential requirement in various marine species. Foods rich in vanadium are mushrooms, shellfish, dill seed, parsley, and black pepper [185]. Vanadium is poorly absorbed and is converted into vanadyl ion in the blood. Similar to chromium, vanadyl is transported by transferrin and albumin to target tissue. There is little long-term systemic toxicity due to vanadium [186]. Modulation of gene expression by vanadium has been described for various cytokines and transcription factors, including macrophage inflammatory protein (MIP)-2, tumor-necrosis factor-α (TNF-α), IL-8, activator protein-1 (AP-1), nuclear transcription factor-κβ (NF-κβ), ras, c-raf-1, MAPK, p53, and p70^{s6k} (see review in Reference 177). One theory is that vanadyl indirectly modulates gene expression via ROS and changes in REDOX potentials [186]. In addition to its effects as an antidiabetic agent, vanadium has been used for lipid-lowering, diuretic, natriuretic effects, vascular effects, and cancer therapy [186]. The insulin-

TABLE 14.9
Summary of Controlled Trials on Vanadium in DM Patients

Design	Evidence			
	Findings	Reference	Effect	Level
Single arm placebo-controlled N=6 T2DM, 3 weeks $VOSO_4$ 100 mg/day	Increased insulin action	Cohen et al. [187]	+	3
Single arm placebo-controlled N=6 T2DM, 3 weeks $VOSO_4$ 100 mg/day	Decreased fasting BG, increased insulin action	Halberstam et al. [188]	+	3
Single arm placebo-controlled N=5 T1DM, 3 weeks $VOSO_4$ 100 mg/day	No change in insulin dose, fructosamine, glucose disposal, insulin action	Aharon et al. [189]	–	3
Single-blind placebo lead trial N=16 T2DM, 6 weeks $VOSO_4$ 75, 150, 300 mg/day	Decreased fasting BG, A1C and improved glucose metabolism	Goldfine et al. [190]	+	3
Single-blind placebo lead trial N=16 T2DM, 6 weeks $VOSO_4$ 75, 150, 300 mg/day	No correlation of fasting BG and euglycemic clamp response with peak V levels	Willsky et al. [191]	+	3

Abbreviations: $VOSO_4$—vanadyl sulfate; BG—blood glucose.

Source: Adapted from References [190–195].

mimetic properties of vanadium compounds result from inhibition of protein tyrosine phosphatases (PTPases), which are inactivators of IRS-1, PI 3-kinase, and insulin receptor function [184].

Clinical trials on the effects of vanadium in T2DM patients are summarized in Table 14.9. Level 3 evidence demonstrates a beneficial effect of vanadium on insulin action in T2DM, but not T1DM patients. Adverse effects include nausea, vomiting, diarrhea, cramps, and green discoloration of the tongue. Chromium, iron (ferrous), and aluminum hydroxide can decrease the absorption of vanadium. There are no typical recommended dosages. In light of the weak clinical evidence and potential for adverse effects, vanadium therapy is not recommended for routine use in diabetes (grade D).

MAGNESIUM

There are several inferential observations that have led to the concept of magnesium supplementation in diabetic and prediabetic patients: (1) magnesium is a cofactor for many biochemical reactions in glucose homeostasis and insulin action [192,193], as well as GSIS and free radical scavenging [194–196]; (2) patients with diabetes have low magnesium levels [193]; (3) magnesium status is inversely related to insulin levels in diabetic and prediabetic patients [197,198]; and (4) magnesium status is inversely related to the risk of developing diabetes [197,199,200]. In a recent study reviewing questionnaire data, Song et al. [201] demonstrated a protective role of higher dietary magnesium intake in reducing the risk for T2DM, especially for overweight women. Therapeutically, magnesium supplementation improves insulin-mediated glucose disposal and insulin secretion [199,202–204] though contradictory studies exist [205–207]. Moreover, even the associations of magnesium status and risk of developing diabetes are questioned due to the paucity of prospective data [200,208]. The clinical evidence does not conclusively support a beneficial role of magnesium in diabetics (see Table 14.10). Even though the adverse effects of magnesium can be

TABLE 14.10
Summary of Clinical Data on Magnesium and Diabetes

	Evidence			
Design	Findings	Reference	Effect	Level
PRCT N=63 T2DM, 16 weeks 25 mEq Mg/day placebo-controlled	Improved insulin sensitivity, improved A1C, improved fasting BG	Rodriquez-Moran et al. [202]	+	2
PRCT, crossover N=9 T2DM, 4 weeks 30 mEq Mg/day Placebo-controlled	Increased glucose oxidation and insulin sensitivity	Paolisso et al. [214]	+	2
PRCT N=40 T2DM, 3 months 60 mEq Mg/day Placebo-controlled	No effect on A1C	Eibl et al. [209]	–	2
PRCT, crossover N=56 T2DM 600 mg Mg/day Placebo-controlled	No effect on glycemic control or lipid status	Eriksson and Kohvakka [210]	–	2
PRCT N=50 T2DM, 3 months 30 mEq Mg/day Placebo-controlled	No effect on glycemic control or lipid status	de Valk et al. [207]	–	2
PRCT N=128 T2DM, 30 days Mg oxide (40–80 mEq Mg/day) Placebo-controlled	Mg depletion with T2DM Higher doses of Mg lowered fructosamine levels	Lima Mde et al. [213]	+	2
PRCT N=28 T1DM, 12 months Mg hydroxide (40–60 mEq Mg/day) Placebo-controlled	No effect on cardiovascular risk factors	Hagg et al. [211]	–	2
PRCT, crossover N=11 T2DM, 8 weeks 360 mg Mg/day Placebo-controlled	No effect on A1C or fructosamine	Johnsen et al. [212]	–	3
Questionnaire	Higher Mg intake reduces T2DM risk	Song et al. [201]	+	3

avoided with lower dosing, the routine administration of magnesium to all diabetic patients merely for the purpose of improving glycemic control is not recommended (grade D).

ZINC

In a placebo-controlled study of 30 patients with T2DM, zinc, 30 mg/day, was associated with decreased markers of oxidative stress, typically increased in diabetes but without any effect on A1C levels [215]. There is no evidence-based rationale for the routine use of zinc to improve glycemic control in patients with diabetes (grade D).

OTHER DS/N-FF

VITAMIN C

Intravenous infusion of ascorbic acid (AA; vitamin C) restores endothelium-dependent vasodilation, which is impaired by ROS formation during periods of hyperglycemia [216]. These results are consistent with the findings by Regensteiner et al. [217] in which oral arginine (9 g/day), vitamin E (1800 mg/day), and AA (1000 mg/day) improved the brachial artery diameter response in patients with T2DM. Also, in a PRCT of 30 patients with T2DM, 500 mg po AA lowered arterial blood pressure and improved arterial stiffness [218]. Since AA enters cells via sodium-dependent facilitated transport (uncharged AA) or via glucose transporter (GLUT) (dihydroascorbate; DHA), it has been postulated that during hyperglycemic states, DHA transport is decreased [219]. This results in impaired intracellular AA-mediated antioxidant activity, resulting in neuropathy, nephropathy, vasculopathy, and retinopathy. This is also the basis for potential benefits of antioxidant therapy in these conditions. Adverse effects of AA in doses of 500–1000 mg daily are rare (grade C).

COENZYME Q10

In a PRCT involving 74 patients with T2DM, conducted by Hodgson et al. [220], coenzyme Q10 (CoQ10), 100 mg orally twice a day for 12 weeks, was associated with reduced A1C (but only $-0.37 \pm 0.17\%$; p = 0.032) and blood pressure levels without reduced oxidative stress (evidence level 3). This single well-designed study fails to demonstrate a clinically significant effect on glycemic control—though additional larger trials with greater power may do so—and therefore does not represent conclusive proof of benefit. Nevertheless, the risks associated with CoQ10 are minimal (primarily GI, with doses greater than 200 mg daily, and CoQ10 may interfere with the action of warfarin) (grade C).

GLUCOSAMINE-CHONDROITIN

In a PRCT of 34 patients with T2DM, glucosamine, 1500 mg daily, and chondroitin, 1200 mg daily, for 90 days, did not affect A1C levels [221]. This negates claims, based on animal data and warnings in the Physician's Desk Reference (PDR) [222], that glucosamine affects glucose metabolism and precautions should be taken in patients with diabetes. There is no reason to recommend either glucosamine or chondroitin for glycemic control in diabetes (grade D).

ORAL AMINO ACIDS

In a randomized, open-label, crossover study, 34 consecutive elderly (age 65–85 years) patients with T2DM and A1C levels > 7% were treated with supplemental oral amino acids (OAA) (8 g/day: leucine [2.5 g/day], lysine [1.3 g/day], isoleucine [1.25 g/day], valine [1.25 g/day], threonine [0.7 g/day], cysteine [0.3 g/day], histidine [0.3 g/day], phenylalanine [0.2 g], methionine [0.1 g], tyrosine [0.06 g/day], and tryptophan [0.04 g/day]; lipid 0.43 g/day; carbohydrate 8.15 g/day; total kcal 449 kcal/day) [223]. Treatment was associated with decreased fasting and postprandial blood glucose, A1C levels, and insulin resistance [223]. Potential mechanisms for this effect include: (1) stimulation of protein synthesis with resultant increased glucose utilization and (2) upregulation of insulin receptor synthesis and autophosphorylation [223]. An additional theoretical advantage of OAA in diabetic patients is the stimulatory effect of branched-chain amino acids on myocardial protein synthesis and reduction in myocardial lactate production [224]. OAA are safe provided they are not ingested in excess (15–20% of total daily energy for patients with diabetes; 134) (grade C).

DIABETIC PERIPHERAL NEUROPATHY

Both T1DM and T2DM patients are at risk for developing peripheral neuropathy. Mechanisms contributing to nerve degeneration in diabetics include increased polyol pathway flux, free radical formation, advanced glycosylation endproduct formation, prostaglandin vasodilator production, and reduced vascular perfusion. Usual therapeutic strategies involve improving glycemic control and pharmaceuticals. Various DS/N-FF have also been studied with respect to diabetic neuropathy, and Halat and Dennehy [235] have conducted a technical review of several agents.

Evening primrose oil (EPO; *Oenothera biennis*) contains the n-6 essential fatty acids γ-linolenic acid (GLA) and linoleic acid. These fatty acids are vital for myelin synthesis and formation of the neuronal cell membrane. Several clinical studies involving diabetic patients have demonstrated benefit from GLA, in an evening primrose oil supplement, with respect to their peripheral neuropathy (see Table 14.11). Potential adverse effects are inhibition of platelet aggregation via increased prostaglandin E_1 (PGE_1) generation and seizures. Taken together, EPO may be used judiciously in patients with mild to moderate peripheral neuropathy who achieve incomplete results from conventional therapies (grade C).

α-lipoic acid (ALA), or thioctic acid, is currently approved for use in patients with diabetic peripheral neuropathy in Germany. α-Lipoic acid is a mitochondrial free radical scavenger and can increase nerve blood flow, distal nerve conduction, and endoneural glucose uptake [233]. Four significant clinical trials demonstrating benefit are also given in Table 14.11, with other clinical studies in the literature being inconclusive [234]. Adverse effects are mild: headache, rash, GI upset, and hypoglycemia. Due to the chelating properties of ALA, patients should be monitored for iron deficiency. In patients who continue to exhibit symptoms or neurologic deficits unresponsive to conventional therapy, ALA may be considered at doses used in the above studies, namely, 1800 mg for a 3-week trial period (grade C).

Other DS/N-FF used for diabetic peripheral neuropathy include:

- Capsaicin (0.075%), an ingredient in chili pepper, is a topical analgesic with four PRCTs demonstrating benefit [235–238] and one demonstrating no effect [239]; some patients experience burning at the application site (grade C).
- Acetyl-L-carnitine (1000 mg/day) improved symptoms in a small [240] and recent large PRCT [241] but not in another large PRCT [242]; there are no significant risks (grade C).
- Vitamin B_6 (25 mg/day) demonstrated benefit in one small study [243] but not in three subsequent PRCTs [244–246]; neurotoxicity is a potential adverse effect (grade D).
- Vitamin E (900 IU/day) demonstrated benefit in a single PRCT of only 21 patients [247]; adverse reactions are rare (grade C).
- St. John's wort (900 mg/day) has antidepressant activity and was found to decrease "shooting" pain but had no effect on other neuropathic symptoms [248]; various drug interactions have been reported (grade C).

CONCLUSIONS

There are hosts of other DS/N-FF, especially a multitude of herbs that have been used in diabetics, but not reviewed here. Several DS/N-FF reviewed in this chapter are supported by clinical evidence, which when coupled with subjective assessments of risk and benefit, result in a recommendation

TABLE 14.11
Clinical Trials of DS/N-FF and Peripheral Neuropathy in Diabetic Subjects

DS/N-FF	Design	Findings	Reference	Effect	Evidence Level
GLA/EPO	PRCT 360 mg/day GLA 6 months N = 22	Improved nerve function	Jamal et al. [226]	+	2
	PRCT 480 mg/day GLA 12 months N = 84	Improved nerve function	Keen et al. [227]	+	2
	PRCT 480 mg/day GLA 12 months N = 51	No effect on vibratory perception	Purewal et al. [228]	–	2
α-Lipoic acid	PRCT 100, 600, 1,200 mg IV/day 3 weeks N = 260	Decreased Sx	ALADIN Ziegler et al. [229]	+	2
	PRCT 600, 1,200 mg po/day 2 years N = 65	Improved nerve conduction	ALADIN II Reljanovic et al. [230]	+	3
	PRCT 600 mg IV × 3 weeks then 1,800 mg po × 6 months N = 377	Improve nerve deficits no effect on Sx	ALADIN III Ziegler et al. [231]	+	2
	PRCT 1,800 mg po/day 3 weeks N = 22	Improved Sx and nerve deficits	ORPIL Ruhnau et al. [232]	+	2

Abbreviations: ALADIN—α-Lipoic Acid in Diabetic Neuropathy; ORPIL—Oral Pilot

grade of C. The best-proven clinical effect of DS/N on glycemic control is a 0.5% A1C reduction, which is less than the least effective approved pharmaceuticals associated with 1.0% A1C reductions. This translates into a rational clinical practice of allowing patients who desire to take DS/N-FF the opportunity to take them, with the understanding that they are aware of potential adverse effects, that they do not represent a replacement for conventional treatment, and that they will continue to follow up with the physician. Routine multivitamin use and vitamin C supplementation may also be included in this category of DS/N-FF with a recommendation grade C. DS/N-FF with a recommendation grade D should not be taken by patients though physicians may comment to their patients that, as new clinical evidence becomes available, recommendation grades may change. However, documentation of risks of specific DS/N-FF in the traditional and alternative medicine literature are generally not as complete as with pharmaceuticals subjected to more extensive clinical trials. In a meta-review of 108 clinical trials, investigating 36 herbs and 9 vitamin/mineral supplements, involving 4565 patients, favorable evidence (> 50% controlled trials suggested efficacy with minimal adverse events) was available for American ginseng (best evidence—grade A), *Coccinia indica* (best evidence—grade A), L-carnitine (best evidence for short-term metabolic trial—grade A), *Trigonella foenum*, nopal, *Gymnema sylvestre*, aloe vera, *Momordica charantia*, chromium, and vanadium [249].

The ultimate judge for the use of DS/N-FF in the management of diabetes ought to be the physician in discussion with the patient. Levels of evidence, adverse effects, anecdote, and recommendation grades simply serve as guidelines for a focused discussion on the matter with the interested patient. If the physician chooses to introduce a DS/N-FF as part of a comprehensive nutritional program for diabetes, risks and benefits must be weighed as with any pharmaceutical. Incomplete data regarding risks and potential shortcomings in the manufacturing process for DS/N-FF must be incorporated in this decision making. Indeed, patients have been empowered by DSHEA to purchase and consume DS/N-FF independently of their physicians. Nevertheless, it is hoped that an unbiased, productive dialogue is practiced with their physician.

REFERENCES

1. Dalen JE, Is integrative medicine the medicine of the future? A debate between Arnold S. Relman, MD, and Andrew Weil, MD, *Arch Int Med*, 159:2122–2126, 1999.
2. Goodman NW, Criticizing evidence-based medicine, *Thyroid*, 10:157–160, 2000.
3. Engel GL, The need for a new medical model: A challenge for biomedicine, *Science*, 196:129–136, 1977.
4. Steel K, Gertman PM,and Crescenzi C et al., Iatrogenic illness on a general medical service at a university hospital, *N Engl J Med*, 304:638–642, 1981.
5. Studdert DM, Eisenberg DM, and Miller FH et al., Medican malpractice implications of alternative medicine, *JAMA*, 280:1610–1615, 1998.
6. Zeisel SH, Regulation of "nutraceuticals," *Science*, 285:1853–1855, 1999.
7. Hasler CM, Functional foods: Their role in disease prevention and health promotion, http://www.nutri-watch.org/04Foods/ff.html, Accessed August 29, 2005.
8. Eisenberg DM, Davis RB, and Ettner SL, et al., Trends in alternative medicine use in the United States, 1990–1997, Results of a follow-up national survey, *JAMA*, 280:1569–1575, 1998.
9. Eisenberg DM, Kessler RC, and Foster C et al., Unconventional medicine in the United States: Prevalence, costs, and patterns of use, *N Engl J Med*, 328:246–252, 1993.
10. Ryan EA, Pick ME, and Marceau C, Use of alternative medicines in diabetes mellitus, *Diabetic Med*, 18:242–245, 2001.
11. Ford ES, Vitamin supplement use and diabetes mellitus incidence among adults in the United States. *Am J Epidemiol*, 153:892–897, 2001.
12. Barringer TA, Kirk JK, and Santaniello AC et al., Effect of a multivitamin and mineral supplement on infection and quality of life, A randomized, double-blind, placebo-controlled trial. *Ann Int Med*, 138:365–172, 2003.
13. Oubré AY, Carlson TJ, and King SR et al., From plant to patient: An ethnomedical approach to the identification of new drugs for the treatment of NIDDM, *Diabetologia* ,40:614–617, 1997.
14. Dey L, Attele AS, and Yuan C-S, Alternative therapies for type-2 diabetes, *Alt Med Rev*, 7:45–58, 2002.
15. Savickiene N, Dagilyte A, and Lukosius A et al., In: Fleming, T, Ed., Importance of biologically active components and plants in the prevention of complications of diabetes mellitus, *Medicina (Kaunas)*, 38:970–975; 2002.
16. PDR for Herbal Medicines, Montvale, NJ: Medical Economics Company, 2000.
17. Grover JK, Yadav S, and Vats V, Medicinal plants of India with anti-diabetic potential, *J Ethnopharmacol*, 81:81–100, 2002.
18. Bailey CJ and Day C, Traditional plant medicines as treatments for diabetes, *Diabetes Care*, 12:553, 1989–564.

19. Adusumilli PS, Ben-Porat L, and Pereira M et al., The prevalence and predictors of herbal medicine use in surgical patients, *J Am Coll Surg,* 198:583–590, 2004.

20. Tomoda M, Shimada K, and Konno C, et al., Partial structure of panaxan A, a hypoglycaemic glycan of Panax ginseng roots, *Planta Med,* 50:436–438, 1984.

21. Konno C, Sugiyama K, and Kano M, et al., Isolation and hypoglycaemic acitivity of panaxans A, B, C, D, and E, glycans of Panax ginseng roots, *Planta Med,* 50:434–436, 1984.

22. Konno C, Murakami M, and Oshima Y et al., Isolation and hypoglycemic acitivity of panaxans Q, R, S, T, and U, glycans of Panax ginseng roots, *J Ethnopharmacol,* 14:69–74, 1985.

23. Yokozawa T, Kobayashi T, and Oura H et al., Studies on the mechanism of the hypoglycemic activity of ginenoside-Rb2 in streptozotocin-diabetic rats, *Chem Pharm Bull (Tokyo),* 33:869–872, 1985.

24. Oshima Y, Konno C, and Hikino H, Isolation and hypoglycemia acitivity of panaxans I, J, K, and L, glycans of Panax ginseng roots, *J Ethnopharmacol,* 14:255–259, 1985.

25. Sotaniemi EA, Haapakoski E, and Rautio A, Ginseng therapy in non-insulin-dependent diabetic patients, *Diabetes Care,* 18:1373–1375, 1995.

26. Vuksan V, Sievenpiper JL, and Koo VY et al., American ginseng (*Panax quinquefolius L*) reduces postprandial glycemia in nondiabetic subjects and subjects with type-2 diabetes mellitus, *Arch Int Med,* 160:1009–1113, 2000.

27. Yuan CS, Wu JA, and Lowell T et al., Gut and brain effects of American ginseng root on brainstem neuronal activities in rats, *Am J Chin Med,* 26:47–55, 1998.

28. Gillis CN, Panax ginseng pharmacology: A nitric oxide link? *Biochem Pharmacol,* 54:1–8, 1997.

29. Kimura M, Waki I, and Chujo T et al., Effects of hypoglycemic components in ginseng radix on blood insulin level in alloxan diabetic mice and on insulin release from perfused rat pancreas, *J Pharmacolcobiodyn,* 4:410–417, 1981.

30. Schulz V, Hansel R, and Tyler VE, Rational phytotherapy, In: *Agents that Increase Resistance to Diseases,* New York, NY: Springer-Verlag, 269–272, 1998.

31. Welihinda J, Karunanayake EH, and Sheriff MH et al., Effect of *Momordica charantia* on the glucose tolerance in maturity onset diabetes, *J Ethnopharmacol,* 17:277–282, 1986.

32. Srivastava Y, Venkatakrishna-Bhatt H, and Verma Y et al., Antidiabetic and adaptogenic properties of *Momordica charantia* extract, An experimental and clinical evaluation, *Phytother Res,* 7:285–289, 1993.

33. Akhtar MS, Athar MA, and Yaqub M, Effect of *Momordica charantia* on blood glucose level of normal and alloxan-diabetic rabbits, *Planta Med,* 42:205–212, 1981.

34. Bailey CJ and Day C, Traditional plant medicines as treatments for diabetes, *Diabetes Care,* 12:553, 1989–564.

35. Murase T, Nagasawa A, and Suzuki J et al., Beneficial effects of tea catechins on diet-induced obesity: Stimulation of lipid catabolism in the liver, *Int J Obes Relat Metab Disord,* 26:1459, 2002–1464.

36. Lapidot T, Walker MD, and Kanner J, Antioxidant and prooxidant effects of phenolics on pancreatic β-cells *in vitro*, *J Agric Food Chem,* 50:7220–7225, 2002.

37. Han MK, Epigallocatechin gallate, a constituent of green tea, suppresses styokine-induced pancreatic β-cell damage, *Exp Mol Med,* 35:136–139, 2003.

38. Chakravarthy BK, Gupta S, and Gambhir SS et al., Pancreatic β-cell regeneration in rats by (-)-epicatechin, *Lancet,* 2:759–760, 1981.

39. Chakravarthy BK, Gupta S, and Gode KD, Functional β-cell regeneration in the islets of pancreas in alloxan-induced diabetic rats by (-)-epicatechin, *Life Sci,* 31:2693–2697, 1982.

40. Indian Council of Medical Research (ICMR), Collaborating Centres, New Delhi, Flexible dose open trial of Vijayasar in cases of newly-diagnosed insulin-dependent diabetes mellitus, *Indian J Med Res,* 108:24–29, 1998.

41. Allen FM, Blueberry leaf extract: Physiological and clinical properties in relation to carbohydrate metabolism, *JAMA,* 89:1577–1581, 1927.

42. Scharrer A and Ober M, Anthrocyanosides in the treatment of retinopathies (author's transl.), *Klin Monatsbl Augenheikd,* 178:386–389 [article in German], 1981.

43. Caselli L, Clinical and electroretinopgraphic study on activity of anthrocyanosides, *Arch Med Int,* 37:29–35, 1985.

44. Cignarella A, Nastasi M, and Cavalli E et al., Novel lipid-lowering properties of *Vaxxinium myrtillus L* leaves, a traditional antidiabetic treatment, in several models of rat dyslipidaemia: A comparison with ciprofibrate, *Thromb Res,* 84:311–322, 1996.

45. Asgary S, Naderi GH, and Sarrafzadegan N et al., Anti-oxidant effect of flavonoids on hemoglobin glycosylation, *Pharm Acta Helv,* 73:223–226, 1999.

46. Chambers BK and Camire ME, Can cranberry supplementation benefit adults with type-2 diabetes? *Diabetes Care,* 26:2695–2696, 2003.

47. Kalderon B, Gutman A, and Levy E et al., Characterization of stages in development of obesity-diabetes syndrome in sand rat (*Psammomys obesus*), *Diabetes,* 35:717–724, 1986.

48. Yaniv Z, Dafni A, and Friedman J et al., Plants used for the treatment of diabetes in Israel, *J Ethnopharmacol,* 19:145–151, 1987.

49. Okyar A, Can A, and Akev N et al., Effect of *Aloe vera* leaves on blood glucose level in type-I and type-II diabetic rat models, *Phytother Res,* 15:157–161, 2001.

50. Rajasekaran S, Sivagnanam K, and Ravi K et al., Hypoglycemic effect of *Aloe vera* gel on streptozocin-induced diabetes in experimental rats, *J Med Food,* 7:61–66, 2004.

51. Can A, Akev N, and Ozsoy N et al., Effect of *Aloe vera* leaf gel and pulp extracts on the liver in type-II diabetic rat models, *Biol Pharm Bull,* 27:694–698, 2004.

52. Bolkent S, Akev N, and Ozsoy N et al., Effect of *Aloe vera* (*L.*) *Burm Fil* leaf gel and pulp extracts on kidney in type-II diabetic rat models, *Indian J Exp Biol,* 42:48–52, 2004.

53. Abdullah KM, Abdullah A, and Johnson ML, et al., Effects of *Aloe vera* on gap junctional intracellular comminuation and proliferation of human diabetic and nondiabetic skin fibroblasts, *J Altern Complement Med,* 9:711–718, 2003.

54. Ghannam N, Kingston M, and Al-Meshaal IA et al., The antidiabetic activity of aloes: Preliminary clinical and experimental observations, *Horm Res,* 24:288–294, 1986.

55. Yongchariyudha S, Rungpitarangsi V, Bunyapraphatsara N, and Chokechaijaroenporn O, Antidiabetic activity of *Aloe vera L.* juice: I, Clinical trial in new cases of diabetes mellitus, *Phytomedicine,* 3:241, 243, 1996.

56. Bunyapraphatsara N, Yongchaiydha S, and Rungpitarangsi V et al., Antidiabetic activity of *Aloe vera L.* juice: II, Clinical trial in diabetic mellitus patients in combination with glibenclamide, *Phytomedicine,* 3:245–248, 1996.

57. Vogler BK and Ernst E. Aloe vera: A systemic review of its clinical effectiveness, *Br J Gen Pract,* 49:823–828, 1999.

58. Cunnane SC, Ganguli S, and Menard C et al., High alpha-linolenic acid flaxseed (*Linum usitatissimum*): Some nutritional properties in humans, *Br J Nutr,* 69:443–453, 1993.

59. Fedorak RN, Cheeseman CI, and Thomson BR et al., Altered glucose carrier expression: Mechanism of intestinal adaptation during streptozotocin-induced diabetic rats, *Am J Physiol,* 261:G585–591, 1991.

60. Szkudelska K, Nogowski L, and Szkudelski T, Genistein affects lipogenesis and lipolysis in isolated rat adipocytes, *J Steroid Biochem Mol Biol,* 75:265–271, 2000.

61. Perez C, Canal JR, and Torres MD, Experimental diabetes treated with *ficus caria* extract: Effect on exidative stress parameters, *Acta Diabetol,* 40:3–8, 2003.

62. Serraclara A, Hawkins F, and Perez C et al., Hypoglycemic action of an oral fig-leaf decoction in type-I diabetes patients, *Diabetes Res Clin Pract,* 39:19–22, 1998.

63. Wadood N, Wadood A, and Nisar M, Effect of *ficus religiosa* on blood glucose and total lipid levels of normal and alloxan diabetic rabbits, *J Ayub Med Coll Abbottabad,* 15:40–42, 2003.

64. Daniel RS, Devi KS, and Augusti KT et al., Mechanism of action of antiatherogenic and related effects of *Ficus bengalensis* linn: Flavonoids in experimental animals, *Ind J Exp Biol,* 41:296–303, 2003.

65. Geetha BS, Mathew BC, and Augustic KT. Hypoglycemic effects of leucodelphinidin derivative isolated from *Ficus bengalensis* (linn), *Indian J Physiol Pharmacol,* 38:220–222, 1994.

66. Frati Munari AC, Vera Lastra O, and Ariza Andraca CR, Evaluation of nopal capsules in diabetes mellitus, *Gac Med Mex,* 128:431–436, 1992.

67. Frati Munari AC, de Leon C, and Ariza-Andraca R et al., Effect of dehydrated extract of nopal (*Opuntia ficus indica mill.*) on blood glucose, *Arch Invest Med (Mex),* 20:211–216, 1989.

68. Frati-Munari AC, Del Valle-Martinez LM, and Ariza-Andraca CR et al., Hypoglycemic action of different doses of nopal (*Opuntia streptacantha Lemaire*) in patients with type-II diabetes mellitus, *Arch Invest Med (Mex),* 20:197–201, 1989.

69. Frati-Munari AC, Gordillo BE, and Altamirano P et al., Hypoglycemic effect of *Opuntia streptacantha Lemaire* in NIDDM, *Diabetes Care,* 11:63–66, 1988.

70. Frati-Munari AC, Fernandez-Harp JA, and de la Riva H et al., Effects of nopal (*Opuntia sp.*) on serum lipids, glycemia, and body weight, *Arch Invest Med (Mex),* 14:117–125, 1983.

71. Ibanez-Camacho R and Roman-Ramos R, Hypoglycemic effect of Opuntia cactus, *Arch Invest Med (Mex),* 10:223–230, 1979.

72. Soto CP, Perez BL, and Favari LP et al., Prevention of alloxan-induced diabetes mellitus in the rat by silymarin, *Comp Biochem Physiol C Pharmacol Toxicol Endocrinol,* 119:125–129, 1998.

73. Velussi M, Cernigoi AM, and de Monte A et al., Long-term (12 months) treatment with an anti-oxidant drug (silymarin) is effective on hyperinsulinemia, exogenous insulin need, and malondialdehyde levels in cirrhotic diabetic patients, *J Hepatol,* 26:871–879, 1997.

74. Lirussi F, Beccarello A, and Zanette G et al., Silybin-beta-cyclodextrin in the treatment of patients with diabetes mellitus and alcoholic liver disease. Efficacy study of a new preparation of an antioxidant agent, *Diabetes Nutr Metab,* 15:222–231, 2002.

75. Matsuda T, Ferreri K, and Todorov I et al., Silymarin protects pancreatic β-cells against cytokine-mediated toxicity: Implication of c-Jun NH2-terminal kinase and Janus kinase/signal transducer and activator of transcription {STAT} pathways, *Endocrinology,* 2004. [Epub ahead of print].

76. Saxena A and Vikram NK, Role of selected Indian plants in management of type-2 diabetes, A review, *J Alt Compl Med,* 10:369–378, 2004.

77. Gupta A, Gupta R, and Lal B, Effect of *Trigonella foenum graecum* (fenugreek) seeds on glycemic control and insulin resistance in type-2 diabetes mellitus, A double-blind controlled study, *J Assoc Physicians India,* 49:1057–1061, 2001.

78. Sharma RD, Raghuram TC and Rao NS, Effect of fenugreek seeds on blood glucose and serum lipids in type-1 diabetes, *Eur J Clin Nutr,* 44:301–306, 1990.

79. Baskaran K, Kizar Ahamath B, and Radha Shanmugasundaram K et al., Antidiabetic effect of a leaf extract from *Gymnema sylvestre* in non-insulin-dependent diabetes mellitus patients, *J Ethnopharmacol,* 30:295–300, 1990.

80. Shanmugasundaram ER, Rajeswari G, and Baskaran K et al., Use of *Gymnema sylvestre* leaf extract in the control of blood glucose in insulin-dependent diabetes mellitus, *J Ethnopharmacol,* 30:281–294, 1990.

81. Shabib BA, Khan LA, and Rahman R, Hypoglycemic activity of *Coccinia indica* and *Momordica charantia* in diabetic rats: Depression of the hepatic gluconeogenic enzymes glucose-6-phosphatase and fructose-1,6-phosphatase and elevation of liver and red-cell shunt enzyme glucose-6-phosphate dehydrogenasse, *Biochem J,* 292 (Part 1):267–270, 1993.

82. Azad Khan AK, Akhtar S, and Mahtab H, *Coccinia indica* in the treatment of patients with diabetes mellitus, *Bangladesh Med Res Council Bull,* 5:60–66, 1979.

83. Khan AK, Akhtar S, and Mahtab H, Treatment of diabetes mellitus with *Coccinia indica, Brit Med J,* 280:1044, 1980.

84. Kamble SM, Kamlakar PL, and Vaidya S et al., Influence of *Coccinia indica* on certain enzymes in glycolytic and lipolytic pathway in human diabetes, *Ind J Med Sci,* 52:143–146, 1998.

85. Platel K and Srinivasan K, Plant foods in the management of diabetes mellitus: Vegetables as potential hypoglycemic agents, *Die Nahrung,* 41:68–74, 1997.

86. Hossain MZ, Shibib BA, and Rahman R, Hypoglycemic effects of *Coccinia indica*: Inhibition of key glucogenic enzyme, glucose-6-phosphatase, *Ind J Exp Biol,* 30:418–420, 1992.

87. Srividya N and Periwal S, Diuretic, hypotensive, and hypoglycemic effects of *Phyllanthus amarus. Indian J Exp Biol,* 33:861–864, 1995.

88. Hsia SH, Bazargan M, and Davidson MB, Effect of pancreas tonic (an Ayurvedic herbal supplement) in type-2 diabetes mellitus, *Metabolism,* 53:1166–1173, 2004.

89. Jia W, Gao W and Tang L, Antidiabetic herbal drugs officially approved in China, *Phytother Res,* 17:1127–1134, 2003.

90. Li WL, Zheng HC, and Bukuru J et al., Natural medicines used in the traditional Chinese medical system for therapy of diabetes mellitus, *J Ethnopharmacol,* 92:1–21, 2004.

91. Lui JP, Zhang M, and Wang WY et al., Chinese herbal medicines for type-2 diabetes mellitus, *Cochrane Database Syst Rev,* CD003642, 2004.

92. Sharma KK, Gupta RK, and Gupta S et al., Antihyperglycemic effect of onion: Effect on fasting blood sugar and induced hyperglycemia in man, *Indian J Med Res,* 65:422–429, 1977.

93. Jain RC, Vyas CR, and Mahatma OP, Letter: Hypoglycemic action on onion and garlic, *Lancet,* 2:1491, 1973.

94. Qidwai W, Qureshi R, and Hasan SN et al., Effect of dietary garlic (Allium sativum) on the blood pressure in humans—a pilot study, *J Pak Med Assoc* 50:204–207, 2000.

95. Sheela CG and Augusti KT, Antidiabetic effects of S-allyl cysteine sulphoxide isolated from garlic Allium sativum Linn, *Indian J Exp Biol,* 30:523–526, 1992.

96. Campos KE, Diniz YS, and Cataneo AC et al., Hypoglycemia and antioxidant effects of onion, *Allium cepa*: Dietary onion addition, antioxidant activity and hypoglycaemic effects on diabetic rats, *Int J Food Sci Nutr,* 54:241–246, 2003.

97. Baluchnejadmojarad T and Roghani M, Endothelium-dependent and -independent effect of aqueous extract of garlic on vascular reactivity on diabetic rats, *Fitoterapia,* 74:630–637, 2003.

98. Khan BA, Abraham A, and Leelamma S, Hypoglycemic action of *Marraya koeingii* (curry leaf) and *Brassica juncea* (mustard): Mechanism of action, *Ind J Biochem Biophys,* 32:106–108, 1995.

99. Iyer UM and Mani UV, Studies on the effects of curry leave supplementation (*Marraya koeingii*) on lipid profile, glycated proteins, and amino acids in non-insulin-dependent diabetic patients, *Plant Foods Hum Nutr,* 40:275–282, 1990.

100. Agrawal P, Rai V, and Singh RB, Randomized placebo-controlled, single blind trial of holy basil leaves in patients with non-insulin-dependent diabetes mellitus, *Int J Clin Pharmacol Ther,* 34:406–409.), 1996.

101. Oya T, Osawa T, and Kawakishi S, Spice constituents scavenging free radicals and inhibiting pento-sidine formation in a model system, *Biosci Biotechnol Biochem,* 61:263–266, 1997.

102. Akhani SP, Vishwakarma SL, and Goyal RK, Anti-diabetic activity of *Zingiber officinale* in strepto-zotocin-induced type-I rats, *J Pharm Pharmacol,* 56:101–105, 2004.

103. Bordia A, Verma SK, and Srivastava KC, Effect of ginger (*Zingiber officinale Rosc.*) and fenugreek (*Trigonella foenumgraecum L.*) on blood lipids, blood sugar, and platelet aggregation in patients with coronary artery disease, *Prostaglandins Leukot Essent Fatty Acids,* 56:379–384, 1997.

104. Broadhurst CL, Polansky MM, and Anderson RA, Insulin-like biological activity of culinary and medicinal plant aqueous extracts *in vitro, J Agric Food Chem,* 48:849–852, 2000.

105. Imparl-Radosevich J, Deas S, and Polansky MM et al., Regulation of PTP-1 and insulin receptor kinase by fractions from cinnamon: Implications for cinnamon regulation on insulin signaling, *Horm Res,* 50:177–182, 1998.

106. Khan A, Safdar M, and Khan MMA et al., Cinnamon improves glucose and lipids of people with type-2 diabetes, *Diabetes Care,* 26:3215–3218, 2003.

107. Anderson RA, Broadhurst CL, and Polansky MM et al.. Isolation and characterization of polyphenol type-A polymers from cinnamon with insulin-like biologic activity, *J Agric Food Chem,* 52:65–70, 2004.

108. Grassi D, Necozione S, and Lippi C et al., Cocoa reduces blood pressure and insulin resistance and improves endothelium-dependent vasdilation in hypertensives, *Hypertension,* 46:398–405, 2005.

109. Grassi D, Lippi C, and Necozione S et al., Short-term administration of dark chocolate is followed by a significant increase in insulin sensitivity and a decrease in blood pressure in healthy persons, *Am J clin Nutr,* 81:611–614, 2005.

110. Brand-Miller J, Holt SH, and de Jong V et al., Cocoa powder increases postprandial insulinemia in lean young adults, *J Nutr,* 133:3149-3152, 2003.

111. Keen CL, Holt RR, and Oteiza PI et al., Cocoa antioxidants and cardiovascular health, *Am J Clin Nutr,* 81(suppl):298–303S, 2005.

112. Zumbe A and Brinkworth RA, Comparative studies of gastrointestinal tolerance and acceptability of milk chocolate containing either sucrose, isomalt or sorbitol in healthy consumers and type II diabetics, *Z Ernahrungswiss,* 31:40–48, 1992.

113. Gee JM, Cooke D, and Gorick S et al., Effects of conventional sucrose-based, fructose-based and isomalt-based chocolates on postprandial metabolism in non-insulin-dependent diabetics, *Eur J Clin Nutr,* 45:561–566, 1991.

114. Osakabe N, Yamagishi M, and Natsume M et al., Ingestion of proanthocyanidins derived from cacao inhibits diabetes-induced cataract formation in rats, *Exp Biol Med,* 229:33–39, 2004.

115. Nguyen NU, Henriet MT, and Dumoulin G et al., Increase in calciuria and oxaluria after a single chocolate bar load, *Horm Metab Res,* 26:383–386, 1994.

116. Broadhurst CL, Polansky MM, and Anderson RA, Insulin-like biological activity of culinary and medicinal plant aqueous extracts *in vitro, J Agric Food Chem,* 48:849–852, 2000.

117. Hosoda K, Wang MF, and Liao ML et al., Antihypertensive effect of oolong tea in type-2 diabetics, *Diabetes Care,* 26:1714–1718, 2003.

118. Waltner-Law ME, Wang XL, and Law BK et al., *Epigallocatechin gallate*, a constituent of green tea, represses hepatic glucose production, *J Biol Chem,* 277:34933–34940, 2002.

119. Watson JM, Jenkins EJ, and Hamilton P et al., Influence of caffeine on the frequency and perception of hypoglycemia in free-living patients with type-1 diabetes, *Diabetes Care,* 23:455-459, 2000.

120. van Dam RM and Feskens EJ, Coffee consumption and risk of type-2 diabetes mellitus, *Lancet,* 360:1477–1478, 2002.

121. Yeomans MR, Caton S, and Hetherington MM, Alcohol and food intake, *Curr Op Clin Nutr Metab Care,* 6:639–644, 2003.

122. Yeomans MR and Phillips MF, Failure to reduce short-term appetite following alcohol is independent of beliefs about the presence of alcohol, *Nutr Neurosci,* 5:131–139, 2002.

123. Raben A, Agerholm-Larsen L, and Flint A et al., Meals with similar energy densities but rich in protein, fat, carbohydrate, or alcohol have different effects on energy expenditure and substrate metabolism but not on appetite and energy intake, *Am J Clin Nutr,* 77:91–100, 2003.

124. Clark JT, Keaton AK, and Sahu A et al., Neuropeptide Y (NPY) levels in alcoholic and food restricted male rats: Implications for site-selective function, *Regul Pept,* 75–76:335–345, 1998.

125. von meyenberg CW, Langhans W, and Hrupka BJ, Evidence for a role of the 5-HT2C receptor in central lipopolysaccharide-, interleukin-1 beta-, and leptin-induced anorexia, *Pharmacol Biochem Behav,* 74:1025–1031, 2003.

126. Chester JA and Cunningham CL, GABA(A) receptor modulation of the rewarding and aversive effects of ethanol, *Alcohol,* 26:131–143, 2002.

127. Widdowson PS and Holman RB, Ethanol-induced increase in endogenous dopamine release may involve endogenous opioids, *J Neurochem,* 59:157–163, 1992.

128. Hwang MY, Glass RM, and Molter J, Benefits and dangers of alcohol, *JAMA,* 281:104, 1999.

129. U.S. Department of Agriculture, Dietary Guidelines for Americans 2005, www.health-ierus.gov/dietaryguidelines.

130. Davies MJ, Baer DJ, and Judd JT et al., Effects of moderate alcohol intake on fasting insulin and glucose concentrations and insulin sensitivity in postmenopausal women, *JAMA,* 287:2559–2562, 2002.

131. Greenfield JR, Samaras K, and Hayward CS et al., Beneficial postprandial effect of a small amount of alcohol on diabetes and cardiovascular risk factors: Modification by insulin resistance, *J Clin Endocrinol Metab,* 90:661–672, 2005.

132. Rimm EB, Chan J, and Stampfer MJ et al., Prospective study of cigarette smoking, alcohol use, and the risk of diabetes in men, *Br Med J,* 310:555–559, 1995.

133. Conigrave KM, Hu BF, and Camargo CA et al., A prospective study of drinking patterns in relation to risk of type-2 diabetes among men, *Diabetes,* 50:2390–2395, 2001.

134. Kao WH, Puddey IB, and Boland LL et al., Alcohol consumption and the risk of type-2 diabetes mellitus: Athesclerosis risk in communities study, *Am J Epidemiol,* 154:748–757, 2001.

135. Carlsson S, Hammar N, and Efendic S et al., Alcohol consumption, Type-2 diabetes mellitus and impaired glucose tolerance in middle-aged Swedish men, *Diabet Med,* 17:776, 2000–781.

136. Wannamethee SG, Camargo CA, Jr, and Manson JE et al., Alcohol drinking patterns and risk of type-2 diabetes mellitus among younger women, *Arch Int Med,* 163:1329–1336, 2003.

137. Dixon JB, Dixon ME, and O'Brien PE, Alcohol consumption in the severely obese: Relationship with the metabolic syndrome, *Obes Res,* 10:245–252, 2002.

138. Vernay M, Balkau B, Moreau JG, Sigalas J, Chesnier MC, Ducimetiere P, and The DESIR and Study Group, Alcohol consumption and insulin resistance syndrome parameters: Associations and evolutions in a longitudinal analysis of the French DESIR cohort, *Ann Epidemiol,* 14:209–214, 2004.

139. Turner BC, Jenkins E, and Kerr D et al., The effect of evening alcohol consumption on next–morning glucose control in type-1 diabetes, *Diabetes Care,* 24:1888–1893, 2001.

140. Harding AH, Sargeant LA, and Khaw KT et al., Cross-sectional association between total level and type of alcohol consumption and glycosylated haemoglobin levels: The EPIC-Norfolk Study, *Eur J Clin Nutr,* 56:882–890, 2002.

141. Gin H, Morlat P, and Ragnaud JM et al., Short-term effect of red wine (consumed during meals) on insulin requirement and glucose tolerance in diabetic patients, *Diabetes Care,* 15:546–548, 1992.

142. Avogara A, Duner E, and Marescotti C et al., Metabolic effects of moderate alcohol intake with meals in insulin-dependent diabetics controlled by artificial endocrine pancreas (AEP) and in normal subjects, *Metabolism,* 32:463–470, 1983.

143. American and Diabetes Association, American Diabetes Association position statement: Evidence-based nutrition principles and recommendations for the treatment and prevention of diabetes and related complications, *J Am Dietetic Assoc,* 102:109–118, 2002.

144. Haut MJ and Cowan DH, The effect of ethanol on hemostatic properties of human blood platelets, *Am J Med,* 56:22–33, 1974.

145. International Life and Sciences Institute, Ethanol stimulates apo A-1 secretion in human hepatocytes: A possible mechanism underlying the cardioprotective effect of ethanol, *Nutr Rev,* 51:151–152, 1993.

146. Castelli WP, Doyle JT, and Gordon T et al., Alcohol and blood lipids: The cooperative lipoprotein phenotyping study, *Lancet,* 2:153–155, 1977.

147. Sile SQ, Neese RA, and Hellerstein MK, *De novo* lipogenesis, lipid kinetics, and whole-body lipid balances in humans after acute alcohol consumption, *Am J Clin Nutr,* 70:928–936, 1999.

148. Krauss R and Burke D, Identification of multiple subclasses of plasma low-density lipoproteins in normal humans, *J Lipid Res,* 23:97–104, 1982.

149. MacDonald I, Ed., *Health Issues Related to Alcohol Consumption,* Oxford UK: Blackwell Sci 2nd ed., 488, 1999.

150. Thun MJ, Peto FRS, and Lopez AD et al., Alcohol consumption and mortality among middle-aged and elderly U.S. adults, *N Engl J Med,* 337:1705–1714, 1997.

151. Rimm EB, Klatsky A, and Grobbee D et al., Review of moderate alcohol consumption and reduced risk of coronary heart disease: Is the effect due to beer, wine, or spirits? *Br Med J,* 312:731–736, 1996.

152. Renaud S and de Lorgeril M, Wine, alcohol, platelets, and the French Paradox for coronary heart disease, *Lancet,* 339:1523–1526, 1992.

153. German JB and Walzem RL, The health benefits of wine, *Annu Rev Nutr,* 20:561–593, 2000.

154. Panganga G, Miller N, and Rice-Evans CA, The polyphenolic content of fruit and vegetables and their antioxidant activities: What does a serving constitute? *Free Rad Res,* 30:153–162, 1999.

155. Maxwell S, Cruickshank A, and Thorpe G, Red wine and antioxidant activity in serum, *Lancet,* 344:193–194, 1994.

156. Mezzano D, Leighton F, and Martinez C et al., Complementary effects of Mediterranean diet and moderate red wine intake on haemostatic cardiovascular risk factors, *Eur J Clin Nutr,* 55:444–451, 2001.

157. Duthie GG, Pedersen MW, and Gardner PT et al., The effect of whiskey and wine consumption on total phenol content and antioxidant capacity from healthy volunteers, *Eur J Clin Nutr,* 52:733–736, 1998.

158. Ceriello A, Bortolotti N, and Motz E et al., Meal-generated oxidative stress in diabetes, The protective effect of red wine, *Diabetes Care,* 22:2084–2085, 1999.

159. Ceriello A, Bortolotti N, and Motz E et al., Red wine protects diabetic patients from meal-induced oxidative stress and thrombosis activation: A pleasant approach to the prevention of cardiovascular disease in diabetes, *Eur J Clin Invest,* 31:322–328, 2001.

160. Tessari P, Bruttomesso, and Pianta A et al., Effects of wine intake on postprandial plasma amino acid and protein kinetics in type-1 diabetes, *Am J Clin Nutr,* 75:856–866, 2002.

161. Jankowski A, Jankowska B, and Niedworok J, The effect of anthocyanin dye from grapes on experimental diabetes, *Folia Med Cracov,* 41:5–15, 2000.

162. Landrault N, Poucheret P, and Azay J et al., Effect of a polyphenols-enriched Chardonnay white wine in diabetic rats, *J Agric Food Chem,* 51:311–318, 2003.

163. Aviram M, Rosenblat M, and Billecke S et al., Human serum paraoxonase (PON 1) is inactivated by oxidized low-density lipoprotein and preserved by antioxidants, *Free Radic Biol Med,* 26:892–904, 1999.

164. Arts IC, Jacobs DR, and Harnack LJ et al., Dietary catechins in relation to coronary heart disease death among postmenopausal women, *Epidemiology,* 12:668–675, 2001.

165. Rhee SJ, Choi JH, and Park MR, Green tea catechin improves microsomal phospholipase A2 activity and the arachidonic acid cascade system in the kidney of diabetic rats, *Asia Pac J Clin Nutr,* 11:226–231, 2002.

166. Rizvi SI and Zaid MA, Intracellular reduced glutathione content in normal and type-2 diabetic erythrocytes: Effect of insulin and (-)epicatechin, *J Physiol Pharmacol,* 52:483–488, 2001.

167. Rizvi SI and Zaid MA, Insulin-like effect of (-)epicatechin on erythrocyte membrane acetylcholinesterase activity in type-2 diabetes mellitus, *Clin Exp Pharmacol Physiol,* 28:776–778, 2001.

168. Matteucci E, Rizvi SI, and Giampietro O, Erythrocyte sodium/hydrogen exchange inhibition by (-) epicatechin, *Cell Biol Int,* 25:771–776, 2001.

169. Corder R, Douthwaite JA, and Lees DM et al., Health: Endothelin-1 synthesis reduced by red wine, *Nature,* 414:863–864, 2001.

170. Chen CK and Pace-Asciak CR, Vasorelaxing activity of resveratrol and quercetin in isolated rat aorta, *Gen Pharmacol,* 27:363–366, 1996.

171. Wallerath T, Poleo D, and Li H et al., Red wine increases the expression of human endothelial nitric oxide synthase, a mechanism that may contribute to its beneficial cardiovascular effects, *J Am Coll Cardiol,* 41:471–478, 2003.

172. da Luz PL and Coimbra SR, Wine, alcohol and atherosclerosis: Clinical evidences and mechanisms, *Brazilian J Med Biol Res,* 37:1275–1295, 2004.

173. Klatsky AL, Armstrong MA, and Friedman GD, Red wine, white wine, liquor, beer, and risk for coronary artery disease hospitalization, *Am J Cardiol,* 80:416–420, 1997.

174. Hendler SS and Rorvik D, *PDR for Nutritional Supplements,* Montvale, NJ: Medical Economics Company, 2001.

175. Vincent JB, Recent advances in the nutritional biochemistry of trivalent chromium, *Proc Nutr Soc,* 63:41–47, 2004.

176. Morris BW, MacNeil S, and Hardisty CA et al., Chromium homeostasis in patients with type-2 (NIDDM) diabetes, *J Trace Elem Med Biol,* 13:57–61, 1999.

177. Rabinowitz MB, Gonick HC, and Levin SR et al., Effects of chromium and yeast supplements on carbohydrate and lipid metabolism in diabetic men, *Diabetes Care,* 6:319–327, 1983.

178. Lee NA and Reasner CA, Beneficial effect of chromium supplementation on serum triglyceride levels in NIDDM, *Diabetes Care,* 17:1449–1452, 1994.

179. Anderson RA, Cheng N, and Bryden NA et al., Elevated intakes of supplemental chromium improve glucose and insulin variables in individuals with type-2 diabetes, *Diabetes,* 46:1786–1791, 1997.

180. Bahijiri SM, Mira SA, and Mufti AM et al., The effects of inorganic chromium and brewer's yeast supplementation on glucose tolerance, serum lipids, and drug dosage in individuals with type-2 diabetes, *Saudi Med J,* 21:831–837, 2000.

181. Althuis MD, Jordan NE, Ludington EA, and Wittes JT, Glucose and insulin responses to dietary chromium supplements, A meta-analysis, *Am J Clin Nutr,* 76:148–155, 2002.

182. Uusitupa MI, Mykkanen L, and Siitonen O et al., Chromium supplementation in impaired glucose tolerance of elderly: Effects on blood glucose, plasma insulin, C-peptide, and lipid levels, *Br J Nutr,* 68:209–216, 1992.

183. Offenbacher EG and Pi-Sunyer FX, Beneficial effects of chromium-rich yeast on glucose tolerance and blood lipids in elderly subjects, *Diabetes,* 29:919–925, 1980.

184. O'Connor JC and Freund GG, Vanadate and rapamycin synergistically enhance insulin-stimulated glucose uptake, *Metabolism,* 52:666–674, 2003.

185. Badmaev V, Prakash S, and Majeed M, Vanadium: A review of its potential role in the fight against diabetes, *J Altern Complement Med,* 5:273–291, 1999.

186. Mukherjee B, Patra B, and Mahapatra S et al., Vanadium—an element of atypical biological significance, *Toxicol Lett,* 150:135–143, 2004.

187. Cohen N, Halberstam M, and Shlimovich P et al., Oral vanadyl sulfate improves hepatic and peripheral insulin sensitivity in patients with non-insulin-dependent diabetes mellitus, *J Clin Invest,* 95:2501–2509, 1995.

188. Halberstam M, Cohen N, and Shlimovich P et al., Oral vanadyl sulfate improves insulin sensitivity in NIDDM but not in obese nondiabetic subjects, *Diabetes,* 45:659–666, 1996.

189. Aharon Y, Mevorach M, and Shamoon H, Vanadyl sulfate does not enhance insulin action in patients with type-1 diabetes, *Diabetes Care,* 21:2194–2195, 1998.

190. Goldfine AB, Patti ME, and Zuberi L et al., Metabolic effects of vanadyl sulfate in humans with non-insulin-dependent diabetes mellitus: *In vivo* and *in vitro* studies, *Metabolism,* 49:400–410, 2000.

191. Willsky GR, Goldfine AB, and Kostyniak PJ et al., Effect of vanadium(IV) compounds in the treatment of diabetes: *In vivo* and *in vitro* studies with vanadyl sulfate and bis(maltolato)oxovanadium(IV), *J Inorg Biochem,* 85:33–42, 2001.

192. Saris NE, Mervaala E, and Karppanen H et al., Magnesium: An update on physiological, clinical, and analytical aspects, *Clin Chem Acta,* 294:1–26, 2000.

193. Barbagallo M, Dominguez IJ, and Galioto A et al., Role of magnesium in insulin action, diabetes and cardio-metabolic syndrome X, *Mol Aspects Med,* 24:39–52, 2003.

194. Suarez A, Pulido N, and Casla A et al., Impaired tyrosine kinase activity of muscle insulin receptors from hypomagnesaemic rats, *Diabetologia,* 38:1262–1270, 1995.

195. Kandeel FR, Balon E, and Scott S et al., Magnesium deficiency and glucose metabolism in rat adipocytes, *Metabolism,* 45:838–843, 1996.

196. Gugliano D, Paolisso G, and Ceriello A, Oxidative stress and diabetic vascular complications, *Diabetes Care,* 19:257–267, 1996.

197. Ma J, Folsom AR, and Melnick SL et al., Associations of serum and dietary magnesium with cardiovascular disease, hypertension, diabetes, insulin, and carotid arterial wall thickness: The ARIC Study, *J Clin Epidemiol,* 48:927–940, 1995.

198. Rosolova H, Mayer O, and Reaven GM, Insulin-mediated glucose disposal is decreased in normal subjects with relatively low plasma magnesium concentrations, *Metabolism,* 49:418–420, 2000.

199. Paolisso G and Barbagallo M, Hypertension, diabetes mellitus, and insulin resistance: The role of intracellular magnesium, *Am J Hypertens,* 10:346–355, 1997.

200. Kao WH, Folsom AR, and Nieto FJ et al., Serum and dietary magnesium and the risk for type-2 diabetes mellitus: The Atherosclerosis Risk in Communities Study, *Arch Int Med,* 159:2151–2159, 1999.

201. Song Y, Manson JE, and Buring JE et al., Dietary magnesium intake in relation to plasma insulin levels and risk of type-2 diabetes in women, *Diabetes Care,* 27:59–65, 2004.

202. Rodriquez-Moran M and Guerrero-Romero F, Oral magnesium supplementation improves insulin sensitivity and metabolic control in type-2 diabetic subjects, A randomized double-blind controlled trial, *Diabetes Care,* 26:1147–1152; Saris et al., 2000, 2003.

203. Balon TW, Gu JL, and Tokuyama Y et al., Magnesium supplementation reduces development of diabetes in a rat model of spontaneous NIDDM, *Am J Physiol,* 269:E745–752, 1995.

204. de Lourdes Lima M, Cruz T, and Carreiro Pousada J et al., The effect of magnesium supplementation in increasing doses on the control of type-2 diabetes, *Diabetes Care,* 21:682–686, 1998.

205. Gullestad L, Jacobsen T, and Dolva LO, Effect of magnesium treatment on glycemic control and metabolic parameters in NIDDM patients, *Diabetes Care,* 17:460–461, 1994.

206. Eibi NL, Kopp HP, and Nowak HR et al., Hypomagnesemia in type-II diabetes: Effect of a 3-month replacement therapy, *Diabetes Care,* 18:188–192, 1995.

207. de Valk HW, Verkaaik R, and van Rijn HJ et al., Oral magnesium supplementation in insulin–requiring type-2 diabetic patients, *Diabet Med,* 15:503–507, 1998.

208. Colditz GA, Manson JE, and Stampfer MJ et al., Diet and risk of clinical diabetes in women, *Am J Clin Nutr,* 55:1018–1023, 1992.

209. Eibl NL, Kopp HP, and Nowak HR et al., Hypomagnesemia in type-II diabetics: Effect of a 3-month replacement therapy, *Diabetes Care,* 18:188–192, 1995.

210. Eriksson J and Kohvakka A, Magnesium and ascorbic acid supplementation in diabetes mellitus, *Ann Nutr Metab,* 39:217–223, 1995.

211. Hagg E, Carlberg BC, and Hillorn VS et al., Magnesium therapy in type-1 diabetes, A double-blind study concerning the effects on kidney function and serum lipid levels, *Magnes Res,* 12:123–130, 1999.

212. Johnsen SP, Husted SE, and Ravn HB et al., Magnesium supplementation to patients with type-II diabetes, *Ugeskr Laeger,* 161:945–948, 1999.
213. Lima Mde L, Cruz T, and Pousada JC et al., The effect of magnesium supplementation in increasing doses on the control of type-2 diabetes, *Diabetes Care,* 21:682–686, 1998.
214. Paolisso G, Scheen A, and Cozzolino D et al., Changes in glucose turnover parameters and improvement of glucose oxidation after 4-week magnesium administration in elderly noninsulin-dependent (type-II) diabetic patients, *J Clin Endocrinol Metab,* 78:1510–1514, 1994.
215. Roussel AM, Kerkeni A, and Zouari N et al., Antioxidant effects of zinc supplementation in Tunisians with type-2 diabetes mellitus, *J Am Coll Nutr,* 22:316–321, 2003.
216. Beckman JA, Goldfine AB, and Gordon MB et al., Ascorbate restores endothelium-dependent vasdilation impaired by acute hyperglycemia in humans, *Circulation,* 103:1618–1623, 2001.
217. Regensteiner JG, Popylisen S, and Bauer TA et al., Oral L-arginine and vitamins E and C improve endothelial function in women with type-2 diabetes, *Vasc Med,* 8:169–175, 2003.
218. Mullan BA, Young IS, and Fee H et al., Ascorbic acid reduces blood pressure and arterial stiffness in type-2 diabetes, *Hypertension,* 40:804–809, 2002.
219. Root-Bernstein R, Busik JV, and Henry DN, Are diabetic neuropathy, retinopathy and nephropathy caused by hyperglycemic exclusion of dehydroascorbate uptake by glucose transporters? *J Theor Biol,* 21:345–359, 2002.
220. Hodgson JM, Watts GF, and Playford DA et al., Coenzyme Q10 improves blood pressure and glycaemic control, Controlled trial in subjects with type-2 diabetes, *Eur J Clin Nutr,* 56:1137–1142, 2002.
221. Scroggie DA, Albright A, and Harris MD, The effect of glucosamine-chondroitin supplementation on glycosylated hemoglobin levels in patients with type-2 diabetes mellitus, *Arch Int Med,* 163:1587–1590, 2003.
222. *Physicians' Desk Reference for Nutritional Supplements,* Montvale, NJ: Medical Economics Co, 186–189 2001.
223. Solerte SB, Gazzaruso C, and Schifino N et al., Metabolic effects of orally administered amino acid mixture in elderly subjects with poorly controlled type-2 diabetes mellitus, *Am J Cardiol,* 93(Suppl 8a):23A–29A, 2004.
224. Aquilani R, Oral amino acid administration in patients with diabetes mellitus: Supplementation or metabolic therapy? *Am J Cardiol,* 93(Suppl 8a):21A–22A, 2004.
225. Halat KM and Dennehy CE, Botanicals and dietary supplements in diabetic peripheral neuropathy, *J Am Board Fam Pract,* 16:47–57, 2003.
226. Jamal GA and Carmichael H, The effect of gamma linolenic acid human diabetic peripheral neuropathy, A double-blind placebo-controlled trial, *Diabet Med,* 7:319–323, 1990.
227. Keen H, Payan J, and Allawi J et al., Treatment of diabetic neuropathy with gamma-linolenic acid. *Diabetes Care,* 16:8–15, 1993.
228. Purewal TS, Evans PMS, and Havard F et al., Lack of effect of evening primrose oil on autonomic function tests after 12 months of treatment, *Diabetologia,* 40(Suppl 1):A556, 1997.
229. Ziegler D, Hanefeld M, and Ruhnau KJ et al., Treatment of symptomatic diabetic peripheral neuropathy with the antioxidant α-lipoic acid, A three-week multicenter randomized controlled trial (ALADIN Study), *Diabetologia,* 38:1425–1433, 1995.
230. Reljanovic M, Reichel G, and Rett K et al., Treatment of diabetic polyneuropathy with antioxidant thioctic acid (α-lipoic acid), A two-year multi-center randomized double-blind placebo-controlled trial, Alpha Lipoic Acid in Diabetic Neuropathy (ALADIN II), *Free Radic Res,* 31:171–179, 1999.
231. Ziegler D, Hanefeld M, and Ruhnau KJ et al., Treatment of symptomatic diabetic polyneuropathy with the antioxidant alpha-lipoic acid, A 7-month multicenter randomized controlled trial (ALADIN III Study), ALADIN III Study Group, Alpha-Lipoic Acid in Diabetic Neuropathy, *Diabetes Care,* 22:1296–1301, 1999.
232. Ruhnau KJ, Meissner HP, and Finn JR et al., Effects of 3-week oral treatment with the antioxidant thioctic acid (alpha–lipoic acid) in symptomatic diabetic polyneuropathy, *Diabet Med,* 16:1040–1043, 1999.
233. Nagamatsu M, Nickander KK, and Schmelzer JD et al., Lipoic acid improves nerve blood flow, reduces oxidative stress, and improves distal nerve conduction in experimental diabetic neuropathy, *Diabetes Care,* 18:1160–1167, 1995.

234. Ziegler D, Reljanovic M, and Mehnert H et al., Alpha-lipoic acid in the treatment of diabetic polyneuropathy in Germany, Current evidence from clinical trials, *Exp Clin Endocrinol Diabetes,* 107:421–430, 1999.

235. Scheffler NM, Sheitel PL, and Lipton MN, Treatment of painful diabetic neuropathy with capsaicin 0.075%, *J Am Podiatr Med Assoc,* 81:288–293, 1991.

236. Chad DA, Aronin N, and Lundstrom R et al., Does capsaicin relieve the pain of diabetic neuropathy? *Pain,* 42:387–388, 1990.

237. The Capsaicin Study Group, Treatment of painful diabetic neuropathy with topical capsaicin— a multicenter, double-blind, vehicle-controlled study, *Arch Intern Med,* 151:2225–2229, 1991.

238. Tandan R, Lewis GA, and Krusinski PB et al., Topical capsaicin in painful diabetic neuropathy, Controlled study with long-term follow-up, *Diabetes Care,* 15:8–14, 1992.

239. Low PA, Opfer-Gehrking TL, and Dyck PJ et al., Double-blind, placebo-controlled study of the application of capsaicin cream in chronic distal painful plyneuropathy, *Pain,* 62:163–168, 1995.

240. Quatraro A, Roca P, and Donzella C et al., Acetyl-L-Carnitine for symptomatic diabetic neuropathy, *Diabetologia,* 38:123, 1995.

241. Sima AAF, Calvani M, and Mehra M et al., The Acetyl-L-Carnitine and Study Group, Acetyl-L-Carnitine improves pain, nerve regeneration, and vibratory perception in patients with chronic diabetic neuropathy, *Diabetes Care,* 28:89–94, 2005.

242. Abbott CA, Vileikyte L, and Williamson S et al., ALCAR Foot Ulcer Study Group, Effect of treatment with acetyl-L-Carnitine on diabetic foot ulceration in patients with peripheral neuropathy, A 1-year prospective multi-centre study, *Diabetologia,* 40(Suppl 1):A556, 1997.

243. Jones CL and Gonzalez V, Pyridoxine deficiency: A new factor in diabetic neuropathy, *J Am Podiatry Assoc,* 68:646–653, 1978.

244. Cohen KL, Gorecki GA, and Silverstein SB et al., Effect of pyridoxine (vitamin B_6) on diabetic patients with peripheral neuropathy, *J Am Podiatry Assoc,* 74:394–397, 1984.

245. Levin ER, Hanscom TA, and Fisher M et al., The influence of pyridoxine in diabetic peripheral neuropathy, *Diabetes Care,* 4:606–609, 1981.

246. McCann VJ and Davis RE, Pyridoxine and diabetic neuropathy, A double-blind controlled study, *Diabetes Care,* 6:102–103, 1983.

247. Tutuncu NB, Bayraktar M, and Varli K, Reversal of defective nerve conduction with vitamin E supplementation in type-2 diabetes, A preliminary study, *Diabetes Care,* 11:915–918, 1998.

248. Sindrup SH, Madsen C, and Bach FW et al., St John's wort has no effect on pain in polyneuropathy, *Pain,* 91:361–365, 2001.

249. Yeh GY, Eisenberg DM, and Kaptchuk TJ et al., Systematic review of herbs and dietary supplements for glycemic control in diabetes, *Diabetes Care,* 26:1277–1294, 2003.

15 Exercise, Nutrition, and Diabetes

Philip Rabito, Jeffrey I. Mechanick, and Elise M. Brett

CONTENTS

INTRODUCTION

Exercise is an important component of healthy lifestyle for the prevention of disease in the general population. Increasing physical activity has also been shown to improve flexibility [1], psychological well-being [2], and longevity [3]. Recommendations for exercise for Americans have recently become more aggressive (see Table 15.1). In diabetes management, there is a complex interplay among physical activity, nutrition, pharmacological intervention, and genomics. In prediabetes and Type-2 diabetes mellitus (T2DM), physical activity is an essential component of treatment as it lowers blood glucose and reduces obesity [4]. In Type-1 diabetes mellitus (T1DM), exercise can result in a complex set of metabolic derangements if careful monitoring and adjustments are not in place. Importantly, exercise plays a role in preventing cardiovascular disease [5] and cerebrovascular disease [6], which are major causes of morbidity and mortality in the diabetic population.

For the following discussion it is necessary to define some important terms. Physical activity is any contraction by skeletal muscles that results in an energy expenditure that is greater than the resting energy expenditure. Exercise involves planned, structured, and repetitive body movements designed to improve fitness and usually occur as part of leisure activity. Aerobic exercise involves continuous, rhythmic, and repeated movements of the same large muscle groups, such as jogging, cycling, and cross-country skiing. Resistance training, such as isotonic weight training and isometrics, improves strength and muscular fitness. Endurance training involves regular aerobic exercise sessions that are frequent enough to improve cardiorespiratory fitness. Eccentric exercise, such as downhill running, downhill skiing, stretching and long jumps, involves lengthening of the muscle fibers as tension develops. Sport is a form of exercise involving a set of rules within a competitive framework and includes soccer, baseball, football, basketball, gymnastics, and track and field.

Exercise intensity correlates with certain physical signs (see Table 15.2). In response to exercise, there is typically a faster heart and respiratory rate, body warmth, swelling of the hands and feet, sweats, and if the person is not well-conditioned, muscular aches for a day or two afterwards [7]. Warning signs of excessive physical exertion warranting medical attention include extreme breathlessness, wheezing, coughing, chest pain or pressure, extreme sweats, dizziness, fainting, light-headedness, nausea, severe muscular pain or cramps, joint pain, and long-standing fatigue [7].

The "$V_{O2\,max}$" is the maximum amount of oxygen (mL) consumed per minute per kg body weight, and is a measure of cardiovascular fitness. The $V_{O2\,max}$ increases as a person becomes more

TABLE 15.1
Exercise Recommendations for the General Population

Aerobic		Resistance (twice a week)	Flexibility (twice a week)
Moderate intensity	40–60% $V_{O2\,max}$/ 50–70% max heart rate Minimum of 30 minutes/day; Up to or over 60 minutes/day in order to achieve a normal weight (BMI < 25 kg/M^2)		

High intensity	35 Minutes/per day
	10 Minutes/day of low-intensity
	  in previously inactive persons and
	  then build up to 30 minutes/day
	Increase routine daily physical activity		

Source: From References [87,113,114].

TABLE 15.2
Exercise Intensity and Physical Signs

Level	Intensity Rating	Physical Signs
0	None	None
1	Minimal	None
2	Barely	Sensation of movement
3	Moderate	More sensation of movement
4	A little hard	Warmth and/or light sweating
5	Hard	Sweating
6	Harder	Moderate sweating
7	Very hard	Moderate sweating, can talk
8	Extremely hard	Heavy sweating, cannot talk
9	Maximum effort	Very heavy sweating, cannot talk
10	Maximum effort	Exhaustion

Source: http://www.betterhealth.vic.gov.au/bhcv2/bhcarticles.nsf/pages/Exercise_intensity?open. Accessed on February 18, 2005 [7].

fit. This can be accomplished by exercising at a moderate (40–60% $V_{O2\,max}$) to vigorous (> 60% $V_{O2\,max}$) intensity, for > 35 minutes 3–5 days/week. This correlates to increases of the heart rate to 50–70% to > 70%, respectively, of its maximum during training (see Table 15.3). The mean $V_{O2\,max}$ for men is 3.5 L/minute and for women, 2.7 L/minute, but varies according to the level of conditioning.

Diabetic patients are at risk for microvascular and macrovascular disease that may be clinically silent and can be unmasked during exercise. Sedentary diabetic patients who are beginning an exercise program should have a medical evaluation to assess their risks. The history and physical examination should focus on the cardiovascular system, the peripheral vascular system, the nervous system, the skin, kidneys, and eyes. A graded exercise test with electrocardiogram (EKG) monitoring should be considered in patients meeting one of the following criteria: (1) over age 35, (2) over age 25 with T2DM for 10 years or T1DM for 15 years, (3) presence of other cardiovascular risk factors, (4) microvascular disease, (5) peripheral vascular disease, or (6) autonomic neuropathy (expert consensus) [8]. The intensity of exercise in patients with autonomic neuropathy should be limited to avoid the potential for arrhythmia and sudden death. Proper footwear prevents soft-tissue injury, orthopedic injury, and infection. Non-weight-bearing exercising, such as swimming or water

TABLE 15.3
Target Heart Rates for Exercise

Age (years)	Target Heart Rate (60–80% maximum; beats/minute)
20	140–170
25	136–165
30	133–162
35	130–157
40	126–153
45	122–149
50	119–145
55	115–140
60	112–136
65	109–132

TABLE 15.4
Metabolic Changes Associated with Exercise

Muscular activity requires 5-adenosine triphosphate (ATP); ATP stores are replenished by phosphocreatine
Mitochondrial physiology replenishes phosphocreatine but this requires fuel (glucose and fat)
Muscle glucose uptake increases, due to:
    Increased perfusion to working muscles
    Increased glucose transporter 4 (GLUT4) translocation via 5'-adenosine monophosphate-activated protein (AMP)
      kinase and nitric oxide (NO)
    Increased glucose phosphorylation via hexokinase II
Muscle glycogen provides fuel during early stages of exertion
Glucose, nonesterified fatty acids (NEFA) and intramuscular triglycerides (TG) provide fuel as exercise continues
Fatty acid oxidation increases
Glycogenolysis shifts to gluconeogenesis to provide glucose as exercise continues
Carbohydrate oxidation increases as exercise continues
These events are regulated by:
    Nutrition
    Hormonal
    Age
    Exercise type
    Physical conditioning
    Exercise intensity and duration.

aerobics, is preferred when there is decreased pain sensation [9]. Patients who have undergone laser photocoagulation for retinopathy should refrain from exercise for 3–6 months (expert opinion) [9].

METABOLIC CHANGES WITH EXERCISE

Exercise sets into motion a complex metabolic response (see Table 15.4) [10–12]. In nondiabetic subjects, exercise-induced muscle glucose uptake (see Figure 15.1) is coupled with endogenous glucose production (EGP). The increase in EGP results from increased counter-regulatory hormones and decreased insulin secretion. These hormonal changes result from fuel deficits, neural feed-forward mechanisms, and blood flow changes [13]. Decreased basal and glucose-stimulated insulin secretion (GSIS) during exercise is associated with decreased concentrations of β-cell glucokinase and proinsulin mRNA [13,14]. Low insulin levels disinhibit the glycogenolytic response. Glucagon stimulates glycogenolysis, gluconeogenesis, hepatic amino acid metabolism, and fatty acid oxidation

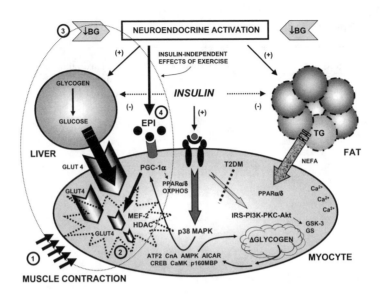

FIGURE 15.1 Molecular mechanism of exercise-induced glucose uptake. Muscular contraction (Step 1) is associated with dissociation of HDAC and activation of MEF-2 and GLUT4 mediated glucose uptake (Step 2; dotted star) [123]. The transient hypoglycemia (Step 3) activates the sympatho-adrenal axis and autonomic nervous system creating a feed-forward loop in which this action is amplified. EPI stimulates PGC-1α expression (Step 4) which enhances mitochondrial biogenesis (phosphocreatine and ATP formation with oxidative phosphorylation), PPAR-α/δ (mediating fatty acid oxidation), MEF-2 and protein expression yielding muscle adaptation to endurance exercise [124]. Additional pathways modulate these events. p38 MAPK activation, which is preserved with T2DM and insulin resistance, enhances PGC-1α stability via various factors, but is not a transcriptional regulator [125]. Atypical PKC may also stimulate GLUT4 activity in response to Erk 1/2 or intracellular calcium [126,127]. Muscular contraction also stimulates the AICAR-AMPK pathway, which inactivates glycogen synthesis and activates p38 MAPK [128]. Glycogen synthesis is also inhibited by the Akt-GSK3 pathway [129]. Thus, in patients with T2DM, exercise circumvents defects in the IRS-PI3K pathway and activates glucose uptake via p38 MAPK, PGC-1α, and MEF-2. In patients with T1DM who are insulin-deficient, hepatic glucose production may exceed muscle glucose uptake and produce hyperglycemia. In patients with T1DM on exogenous insulin, muscle glucose uptake may exceed hepatic glucose production and produce hypoglycemia. Abbreviations: HDAC—histone deacetylase; MEF-2—myocyte enhancer factor-2; GLUT4—glucose transporter 4; EPI—epinephrine; PGC-1α—peroxisome proliferator activated receptor γ co-activator 1α; OXPHOS—oxidative phosphorylation; PPAR-α/δ—peroxisome proliferator activated receptor α/δ; MAPK—mitogen-activated protein kinase; PKC—protein kinase C; Erk 1/2—extracellular regulated protein kinase 1/2; AICAR—5′-aminoimidazole-4-carboxamide (AICA)-riboside; AMPK—5′-AMP-activated protein kinase; IRS—insulin receptor substrate; PI3K—phosphatidylinositol-3-kinase; Akt—protein kinase B; GSK3—glycogen synthase kinase-3; ATF-2—activating transcription factor-2; CnA—calcineurin; CREB—cAMP response element binding protein; CaMK—calmodulin-dependent kinase; p160MBP—p160 myb binding protein.

to provide metabolic fuel. Without this adaptive reflex that augments EGP, hypoglycemia would result with exercise. During intense exercise ($V_{O2\ max} > 80\%$), catecholamines play a greater role in augmenting EGP [15], particularly by mobilizing muscle glycogen. Furthermore, it has been suggested that there are exercise-specific stimuli to hepatic glucose release independent of pancreatic hormone and hepatic catecholamine action, such as involving the carotid bodies [16].

Acute exercise increases the action of insulin during and for hours after the exercise session in nondiabetic subjects [17]. It is interesting that during exercise, glucose uptake may be independent of insulin receptor activation, insulin receptor substrate (IRS) 1/2 phosphorylation, and phosphatidylinositol-3-kinase (PI3K) phosphorylation [18]. Nevertheless, there are synergistic effects of exercise and insulin on glucose uptake. The mechanism of this synergism is related to increased perfusion and insulin delivery to the muscles, insulin suppression of non-esterified fatty acids (NEFA), and insulin activation of post-insulin receptor signal transduction [18,19]. Exercise shifts insulin-stimulated glucose disposal from nonoxidative to oxidative metabolism [13]. This effect is most pronounced during the postprandial state (high endogenous insulin levels) and with insulin therapy [13].

Endurance training increases insulin sensitivity and insulin mediated glucose uptake in nondiabetic humans [20]. One mechanism by which this occurs is that regular exercise potentiates the insulin-stimulated IRS1/2-PI3K pathway in skeletal muscle [21]. In addition, muscle GLUT4 content is increased with training [22]. Training also enhances insulin sensitivity of glucose uptake and lipolysis in adipose tissue in humans [23]. The increased insulin responsiveness in adipocytes appears to be modulated by the IRS/PI3K/Akt pathway [24]. Endurance-trained individuals oxidize more fat from adipose and intramuscular triglycerides than untrained individuals at the same exercise intensity, thus sparing glucose [25]. Resistance training has also been shown to increase insulin action and reduce hyperinsulinemia in normal subjects [26].

Interestingly, after marathon running, insulin sensitivity is decreased in healthy subjects [27] despite low glycogen content and enhanced glycogen synthase activity. This is thought to be due to increased lipid oxidation and the inhibitory effect of fat utilization on glucose disposal ("Randle cycle"). Insulin clearance is enhanced after marathon running, which further spares glucose and allows enhanced lipid oxidation [28]. Eccentric exercise, which typically results in muscle damage, also induces a transient insulin resistance [29].

Other adaptations that occur with aerobic exercise include an increase in cardiac output and density of muscle capillaries [30], improvement in oxidative capacity of type-1 slow-twitch fibers [31], increase in muscle mitochondria, enhanced glycogen synthase and hexokinase activity, and increase in the GLUT4 receptors [32]. Under anaerobic conditions with rigorous exercise, lactate accumulates and leads to muscle fatigue and decreased exercise capacity. Physical training improves the capacity for oxygen delivery and restrains lactate production.

Carbohydrate availability during sustained (> 1–1.5 hours) exercise influences muscle physiology and physical performance. Carbohydrate ingestion during prolonged exercise improves endurance by slowing the mobilization of endogenous fuels, thus preserving muscle glycogen [13]. However, muscle glycogenolysis is not completely spared with carbohydrate ingestion [33]. Adopo et al. [34] found that approximately 40% of a 50 g glucose load ingested at the start of a moderate exercise session is metabolized during the first hour. In addition, since glucose and fructose absorption and metabolism differ to some degree, ingesting a combination of these hexoses results in greater oxidation than if ingested individually [34]. Carbohydrate ingestion has little influence on oxidation rates during periods of low- or high-intensity work [35,36].

After an exercise session, a series of coordinated adaptive events replenish fuel stores, especially muscle and liver glycogen. This is activated by muscle contraction and mediated by various downstream pathways involved with insulin receptor signaling distal to the IRS1/2-PI3K cascade (see Table 15.5). During recovery, insulin levels rise and glucose remains in the normal range. In addition, there is a decrease in carbohydrate oxidation and pyruvate dehydrogenase (PDH) activation and an increase in lipid oxidation [37]. Plasma fatty acids, very low-density lipoprotein cholesterol (VLDL-c), and intramuscular acetylcarnitine stores, but not intramuscular triglycerides, appear to be important fuels for aerobic energy [37]. Moreover, glycogen synthase kinase-3 (GSK3) is deactivated with muscle contraction leading to gene transcription, protein synthesis, and glycogen synthesis during recovery [38,39]. There is an initial phase of rapid glycogen synthesis lasting 30–60 minutes, which does not require insulin and is the result of exercise induced translocation of GLUT4 to the cell surface [40]. This is followed by a slower second phase lasting several hours which is insulin-dependent. The availability of carbohydrate is a rate-limiting factor for glycogen synthesis [40]. Glycogen synthesis is faster when carbohy-

TABLE 15.5
Metabolic Pathways Activated by Muscle Contraction That Lead to Recovery of Fuel Stores after Exercise

Pathway (Reference)[a]	Action
Akt [115]	Insulin-like
AMP kinase [116]	Decreases anaerobic glycogen metabolism,
	increases aerobic glucose and fatty acid metabolism,
	upregulates mitochondrial content with endurance,
	activated by metformin
GLUT4 [117]	Glucose uptake
Glycogenin [118]	Generates primer for glycogen synthesis
Hexokinase II [119]	Functionally couples glycolysis with mitochondrial energy metabolism
MAP kinases [120,121]	Transcriptional regulation which alters muscle phenotype
	p38
	c-Jun N-terminal (JNK)
	Extracellular signal regulated (ERK)
p70[s6k] [122]	Activation of protein synthesis
	Enhanced by dietary branched-chain amino acids

[a] See text and Appendix 1 for abbreviations.

drate is consumed post-exercise, a phenomenon known as "supercompensation." Supplementing carbohydrate at 1.2 g/kg/hour at 30-minute intervals for up to 5 hours post-exercise appears to maximize the rate of glycogen resynthesis [41]. The addition of protein and amino acids to a carbohydrate-containing solution can accelerate glycogen synthesis when carbohydrate intake is lower at 0.8 g/kg/hour [41] but has no effect when the higher amount of carbohydrate is ingested [42]. Rates of glycogen resynthesis are higher after short-term high-intensity exercise than prolonged exercise or resistance exercise [43]. This is thought to be due to (1) the higher levels of lactate and glycolytic intermediates after high-intensity exercise as well as (2) the greater glycogen depletion in fast-twitch fibers which have a higher level of glycogen synthase activity as compared with slow-twitch fibers. Glycogen resynthesis is further delayed after resistance exercise with an eccentric component.

Exercise also triggers a set of metabolic, hormonal, humoral, and enzymatic events that ultimately exert transcriptional and translational control over genomic expression. Several lines of pre-clinical evidence support this concept but a cohesive and integrated framework in humans remains unsolved. Various genomic mutations and polymorphisms modulate the metabolic response to exercise. For example, the Gln27Glu and Gly16Arg polymorphism in the β_2-adrenoceptor (BAR-2) gene coding sequence, which controls adipose tissue lipolysis with exercise, is associated with obesity and the metabolic syndrome [44–46]. Beneficial effects of exercise have been observed on ob [47], leptin [48], lipoprotein lipase [49], apolipoprotein A1 [50], low-density lipoprotein cholesterol (LDL-c) receptor [50], high-density lipoprotein cholesterol (HDL-c) scavenger receptor [51], manganese superoxide dismutase [52], catalase [52], and glutathione peroxidase [52] gene expression.

EXERCISE IN TYPE-1 DIABETES MELLITUS

Although exercise is important for cardiovascular fitness in people with T1DM, it does not improve glycemic control [53,54]. In fact, people with T1DM who participate in competitive sports often exhibit worse glycemic control than sedentary patients [55]. Exercise, including Olympic-level sports or marathon running, can be safely performed although carbohydrate intake and insulin administration must be carefully adjusted to avoid metabolic deterioration. The cardiac output, respiratory capacity and $V_{O2\,max}$ are similar between patients with T1DM and nondiabetic patients

[56]. However, the metabolic response to exercise is abnormal in patients with T1DM. Unlike normal individuals where insulin levels decrease markedly during exercise, people with T1DM have a relative hyperinsulinemia during exercise due to exogenously administered insulin [57]. As a result, hepatic glucose production is attenuated, increasing the risk of hypoglycemia.

Increased glucagon secretion is the major defense against hypoglycemia during exercise, with catecholamines playing an important role with intense exercise [15]. Feed-forward circuits create a vicious cycle wherein exercise induces transient hypoglycemia, activating neuroendocrine and autonomic counter-regulatory pathways, which then improve glucose uptake and potentially exacerbate the hypoglycemia [58]. Patients with T1DM may have a reduced counter-regulatory response to exercise-induced hypoglycemia [59]. Deficient release of catecholamines reduces lipolysis in muscle and adipose. This leads to decreased glycerol availability via gluconeogenesis for conversion to glucose, and contributes to hypoglycemia [60]. Moreover, previous-day hypoglycemia can further blunt the counter-regulatory response in diabetics during subsequent prolonged moderate-intensity exercise [61]. Conversely, repeated episodes of prolonged exercise of low- to moderate- intensity blunt counter-regulatory responses to next day hypoglycemia [62].

In T1DM, the normal increase in insulin-induced muscle glucose uptake with exercise is not observed [63]. This is likely due to a defect in the insulin signaling pathway [60] and not an impairment of exercise-induced skeletal muscle blood flow [64]. With training, glycogen synthase activity increases in T1DM but insulin receptor function remains unchanged [65]. After marathon running, insulin sensitivity is unchanged and insulin clearance is enhanced, similar to normal individuals [66].

The type of insulin used and location of the insulin injection can potentially contribute to exercise-related hypoglycemia in T1DM. Insulin absorption is accelerated when administered near the working skeletal muscle because of increased local blood flow [67]. Hypoglycemia can be particularly pronounced if exercise occurs soon after administration of a short- or rapid-acting insulin and even more if the insulin is accidentally injected directly into the muscle instead of the subcutaneous tissue. However, intense exercise does not increase the absorption rate of subcutaneously injected basal long-acting insulin glargine [68].

Exercise can also exacerbate hyperglycemia and ketonemia in T1DM, particularly in those patients who are underinsulinized and already hyperglycemic before the exercise session begins. This is due to low pyruvate dehydrogenase activity, elevated lipolysis, and elevated non-esterefied fatty acids (NEFA) production rates. In addition, the counter-regulatory surge associated with exercise is unopposed, in the setting of insulinopenia, so that EGP is further increased while muscle glucose uptake is low. Therefore, it is best to avoid exercising during severe hyperglycemia to avoid worsening glucose control and ketosis. If glucose is markedly elevated >300 mg/dL or ketones are present, exercise should be deferred. Exercise does not need to be postponed with milder hyperglycemia, but it may be necessary to take a "correction" dose of short- or rapid-acting insulin prior to exercise. Ideally, people with T1DM should check their capillary blood glucose levels before, during (if exercise is prolonged > 45 minutes), immediately after, and 1–2 hours after an exercise session. The routine use of noninvasive glucose monitors is currently unreliable during moderate to intense exercise, [69] but improvement in such devices may eventually serve to assist with monitoring.

Strategies for avoiding hypoglycemia during exercise involve decreasing mealtime insulin before exercising, decreasing basal insulin if using continuous subcutaneous insulin infusion (CSII), or increasing carbohydrate intake. Rabasa-Lhoret et al. [70] studied the glucose response to exercise of different intensities and durations in 8 men with T1DM on a basal-bolus regimen. Exercise was performed 90 minutes after a meal, and pre-meal insulin doses were lowered based on planned exercise to avoid hypoglycemia (see Table 15.6). It should be noted that while effective, such an approach necessitates mild hyperglycemia after the meal and before exercise. Grimm et al. [71] demonstrated less hypoglycemia when carbohydrate intake was appropriately increased as compared with adjustments in insulin dosage.

EXERCISE AND PREDIABETES

An evidence-based technical review on physical activity and exercise in the T2DM patient was published by the American Diabetes Association (ADA) in 2004 [9] and is based on recent basic and clinical studies that demonstrate (1) lifestyle interventions including exercise reduce the incidence of T2DM in persons with impaired glucose tolerance (IGT), (2) meta-analyses demonstrating the beneficial effects of exercise on hemoglobin A1C (A1C) levels independent of body weight, (3) large cohort studies linking decreased fitness with increased risk of cardiovascular disease (CVD) mortality in diabetic patients, and (4) safety and efficacy of progressive resistance training on glycemic control and CVD risk.

The increasing incidence of obesity and sedentary lifestyle, due to urbanization and industrialization of society, are coincident with the meteoric rise in diabetes and prediabetes. For every 2-hour increment in television viewing daily, the incidence of obesity and diabetes increases 23% and 14%, respectively [72]. Diabetic subjects have a two- to fourfold higher cardiovascular mortality than nondiabetic subjects. Regular exercise can reduce this cardiovascular mortality [73]. This is consistent with observations that exercise reduces hypertension [74], LDL-c levels (with increases in HDL-c) [75], and insulin levels [76] while improving insulin sensitivity and glycemic control [77]. Exercise also improves resting fibrinolytic activity in diabetics [78].

The Finnish Diabetes Prevention Study followed overweight subjects with IGT who lost $\geq 5\%$ body weight, adhered to a moderate-intensity exercise program of > 30 minutes/day, limited total and saturated fat to $< 30\%$ and $< 10\%$, respectively, and consumed at least 15 g/1000 kcal fiber [79]. The U.S. Diabetes Prevention Program followed subjects with IGT who achieved and maintained $\geq 7\%$ weight loss with a low-calorie, low-fat diet, and engaged in moderate-intensity exercise for ≥ 150 minutes/week [80]. In both of these prospective, randomized, controlled trials, there was a 58% reduction in the relative risk of diabetes with the lifestyle interventions that incorporated exercise. Additional studies have confirmed these findings and are reviewed in the ADA Technical Review [9]. Therefore, based on the clinical evidence, persons with IGT should participate in a weight control program incorporating moderate-to-vigorous exercise ≥ 150 minutes/week and a healthy energy-restricted diet (evidence level 1) [9].

EXERCISE AND TYPE-2 DIABETES MELLITUS

In contrast with T1DM patients, who generally have normal exercise capacity, T2DM patients have reduced oxidative capacity [81], impaired mitochondrial activity [81], and decreased peripheral O_2 extraction with exercise [82]. Even though patients with T2DM are more likely to be obese and have a lower $V_{O2\ max}$ than nondiabetics [83], $V_{O2\ max}$ increases normally during endurance training. Importantly, insulin sensitivity is improved in T2DM after one exercise session [84] and this effect can last 24 to over 72 hours [85,86]. This duration justifies an exercise prescription of 3 times/week though daily exercise programs may offer greater benefit [87].

In T2DM, exercise is associated with a decrease in blood glucose due to suppression of EGP and an increase in muscle glucose uptake. Exercise mediated glucose uptake is not reduced despite insulin resistance. People with T2DM are able to take up glucose during exercise via an insulin-independent mechanism and the glucose uptake can even be greater than nondiabetics due to the ambient hyperglycemia [88]. Moderate exercise after a meal reduces postprandial glycemia in patients with T2DM, but the effect does not persist for the subsequent meal [89].

Both resistance training [90,91] and aerobic exercise [92] improve glycemic control and insulin action and lower fasting insulin in patients with T2DM. In one study [93], there was a dose-response relationship between exercise intensity (up to $> 75\%$ $V_{O2\ max}$) and both cardiorespiratory fitness and A1C levels. This effect is independent of significant total body weight reduction but is associated with both visceral and subcutaneous fat loss [93]. In obese, but not lean, patients with T2DM, exercise-induced fat metabolism is characterized by decreased NEFA and increased intra-

TABLE 15.6

Guidelines for Reduction in Pre-Meal Rapid-Acting Insulin Dose before Exercise

Exercise Intensity (% $V_{O2\ max}$)	% Dose Reduction	
	30 Minutes of Exercise	60 Minutes of Exercise
25	25	50
50	50	75
75	75	—

Source: From Reference [70] with permission.

muscular TG utilization [94,95]. GLUT-4 expression and glycogen synthase activity but not insulin signaling are increased in overweight nondiabetic and type-2 diabetic patients after aerobic exercise training [96]. Strength training is associated with increased GLUT4, insulin receptor, protein kinase B- alpha/beta, and glycogen synthase activity [97].

Patients with diet-controlled T2DM or those taking insulin sensitizers alone, experience increased muscle glucose uptake, reduced EGP, and a lowering of blood glucose without risk of symptomatic hypoglycemia. In one study, glucose decreased by 35 mg/dL after 45 minutes of exercise on a cycle ergometer in diet-controlled diabetic patients who started the exercise hyperglycemic [98]. Pre-exercise precautions are not generally necessary in patients with T2DM taking only insulin sensitizers or α-glucosidase inhibitors. In contrast, patients taking a sulfonylurea or insulin have supraphysiologic insulin levels, enhanced peripheral glucose utilization, enhanced suppression of EGP, and increased risk for hypoglycemia [99].

Exercise should be coupled with dietary strategies for weight loss, that is, balanced calorie restriction. Many clinical studies and successful weight loss programs have buttressed this approach [100]. Exercise programs alone produce only mild weight loss as obese patients (1) cannot produce a sufficient energy deficit with exercise alone, (2) eat more when exercising, and (3) become less active when not exercising [100]. However, in one randomized trial of moderate-intensity exercise vs. diet, with both producing the same 700 kcal/day energy deficit, fat loss was comparable [101]. Thus, patients with T2DM should exercise at the highest intensity that is tolerated. Ideally, this would entail at least 4–7 hours, divided into 3–7 sessions of moderate- to high-intensity aerobic exercise per week [87,102]. The upper limits of this range and intensity are best for long-term maintenance of major weight loss (levels 1–2 evidence) [9].

Based on the clinical evidence, resistance training should be included in any exercise program for patients with T2DM. The advantages of incorporating resistance training include (1) breaking the monotony of aerobic routines; (2) increasing muscle mass, strength, and functional status; (3) improving body composition; and (4) reversing age-related sarcopenia. In the absence of any contraindications, patients with T2DM should engage in progressive resistance training 3 times/week, involving all major muscle groups, and advance to 3 sets of 8–10 repetitions at a weight that cannot be lifted > 8–10 times (evidence level 1) [87]. Ideally, patients new to weight training should be supervised by a qualified exercise trainer.

EXERCISE IN GESTATIONAL DIABETES

The therapeutic goal for managing gestational diabetes (GDM) is to achieve euglycemia in order to avert fetal-maternal complications. Dietary manipulations are the mainstay of treatment. However, up to 39% of patients with GDM will require insulin during pregnancy [103]. Exercise is a safe and effective adjunct in the treatment of GDM. The American College of Obstetricians and Gynecologists (ACOG) recommends approximately 30 minutes or more of moderate exercise per day with pregnancy unless there are medical or obstetrical complications [104]. This recommendation has been applied to women with GDM and is endorsed by the ADA [105]. Various forms of exercise, including circuit-type resistance training [106], light recumbent bicycling (50% $V_{O2\ max}$) [107], and arm ergometry [108] have been shown to be safe and may obviate the need for insulin in GDM. Even walking at a leisurely pace after meals has been shown to significantly improve postprandial hyperglycemia [109].

In a literature review on exercise and pregnancy, Wolfe and Weissgerber [110] concluded that (1) $V_{O2\ max}$ was preserved in pregnancy with physical activity but anaerobic working capacity may be reduced in late gestation; (2) heart rate reserve was decreased; and (3) strenuous exercise was associated with fetal heart rate variability and reduced fetal glucose availability. Therefore, some of the hesitance in prescribing exercise in GDM has been the concern for the safety of the patient and the developing fetus. Exercise has also been implicated in stimulating uterine contractions and possibly causing pre-term labor because of the catecholamine surge associated with exercise [111]. One study showed that employing upper arm ergometric exercises at moderate intensity resulted in a lower incidence of uterine contractions when compared to lower extremity exercises and also significantly reduced fasting and postprandial blood glucose levels [108]. If contractions are experienced in any exercise, the activity should immediately be terminated. Swimming and other aquatic exercises are beneficial in GDM [112]. The buoyant properties of water lower the risk of musculoskeletal injury and hyperthermia and any resulting fetal ischemia is reduced by the cooling effect of water. In general, non-weight-bearing exercises including swimming, cycling, and upper arm ergometrics are recommended over weight-bearing activities such as jogging or aerobics classes because of the reduced stress on the joints and lower risk of injury. Resistance training is not recommended in pregnancy because of the potential for uterine contractions from the valsalva maneuver.

REFERENCES

1. American College of Sports Medicine Position Stand, The recommended quantity and quality of exercise for developing and maintaining cardiorespiratory and muscular fitness and flexibility in healthy adults, *Med Sci Sports Exerc,* 30:975-991, 1998.
2. Bass MA, Enochs WK, and DiBrezzo R, Comparison of two exercise programs on general well-being of college students, *Psychol Rep,* 91:1195–1201, 2002.
3. Paffenbarger RS, Jr, Hyde RT, and Wing AL et al., The association of changes in physical activity level and other lifestyle characteristics with mortality among men, *N Engl J Med,* 28:538–545, 1993.
4. Holcomb CA, Heim DL, and Loughin TM, Physical activity minimizes the association of body fatness with abdominal obesity in white, premenopausal women, Results from the Third National Health and Nutrition Examination Survey, *J Am Diet Assoc,* 104:1859–1862, 2004.
5. Berlin JA and Colditz GA, A meta-analysis of physical activity in thr prevention of coronary heart disease, *Am J Epidemiol,* 132:612–628, 1990.
6. Fletcher GF, Exercise in the prevention of stroke, *Health Rep,* 6:106–110, 1994.
7. http://www.betterhealth.vic.gov.au/bhcv2/bhcarticles.nsf/pages/Exercise_intensity?open, Accessed on February 18, 2005.
8. Zinman B, Ruderman N, and Campaigne BN et al., American Diabetes Association, Physical activity/exercise and diabetes mellitus, *Diabetes Care,* 26:S73–77, 2003.
9. Sigal RJ, Kenny GP, and Wasserman DH et al., Physical activity/exercise and type-2 diabetes, *Diabetes Care,* 7:2518–2539, 2004.
10. Wasserman DH, Davis SN, and Zinman B, Fuel metabolism during exercise in health and diabetes, In: *Handbook or Exercise in Diabetes,* Ruderman N, Devlin JT, and Scheider SH, Eds., Alexandria, VA: American Diabetes Association, 2002:63–99.
11. Ivy JL, Exercise physiology and adaptations to training, In: *Handbook or Exercise in Diabetes,* Ruderman N, Devlin JT, and Scheider SH, Eds., Alexandria, VA: American Diabetes Association, 2002:23–62.

12. Goodyear LJ and Horton ES, Signal transduction and glucose transport in muscle, In: *Handbook or Exercise in Diabetes*, Ruderman N, Devlin JT, and Scheider SH, Eds., Alexandria, VA: American Diabetes Association, 2002:63–99.

13. Wasserman DH and Cherrington AD, Regulation of extramuscular fuel sources during exercise, In: *Handbook of Physiology*, Rowell LB and Shepherd JT, Eds., Columbia, MD: Bermedica Production, 1036–1074, 1996.

14. Koranyi LI, Bourney RE, and Slentz CA et al., Coordinate reduction of rat pancreatic islet glucokinase and proinsulin mRNA by exercise training, *Diabetes,* 40:401–404, 1991.

15. Sigal RJ, Purdon C, and Bilinski D et al., Glucoregulation during and after intense exercise: Effects of beta-blockade, *J Clin Endocrinol Metab,* 78:359–366, 1994.

16. Coker RH, Yoshiharu Koyama, and Denny JC et al., Prevention of overt hypoglycemia during exercise, *Diabetes,* 1:1310–1318, 2002.

17. Wojtaszewski JF, Hansen BF, and Kiens B et al., Insulin signaling in human skeletal muscle: Time course and effect of exercise, *Diabetes,* 6:1775–1781, 1997.

18. Goodyear LJ, Giorgino F, and Balon TW et al., Effects of contractile activity on tyrosine phosphoproteins and PI 3-kinase activity in rat skeletal muscle, *Am J Physiol,* 268:E987–995, 1995.

19. Richter EA, Glucose utilization, In: *Handbook of Physiology*, Rowell LB and Shepherd JT, Eds., New York: Oxford University Press, 1996:912–951.

20. Dela F, Mikines KJ, and von Linstow M et al., Effect of training on insulin-mediated glucose uptake in human muscle, *Am J Physiol,* 63:E1134–1143, 1992.

21. Kirwan JP, del Aguila LF, and Hernandez JM et al., Regular exercise enhances activation of IRS-1-associated PI3-kinase in human skeletal muscle, *J Appl Physiol,* 88:797–803, 2000.

22. Houmard JA, Shinebarger MH, and Dolan PL et al., Exercise training increases GLUT-4 protein concentration in previously sedentary middle aged men, *Am J Physiol,* 64;E896–901, 1993.

23. Stallknecht B, Larsen JJ, and Mikines KJ et al., Effect of training on insulin sensitivity of glucose uptake and lipolysis in human adipose tissue, *Am J Physiol Endocrinol Metab,* 79:E376–385, 2000.

24. Peres SB, de Moraes SM, and Costa CE et al., Endurance exercise training increases insulin responsiveness in isolated adipocytes through IRS/PI3 kinase/Akt pathway, *J Appl Physiol,* 8:1037–1043, 2005.

25. Coggan AR, Raguso CA, and Gastaldelli A et al., Fat metabolism during high-intensity exercise in endurance trained and untrained men, *Metabolism,* 9:122–128, 2000.

26. Ryan AS, Pratley RE, and Goldberg AP et al., Resistive training increases insulin action in postmenopausal women, *J Gerontol A Biol Sci Med Sci,* 1:M199–205, 1996.

27. Tuominen JA, Ebeling P, and Bourey R et al., Postmarathon paradox: Insulin resistance in the face of glycogen depletion, *Am J Physiol,* 70:336–343, 1996.

28. Tuominem JA, Ebeling P and Koivisto VA, Exercise increases insulin clearance in healthy man and insulin-dependent diabetes mellitus patients, *Clin Physiol,* 7:19–30, 1997.

29. Kirwan JP, Hickner RC, and Yarasheski KE et al., Eccentric exercise induces transient insulin resistance in healthy individuals, *J Appl Physiol,* 2:2197–2202, 1992.

30. Saltin B and Rowell LB, Functional adaptations to physical activity and inactivity, *Fed Proc,* 39:1506–1513, 1980.

31. Saltin B, Henriksson J, and Nyaard E et al., Fiber types and metabolic potentials of skeletal muscles in sedentary man and endurance runners, In: *The Marathon: Physiological, Medical, Epidemiological, and Psychological Studies,* Vol. 301, Milvy P, Ed., New York, NY: Annals of the New York Academy of Sciences, 3–29, 1977.

32. Hayashi T, Wojtaszewski JF, and Goodyear LJ, Exercise regulation of glucose transport in skeletal muscle, *Am J Physiol,* 273:E1039–1051, 1997.

33. Coyle EF, Coggin AR, and Hemmert MK et al., Muscle glycogen utilization during prolonged strenuous exercise when fed carbohydrate, *J Appl Physiol,* 61:165–172, 1986.

34. Adopo E, Peronnet F, and Massicotte D et al., Respective oxidation of exogenous glucose and fructose given in the same drink during exercise, *J Appl Physiol,* 76:1014–1019, 1994.

35. Pirnay F, Crielaard JM, and Pallikarakis N et al., Fate of exogenous glucose during exercise of different intensities in humans, *J Appl Physiol,* 43:258, 1982–2261.

36. Duchman SM, Ryan AJ, and Schedl HP et al., Upper limit for intestinal absorption of a dilute glucose solution in men at rest, *Med Sci Sports Exerc,* 29:482–488, 1997.

37. Kimber NE, Heigenhauser GJ, and Spriet LL et al., Skeletal muscle fat and carbohydrate metabolism during recovery from glycogen-depleting exercise in humans, *J Physiol,* 48:919–927, 2003.

38. Markuns JF, Wojtaszewski JFP, and Goodyear LJ, Insulin and exercise decrease glycogen synthase kinase-3 activity by different mechanisms in rat skeletal muscle, *J Biol Chem,* 274:24896–249000, 1999.

39. Sakamoto K and Goodyear LJ, Intracellular signaling in contracting skeletal muscle, *J Appl Physiol,* 93:369–383, 2002.

40. Jentjens R and Jeukendrup A, Determinants of post-exercise glycogen synthesis during short-term recovery, *Sports Med,* 3:117–144, 2003.

41. van Loon LJ, Saris WH, and Kruijshoop M et al., Maximizing postexercise muscle glycogen synthesis: Carbohydrate supplementation and the application of amino acid or protein hydrolysate mixtures, *Am J Clin Nutr,* 2:106–111, 2000.

42. Jentjens RL, van Loon LJ, and Mann CH et al., Addition of protein and amino acids to carbohydrates does not enhance postexercise muscle glycogen synthesis, *J Appl Physiol,* 1:839–846, 2001.

43. Pascoe DD and Gladden LB, Muscle glycogen resynthesis after short term, high-intensity exercise and resistance exercise, *Sports Med,* 1:98–118, 1996.

44. Large V, Hellstrom L, and Reynisdottir S et al., Human beta-2 adrenoceptor gene polymorphisms are highly frequent in obesity and associate with altered adipocyte beta-2 adrenoceptor function, *J Clin Invest,* 100:3005–3013, 1997.

45. Dallongeville J, Helbecque N, and Cottel D et al., The gln16 → Arg16 and Gln27 → Glu27 polymorphisms of beta2-adrenergic receptor are associated with metabolic syndrome in men, *J Clin Endocrinol Metab,* 88:4862–4866, 2003.

46. Meirhaeghe A, Helbecque N, and Cottel D, β2-adrenoceptor gene polymorphism, body weight, and physical activity, *Lancet,* 353:896, 1999.

47. Zhang D, Wooter MH, and Zhou Q et al., The effect of exercise on ob gene expression, *Biochem Biophys Res Commun,* 225:747–750, 1996.

48. Jeffrey JZ, Stephen LH, and Steven RS et al., Voluntary wheel running decreases adipose tissue mass and expression of leptin mRNA on Osborne-Mendel rats, *Diabetes,* 46:1159-1166, 1997.

49. Seip RL, Angelopoulos TJ, and Semenkoveih CF, Exercises induce human lipoprotein lipase gene expression in skeletal muscle but not adipose tissue, *Am J Physiol,* 268:E229–236, 1995.

50. Cai L and Chen JD, Molecular mechanism of aerobic exercise on the prevention of hyperlipidemia for high-fat diet rats, *Cin J Sports Med,* 18:314–316, 1999.

51. Li CY and Chen JD, Reverse transference of cholesterol and high-density lipoprotein receptor (HDL–R), *Chin J Sports Med,* 19:71–73, 2000.

52. Somani SM and Rybak LP, Comparative effects of exercise training on transcription of antioxidant enzyme and the activity in old rat heart, *Indian J Physiol Pharmacol,* 40:205–212, 1996.

53. Ligetenberg PC, Blans M, and Hoekstra JB et al., No effect of long-term physical activity on the glycemic control in type-1 diabetes patients, A cross-sectional study, *Neth J Med,* 5:59–63, 1999.

54. Roberts L, Jones TW, and Fournier PA, Exercise training and glycemic control in adolescents with poorly controlled type-1 diabetes mellitus, *J Pediatr Endocrinol Metab,* 5:621–627, 2002.

55. Ebeling P, Tuominen JA, and Bourey R et al., Athletes with IDDM exhibit impaired metabolic control with increased lipid utilization with no increase in insulin sensitivity, *Diabetes,* 4:471–477, 1995.

56. Nugent AM, Steele IC, and al-Modaris F et al., Exercise responses in patients with IDDM, *Diabetes Care,* 20:1814–1821, 1997.

57. Richter EA and Galbo H, Diabetes and exercise, *International Diab Monitor,* 16:1–9, 2004.

58. Ertl AC and Davis SN, Evidence for a vicious cycle of exercise and hypoglycemia in type-1 diabetes mellitus, *Diabetes Metab Res Rev,* 20:124–130, 2004.

59. Schneider SH, Vitug A, and Ananthakrishnan R et al., Impaired adrenergic response to prolonged exercise in type-I diabetes, *Metabolism,* 40:1219–1225, 1991.

60. Enoksson S, Caprio SK, and Rife F et al., Defective activation of skeletal muscle and adipose tissue lipolysis in type-1 diabetes mellitus during hypoglycemia, *J Clin Endocrinol Metab,* 8:1503–1511, 2003.

61. Galassetti P, Tate D, and Neill RA et al., Effect of antecedent hypoglycemia on counterregulatory responses to subsequent euglycemic exercise in type-1 diabetes, *Diabetes,* 2:1761–1769, 2003.

62. Sandoval DA, Guy DL, and Richardson MA et al., Effects of low and moderate antecedent exercise on counterregulatory responses to subsequent hypoglycemia in type-1 diabetes, *Diabetes,* 3:1798–1806, 2004.

63. Peltoniemi P, Yki-Jarvinen H, and Oikonen V et al., Resistance to exercise-induced increase in glucose uptake during hyperinsulinemia in insulin-resistant skeletal muscle of patients with type-1 diabetes, *Diabetes,* 0:1371–1377, 2001.

64. Skyrme-Jones RA, Berry KL, and O'Brien RC et al., Basal and exercise-induced skeletal muscle blood flow is augmented in type-I diabetes mellitus, *Clin Sci,* 8:111–120, 2000.

65. Bak JF, Jacobsen UK, and Jorgensen FS et al., Insulin receptor function and glycogen synthase activity in skeletal muscle biopsies from patients with insulin-dependent diabetes mellitus: Effects of physical training, *J Clin Endocrinol Metab,* 9:158–164, 1989.

66. Tuominen JA, Ebeling P, and Vuorinen-Markkola H et al., Post-marathon paradox in IDDM: Unchanged insulin sensitivity in spite of glycogen depletion, *Diabet Med,* 4:301–308, 1997.

67. Zinman B, Murray FT, and Vranic M et al., Glucoregulation during moderate exercise in insulin-treated diabetics, *J Clin Endorinol Metab,* 5:641–652, 1977.

68. Peter R, Luzio SD, and Dunseath G et al., Effects of exercise on the absorption of insulin glargine in patients with type-1 diabetes, *Diabetes Care,* 8:560–565, 2005.

69. Nunnold T, Colberg SR, and Herriott MT et al., Use of the noninvasive Gluco Watch Biographer during exercise of varying intensity, *Diabetes Technol Ther,* 6:454–62, 2004.

70. Rabasa-Lhoret R, Bourque J, and Ducross F et al., Guidelines for premeal insulin dose reduction for postprandial exercise of different intensities and durations in type-1 diabetic subjects treated intensively with a basal-bolus insulin regimen (ultralente-lispro), *Diabetes Care,* 4:625–630, 2001.

71. Grimm JJ, Ybarra J, and Berne C et al., A new table for prevention of hypoglycemia during physical activity in type-1 diabetic patients, *Diabetes Metab,* 0:465–470, 2004.

72. Hu FB, Li TY, Colditz GA, Willet WC, and Manson JE, Television watching and other sedentary behaviors in relation to risk of obesity and type-2 diabetes mellitus in women, *JAMA,* 289:1785–1791, 2003.

73. Hu FB, Stampfer MJ, and Solomon C et al., Physical activity and the risk of cardiovascular events in diabetic women, *Ann Intern Med,* 34:96–105, 2001.

74. Fagard RH, Physical activity in the prevention and treatment of hypertension in the obese, *Med Sports Exerc,* 19(Suppl 11):S624–618, 1999.

75. Wood PD, Stefanick ML, and Williams PT et al., The effects on plasma lipoprotein of a prudent weight-reducing diet, with or without exercise, in overweight men and women, *N Engl J Med,* 325:461–466, 1991.

76. Mayer-Davis EJ, D'Agostino R, Jr, and Karter AJ et al., Intensity and amount of physical activity in relation to insulin: The Insulin Resistance Atherosclerosis Study, *JAMA,* 279:669–674, 1998.

77. Boule NG, Haddad E, and Kenny GP et al., Effects of exercise on glycemic control and body mass index in type-2 diabetes mellitusm, A meta-analysis of controlled clinical trials, *JAMA,* 286:1218–1227, 2001.

78. Schneider SH, Kim HC, and Khachadurian AK et al., Impaired fibrinolytic response to exercise in type-II diabetes: Effects of exercise and physical training, *Metabolism,* 37:924–929, 1988.

79. Tuomilehto J, Lindstrom J, and Eriksson JG et al., Prevention of type-2 diabetes mellitus by changes in lifestyle among subjects with impaired glucose tolerance, *N Engl J Med,* 344:1343–1350, 2001.

80. Diabetes Prevention Program Research Group, Reduction in the incidence of type-2 diabetes with lifestyle intervention or metformin, *N Engl J Med,* 346:393–403, 2002.

81. Schrauwen P and Hesselink MKC, Oxidative capacity, lipotoxicity, and mitochondrial damage in type-2 diabetes, *Diabetes,* 3:1412–1417, 2004.

82. Baldi J, Aoina JL, and Oxenham HC et al., Reduced exercise arteriovenous O_2 difference in type-2 diabetics, *J Appl Physiol,* 4:1033–1038, 2003.

83. Schneider SH, Khachadurian AK, and Amorosa LF et al., Ten-year experience with an exercise-based outpatient life-style modification program in the treatment of diabetes mellitus, *Diabetes Care,* 5:1800–1810, 1992.

84. Schneider SH and Elouzi EB, The role of exercise in type-II diabetes mellitus, *Prev Cardiol,* 3:77–82, 2000.

85. Wallberg-Henriksson H, Rincon J, and Zierath JR, Exercise in the management of non-insulin-dependent diabetes mellitus, *Sports Med,* 25:25–35, 1998.

86. Zachwieja JJ, Toffolo G, and Cobelli C et al., Resistance exercise and growth hormone administration in older men: Effects on insulin sensitivity and secretion during a stable-label intravenous glucose tolerance test, *Metabolism,* 45:254–260, 1996.

87. Blair SN, LaMonte MJ, and Nichaman MZ, The evolution of physical activity recommendations: How much is enough? *Am J Clin Nutr,* 79(Suppl 5):913S–920S, 2004.

88. Kennedy JW, Hirshman MF, and Gervino EV et al., Acute exercise induces GLUT4 translocation in skeletal muscle of normal human subjects and subjects with type-2 diabetes, *Diabetes,* 48:1192–1197, 1999.

89. Larsen JJ, Dela F, and Kjaer M et al., The effect of moderate exercise on postprandial glucose homeostasis in NIDDM patients, *Diabetologia,* 40:447–453, 1997.

90. Fenicchia LM, Kanaley JA, and Azevedo JL, Jr, et al., Influence of resistance exercise training on glucose control in women with type-2 diabetes, *Metabolism,* 3:284–289, 2004.

91. Baldi JC and Snowling N, Resistance training improves glycaemic control in obese type-2 diabetic men, *Int J Sports Med,* 4:419–423, 2003.

92. Tokmakidis SP, Zois CE, and Volaklis KA et al., The effects of a combined strength and aerobic exercise program on glucose control and insulin action in women with type–2 diabetes, *Eur J Appl Physiol,* 2:437–442, 2004.

93. Mourier A, Gautier JF, and de Kerviler E et al., Mobilization of visceral adipose tissue related to the improvement in insulin sensitivity in response to physical training in NIDDM: Effects of branched-chain amino acid supplements, *Diabetes Care,* 20:385–391, 1997.

94. Blaak EE, van Aggel-Leijssen DP, and Wagenmakers AJ et al., Impaired oxidation of plasma-derived fatty acids in type-2 diabetic subjects during moderate-intensity exercise, *Diabetes,* 49:2102–2107, 2000.

95. Borghouts LB, Wagenmakers AJ, and Goyens PL et al., Substrate utilization in non-obese type-II diabetic patients at rest and during exercise, *Clin Sci (Lond),* 103:559–566, 2002.

96. Christ-Roberts CY, Pratipanawatr T, and Pratipanawatr W et al., Exercise training increases glycogen synthase activity and GLUT4 expression but not insulin signaling in overweight nondiabetic and type-2 diabetic subjects, *Metabolism,* 3:1233–42, 2004.

97. Holten MK, Zacho M, and Gaster M et al., Strength training increases insulin-mediated glucose uptake, GLUT4 content, and insulin signaling in skeletal muscle in patients with type-2 diabetes, *Diabetes,* 3:294–305, 2004.

98. Minuk HL, Vranic M, and Hanna AK et al., Glucoregulatory and metabolic response to exercise in obese noninsulin-dependent diabetes, *Am J Physiol,* 240:E458–464, 1981.

99. Larsen JJ, Dela F, and Madsbad S et al., Interaction of sulfonylureas and exercise on glucose homeostasis in type-2 diabetic patients, *Diabetes Care,* 2:1647–1654, 1999.

100. Wing RR, Exercise and weight control, In: *Handbook of Exercise in Diabetes*, 2nd ed., Ruderman N, Devlin JT, and Schneider SH et al., Eds., Alexandria, VA: American Diabetes Association, 2002:355–364.

101. Ross R, Dagnone D, and Jones PJH et al., Reduction in obesity and related comorbid conditions after diet-induced weight loss or exercise-induced weight loss in men, A randomized, controlled trial, *Ann Int Med,* 133:92–103, 2000.

102. Klem ML, Wing RR, and McGuire MT et al., A descriptive study of individuals successful at long-term maintenance of substantial weight loss, *Am J Clin Nutr,* 66:239–246, 1997.

103. Langer O, Berkus M, and Brustman L et al., Rational for insulin management in gestational diabetes, *Diabetes,* 40(Suppl 2):186–190, 1991.

104. ACOG Committee Opinion No. 267, Exercise during pregnancy and the postpartum periods, *Obstet Gynecol,* 99:171–173, 2002.

105. American Diabetes Association, Gestational diabetes mellitus, *Diabetes Care,* 27:S88–90, 2004.

106. Brankston GN, Mitchell BF, and Ryan EA et al., Resistance exercise decreases the need for insulin in overweight women with gestational diabetes mellitus, *Am J Obstet Gynecol,* 190:188–193, 2004.

107. Bung P, Artal R, and Khodiguian N et al., Exercise in gestational diabetes: An optional therapeutic approach? *Diabetes,* 40(Suppl 2):182–185, 1991.

108. Jovanovic-Peterson L and Peterson CM, Is exercise safe or useful for gestational diabetic women? *Diabetes,* 0(Suppl 2):179–181, 1991.

109. Garcia-Patterson A, Martin E, and Ubeda J et al., Evaluation of light exercise in the treatment of gestational diabetes, *Diabetes Care,* 4:2006–2007, 2001.

110. Wolfe LA and Weissgerber TL, Clinical physiology of exercise in pregnancy, A literature review, *J Obstet Gynaecol Can,* 25:473–483, 2003.

111. Jovanovic L, Kessler A, and Peterson CM, Human maternal and fetal response to graded exercise, *J Appl Physiol,* 8:1719–1722, 1985.

112. Hartman S and Bung P, Physical exercise during pregnancy—physiological considerations and recommendations, *J Perinat Med,* 27:204–215, 1999.

113. Dietary Guidelines Advisory Committee, Nutrition and your health: Dietary guidelines for Americans, 2005, http://www.health.gov/ dietaryguidelines/dga2005/report/, Accessed on February 20, 2005.

114. Klein S, Sheard NF, and Pi-Sunyer X et al., Weight management through lifestyle modification for the prevention and management of type-2 diabetes: Rationale and strategies, *Am J Clin Nutr,* 80:257–263, 2004.

115. Sakamoto K, Hirshman MF, and Aschenbach WG et al., Contraction regulation of Akt in rat skeletal muscle, *J Biol Chem,* 277:11910–11917, 2002.

116. Iglesias MA, Ye JM, and Frangioudakis G et al., AICAR administration causes an apparent enhancement of muscle and liver insulin action in insulin-resistant high-fat-fed rats, *Diabetes,* 51:2886–2894, 2002.

117. Ren JM, Semenkovich CF, and Gulve EA et al., Exercise induces rapid increases in GLUT4 expression, glucose transport capacity, and insulin-stimulated glycogen storage in muscle, *J Biol Chem,* 269:14396–14401, 1994.

118. Kraniou Y, Cameron-Smith D, and Misso M et al., Effects of exercise on GLUT-4 and glycogenin gene expression in human skeletal muscle, *J Appl Physiol* 88:794–796, 2000.

119. O'Doherty RM, Bracy DP, and Osawa H et al., Rat skeletal muscle hexokinase II mRNA and activity are increased by a single bout of acute exercise, *Am J Physiol,* 266:E171–178, 1994.

120. Sherwood DJ, Dufresne SD, and Markus JF et al., Differential regulation of MAP kinase, p70(s6k) and akt by contraction and insulin in rat skeletal muscle, *Am J Physiol,* 276:E870–878, 1999.

121. Osman AA, Pendergrass M, and Koval J et al., Regulation of MAP kinase pathway activity *in vivo* in human skeletal muscle, *Am J Physiol,* 278:E992–999, 2000.

122. Karlsson HKR, Nilsson PA, and Nilsson J et al., Branched-chain amino acids increase p70[sk6] phosphorylation in human skeletal muscle after resistance exercise, *Am J Physiol Endocrinol Metab,* 287:E1–7, 2004.

123. McGee SL and Hargreaves M, Exercise and myocyte enhancer factor 2 regulation in human skeletal muscle, *Diabetes* 53:1208–1214, 2004.

124. Akimoto T, Pohnert SC, and Li P et al., Exercise stimulated PGC-1α transcription in skeletal muscle through activation of the p38 MAPK pathway, *J Biol Chem,* 2005 [Epub ahead of print].

125. Watt MJ, Southgate RJ, and Holmes AG et al., Suppression of plasma free fatty acids upregulates peroxisome proliferator-activated receptor (PPAR-) alpha and delta and PPAR coactivator 1alpha in human skeletal muscle, but not lipid regulatory genes, *J Mol Endocrinol,* 33:533–544, 2004.

126. Nielsen JN, Frosig C, and Sajan MP et al., Increased atypical PKC activity in endurance-trained human skeletal muscle, *Biochem Biophys Res Commun,* 312:1147–1153, 2003.

127. Richter EA, Nielsen JN, and Jorgensen SB et al., Signalling to glucose transport in skeletal muscle during exercise, *Acta Physiol Scand,* 178:329–335, 2003.

128. Jorgensen SB, Neilsen JN, and Birk JB et al., *Diabetes,* 53:3074–3081, 2004.

129. Sakamoto K, Arnolds DE, and Ekberg I et al., Exercise regulates Akt and glycogen synthase kinase-3 activities in human skeletal muscle, *Biochem Biophys Res Commun,* 319:419–425, 2004.

Appendix 1
Abbreviations

A1C	hemoglobin A1C
AA	ascorbic acid
AACE	American Association of Clinical Endocrinologists
ACC	acetyl-CoA carboxylase
ACE	American College of Endocrinology
ACE-I	angiotensin-converting enzyme inhibitor
ACOG	American College of Obstetricians and Gynecologists
Ach	acetylcholine
ACSM	American College of Sports Medicine
ADA	American Diabetes Association
ADH	alcohol dehydrogenase
ADM	atypical diabetes mellitus (of African-Americans)
ADP	5-adenosine diphosphate
AFGF	acidic fibroblast growth factor
AGE	advanced glycation endproducts
AGM_1	N-acetylglucosamine-phosphate mutase
AgRP	agouti-related peptide
AICAR	5-aminoimidazole-4-carboxamide ribofuranoside
AIF	apoptosis inducing factor
Akt	protein kinase B
ALA	lipoic acid
ALDH2	aldehyde dehydrogenase-2
AMP	5-adenosine monophosphate
AMPK	5-adenosine monophosphate-activated protein kinase
ANT	adenine nucleotide translocator
AP-1	activator protein-1
Apaf-1	apoptosis protease-activating factor-1
AQP2	aquaporin-2
AR	aldose reductase
ARB	angiotensin receptor blocker
ASK1	apoptosis signal-regulating kinase-1
ATF-2	activating transcription factor-2
ATP	5-adenosine triphosphate
ATP II / III	Adult Treatment Panel II/III
AVP	arginine vasopressin
BAD	BH-3 only subgroup molecule, of the Bcl-2 family, pro-apoptotic
BAR-2, -3	$\beta(2)$-, $\beta(3)$-adrenergic receptor
BAX	Bcl-2 family member, multi-domain, pro-apoptotic
BB	BioBreeding rat
Bcl-2	Bcl-2 family member, anti-apoptotic
BCM	body cell mass
BETA2	β-cell E box transactivator 2
BFGF	basic fibroblast growth factor
BH-3	Bcl-2 homology-3
BMI	body mass index

CABG	coronary artery bypass graft
CACT	carnitine-acyl-carnitine translocase
CAD	coronary artery disease
CaM	calmodulin
CAM	complementary and alternative medicine
CaMKIV	calcium/calmodulin-dependent protein kinase IV
cAMP	adenosine 3,5-cyclic phosphate
CAP	c-cbl-associated protein
CAPS	Ca^{++}-dependent activator protein for secretion
CART	cocaine- and amphetamine-regulated transcript
CBP	CREB-binding protein
CCK	cholecystokinin
CDE	certified diabetes educator
C/EBP-α,β	CCAAT/enhancer-binding protein-α,β
cGMP	guanosine 3,5-cyclic phosphate
CGMS	continuous glucose monitoring systems
CGRP	calcitonin gene-related peptide
CHD	coronary heart disease
CHF	congestive heart failure
CKD	chronic kidney disease
CML	N-carboxymethyl-lysine
CnA	calcineurin
CoQ10	coenzyme Q10
COX	cytochrome c oxidase
CPEO	chronic progressive external ophthalmoplegia
CPT-I	carnitine palmitoyltransferase I
CPT-II	carnitine palmitoyltransferase II
CRABP-II	cellular retinoic acid-binding protein-II
CREB	cAMP-response element binding protein
CREM	cAMP-response element modulator
CRP	C-reactive protein
CRT	creatine transport system
CSII	continuous subcutaneous insulin infusion
CVD	cardiovascular disease
DASH	Dietary Approaches to Stop Hypertension
DAG	diacylglycerol
DCCT	Diabetes Control and Complications Trial
DHA	dihydroascorbic acid
DIDMOAD	diabetes insipidus, diabetes mellitus, optic atrophy, deafness
DKA	diabetic ketoacidosis
DPP	diabetes prevention program
DPP-IV	dipeptidyl peptidase IV
DSHEA	Dietary Supplement Health and Education Act
DS/N-FF	dietary supplements, nutraceuticals and functional foods
EGCG	epigallocatechin gallate
EGF	epidermal growth factor
EGP	endogenous glucose production
EN	enteral nutrition
EN-RAGE	extracellular newly identified receptor for AGE binding protein
eNOS	endothelial nitric oxide synthase
EPA-E	eicosapentaenoic acid ethyl ester
EPO	evening primrose oil
ERK	extracellular-regulated kinase
ESRD	end stage renal disease
ET-1	endothelin-1

ETC	electron transport chain
FAD	flavin adenine dinucleotide
FADH	flavin adenine dinucleotide, reduced form
Fas	member of tumor-necrosis factor receptor family, pro-apoptotic
FasL	Fas ligand, membrane protein
FBG	fasting blood glucose
FDA	Food and Drug Administration
FFA	free fatty acid
FGF-2	fibroblast growth factor-2
FMN	flavin mononucleotide
G6P	glucose-6-phosphate
GABA	γ-aminobutyric acid
GAD	glutamic acid decarboxylase
GAPDH	glyceraldehyde-3-phosphate dehydrogenase
GC	glucocorticoids
GDH	glutamate dehydrogenase
GDM	gestational diabetes
GDP	guanosine 5'-diphosphate
GERD	gastroesophageal reflux disease
GFR	glomerular filtration rate
GI	glycemic index
GIP	gastric inhibitory polypeptide; glucose-dependent insulinotropic polypeptide
GK	glucokinase; hexokinase IV
GL	glycemic load
GLA	linolenic acid
GLP-1, -2	glucagon-like peptide-1, -2
GLUT1, 2, 3, 4	glucose transporter 1, 2, 3, 4
GMP	guanosine 5-monophosphate
GRP	gastrin-releasing peptide
GS4	*Gymnema sylvestre* extract
GSIS	glucose-stimulated insulin secretion
GSK3	glycogen synthase kinase-3
GTF	glucose tolerance factor
GTP	guanosine 5-triphosphate
HAIR-AN	hyperandrogenism, insulin resistance, acanthosis nigricans syndrome
HCS	holocarboxylase synthetase
HD	hemodialysis
HDAC	histone deacetylase
HDL	high-density lipoprotein
HFCS	high-fructose corn syrup
HFHA	high-fat, high-amino acid
HKII	hexokinase II; binds to VDAC and inhibits apoptosis
HKIV	hexokinase IV; glucokinase; high affinity, mutated in MODY-2
HIV	human immunodeficiency virus
HLA	human leukocyte antigens
HLH	helix-loop-helix (protein)
HMG CoA	3-hydroxy-3-methylglutaryl coenzyme A
hmGPD	human mitochondrial glycerol-3-phosphate dehydrogenase
HNE	4-hydroxynonenal
HNF	hepatic nuclear factor
HOMA	homeostasis-model assessed
5-HT	5-hydroxytryptamine (serotonin)
IAP	inhibitor of apoptosis protein
ICAM	intracellular adhesion molecule-1

ICU	intensive care unit
IDPN	intradialytic parenteral nutrition
IFG	impaired fasting glucose
IFN-γ	interferon-γ
IGF-1	insulin-like growth factor 1
IGT	impaired glucose tolerance
IKK	inhibitor B kinase
IκB-(α)	inhibitory κB-(α)
IL-1(β), -6, -18	interleukin-1β, -6, -18
IM	inner mitochondrial membrane
iNOS	inducible nitric oxide synthase
IOM	Institute of Medicine
IPF-1	insulin promoter factor-1
IRAS	Insulin Resistance Atherosclerosis Study
IRS	insulin resistance syndrome
IRS (-1, -2)	insulin receptor substrate (-1, -2)
ISF	insulin sensitivity factor
IVGTT	intravenous glucose tolerance
JAK	Janus kinases
JNK	c-Jun N-terminal kinase, member of the MAPK subfamily
Jun	member of activator protein-1 family of transcription factors
KGF	keratinocyte growth factor
Kir6.2	inwardly rectifying K$^+$ channel
KSS	Kearns Sayre syndrome
LA	α-lipoic acid
LDL	low-density lipoprotein
LHON	Leber's hereditary optic neuropathy
LPS	lipopolysaccharide
L-VDCC	L-type voltage-dependent Ca^{++} channel
MAPK	mitogen-activating protein kinase
MC -3, -4	melanocortin-3, -4
MCC	methylcrotonyl CoA carboxylase
MCH	melanin-concentrating hormone
MCP-1	monocyte chemotactic protein-1
MDI	multiple daily injections
MDRD	Modification of Diet in Renal Disease Study
MEF-2	myocyte enhancer factor-2
MELAS	mitochondrial encephalopathy, lactic acidosis, and stroke-like episodes
MEOS	microsomal ethanol oxidizing system
MERRF	myoclonic epilepsy and ragged red fiber disease
MG	methylglyoxal
MHC	major histocompatibility complex
MIA	malnutrition, inflammation, and atherosclerosis syndrome
MIDD	maternally inherited diabetes and deafness syndrome
MiMyCa	maternally inherited myopathy with cardiac involvement
MIP-2	macrophage inflammatory protein – 2
MMP	matrix metalloproteinase
MNGIE	mitochondrial neurogastrointestinal encephalopathy
MNT	medical nutrition therapy
mPTP	mitochondrial permeability transition pore
MODY	maturity-onset diabetes of the young
α-MSH	alpha-melanocyte stimulating hormone
MtCK	mitochondrial creatine kinase
MTDM	mitochondrial diabetes
mtDNA	mitochondrial DNA

MTE	multiple trace element
MTE-1	mitochondrial thioesterase
mtTERF	mitochondrial transcription termination factor
mtTFA	mitochondrial transcription factor A
MUFA	monounsaturated fatty acids
n-3 FA	omega-3 fatty acids
NA	nicotinic acid
NAD	nicotinamide adenine dinucleotide
NADH	nicotinamide adenine dinucleotide, reduced form
NADP	nicotinamide adenine dinucleotide phosphate
NADPH	nicotinamide adenine dinucleotide phosphate, reduced form
NAFLD	nonalcoholic fatty liver disease
NAPRT	nicotinamide phosphoribosyltransferase
NARP	neurogenic weakness, ataxia and retinitis pigmentosa
NAASO	North American Association for the Study of Obesity
NBD	nucleotide binding domains
NCEP	National Cholesterol Education Program
ND (1, 2, 3, 4, 5, 6)	NADH dehydrogenase (1, 2, 3, 4, 5, 6)
NDDG	National Diabetes Data Group
nDNA	nuclear DNA
NEFA	non-esterified fatty acids
NEUROD1	neurogenic differentiation factor-1
NF-$\kappa\beta$	nuclear transcription factor-$\kappa\beta$
NHANES (III)	(Third) National Health and Nutrition Examination Survey
NHLBI	National Heart, Lung, and Blood Institute
NO	nitric oxide
NOD	nonobese diabetic mouse
NPH	neutral pH–protamine–Hagedorn insulin
nPNA	normalized protein nitrogen appearance
NPY	neuropeptide Y
NRF-1	nuclear respiratory factor-1
OAA	oral amino acids
ODA	oral diabetes agent
OGTT	oral glucose tolerance test
OM	outer mitochondrial membrane
Oxm	oxyntomodulin
OTC	over-the-counter
OXPHOS	oxidative phosphorylation
p160MBP	p160 myb binding protein
PAI-1	plasminogen activator inhibitor-1
PARP	poly(ADP-ribose) polymerase
PC	pyruvate carboxylase
PCC	propionyl CoA carboxylase
PCOS	polycystic ovary syndrome
PD	peritoneal dialysis
PDF	peritoneal dialysis fluid
PDX-1	pancreatic duodenal homeobox-1
PDGF	platelet-derived growth factor
PDGFR	platelet-derived growth factor β receptor
PDH	pyruvate dehydrogenase
PEM	protein-energy malnutrition
PEO	progressive external ophthalmoplegia
PEPCK	phosphoenolpyruvate carboxykinase
PGC1α	peroxisome proliferators-activated receptor γ coactivators 1α
PGE$_2$	prostaglandin E$_2$

PI3K	phosphatidylinositol-3-kinase
PKA	protein kinase A
PKB	protein kinase B
PKC	protein kinase C
PGC-1()	peroxisome proliferators-activated receptor γ coactivator-1()
PGI$_2$	prostacyclin
PN	parenteral nutrition
POMC	pro-opiomelanocortin
PP	pancreatic polypeptide
PP1	protein phosphatase 1
PPAR-(α ,γ, δ)	peroxisome proliferators-activated receptor-(α, γ, δ)
PPG	postprandial glucose
PRCT	prospective randomized controlled trial
PTDM	post-transplant diabetes
PTH	parathyroid hormone
PTP(-1)	protein-tyrosine phophatase(-1)
PYY	peptide YY
PUFA	polyunsaturated fatty acids
RAGE	AGE receptor
RAR	retinoic acid receptor
RD	registered dietician
REE	resting energy expenditure
Rf	riboflavin
RHI	regular human insulin
RIPE-3b1	rat insulin promoter element-3b1
ROS	reactive oxygen species
RR-MAD	riboflavin-responsive, multiple acylcoenzyme A dehydrogenase
RTK	receptor tyrosine kinases
RXR	retinoid X receptor
SCO2	cytochrome c oxidase assembly gene
Sco2	protein encoded by SCO2 gene
SERCA2a	sarcoendoplasmic reticulum Ca^{2+} ATPase
sICAM	soluble intercellular adhesion molecule
SH	stress hyperglycemia
SMBG	self-monitoring of blood glucose
SMC	smooth muscle cell
SOCS	suppressor of cytokine signaling
SOD	superoxide dismutase
SNRI	serotonin and norepinephrine reuptake inhibitor
SSRI	selective serotonin reuptake inhibitor
STAT	signal transducers and activators of transcription
STF-1	somatostatin transcription factor-1
SU	sulfonylurea
SUR	sulfonylurea receptor
sVCAM	soluble vascular cellular adhesion molecule
T1DM	type-1 diabetes
T2DM	type-2 diabetes
TDD	total daily dose
TEE	total energy expenditure
TF	tissue factor
TFA	trans-fatty acids
TG	thyroglobulin
TGF-β	transforming growth factor-β
TLC	therapeutic lifestyle changes
TNF-α	tumor-necrosis factor-α

TOS	α-tocopherol succinate
TP	thymidine phosphorylase
tPA(-1)	tissue plasminogen activator(-1)
TPN	total parenteral nutrition
TPO	thyroid peroxidase
γ-TQ	γ-tocopheryl quinine
TRAP	total radical-trapping antioxidant parameter
TRIGR	Trial to Reduce Insulin Dependent Diabetes in the Genetically at Risk
TRIPOD	Troglitazone in the Prevention of Diabetes
TZD	thiazolidinedione(s)
UCP1, UCP2, UCP3	uncoupling protein (1, 2, 3)
UKPDS	United Kingdom Prospective Diabetes Study
uPA	urokinase-type plasminogen activator
USDA	United States Department of Agriculture
UUN	urine urea nitrogen
VCAM-1	vascular cell adhesion molecule-1
VDAC	voltage-dependent anion channel
VEGF	vascular endothelial growth factor
VLDL	very low-density lipoproteins
WAVE-1	Wiskott–Aldrich family member, kinase anchoring protein
WHO	World Health Organization

Appendix 2
Levels of Evidence and Recommendation Grades Used for Technical Reviews

Evidence Level	Recommen- dation Grade	Description	References
1		Well-controlled, generalizable, randomized trial	ADA, DS/N, OB
		Adequately powered	ADA, DS/N
		Well-controlled multi-center trial	ADA, DS/N
		Large meta-analyses with quality ratings	ADA, DS/N
		All-or-none evidence	ADA, DS/N
2		Randomized controlled trial—limited body of data	DS/N, OB
		Well-conducted prospective cohort study	ADA, DS/N
		Well-conducted meta-analysis of cohort studies	ADA, DS/N
3		Flawed randomized clinical trials	ADA, DS/N, OB
		Observational studies	ADA, DS/N, OB
		Case series or case reports	ADA, DS/N
		Conflicting evidence with weight of evidence	
		Supporting the recommendation	ADA
4		Expert consensus	ADA, DS/N, OB
		Expert opinion based on experience	ADA, DS/N, OB
		Theory-driven conclusions	DS/N
		Unproven claims	DS/N
	A	Homogeneous evidence from multiple well-designed randomized controlled trials with sufficient statistical power	AGA
		Homogeneous evidence from multiple well-designed cohort controlled trials with sufficient statistical power	AGA
		≥ One conclusive Level I publication demonstrating benefit >> risk	DS/N
	B	Evidence from at least one large well-designed clinical trial, cohort or case-controlled analytic study, or meta-analysis	AGA
		No conclusive Level I publication; ≥ one conclusive	DS/N
		Level II publication demonstrating benefit >> risk	AGA
	C	Evidence based on clinical experience, descriptive studies, or expert consensus opinion	
		No conclusive Level I or II publication; ≥ one	DS/N

Evidence Level	Recommen-dation Grade	Description	References
		conclusive Level III publication demonstrating benefit >> risk	
		No conclusive risk at all and no conclusive benefit demonstrated by evidence	DS/N
	D	Not rated	AGA
		No conclusive Level I, II, or III publication demonstrating benefit >> risk	DS/N
		Conclusive Level I, II, or III publication demonstrating risk >> benefit	DS/N

Abbreviations: ADA—American Diabetes Association (2004), DS/N—Mechanick et al., (2003), OB—NHLBI (1998), AGA—American Gastroenterological Association (2003).

Sources: American Diabetes Association, ADA clinical practice recommendations: Introduction, *Diabetes Care,* 27:S1–S2, 2004.

American Gastroenterological Association, AGA technical review on osteoporosis in hepatic disorders, *Gastroenterol,* 125: 941–966.

Mechanick JI, Brett EM, Chausmer AB, Dickey RA, and Wallach S, American Association of Clinical Endocrinologists Medical Guidelines for the Clinical Use of Dietary Supplements and Nutraceuticals, *Endocr Pract,* 9:417–470. NHLBI Obesity Education Initiative Expert Panel on the Identification, Evaluation, and Treatment of Overweight and Obesity in Adults, Clinical guidelines on the identification, evaluation, and treatment of overweight and obesity in adults, NIH Publication No. 98-4093, September 1998.

Appendix 3
Dietary Reference Intakes of Relevant Nutrients for the Adult Diabetic or Prediabetic Patient

DEFINITIONS

1. Recommended dietary allowance (RDA)—average nutrient intake level sufficient to meet needs of 97–98% of healthy individuals according to gender and life stage.
2. Adequate intake (AI)—recommended nutrient intake based on approximations when an RDA cannot be determined.
3. Tolerable upper intake level (UL)—highest level of daily nutrient intake unlikely to pose risk to nearly all persons in the general population.
4. Estimated average requirement (EAR)—daily nutrient intake that meets needs of 50% of healthy persons according to gender and life stage and is the basis for the RDA.
5. Acceptable macronutrient distribution range (AMDR)—range of intake (as percentage) associated with reduced risk of chronic disease while providing essential nutrient intake.

Nutrient[a]	RDA	AI	UL	EAR	AMDR (%)
WATER AND ELECTROLYTES					
Water (L/day)		2.1–3.3			
Sodium (g/day)		1.2–1.5	2.2–2.3		
Potassium (g/day)		4.5–4.7			
MACRONUTRIENTS					
Protein (g/day)	34–56				10–35
Carbohydrate (g/day)[b]	130				45–65
Fiber (g/day)		21–38			
Fat (g/day)					25–35
n-6 PUFA (g/day)		10–17			5–10
n-3 PUFA (g/day)		1.0–1.6			0.6–1.2
VITAMINS					
Biotin (µg/day)		20–30			
Choline (mg/day)		375–550	2000–3500		
Folate (µg/day)	300–400		600–1000		
Niacin (mg/day)	12–14		20–35		
Pantothenic acid (mg/day)		4–5			
Riboflavin (mg/day)	0.9–1.3				
Thiamin (mg/day)	0.9–1.1				
Vitamin A (µg/day)	600–900		1700–3000		
Vitamin B6 (mg/day)	1.0–1.7		60–100		
Vitamin B12 (µg/day)	1.8–2.4				
Vitamin C (mg/day)	45–90		1200–2000		

Nutrient[a]	RDA	AI	UL	EAR	AMDR (%)
Vitamin D (μg/day)[d]	5–15		50		
Vitamin E (mg/day)	11–15		600–1000		
Vitamin K (μg/day)		60–120			
ELEMENTS					
Boron (mg/day)			11–20		
Calcium (mg/day)		1000–1300	2500		
Copper (μg/day)	700–900		5,000–10,000		
Iron (μg/day)	120–150		600–1100		
Magnesium (mg/day)	240–420		350[c]		
Manganese (mg/day)		1.6–2.3	6–11		
Molybdenum (μg/day)	34–45		1100–2000		
Phosphorus (mg/day)	700–1250		3000–4000		
Selenium (mg/day)	40–55		280–400		
Vanadium (mg/day)			1.8		
Zinc (mg/day)	8–11		23–40		

[a] Values in table exclude pregnant or lactating women; values reflect ranges for gender and varying age groups. See Food and Nutrition Information Center at http://www.nal.usda.gov/fnic/etext/000105.html.

[b] Total digestible carbohydrate; maximal intake of added sugars should be < 25% energy.

[c] UL for magnesium only applies to pharmacologic intake.

[d] 1 μg = 40 IU vitamin D.

Appendix 4
Diabetes Management Patient Record Handout

Patient Name:_____

Diagnosis: _____ type-1 diabetes _____ type-2 diabetes

Current Weight: _____lbs/kg Height_____in/cm BMI: _____

Ideal Weight: _____Goal Weight: _____ by date: _____

Current HbA1C: _____ Target HbA1C: _____

Target fasting glucose: _____ Target postprandial glucose: _____

Recommended total calories/day _____

Total grams of carbohydrate/day _____

Total grams of fat/day _____

Total grams of protein/day _____

	Breakfast	Snack	Lunch	Snack	Dinner	Snack	Total
Carb (servings/grams)							
Insulin:Carb Ratio							
Insulin Sensitivity Factor							

	Current Lipid Profile	Target Lipid Profile
Total cholesterol	_____ mg/dL	_____ mg/dL
LDL cholesterol	_____ mg/dL	_____ mg/dL
HDL cholesterol	_____ mg/dL	_____ mg/dL
Triglycerides	_____ mg/dL	_____ mg/dL

Exercise prescription: days per week_____

Minutes per session: aerobic_____ strength training _____

Appendix 5
Dietary Tips for Pregnancy and Diabetes

Claudia Shwide-Slavin

Your diet is very important before, during, and after pregnancy. The primary goal is normal blood sugar to produce a healthy baby. Your physician or registered dietitian will determine the calories for an individualized meal plan based on your pre-pregnancy weight. Blood glucose monitoring when you wake up and 1–2 hours after each meal will determine how to adjust your diet and medication needs throughout your pregnancy. Exercise can help to lower your blood sugar and insulin requirements. Start walking or speak with your clinician about continuing your usual exercise regimen.

WHY SHOULD I EAT A HEALTHY DIET?

- Choosing healthy foods helps to control weight gain, providing the extra calories, vitamins, and minerals that you need during pregnancy. Healthy foods reduce chances of problems in your pregnancy and the use of nonnutritive sweeteners is acceptable during pregnancy because no adverse effects have been reported.
- Protein is needed to help your baby build a healthy immune system, muscles, cells, and hormones.
- Carbohydrates provide energy for your body. The effect of carbohydrate on blood glucose depends on your body. Testing your blood sugar 1–2 hours after eating helps to understand the effect of your food choices. Your goal is to keep blood glucose between 60–120 mg/dL. Reading the nutrition facts label will tell you how much carbohydrate you are choosing.
- Each person requires a different percentage of energy from fat, based on body weight and metabolic profile.
- Unpasturized cheese, hot dogs, and cold cuts that are not microwaved must be avoided because the food may contain the bacteria listeria. Listeria is dangerous to your baby.
- 400 μg folate is recommended each day starting 1 month prior to pregnancy to prevent neural tube defects.
- 1500 mg calcium plus 500–600 IU vitamin D for calcium absorption is recommended each day during pregnancy to build strong bones.
- 28 g/day total fiber is recommended during all three trimesters. Fiber-containing foods also contain vitamins, minerals, and other healthy ingredients.
- 30 mg/ day iron supplement is often recommended during the second and third trimesters to help maintain iron stores and prevent anemia.
- Some herbal therapies taken as supplements have the potential to cause problems during pregnancy and lactation. Avoid chromium, *Gymnema sylvester*, fenugreek, bitter melon, and cinnamon supplements. Discuss the use of any dietary supplement with your doctor before taking it.

WHAT SHOULD I EAT?

- Eat small frequent meals and snacks.
- You may add nonnutritive sweeteners to make limited diets more palatable. These sweeteners include: saccharin, called Sweet'N Low®, Sweet Twin®, and Necta Sweet®; aspartame called Nutrasweet®, Equal®, and Sugar Twin™; acesulfame-K called Sunett®, Sweet & Safe, Sweet One®; and sucralose called Splenda®.
- Eat at least 7–9 oz of protein daily. Protein is found in meat, chicken, turkey, fish, eggs, cheese, peanut butter, and tofu. Some protein-containing foods raise blood glucose levels because they also contain carbohydrates. Examples are milk, yogurt, peanut butter, dried peas, and beans.
- Limit fish to 12 oz/week, choosing shrimp, canned light tuna, wild salmon, pollock, and catfish (including up to 6 oz tuna/week). If you eat a lot of fish one week, you can cut back for the next week or two. Just make sure to average the recommended amount per week.
- Some fish must be avoided because they may harm an unborn fetus and their developing nervous system. Do not eat shark, swordfish, king mackerel, and tilefish during your pregnancy due to their high levels of methyl mercury.
- Avoid raw fish and farmed fish because it may contain viral and bacterial contaminants.
- Every time you eat, include at least one food with carbohydrate. Carbohydrates are found in all fruits, milk, yogurt, starchy vegetables, bread, grains, cereals, beans, pasta and sweets.
- Eat foods with healthy fats. These foods include vegetable oils (olive oil, canola oil, flaxseed oil, soybean oil), nuts, seeds, fish (salmon, tuna, white fish, shrimp), avocados, peanut butter, walnuts, broccoli, spinach, and pinto beans.
- If your cholesterol is running high, eating plant stanols and sterols in Benecol® or Take Control® helps to lower your cholesterol.
- Limit saturated fats, which are found in meat, poultry, butter, 1%, 2%, and 4% (whole) milks or yogurt, cheese, ice cream, egg yolks, coconut oil, and chocolate. Trans-fatty acids and hydrogenated fats are similar to saturated fats and should also be avoided.
- Foods containing folic acid include legumes, green leafy vegetables, liver, citrus fruit, juices, and whole wheat bread. Folic acid is best absorbed from fortified cereals and grains and supplements.
- Calcium is found in all cheese including low-fat types, milk, Lactaid®, and yogurt or in a supplement form. Four servings of these foods will meet your daily needs.
- Dietary fiber is found in bran, grains, vegetables, legumes, seeds, and nuts. Adequate fiber is needed to maintain regularity.
- Iron is found in lean red meat, fish, poultry, dried fruits, and iron-fortified cereals. Eating foods with vitamin C helps the absorption of iron.
- Dietary sources containing chromium are healthy; include broccoli and unprocessed foods in your diet.
- *Gymnema sylvestre* may cause low blood glucose and should be used with caution during pregnancy.
- Fenugreek should be avoided during pregnancy due to its effects on the uterus. For women requiring coumadin there is a negative drug interaction with fenugreek.
- Bitter melon should also be avoided during pregnancy because it promotes bleeding, contractions and may cause the pregnancy to abort.
- Cinnamon has the potential to reduce insulin doses and may cause hypoglycemia in large doses. A small amount of cinnamon used as a spice in a recipe is not harmful.

HOW AND WHEN SHOULD I TEST MY BLOOD?

- You will be testing your blood four or more times a day, using only the sides of your fingertips. Do not test using alternative sites because low blood sugars are not accurately reported.
- Normal blood sugar levels are between 60 mg/dL–90 mg/dL when you wake up and before each meal. When the blood sugar is higher than 90 mg/dL when you wake up, it is not healthy for your baby. Diet and/or medication will need to be adjusted until normal blood sugars are resumed.
- Normal blood sugar levels 1 hour after each meal are under 120 mg/dL. When the blood sugar is higher than 120 mg/dL you may need to cut down on the carbohydrate amounts or carbohydrate choices eaten at the meal. When dietary changes are not recommended, insulin doses are adjusted until blood sugar goals are achieved.
- Blood glucose meters that require a small amount of blood and give results in plasma values are preferred for accuracy and reliability during pregnancy.

Appendix 6
Case Study: Office-Based Nutritional Counseling

Don Smith

Physicians often avoid discussing nutritional management with their diabetic or prediabetic patients. Frequently, this is due to a fear that such a dialogue will consume too much time or a false assumption that patients know basic nutritional facts. What follows is an example of several brief dialogues (less than 5 minutes each) that ascertain the salient points that will guide medical nutritional therapy over the course of multiple office visits for the prediabetic patient. The use of patient handouts for home reading and self-monitoring proves to be a valuable and efficient tool.

Mrs. F is a 48-year-old lawyer with two children ages 16 and 18. Her father had a myocardial infarction at age 57 and her mother has had type-2 diabetes mellitus (T2DM) since age 62. She does not smoke nor does she have a history of hypertension. On physical exam, she is 5 feet 2 inches tall and weighs 147 lb (120 lb is her ideal body weight). She is overweight with a body mass index (BMI) of 27 kg/M^2 and her blood pressure (BP) is 144/82 mm Hg. Her waist circumference is 34 inches. Her fasting lipid profile is as follows:

	mg/dL	mM/L
Total cholesterol	260	6.7
Triglycerides	426	4.8
HDL-c	50	1.3
LDL-c	124	3.2
Total/HDL-c	5.2	5.2
Fasting glucose	112	6.2

See Appendix 1 for abbreviations.

She has three out of five criteria for a diagnosis of metabolic syndrome, a prediabetes condition, according to National Cholesterol Education Program guidelines: triglycerides > 150 mg/dL (1.7 mM/L), blood pressure > 130/85, and glucose > 110 mg/dL (6.1 mM/L). In addition, she has a mildly depressed HDL-c, and is overweight. She is at increased risk to develop frank diabetes mellitus (DM) and coronary heart disease (CHD). She is a very conservative woman, who at 48 years of age, absolutely refuses to consider taking any life-long medication: **"Can't I do anything with diet and exercise?"**

"Certainly, tell me quickly what you typically have for breakfast, lunch, and dinner?"

She continues gratefully: **"For breakfast I have whole-grain bread with margarine and some marmalade. And, of course, my coffee, usually 3 cups per day. Lunch is in the cafeteria where I work, or out with clients. Usually, I have iced tea with a sandwich and some JELL-O®, which I love. I'm so busy at night after my 45 minutes at the gym that I generally have to bring in some takeout food, such as Chinese, pizza, fried chicken, or I make hot dogs and**

macaroni and cheese for the kids, which we all eat. For dessert, we have ice cream maybe twice a week, or some fruit pie, or fruit cocktail."

These items are quickly written in the chart in three columns representing breakfast, lunch, and dinner. Only one aspect of this diet can be focused on in the short time available for this visit: lowering sweets and total calories to normalize triglycerides and glucose. Continuing the dialogue: "What do you put in your coffee? And, do you have any juice to drink with your breakfast?"

"Skim milk and sugar, a teaspoon. And yes I forgot, I love orange juice to start off the morning."

"Do you put a teaspoon of sugar in your iced tea at lunch as well?"

"Certainly ... I grew up in the South, and that's the way we always had it ... with sugar and lemon."

"And after the exercise in the gym, do you eat or drink anything?"

"Gatorade® is all I seem to need."

"And JELL-O, which you also love—is that regular or sugar-free JELL-O?"

"I guess they sell regular JELL-O in the cafeteria; it doesn't say."

"Is your fruit cocktail in the evening reduced-calorie?"

"No, the children seem underweight and they need the calories."

"Look, Mrs. F, I think we can improve your high triglycerides and your prediabetic glucose level with just a few simple changes in your diet. You are having too much sugar, which is turning on the production of triglycerides in your liver. If we could just remove that in your diet, you would find your triglycerides dramatically decrease, and without doing anything else, you would lose a few pounds. Could you use a sugar substitute like Sweet'N Low®, or Equal®, or Splenda® in your coffee and iced tea? I hear they are even doing that in the South now, especially with all the sugar-free iced tea powders people use. Most people can do that without too much misery."

"That's easy if you really think it would help."

"How about cutting out orange juice in the morning? That's a little tougher. Even though there is no table sugar added, fruit juice has fructose, which raises triglycerides, too. But you could eat fruit; for example, an orange or half a grapefruit. Or, you could have low-carb fruit juices such as Hood's Carb Countdown® orange juice or Ruby Red grapefruit beverages, with only 2 grams vs. 22 grams of sugar per 8 ounces. Here's what it looks like and here is a copy of the carton so you can find it in the supermarket. If you must have real orange juice, even Tropicana® has a reduced-sugar version with half the sugar grams of regular orange juice. Try to stick to drinking only 4 ounces."

"Sounds interesting, I should be able to manage this some way."

"And have you ever tried sugar-free JELL-O? It tastes just as good and doesn't have the extra sugar and calories. At work, if you could substitute a low-fat milk product for the JELL-O, such as low-fat yogurt, it might help with keeping your blood pressure lower than it is even now."

"I'll think about it. Anything else?"

"Well, the Gatorade; unfortunately, the sugars in it have caused high triglycerides in more athletes than just you. A sports drink is not essential for a 45-minute workout. Cold water would be sufficient, and wouldn't have those dreaded calories. Finally, I would suggest you consider fresh fruit salad instead of the canned fruit cocktail. Many grocery stores sell the fruit already cut up."

"Doctor, you are treating me like I have diabetes; you forget that I am not my mother."

"I know, but unfortunately, foods that raise sugar levels in diabetics, can do the same in those with prediabetes, like you, and simultaneously can raise triglycerides in those who have a genetic tendency for that. Look, here is my scribbled list of things to keep in mind; let my medical assistant copy it for you. Do what you can. You may be surprised at the good results. Let's give you 2 months and then measure your glucose and lipid profile again."

Two months later Mrs. F returns, having lost 4 lb to 143 lb, with a BMI now of 26.2 kg/M² and a blood pressure of 130/74. Her waist circumference is 33 inches. Her fasting lipid profile has improved:

	Baseline (mg/dL)	(mM/L)	2 Months Later (mg/dL)	(mM/L)
Total cholesterol	260	(6.7)	229	(5.9)
Triglycerides	426	(4.1)	145	(1.6)
HDL-c	50	(1.3)	55	(1.4)
LDL-c	124	(3.2)	145	(3.7)
Total/HDL-c	5.2		4.2	
Glucose	112	(6.2)	102	(5.7)

She has started diluting 2 oz of orange juice in the morning with another 2 oz of cold water, drinks water rather than Gatorade after exercising, and now uses a sugar substitute in her coffee and iced tea. She can't give up the JELL-O at work but takes a smaller portion and has made an easy switch to fresh fruit salad. Heartened by success, she now wishes her LDL-c level to be less than 130 mg/dL (3.4 mM/L). She explains, **"I wish to live to 90 without having any cardiovascular events or procedures, wouldn't you?"**

"Well, let's go over your new breakfast, lunch, and dinner quickly and see if there are any further suggestions I can make."

"For breakfast I have a small taste of orange juice with water, my whole-wheat toast with margarine and a tiny bit of marmalade, and coffee with skim milk and a sweetener. I'll have a cookie mid-morning since the boss has brought them into the office. For lunch, I stick with artificially sweetened iced tea, a sandwich and small amounts of JELL-O. For dinner, it's pretty much the same—take-home fried chicken, pizza, hot dogs with macaroni and cheese, occasional hamburgers and pork chops, twice-weekly ice cream and sometimes cherry or apple pie."

"What sort of margarine do you use in the morning?"

"I prefer the stick margarine; I think it tastes better."

"Well one thing you might consider is changing to tub margarine. Stick margarine is filled with partially-hydrogenated, or trans-fatty acids. Not only do trans-fatty acids raise LDL-c levels, but they will also lower your HDL-c. Any tub margarine is better than stick margarine because they have less trans-fatty acids. The trans-fatty acids in stick margarine raise LDL-c equal to the saturated fat in butter, but they simultaneously lower HDL-c while the saturated fat in butter raises HDL-c. That combined bad effect in stick margarine is why they say stick margarine is worse than butter. There are now margarines with stanol esters added. These were developed in Finland where they enjoy butter as much as you but the heart attack rate was one of the highest in the world, so they developed these stanol-ester margarines to replace the butter. Stanol esters are the plant equivalent to human cholesterol. Stanol esters look so much like cholesterol that they compete with the cholesterol in the intestine for the cholesterol receptors. Since the intestinal cholesterol receptors are partially blocked with stanol esters, less cholesterol is absorbed and thus LDL-c levels drop in the blood stream. The studies show you that you can decrease LDL-c in the blood stream by up to 14% if you use these stanol-ester margarines twice daily, perhaps with toast in the morning and on vegetables at dinner. Here's a paper with the names. Look for them; you should probably try them at least in the morning. What sort of sandwich do you eat at lunch?"

"Either ham and cheese or my favorite ... a BLT—bacon, lettuce, and tomato with mayonnaise."

"Well, the lean ham is OK as long as it isn't packed on too much, but you might want to get rid of the cheese, ask for a little less ham, and simply add more mustard. If you eat bacon too frequently, the saturated fat will raise your LDL-c. How about a BLT once every 2 weeks, and choose a turkey or grilled chicken sandwich more often. Other good choices would be a non-cream-based soup with soda crackers or a salad with olives, tomatoes, a low-fat cheese, and an oil-and-vinegar dressing."

"Well, I'll try and see what I can find; some of my friends eat those things."

"Finally, let's talk about how we can make your dinners healthier. If you want the hamburgers, make sure it's the leanest beef. Trim the fat off the pork chops, slice them thin, and stick with one per dinner. Pizza should be considered an occasional 'treat' if you like it, but not a 'staple dinner'. When eating pizza, limit it to 1 slice only, perhaps with a green salad. Chicken cooked over a rotisserie with the skin removed is lower in saturated fat and calories than the quick takeout chicken with the skin on and fried in trans-fatty acids, and you can find these already cooked at many supermarkets. You might consider substituting a tomato-based or olive oil-based sauce, such as a pesto, on spaghetti for the macaroni and cheese. And I agree hot dogs are tasty and easy to cook; just make sure you look for the lowest-fat ones even if made from turkey or soy products. If you order Chinese food, choose a steamed entrée with lots of vegetables and a little sauce on the side. Would you consider lower-fat desserts? There are dozens of low-fat ice creams and yogurts. Although low in fat, you particularly need to avoid sherbets and sorbets because of their high sugar content, which may raise your triglycerides again if eaten too often. Pies and cookies are tasty, but you've got to know that commercial pastry products are generally loaded with trans-fatty acids. Unsweetened applesauce may be a good substitute for apple pie at times. And there are lower-fat cookies. Look, these are just a few ideas; here's a two-sided handout I've written just so you can remember what we've talked about with other tips we haven't had time to discuss. Just think of a few of these changes and you should do well in lowering your LDL-c."

"Well, doctor, you've overwhelmed me again, but let me think about a few things and I'll see what I can do. Thanks for the time you've given me. I'll try to make a few changes, repeat my blood tests in 2 months, and we'll talk one more time."

Mrs. F returns in another 2 months with the following changes. She has lost another 4 lb to 139 lbs with a BMI of 25.5 kg/M^2 and her blood pressure is now 128/72. Her waist circumference is 32 inches. Her repeat lipid profile has improved even further:

	Before		2 Months Later		4 Months Later	
	mg/dL	(mM/L)	mg/dL	(mM/L)	mg/dL	(mM/L)
Total cholesterol	260	(6.7)	229	(5.9)	220	(5.6)
Triglycerides	426	(4.1)	145	(1.6)	148	(1.7)
HDL-c	50	(1.3)	55	(1.4)	58	(1.5)
LDL-c	124	(3.2)	145	(3.7)	132	(3.4)
Total/HDL-c	5.2		4.2		3.8	
Glucose	112	(6.2)	102	(5.7)	96	(5.3)

She has significantly improved her fasting glucose, triglyceride level, and blood pressure. She loves the idea and taste of her new stanol-ester margarine which she uses in the morning on her toast and occasionally for dinner. Although her kids haven't yet moved from their macaroni and cheese to the pesto on spaghetti with some Parmesan cheese sprinkled on top, she loves it as does her husband. The skin has now come off almost all the chicken the family eats. She has found some low-fat frozen yogurts for desserts. BLTs have become a twice-a-month treat and her ham and cheese sandwiches have less ham and contain cheese only occasionally. She is especially pleased that she has been able to improve her lipid profile on her own without having to rely on medications. She is told that in the future, especially following menopause, her LDL-c may rise sufficiently to necessitate lipid-lowering medications, but that time is far away.

This sequence is rather ideal and a bit lengthy, but with most patients and certainly with motivated ones, some specific, targeted, nutritional suggestions can actually be made. Others, such as the use of soluble fiber to lower LDL cholesterol, can be saved for a future visit, such as in this case. The main idea is to rapidly ask about the patient's eating habits through a typical day. Usually one focuses on just one or two of the most important items in the diet for change, gives and keeps a note of them to be able to reinforce them next time through inquiry, and then moves to more suggestions during future visits. Nutritional suggestions that are discussed can be written up by the physician on a single page and be given as a personalized handout.

Index

A

A3243G mutation, 17–18
Acacia arabica, 269
Acacia catechu, 269, 270
acanthosis nigricans, 18
acceptable macronutrient distribution range (AMDR), 323
acesulfame potassium, 89
acetaldehyde, 276
acetylglucosamines, 26
acetyl-L-carnitine, 284
Achillea fragrantissima, 271
acidic fibroblast growth factor (AFGF), 201
acidosis, 30
aconitase deficiency, 223
acromegaly, 18
activating transcription factor-2 (ATF-2), 300
acute illness and nutrition, 4–7
acute wounds, 194
acylcarnitine, 238
acyl-CoA carboxylase (ACC), 241
ADA diet, 175
adenine-nucleotide translocator (ANT), 222
adequate intake (AI), 323
adiponectins, 22
adrenergic antagonists, 19
adrenocorticotropic hormone, 19
advanced glycosylated endproducts (AGEs), 27–28
Aegle marmelose, 269, 273
aerobic exercise, 301
African Americans, 67, 138
Agaricus bisporus, 269
agouti-related peptide (AgRP), 9
Agropyron repens, 270
alanine, 127
albumin, 156–157
albuminuria, 150, 156
alcohol dehydrogenase (ADH), 276
alcohol intake, 276–279
    and medical nutrition therapy, 130
    and risk of type 2 diabetes, 50, 88
alcoholic beverages, 275–279
aldehyde dehydrogenase-2 (ALDH2), 276
aldose, 24
aldose reductase, 24, 25–26
alfalfa, 269
Alitraq®, 176
Allium cepa, 268, 273
Allium sativum, 268, 273
allspice, 269
almonds, fatty acids in, 236
aloe vera, 268, 271
Alpers' disease, 223
alpine ragwort, 269

Alström syndrome, 18
alternative medicines, 266
Alzheimer's disease, 12
Amadori product, 27
amarta, 269
amino acid-containing peritoneal dialysis fluid, 158
amino acids, 233–234
    daily intake for hospitalized patients, 178
    oral, 283–284
    in protein-restricted diets, 156
amlodipine, 151
Ammi visnaga, 271
amylin, 32
anabolic agents, 159–160
androgen therapy, 159
Anemarrhena asphodeloides, 274
anencephalus, 136
angiotensin receptor blocker (ARB), 151–152
angiotensin-converting enzyme inhibitor (ACE-I), 151–152
anjani, 269
anthocyanins, 277, 278
anticonvulsants, 19
anti-diabetic botanicals, 267–279
    alcoholic beverages, 275–279
    Ayurveda, 272–273
    Chinese medicine, 273–274
    culinary, 273–275
    herbs, 268–272
    tea, 275
    wine, 275–279
antihypertensive agents, 19
antineoplastic agents, 19
antioxidants, 50
    effects of, 88
    for hemodialysis
        patients, 160–161
    and metabolic syndrome, 232
antiprotozoal agents, 19
Apidra®, 129
Apo-E gene, 12
apoptosis, 222, 224, 228
appetite stimulants, 159–160
aquaporin-2 (AQP2), 22
arachidonic acid, 96
Areca catechu, 269
Aretaeus of Cappadocia, 11
arginine, 182, 204, 233
arginine-vasopressin (AVP), 22
Aronia melanocarpa, 271
Artemisia pallens, 269
artificial sweeteners, 89
ascorbic acid, 243–244, 283
asparaginase, 19

337

POINT LOMA NAZARENE UNIVERSITY
RYAN LIBRARY